Renal Biopsy Pathology
with Diagnostic and Therapeutic Implications

Renal Biopsy Pathology with Diagnostic and Therapeutic Implications

BENJAMIN H. SPARGO, M.D.
Professor of Pathology, The University of Chicago Pritzker School of Medicine
Recipient of Research Career Award from the National Heart Institute
Chicago, Illinois

ANTHONY E. SEYMOUR, M.B., B.S., F.R.C.P.A.
Head of Renal Pathology, Institute of Medical and Veterinary Science
Consultant in Renal Pathology, Royal Adelaide Hospital
Associate Pathologist, Adelaide Children's Hospital
Adelaide, South Australia

NELSON G. ORDÓÑEZ, M.D.
Assistant Professor of Pathology, The University of Texas System Cancer Center
Assistant Pathologist, M. D. Anderson Hospital and Tumor Institute
Houston, Texas

A WILEY MEDICAL PUBLICATION
JOHN WILEY & SONS
New York • Chichester • Brisbane • Toronto

*To Barbara and Wendy, without whose patience, forbearance, and support
this book would not have been written, and to the memory of Itsmenia.*

Library of Congress Cataloging in Publication Data:

Spargo, Benjamin H
   Renal biopsy pathology with diagnostic and therapeutic implications.

   (A Wiley medical publication)
   Includes index.
   1. Kidneys—Biopsy. 1. Seymour, Anthony E.,
joint author. II. Ordóñez, Nelson G., Joint
author. III. Title. [DNLM: 1. Biopsy. 2. Kidney diseases—Pathology. WJ300.3 S736r]
RC904.S68   616.6′1′0758   79-24603
ISBN 0-471-03119-4

Printed in the United States of America

10 9 8 7 6 5 4 3 2 1

There are two kinds of confidence which a reader may have in his author . . . . . there is a confidence in facts and a confidence in vision. . . . The former requires simple faith. The latter calls upon you to judge for yourself and form your own conclusions.

Anthony Trollope

Preface

If it were possible to arrive at a perfect solution of these questions, we might hope to obtain the highest reward which can repay our labours—an increased knowledge of the nature of disease, and improvement in the means of its treatment.

Richard Bright

The great contribution of Richard Bright was to correlate structure and function by meticulous clinicopathologic examination. Yet he was not satisfied by the mere recognition of morphologic abnormalities. More important was the necessity to elucidate the underlying nature of kidney disease and provide guides to the development of therapy. Now, more than 150 years later, the aim remains the same. Morphologic examination is one of many methods for the study of kidney disease and remains an avenue to knowledge, not an end in itself.

A book on renal pathology is of little value if it does no more than catalogue the many changes encountered in renal biopsy specimens. Indeed, to do so would be impossible. The pathologist recognizes patterns of morphologic change and interprets them in the light of clinical and immunopathologic data to establish diagnostic categories. Our aim in this book is to define some of these morphologic and pathogenetic patterns of disease and to show how their recognition can provide clues for further investigation while contributing to the assessment of therapy and prognosis.

This book is an expression of our approach to renal disease as well as an exposition of the major features seen in renal biopsy specimens. Much of the credit—although certainly none of the blame—for our approach must go to our physician colleagues whose stimulation and criticism has guided our labors. We thank them and also Richard Bright, who inspired the morphologic study of renal disease and laid down the guidelines that remain the foundations of morphologic study.

Contents

1
Introduction

The introduction of needle biopsy of solid organs in 1939 and its later application to the kidney marked the beginning of a new era in nephrology (1). Previously, the causes and natural histories of many renal lesions had been, perforce, deduced from the appearances of the kidneys at autopsy. The opportunity to examine biopsy material completely changed the role of the pathologist in the study of renal disease. Instead of acting as a final arbiter on a selected group of necessarily fatal conditions, the pathologist became an active member of the investigative team. Thus, the morphologic features of transient conditions and the evolution of progressive diseases could be analyzed for the first time. This drastic change coincided with the development of new and sophisticated techniques, which allowed more detailed examination of human and experimental renal diseases.

Inevitably, the characteristics of human diseases were compared with those of experimentally induced lesions in animals, and new concepts of pathogenesis were developed and investigated. The pathologist remains intimately concerned with the elucidation of disease mechanisms, but has the additional responsibility of delineating the morphologic and prognostic features of individual lesions. This dichotomy between progress and pragmatism has sometimes produced unfortunate and unnecessary conflicts between experimental and diagnostic pathologists. Neither approach is, in fact, entirely effective in isolation and each is mutually contributory. The diagnostic pathologist must chart a careful course between the traditional method of prediction by precedent on the one hand and extrapolation from experimental data on the other. This book attempts to outline a coherent and practical approach to the interpretation of renal lesions in the light of our present knowledge of pathogenetic mechanisms and to predict changes in emphasis that are likely to occur in the future. By necessity, discussion is largely restricted to glomerular diseases since these are the usual causes of symptoms leading to renal biopsy and have been most carefully studied in both humans and experimental systems.

TECHNIQUE

Most renal biopsy is now done via the percutaneous route, using either a cutting needle (2) or simple aspiration (3), but some clinics still prefer to sample the exposed kidney directly at open operation. Whatever the procedure, the biopsy tissue is best collected from the operator by a technician experienced in tissue preparation. We believe that there is no longer any justification for examination of renal biopsy specimens by light microscopy alone (4). Thus, the tissue must be immediately divided into portions for light, electron, and immunofluorescence preparation. The selection of material containing glomeruli for each technique is a perennial problem that has not been solved, in spite of the use of a variety of procedures, and ultimately it depends on careful sampling by an experienced technician. The most satisfactory results are obtained when two biopsy cores are taken. From the first core, two or three samples measuring 0.5 to 1 mm in diameter are immediately taken from each end with a fresh razor or scalpel blade and are immersed in fixative for electron microscopy, while the remainder is placed in saline. Providing the second core is adequate, samples are again taken from each end for electron microscopy, and the remainder is snap frozen for immunofluorescence, the tissue in saline being transferred to fixative for light microscopy. If only one core is obtained, material is taken from each end for electron microscopy, and the central portion is longitudinally divided into two components for light and immunofluorescence microscopy. This procedure may be modified if the biopsy specimen is very small or if samples are required for other procedures. When only a small amount of tissue can be obtained, consultation with the nephrologist performing the procedure will allow the technician to decide which techniques are most likely to provide diagnostic information. Generally, conventional light microscopic preparation can be omitted in such situations, since considerable information can be derived from light microscopic examination of plastic-embedded tissue, and the tissue can be apportioned to only electron and immunofluorescence preparation.

Light Microscopy

Accurate assessment of renal biopsy specimens requires good fixation, careful processing, and thin sections. These standards cannot be achieved if the biopsy specimens are processed and cut with general surgical material. The best results are obtained by an experienced technician using a manual processing procedure and special paraffin wax (5). A variety of fixatives has been recommended for renal biopsy material, but most pathologists feel that mercuric solutions provide the best architectural and cytologic detail. Zenker's fixative is widely used, but corrosive formol is equally effective and has the added advantage of producing complete fixation of biopsy cores in only 30 to 45 minutes. After this time, the core should be processed and stored in either 70% alcohol or 10% formol saline, since longer periods of fixation cause excessive hardening of the tissue. Experience with renal biopsy interpretation has convinced most workers that examination of only two or three sections is inadequate, because a wide range of appearances may be seen in a single biopsy core. Our practice is to cut through the core and to place three or four sections on each slide. At intervals of five, adjacent slides are stained with hematoxylin and eosin (H&E) and periodic acid-Schiff (PAS), a selection of the remainder being stained with PAS-methenamine silver (PASM) (5,6), PASM-chromotrope (7), and Masson trichrome (8). Ideally, the sections should be no more than 2 μ thick. To achieve consistently thin sections of this type, either special paraffin or plastic embedding materials must be used. Standard stains can be used on plastic-embedded material (9), but the preparation of multiple sections at various levels is extremely time consuming. Excellent preparations can be obtained by minor modifications of the paraffin wax, by preliminary cooling of the blocks, and by intermittent cooling of both knife and block with a high-pressure stream of carbon dioxide during the cutting procedure. This protocol, which routinely produces sections in six hours and can be reduced in urgent situations to two hours, is described in detail elsewhere (5).

Electron Microscopy

There is a wide spread misconception that tissue preparation for electron microscopy is a long and complex process. This belief has done much to downgrade the value of electron microscopic analysis, since the major prognostic and therapeutic decisions too often have been made by the time ultrastructural data become available. In fact, the processing time can routinely be reduced to 24 hours without detracting from tissue preservation, and satisfactory results have been reported with protocols requiring less than 5 hours (10). Many fixatives are available and all have varying advantages. We prefer primary fixation in osmium tetroxide for optimal demonstration of deposits and membrane structure, but glutaraldehyde is preferable if the integrity of cytoplasmic organelles is crucial. Osmium tetroxide is a toxic chemical, and primary glutaraldehyde fixation, with secondary osmication, is recommended if the solutions are to be handled by inexperienced personnel. Similarly, several epoxy resins with comparable characteristics are available and selection between them is largely a matter of personal preference. In our laboratories epon and Spurr's resins give satisfactory results.

The cubes of biopsy tissue are immediately immersed in cold 1% osmium tetroxide in S-collidine or cacodylate buffer. After fixation for 45 minutes, the tissue is washed in buffer, dehydrated in either graded alcohols or acidified 2,2-dimethoxypropane, embedded in the epoxy resin, and polymerized at 80°C overnight (11). The next morning, the blocks are removed from the plastic capsules, and 1-μ survey sections are cut with a glass knife onto glass slides that are then stained with toluidine blue. These sections reveal extensive structural detail and repay careful examination (1). Relatively small deposits can be recognized with the oil-immersion lens, and some authors have suggested that light microscopic examination of survey sections can replace electron microscopy in selected cases (12). In general, however, the main purpose of these sections is to select appropriate areas for electron microscopic examination. The selected blocks are then trimmed, and sections are cut with a diamond or glass knife and picked up on rhodium-plated copper grids. Double-staining with uranyl acetate and Reynolds lead citrate demonstrates most features satisfactorily, but methods for PASM-staining of ultrastructural material are available (13) and are of particular value in some forms of mesangiocapillary glomerulonephritis (14).

Occasionally, no glomeruli are included in the material selected for electron microscopic preparation. In this situation, adequate examination of deposits and membrane structures is possible in tissue taken from paraffin blocks (15), even some years after the original biopsy (16), or from portions of sections already mounted on glass slides (17). Similarly, valuable information can be obtained from ultrastructural examination of autopsy tissues (15,18). The electron microscopic features of each disease are reviewed in the appropriate sections of this book, but recent reviews of the subject may be consulted for a general introduction (18,19). Special refinements of electron microscopic techniques, such as scanning electron microscopy (20), have proved useful in the investigation of some human and experimental diseases but have not yet found a place in routine assessment.

Immunofluorescence Microscopy

Direct immunofluorescence is the most satisfactory technique for routine examination, but the indirect method may be used for extra sensitivity or to search for particular antigens or antibodies. The portion of the biopsy specimen selected for immunofluorescence is oriented in standard frozen section embedding compound on a piece of cork and is snap frozen by immersion in a beaker of isopentane surrounded by liquid nitrogen or dry ice. Loss of specific fluorescence and accentuation of background staining occur if the tissue is allowed to thaw, and it is important to maintain the surrounding temperature at -20 to $-40°C$. However, frozen tissue can be safely transported across large distances by packaging with large quantities of dry ice. Frozen sections of $2-4$ μ are cut in a cryostat at $-20°C$ and the air-dried slides are washed for five minutes in phosphate-buffered saline (PBS) to remove entrapped proteins. The sections, either unfixed or after immersion for 10 minutes in 1:1 ether:95% ethanol followed by 20 minutes in 95% ethanol and appropriate washing in PBS, are then overlain with monospecific antisera and are left in a moist chamber for 30 minutes at room temperature. After staining, the sections are washed in several changes of PBS to remove excess reagent and are coverslipped with 90% glycerol in PBS at pH 9.6. Sections prepared in this way may be stored at 4°C for many months without deterioration, but improved storage capacity has been claimed with the use of semipermanent mounting media (21). The sections are examined in ultraviolet light, using either transmitted or incident illumination, and the reactions are graded subjectively, 0 to 4+, and recorded by photography.

The specific antisera most commonly used are for IgG, IgA, IgM, Clq, C3, C4, and fibrinogen or fibrin. A variety of other complement (22) or coagulation (23) factors may be used, and antisera are available for both IgD (24) and IgE (25), but these do not contribute to routine diagnosis in the majority of cases. Commercially available antisera are generally satisfactory but should be checked for monospecificity by establishing lines of identity with known pure components by immunodiffusion or by staining myeloma cells of known immunoglobulin type. Unwanted or background fluorescence may be quenched by appropriate dilution of the reagents and by washing the sections with bovine serum albumin. Known positive and negative controls are probably necessary in laboratories processing few biopsy specimens, but controls are not required if large numbers of cases are examined and antisera are routinely checked for monospecificity and activity. However, the routine use of control reagents for nonimmune proteins, such as α_2-macroglobulin and albumin, is valuable to determine the immune specificity of reactions, and examination of unstained sections allows the identification of autofluorescent material.

An alternative to fluorescein conjugation and darkfield illumination is the technique of peroxidase labeling, by which brown granular precipitates outlining the immune reactions can be recognized by conventional light microscopy (26). This technique is readily applicable to renal biopsy material (27) and has the advantage of producing permanent preparations. However, it may not be as sensitive for weak reactions and has not yet found widespread acceptance. Either the immunofluorescence or immunoperoxidase technique can be applied to fixed and paraffin-embedded material, especially after treatment of sections by proteolytic enzymes, but mercury fixation abolishes the reactions, and complement components cannot be demonstrated (28,29). The typical reaction patterns in various diseases are reviewed below and described in more detail in the appropriate chapters, but recent reviews may be consulted for an introduction to techniques and the interpretation of reactions in both glomeruli (30,31) and extraglomerular tissues (32) in active disease and in severely damaged kidneys (33).

PATHOGENESIS

Most forms of glomerulonephritis are produced by immune mechanisms. There are two forms of immune-mediated glomerular disease: the deposition of preformed immune complexes and the interaction of circulating antibodies with glomerular antigens (34,35). Immune complex disease is characterized by a granular or discontinuous pattern of immunofluorescence, with the size of the complexes and a number of other factors determining whether deposition is predominantly in mesangia or along capillary walls. In contrast, the interaction of circulating antibodies with glomerular basement membrane antigens produces a quite distinct pattern of linear or continuous immunofluorescence. Varying distributions of these two reaction patterns have traditionally been the basis for the immunofluorescent classification of immune-mediated glomerulonephritis. This classification was originally based on assumptions derived from carefully studied experimental models but has now been confirmed in man by a variety of serologic and tissue studies. Generally, the pattern of granular immunofluorescence correlates closely with the demonstration by electron microscopy of dense deposits in various locations, and the presence of ultrastructural deposits is, therefore, regarded as presumptive evidence for immune complex disease.

Brief reviews of pathogenetic mechanisms are included with the discussions of each disease elsewhere in this book, and further details need not be given here. As a general principle, however, it may be stated that predominantly mesangial deposition of large immune complexes causes mesangial proliferative glomerulonephritis, whereas capillary wall localization of smaller complexes is associated with diffuse glomerular proliferation. Continuous immune complex deposition may overload the glomerular capacity for disposal and may lead to extraglomerular deposition with consequent interstitial inflammation (36). Similarly, antiglomerular basement membrane antibodies may localize both in glomerular and tubular membranes, but the pattern of inflammation is, curiously, often irregular. Whatever the mechanism inducing immune glomerular damage, the development of inflammatory changes is mediated by common pathways that do not differ from those causing inflammation in other tissues (37). Immune complexes, whether preformed or produced by the combination of antigen and circulating antibody, cause activation of the complement (38), coagulation (39), and kinin (37) systems with resultant increase in capillary permeability, chemotaxis, and tissue damage. Damage to glomerular constituents may be minor or very severe, with necrosis of capillary walls, leakage of plasma constituents into Bowman's space, and the formation of crescents. Particular diseases are characterized by relatively constant patterns of immunofluorescence reactions and glomerular inflammation that are the basis for pathologic diagnosis.

Glomerulonephritis may be associated with clinical and morphologic evidence of damage in other organs in such disorders as systemic lupus and Goodpasture's disease. The lack of extrarenal manifestations in many apparently primary forms of glomerulonephritis remains a cause for speculation. In some immune complex diseases, such as membranous nephropathy, there is some evidence for in situ formation of complexes but, in others, circulating complexes have been demonstrated in both blood and extrarenal tissues. The glomerulus may be especially vulnerable to the localization of complexes by virtue of its abundant circulation, high intraluminal pressure, and phagocytic capacity. Sequestration of immune complexes may also be favored by combination of complement in the complexes with C3b receptors in the glomerulus. These receptors are, however, present only on visceral epithelial cells and may play no significant role in the localization of intracapillary complexes (40,41). There is considerable speculation over the mechanisms causing formation of nephritogenic complexes, whatever is the mechanism for their deposition. People with deficiencies of several components of the complement pathway are particularly prone to develop glomerulonephritis, and hypocomplementemia produced by other mechanisms may also predispose to glomerulonephritis (38,42). There is evidence for immune deficiency in systemic lupus, and the frequency of glomerulonephritis in patients with cirrhosis suggests that bypassing of the reticuloendothelial system may reduce clearance of potentially phlogistic complexes. The next phase of investigation into immune-mediated glomerulonephritis is likely to be an attempt to elucidate the mechanisms by which nephritogenic immune complexes are formed and allowed to remain in the circulation.

CLASSIFICATION OF GLOMERULAR DISEASE

Glomerulonephritis may be classified by clinical, morphologic, immunopathologic, or prognostic criteria (18,43,44) (Table 1-1). The pathologist requires a basic morphologic framework on which other information can be superimposed. Such a framework facilitates a conventional diagnostic approach—from recognized patterns to specific clinicopathologic entities—and may allow the identification of morphologic patterns that are prognostically favorable regardless of their pathogenesis. Morphologic classification is based on subdivisions created by variations in either the distribution or character of glomerular lesions. There is general agreement over the definitions applied to

Table 1-1. Classification of Glomerular Disease Using Light and Electron Microscopy with Immunofluorescence, with Emphasis on Prognosis

---

Epithelial cell involvement
    Epithelial cell disease
    Focal segmental glomerulosclerosis
    Congenital nephrosis

Membranous glomerulonephropathy
    Idiopathic membranous glomerulonephropathy
    Secondary to drug, infection, neoplasm

Changes in capillary wall in absence of deposits
    Benign familial nephropathy
    Progressive hereditary nephropathy

Glomerular inflammatory disease
    Postinfectious glomerulonephritis (acute and postacute phase)
    Mesangiocapillary (membranoproliferative) glomerulonephritis
      Type I
      Type II
      Type III
    Focal and segmental glomerulonephritis
    Crescentic (rapidly progressive) glomerulonephritis
    Chronic glomerulonephritis

---

the distribution of glomerular disease (Table 1-2), but more specific categorization has excited considerable controversy.

Recently, an international committee convened by the World Health Organization devised a classification of glomerular disease that is likely to be accepted by most pathologists (Table 1-3) (45). This classification is based on a primary subdivision according to the overall pattern of glomerular change and a secondary categorization of the type and distribution of superimposed lesions. While appearing cumbersome at first sight, this approach is necessary because of the frequent coexistence of several disease patterns in individual biopsy specimens. Segmental changes are especially prone to be superimposed on diffuse diseases,

Table 1-2. Classification of Glomerular Disease by Distribution

---

Classification by distribution of disease among many glomeruli
    Focal: disease affecting some but not all glomeruli
    Diffuse: disease affecting all or nearly all glomeruli

Classification by distribution of disease in individual glomeruli
    Segmental: a lesion involving only a portion of a glomerulus (note that the remainder
      of the glomerulus need not be completely normal)
    Global: a lesion involving the entire glomerulus

---

and undue emphasis on the secondary, segmental patterns may lead to erroneous diagnoses with inappropriate diagnostic implications. Segmental sclerosis and hyalinosis, for example, are common and nonspecific features in a wide range of glomerular diseases, while a substantial proportion of biopsy specimens previously categorized as focal glomerulonephritis is now recognized as having significant diffuse abnormalities. Similarly, crescents are merely expressions of severe glomerular damage and, except in catastrophic crescentic disease when the original disease may be unrecognizable, the nature of the underlying lesion is often of major prognostic importance. Classification, therefore, depends on initial examination of all glomeruli to determine the presence or absence of diffuse disease and subsequent categorization of superimposed focal or diffuse lesions. Inevitably, the changes in some biopsy specimens defy classification in our present state of knowledge, and the damage in other specimens is so advanced that only the nonspecific categorization of chronic sclerosing glomerulonephritis can be applied.

This morphologic approach is applicable to all patterns of glomerular disease, but further categorization may be possible on the basis of specific clinical, light, electron, or immunofluorescence microscopic characteristics. In the following chapters, the general patterns of glomerular change are discussed in the order shown in Table 1-3, and diseases with specific features are discussed separately. Whenever possible, the occurrence of a general pattern of morphologic change in a specific clinicopathologic entity is noted so the reader may refer to the appropriate section for a more complete discussion. A subdivision into "primary" and "secondary" types of glomerular disease is not attempted since it is now quite clear that the vast majority of glomerular diseases are secondary to either overt or occult systemic immune disturbances.

BIOPSY INTERPRETATION

Many pathologists regard the interpretation of renal biopsy specimens as extraordinarily difficult. This view has been fostered by constantly changing approaches to classification and the necessity for immunofluorescence and electron microscopic data. In fact, diagnosis from renal biopsy specimens relies on the same foundations of careful observation and clinicopathologic correlation as do all other areas of diagnostic pathology. A knowledge of normal structure is clearly essential, and diagnoses are achieved by the identification of variations from normality in each nephron component. Systems of grading each abnormality have been proposed (46) and are useful for studies of particular diseases, but the basic diagnostic principle is deductive reasoning from established patterns of change. To facilitate this approach, a checklist of features for examination is shown in Table 1-4, and the discussion in subsequent chapters is based on clearly recognizable abnormalities.

There has been considerable discussion over the criteria for acceptance of a renal biopsy specimen as adequate for diagnosis. Early studies comparing needle biopsy specimens and large blocks of the same kidney at autopsy concluded that representative features could be recognized in biopsy specimens containing as few as four glomeruli (47). More extensive use of electron and immunofluores-

Table 1-3. Histologic Classification of Glomerular Lesions by Light Microscopy[a]

Major classification
A.   Minor or no glomerular abnormality
B.   Focal and/or segmental lesions with minor or no lesions in other glomeruli (see supplementary classification)
C.   Diffuse glomerulonephritis
     Mesangial proliferative glomerulonephritis
     Proliferative endocapillary glomerulonephritis
     Mesangiocapillary glomerulonephritis
     Dense deposit glomerulonephritis
     Membranous nephropathy
     Crescentic glomerulonephritis
     Chronic sclerosing glomerulonephritis
     Unclassified glomerulonephritis

Supplementary classification of other significant glomerular features
     None
     Segmental mesangial/endocapillary proliferation
     Segmental hyalinosis
     Segmental sclerosis
     Segmental capillary thrombosis
     Segmental necrosis
     Cellular/fibrocellular crescents
     Segmental capillary wall abnormalities
     Global sclerosis
     Leukocytic infiltration
     Subepithelial deposits
     Transmembranous deposits
     Subendothelial deposits ("wire-loops")
     Mesangial deposits
     Mesangial matrix increase
     Other (specify)

[a]Slightly modified from Churg et al. (45) and reproduced with the permission of Igaku-Shoin Ltd.

cence microscopy has since reduced this figure even further in such diffuse disorders as membranous nephropathy and amyloidosis. The definition of adequacy is, therefore, largely dependent on the disease under consideration. In diseases characterized by irregular or crescentic proliferation, we prefer to base assessment on 10 or more glomeruli, whereas, in diffuse disorders, the recognition of specific features in only one glomerulus may be sufficient for diagnosis. The characteristic ultrastructural features of most lesions are readily recognizable in one glomerulus, but there is often some variation between glomeruli, and we routinely examine two or more glomeruli if these are available.

The assessment of irregular lesions, such as crescents, is best accompanied by a numerical description of the proportion of involved glomeruli. The presence of small crescents in only 1 or 2 of 20 glomeruli may, for example, be of little prognostic or therapeutic importance, whereas circumferential involvement of more than half of the glomeruli is an indication for urgent action. Similarly,

Table 1-4. Checklist for Biopsy Interpretation

	Light Microscopy	Electron Microscopy	Immunofluorescence Miscroscopy

Glomeruli	Size and cellularity
	Mesangia
	Capillary walls
	Deposits and site
	Segmental changes: type and %
	Crescents: type and %
	Polymorphs
		Cellular changes
		Mesangia
		Glomerular basement membrane:
		  width, contour, density
		Deposits—site and character
		Cellular inclusions
		  (e.g. tubulovesicular bodies)
			Reactions and pattern
			Linear/granular
			Mesangial/capillary wall/mixed
			Reagent
			Intensity

Tubules	Dilatation
	Atrophy
	Cellular changes
	  Necrosis
	  Repair
	  Vacuolation
	Casts and type
	Basement membrane
	Inclusion droplets
		Cellular changes
		Inclusions
		Casts
		Basement membrane deposits
			Basement membrane reactions
			  and pattern
			Antinuclear antibody
			Inclusion droplets

Interstitium	Edema Inflammation and type Scarring—%	Deposits Cellular infiltrates	Reactions and distribution
Blood vessels	Medial hypertrophy Elastica changes Hyalinosis Intimal thickening and type Necrosis Vasculitis Juxtaglomerular apparatus	Intimal and medial changes	Reactions and distribution

grading on a percentage basis of the extent of interstitial scarring allows the physician to assess more precisely the outlook for continued renal function. In the assessment of scarring, some care must be taken if biopsy specimens have previously been taken from the same kidney, since significant damage may result from either direct needle trauma or from vascular obliteration (48). The possibility of biopsy-induced scarring needs consideration if interstitial damage seems to be out of proportion to renal functional alterations or if hemosiderin can be demonstrated in the abnormal area. A variety of other quantitative techniques may be applied to renal biopsies, but few are of routine diagnostic value.

SUMMARY

Renal biopsy diagnosis depends on careful examination of satisfactory light, electron, and immunofluorescence preparations in conjunction with a consideration of the clinical features. The pathologist interpreting renal biopsy specimens is an integral part of the team investigating patients with renal disease and cannot work satisfactorily in isolation. Accurate diagnosis is based on recognition of basic patterns of reaction by light microscopy and on identification of underlying mechanisms by other techniques. Correlation of the data obtained by these various approaches provides both quantitative and qualitative information that is of crucial value in the management of patients with renal disease. Although the specialist in renal pathology is best equipped to obtain maximal information from each biopsy specimen, the essential features can almost always be recognized by inexperienced pathologists if satisfactory material is thoroughly examined using a standard approach. The basic elements in the preparation of biopsy material and the approaches to diagnosis having been reviewed, the following chapters outline the characteristics of discrete disease entities.

REFERENCES

1. Seymour AE, Spargo BH, Penska R: Contributions of renal biopsy studies to the understanding of disease. *Am J Pathol* 65:549, 1971.
2. Deeley TJ: *Needle biopsy.* London, Butterworths, 1974.
3. Pasternack A, Helin H, Törnröth T, et al: Aspiration biopsy of the kidney with a new fine needle: a way to obtain glomeruli for morphologic study. *Clin Nephrol* 10:79, 1978.
4. Spargo BH: Practical use of electron microscopy for diagnosis of glomerular disease. *Human Pathol* 6:404, 1975.
5. Meadows, R, Schoemaker H: Improved processing technique for renal biopsies for light microscopy. *J Clin Pathol* 23:548, 1970.
6. Jones DB: Nephrotic glomerulonephritis. *Am J Pathol* 33:313, 1957.
7. Ehrenreich T, Espinosa T: Chromotrope silver methenamine stain of glomerular lesions. *Am J Clin Pathol* 56:448, 1971.
8. Cohen AH: Masson's trichrome stain in the evaluation of renal biopsies: an appraisal. *Am J Clin Pathol* 65:631, 1976.
9. Xipell JM, Gladwin RC: Routine rapid preparation of thin epoxy resin-embedded sections of renal biopsies for light microscopy. *Am J Clin Pathol* 58:469, 1972.

10. Johanssen JV: Rapid processing of kidney biopsies for electron microscopy. *Kidney Int* 3:46, 1973.

11. Luft JH: Improvements in epoxy resin embedding methods. *J Biophys Biochem Cytol* 9:409, 1961.

12. Heaton JM, Turner DR, Cameron JS: Localization of glomerular "deposits" in Henoch-Schönlein nephritis. *Histopathol* 1:93, 1977.

13. Doyle GD, Campbell E: The periodic Schiff-methenamine (PASM) staining of renal biopsies—a light and electron microscopic study. *Irish J Med Sci* 145:127, 1976.

14. Anders D, Agricola B, Sippel M, et al: Basement membrane changes in membrano-proliferative glomerulonephritis: II. Characterization of a third type by silver impregnation. *Virchows Arch (A) Path Anat Histol* 376:1, 1977.

15. Johanssen JV: Use of paraffin material for electron microscopy. *Pathol Annu* 12:189, 1977.

16. Collan Y, Klockars M, Heino M: Revision of light-microscopic kidney biopsy diagnosis in glomerular disease. *Nephron* 20:24, 1978.

17. González-Angulo A, De Chavel IR, Castañeda M: A reliable method for electron microscopic examination of specific areas from paraffin-embedded tissue mounted on glass slides. *Am J Clin Pathol* 70:697, 1978.

18. Spargo BH, Seymour AE: The value of electron microscopy in the study of glomerular disease, in Black DAK (ed): *Renal Disease,* ed 3. Oxford, Blackwell Scientific Publications, 1972, p 155.

19. Churg J, Grishman E: Ultrastructure of glomerular disease: a review. *Kidney Int* 7:254, 1975.

20. Jones DB: Correlative scanning and transmission electron microscopy of glomeruli. *Lab Invest* 37:569, 1977.

21. Couser WG, Lewis EJ: Laboratory suggestion: a method of preservation of immunofluorescence in renal tissue. *Am J Clin Pathol* 61:873, 1974.

22. Verroust PJ, Wilson CB, Cooper NR, et al: Glomerular complement components in human glomerulonephritis. *J Clin Invest* 53:77, 1974.

23. Hoyer JR, Michael AF, and Hoyer LW: Immunofluorescent localization of antihemophilic factor antigen and fibrinogen in human renal diseases. *J Clin Invest* 53:1375, 1974.

24. Katz A, Pruzanski W: IgD deposition in glomerulonephritis: an immunopathological study. *Am J Clin Pathol* 63:291, 1975.

25. Robertson MR, Potter EV, Roberts ML, et al: Immunoglobulin E in renal disease. *Nephron* 16:256, 1976.

26. Mesa-Tejada R, Pascal RR, Fenoglio CM: Immunoperoxidase: a sensitive immunohistochemical technique as a "special stain" in the diagnostic pathology laboratory. *Human Pathol* 8:313, 1977.

27. Turner DR, Wilson CM, Lake A, et al: An evaluation of the immunoperoxidase technique in renal biopsy diagnosis. *Clin Nephrol* 11:13, 1979.

28. Huang S-N, Minassian H, More JD: Application of immunofluorescent staining on paraffin sections improved by trypsin digestion. *Lab Invest* 35:383, 1976.

29. Curran RC, Gregory J: Demonstration of immunoglobulin in cryostat and paraffin sections of human tonsil by immunofluorescence and immunoperoxidase techniques: effects of processing on immunohistochemical performance of tissues and on the use of proteolytic enzymes to unmask antigens in sections. *J Clin Pathol* 31:974, 1978.

30. Wilson CB, Dixon FJ: Diagnosis of immunopathologic renal disease. *Kidney Int* 5:389, 1974.

31. Albini B, Brentjens JR, Andres GA: The immunopathology of the kidney. *Current Topics Immunol* 11:106, 1979.

32. Lehmann DH, Wilson CB, Dixon FJ: Extraglomerular immunoglobulin deposits in human nephritis. *Am J Med* 58:765, 1975.

33. Velosa J, Miller K, Michael AF: Immunopathology of the end-stage kidney: immunoglobulin and complement component deposition in nonimmune disease. *Am J Pathol* 84:149, 1976.

34. Wilson CB, Dixon FJ: The renal response to immunological injury, in Brenner BM, Rector FC Jr, (eds): *The Kidney.* Philadelphia, WB Saunders Co, 1976, Vol II, p 838.

35. Germuth FG Jr, Rodriguez E: *Immunopathology of the Renal Glomerulus: Immune Complex Deposit and Antibasement Membrane Disease.* Boston, Little, Brown and Company, 1973.

36. Brentjens JR, O'Connell DW, Pawlowski IB, et al: Extra-glomerular lesions associated with deposition of circulating antigen-antibody complexes in kidneys of rabbits with chronic serum sickness. *Clin Immunol Immunopathol* 3:112, 1974.

37. Ryan GB, Majno G: Acute inflammation: a review. *Am J Pathol* 86:183, 1977.

38. Ruddy S, Gigli I, Austen KF: The complement system of man. *N Engl J Med* 287:489, 545, 590, 641, 1972.

39. Vassalli P, McCluskey RT: The pathogenetic role of the coagulation process in glomerular diseases of immunologic origin. *Adv Nephrol* 1:47, 1971.

40. Shin ML, Gelfand MC, Nagle RB, et al: Localization of receptors for activated complement on visceral epithelial cells of the human renal glomerulus. *J Immunol* 118:869, 1977.

41. Burkholder PM, Oberley TD, Barber TA, et al: Immune adherence in renal glomeruli: complement receptor sites on glomerular capillary epithelial cells. *Am J Pathol* 86:635, 1977.

42. Peters DK, Williams DG: Complement and mesangiocapillary glomerulonephritis: role of complement deficiency in the pathogenesis of nephritis. *Nephron* 13:189, 1974.

43. Witting C: The terminology of nephritis: a review. *Current Topics Pathol* 61:45, 1976.

44. Kashgarian M, Hayslett JP, Spargo BH: Teaching monograph: renal disease. *Am J Pathol* 89:187, 1977.

45. Churg J, et al: *Histological Classification of Renal Diseases.* Tokyo, New York, Igaku-Shoin Ltd, in press.

46. Pirani CL, Salinas-Madrigal L: Evaluation of percutaneous renal biopsy. *Pathol Annu* 3:249, 1968.

47. Kellow WF, Cotsonas NJ, Chomet B, et al: Evaluation of the adequacy of needle-biopsy specimens of the kidney. *Arch Intern Med* 104:353, 1959.

48. Osborne CA, Low DG, Jessen CR: Renal parenchymal response to needle biopsy. *Invest Urol* 9:463, 1972.

2
Normal Renal Structure

The kidneys are complex structures performing many functions. Among the most important of these functions is the production of urine, for which the nephron is the basic functional unit. Both kidneys contain approximately 1 million nephrons, each consisting of a glomerulus and its subtended proximal and distal tubules with the intervening loop of Henle. An ultrafiltrate of plasma crosses the glomerular capillary wall and passes into the tubules, where the secretory and absorptive activities of the lining cells concentrate and modify the filtrate into urine. At the termination of the nephron, the distal tubular contents flow into the collecting tubular system and thence to the renal pelvis, ureter, and bladder. Renal biopsies usually sample only the cortex, and the morphologic study of biopsy tissue is most valuable for the assessment of glomerular disease. This brief review of the normal structure, therefore, concentrates on the glomerulus and provides only a superficial description of the tubules and other components of the kidney.

THE GLOMERULUS

There are two populations of glomeruli. The juxtamedullary glomeruli are larger than those situated more peripherally, and knowledge of the location from which the biopsy specimen is taken is important when assessing glomerular size (1). In either location, the glomerulus consists of a tuft of peculiarly specialized and branching capillaries that arise from the afferent arteriole to form lobules and rejoin the vascular pole to drain into the efferent arteriole. The lobules are poorly defined in normal glomeruli and consist of congeries of capillaries centered on a complex supporting structure, the mesangium. The tuft lies within Bowman's space, which is lined on its parietal aspect by a layer of attenuated epithelial cells overlying the thick basement membrane of Bowman's capsule. This capsule is continuous at the vascular pole with the membranes of the arterioles, and at the urinary pole it merges with the basement membrane of the proximal tubule (Figs. 2-1 to 2-5). Minor degrees of irregular thickening of Bowman's capsule, often with calcification and intramembranous deposit, are common in otherwise normal biopsy specimens and appear to have no significance. The parietal epithelium may be hypertrophied, so it resembles that of the proximal tubule, and degeneration of these cells may produce an artefactual appearance of proteinaceous precipitate in Bowman's space.

The glomerular capillary wall is composed of endothelial and epithelial cells

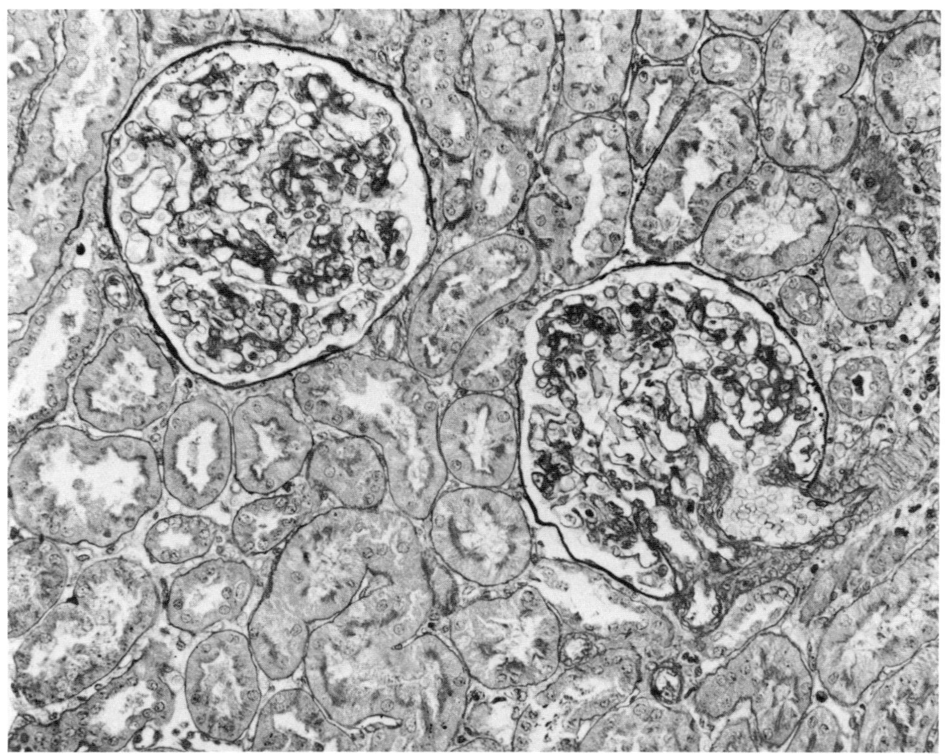

Figure 2-1. Normal renal cortical tissue (PAS stain, ×300).

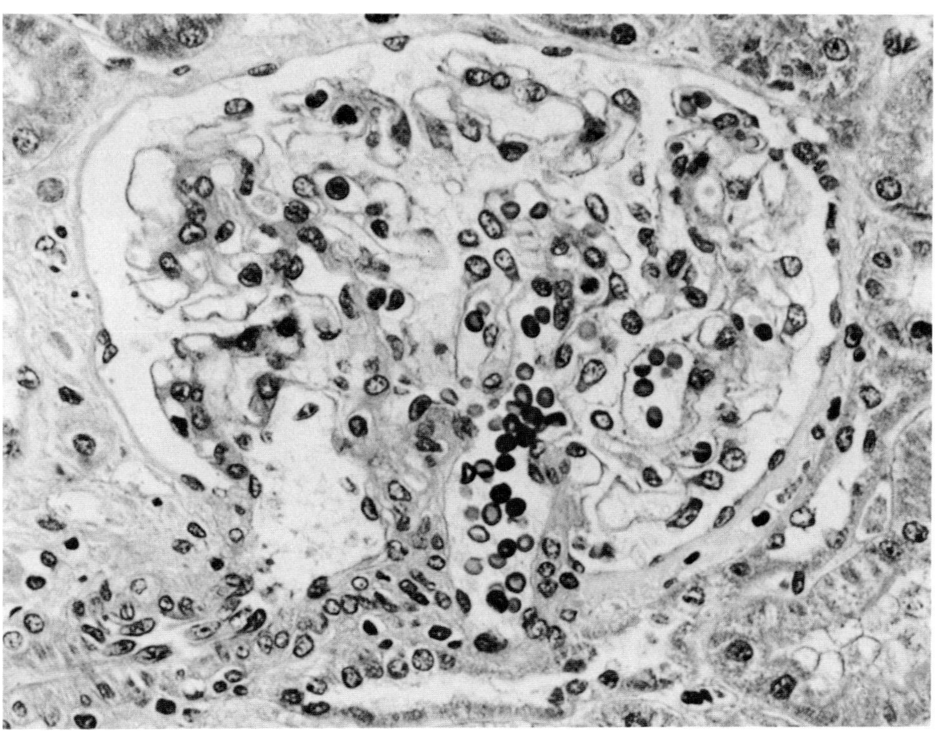

Figure 2-2. A normal glomerulus with afferent and efferent arterioles. The basement membrane is thin and delicate (H&E stain, ×450).

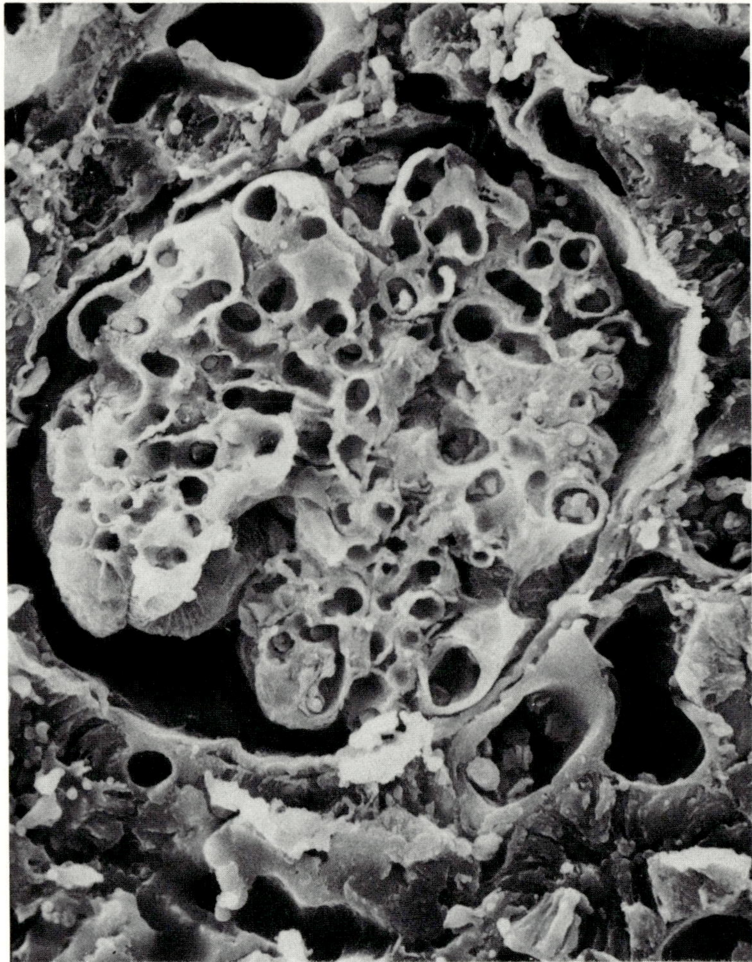

Figure 2-3. Scanning electron micrograph showing glomerular capillary tuft surrounded by Bowman's capsule (×750).

separated by basement membrane. These structures cannot be distinguished in sections stained with H&E, and light microscopic assessment of the capillary components requires PAS or PASM stained sections. Thorough examination of the glomerular capillary is only possible by electron microscopy. The endothelial cells form a thin, fenestrated layer 300–1000 Å in width with the nuclei located at the mesangial aspect (Figs. 2-6, 2-7). Cytoplasmic organelles are sparse in these cells, and the capillary lining is interrupted by round or polygonal pores measuring 500–800 Å in diameter (Fig. 2-8). No limiting membrane spans these pores, and the contents of the capillary in these regions are, therefore, in direct contact with the glomerular basement membrane. The large size of the pores precludes any significant role for the endothelium in the maintenance of glomerular permeability save for restriction of the cellular elements of the blood (Figs 2-7, 2-8).

The glomerular basement membrane does not surround the entire capillary

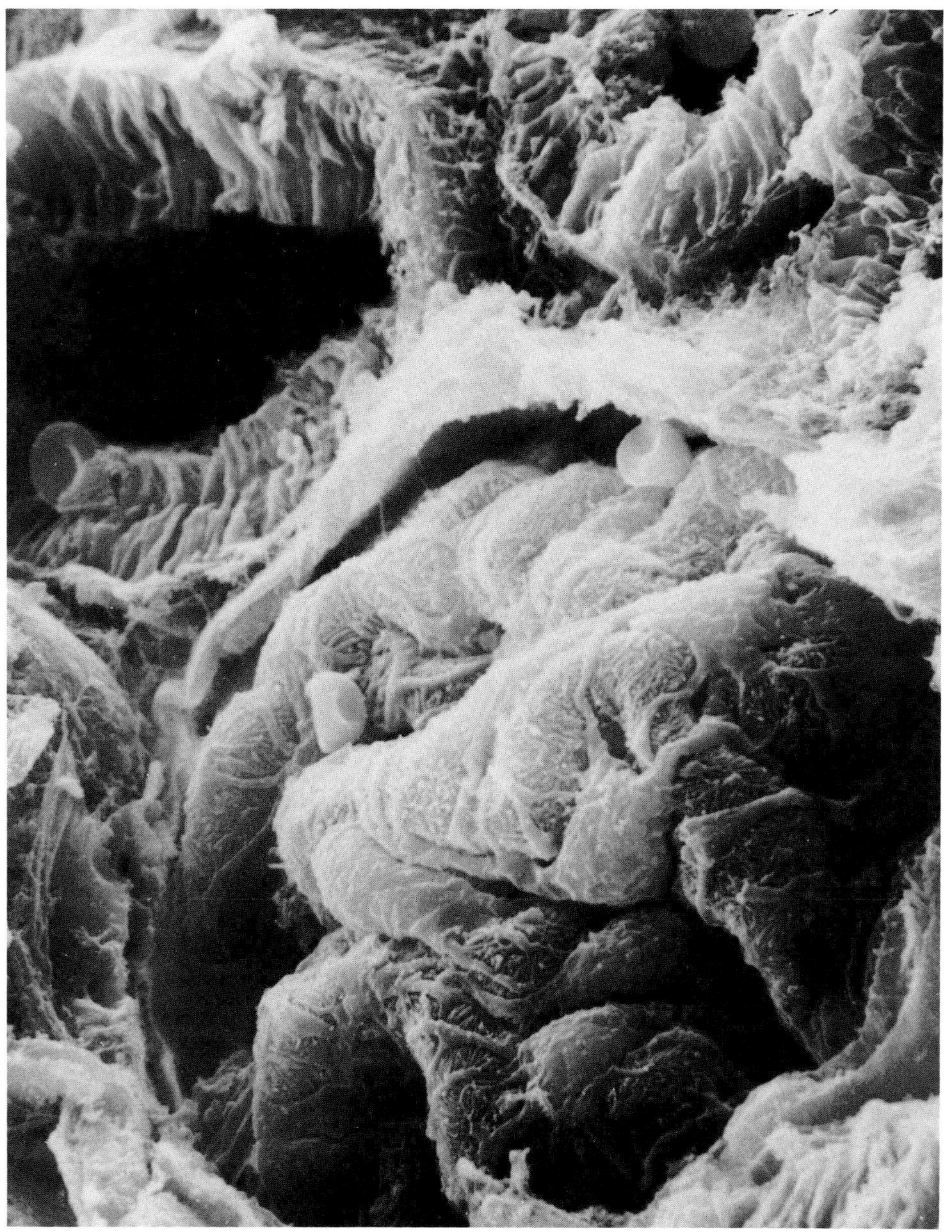

Figure 2-4. Scanning electron micrograph of renal cortex. The capillary loops are covered by epithelial cells (×550).

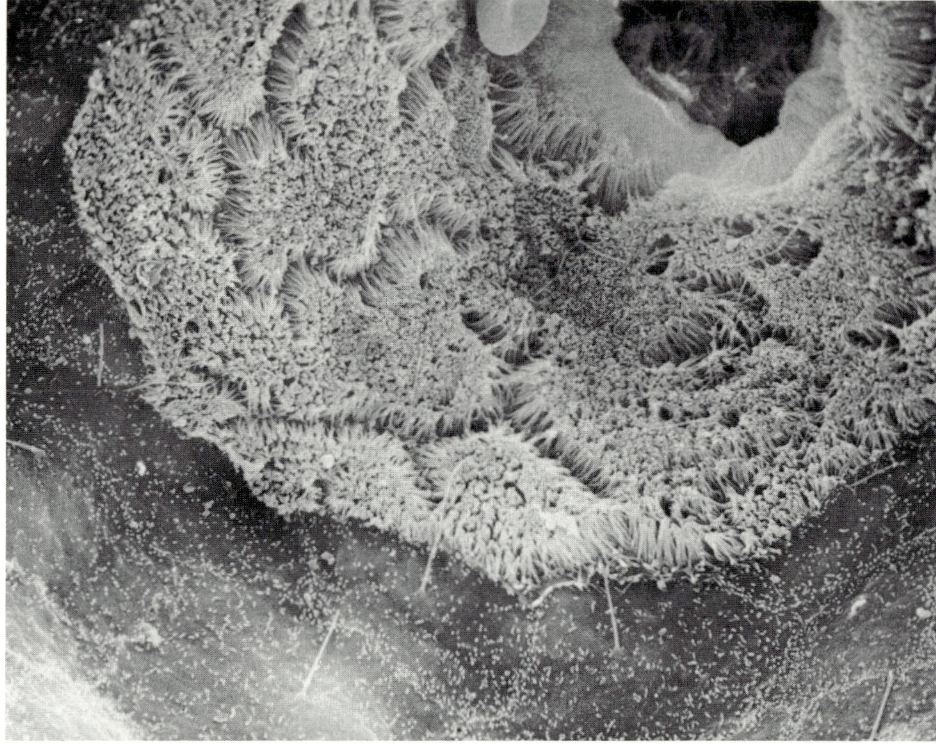

Figure 2-5. Scanning electron micrograph of the urinary pole. The Bowman's capsule is lined by flattened epithelial cells covered by sparse, small microvilli and centrally located cilia. Notice the abrupt beginning of the proximal tubule with conspicous brush border (×2,500).

lumen. Instead, the lumen is bounded centrally by the mesangium, providing a direct path for the disposal of macromolecular substances barred from filtration by the basement membrane. In healthy adults, the membrane is approximately 3,400Å wide, as measured by a variety of techniques (2,3), and it is somewhat narrower in children. Probably because of differences in the perfusion of different lobules at the time of biopsy, moderate variation in membrane width may exist within the same glomerulus. The membrane has a trilaminar structure with a central lamina densa bordered by two narrower layers of decreased density, the laminae rara interna and externa. Generally, the contour, width, and density of the membrane are relatively uniform, but tangential sectioning may produce an appearance of irregular thickening, especially near the mesangial regions, and there may normally be sporadic areas of subendothelial lucency. Normally no dense deposits are visible along the membrane, but subepithelial nodules are occasionally present near the hilus and two patterns of localized subepithelial change may confuse interpretation. Craterlike formations, frequently containing membranous profiles (striated membranous bodies), are sometimes seen on the convexity of capillary loops, and collections of microvesicular bodies may accumulate over mesangia (4−6). Each of these anomalous structures occurs more commonly in damaged glomeruli, but each may be seen in biopsy specimens

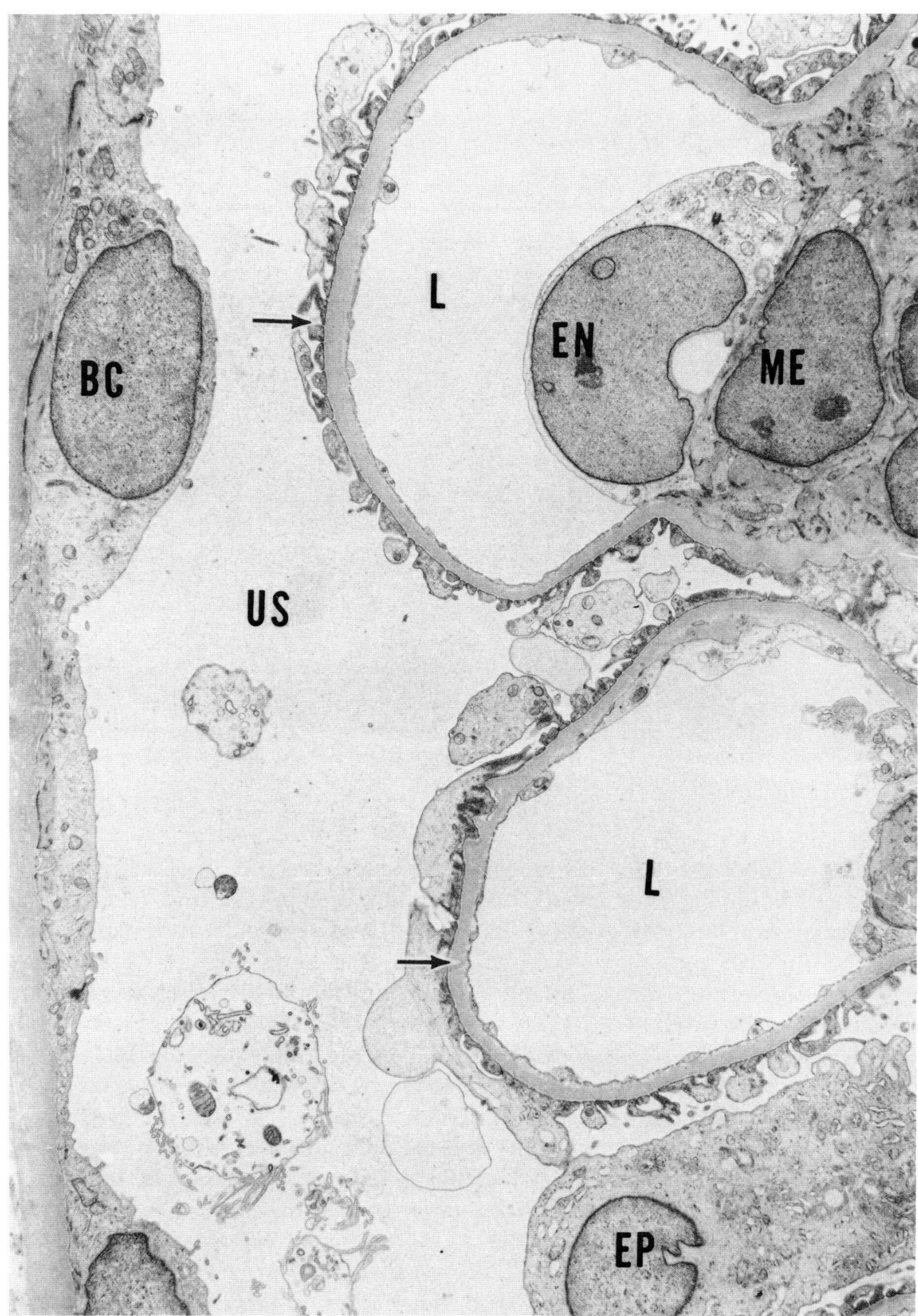

Figure 2-6. Electron micrograph of a normal glomerulus, demonstrating the relation of different cell types. The epithelial aspect of the basement membrane (arrows) appears covered by the foot processes. EN, endothelial cell; ME, mesangium; EP, visceral epithelial cell; BC, Bowman's capsule with parietal epithelial cells; US, urinary space; L, capillary lumen (×9,500).

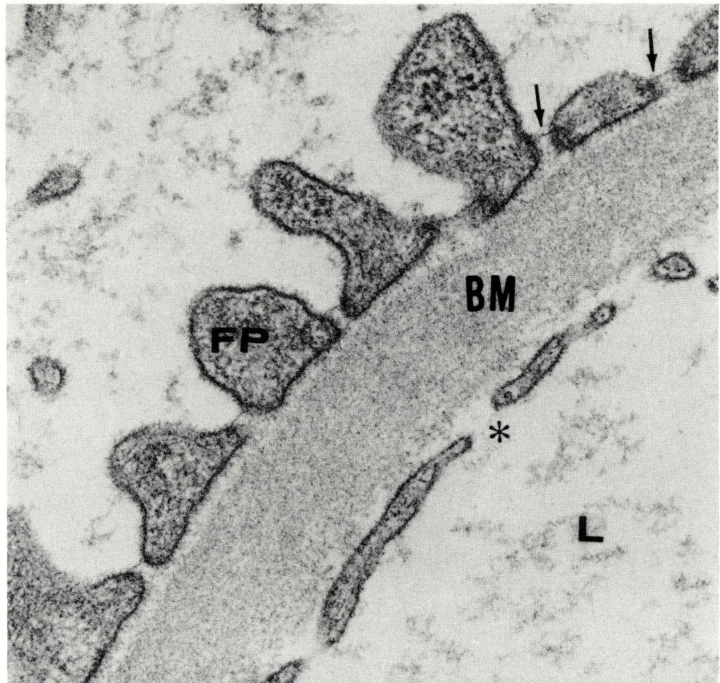

Figure 2-7. Electron micrograph of glomerular capillary loop, demonstrating epithelial foot processes (FP), fenestrated endothelium (⋆), basement membrane (BM), and slit-pore membrane (arrows). L, capillary lumen (×50,000).

showing no other evidence of glomerular disease, especially in older patients.

Visceral epithelial cells cover the basement membranes and encircle the glomerular capillaries (Fig. 2-6). Their cytoplasm contains endoplasmic reticulum, fine ribosomes, small mitochondria, and Golgi profiles. Many microvesicles are present near the cell surface, and both microtubules and fine filaments may be prominent in and around the foot processes. Although a contractile role has been suggested for these filaments, motility of epithelial cells has not yet been demonstrated. The cells are surrounded by a triple-layered cell membrane with a rough surface coating of acid mucosubstances, the glycocalyx, which is rich in sialic acid and has been implicated in the control of permeability (7). Scanning electron microscopy has elucidated the complex structure of the epithelial foot processes by providing a three-dimensional view of their relationship to the capillary wall. The cell body gives off major cytoplasmic extensions, which branch into interdigitating foot processes (8.9). Adjacent foot processes arise from different epithelial cells and, depending on the method of fixation, are situated approximately 400 Å apart with a connecting slit-pore diaphragm 70 Å wide (Figs, 2-4, 2-9). The pattern of foot process "fusion" is produced by swelling of the cell body with retraction of the processes rather than by actual coalescence of adjacent processes, and is better described as foot process obliteration (9). Small foci of obliteration are common in otherwise normal glomeruli, especially over mesangial regions, and have no significance. The osmiophilic

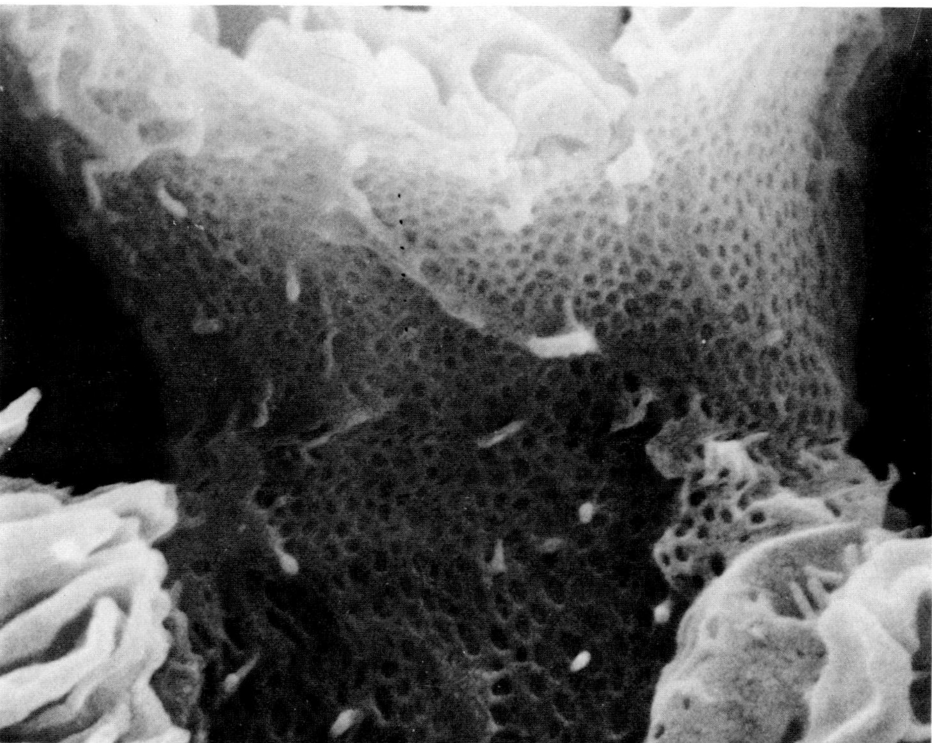

Figure 2-8. Scanning electron micrograph showing fenestrated endothelium of a glomerular capillary loop. Notice the presence of small villi (×22,000).

material normally present in the processes may become irregularly dispersed in areas of obliteration and appear superficially similar to subepithelial deposits.

The visceral epithelial cells are a major source of basement membrane renewal (10), but their role in the maintenance of glomerular permeability is controversial. Normally, water and ions are freely filtered across the capillary wall, but only small quantities of albumin reach Bowman's space and larger molecules are retained. Albumin is, therefore, regarded as the upper limit of the glomerular filter (11). Permeability, however, depends on a variety of other factors, including the charge, rigidity, and configuration of molecules and the hydraulic pressure and rapidity of flow within the capillary (12). A complex, zipperlike arrangement of the epithelial slit-pore membrane has been proposed as the final filtering area (13), but such a mechanism appears to be hydraulically unsound. Instead, the basement membrane is probably the major area of permeability control, filtration being achieved by the convoluted and interconnected arrangement of molecules within the membrane (14,15).

The central portions of glomerular lobules are occupied by the mesangium. This region was regarded for many years as an extension of the endothelium from either adjacent capillaries or hilar arterioles and, for this reason, was ignored in a number of the early studies of glomerular disease. There is now no doubt that the mesangium is a specialized and distinct phagocytic structure of

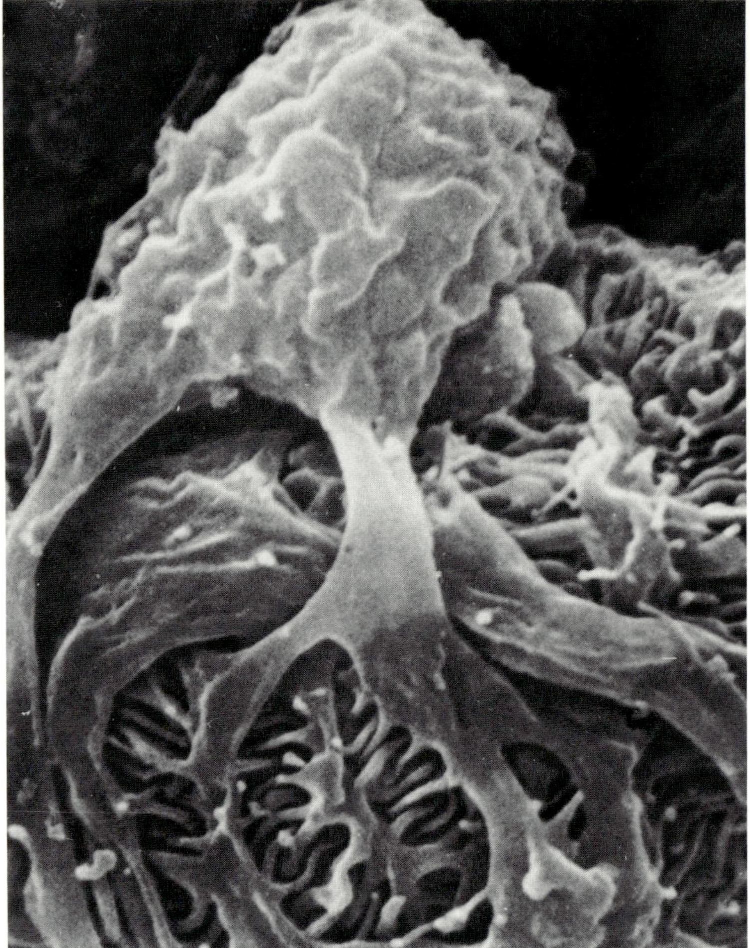

Figure 2-9. Scanning electron micrograph from a normal rat kidney glomerulus, showing cell processes and interdigitating foot processes along the surface of the capillary wall (×15,000).

the glomerulus with no relationship to either endothelium or the reticuloendothelial system (16,17). Macromolecular substances accumulate in the mesangium and are disposed of via a complex canalicular system through the hilus into the distal tubule (18). Mesangial cells have elongated, irregular nuclei and branching cytoplasmic processes that are interspersed with mesangial matrix. Phagolysosomes are frequently visible within the cytoplasm, and there are numerous microfilaments that have been shown to be composed of actomyosin (19,20). Contractile activity of these cells, which has been demonstrated in tissue culture, may be mediated by angiotensin receptors and could be involved in the regulation of glomerular blood flow (20,21). The matrix has an amorphous structure with electron density similar to that of the glomerular basement membrane but with different antigenic characteristics, and it is dispersed throughout the axial region to provide mechanical support. The canalicular component of the matrix may impart a fibrillar pattern, which is occasionally difficult to differentiate from extraneous fibrillar deposits such as amyloid. Mesangial matrix increases progressively with age so that the axial portions of glomeruli from older people usually appear more solid than in children or adolescents. Careful study of mesangial regions may disclose rare and small deposits, especially near the hilus, which probably represent normal disposal of macromolecules and do not necessarily indicate glomerular disease.

PROXIMAL TUBULE

The proximal tubule has two parts (22). The convoluted portion (pars convoluta) arises from the urinary pole of the glomerulus and continues into the straight region (pars recta). The cells of the pars convoluta are cuboidal with eosinophilic cytoplasm and a round basal nucleus. In PAS-stained sections, a magenta apical zone corresponds to the glycocalyx, covering a luxuriant outgrowth of microvilli that increase the surface area of the cell by a factor of 40. Within this apical area is an antigenic component (renal tubular antigen) that has been detected in the deposits of a number of glomerular diseases (23). Many pinocytotic vesicles are present in the subapical region, and prominent tight junctions join the cells near their luminal surfaces. The basal plasma membrane is deeply convoluted, to facilitate tubular transport and is in close contact with elongate mitochondria.

Rough endoplasmic reticulum and ribosomes are prominent throughout the cells, and there are well-developed Golgi profiles near the nuclei. Cytosomes and segrosomes are common in addition to protein transport droplets which are probably concerned with the conservation of filtered albumin (24,25). The cells of the pars recta are rather lower than those more proximally and have a slightly shorter brush border (Figs. 2-10 to 2-13). Clear cell tumors of the renal cortex arise from the proximal tubule (26).

THIN LOOP OF HENLE

The beginning of the thin loop of Henle is marked by an abrupt change in cell type from the cuboidal pattern of the proximal tubule to a flattened, simple epithelium (Fig. 2-10). The length of Henle's loops varies with the positions of the related glomeruli in the cortex. Nephrons in the outer cortex have relatively short loops, whereas those nearer the corticomedullary junction subtend longer loops, which may reach the papillary tip. The lining cells contain sparse organelles and have few surface microvilli (Fig. 2-14). In the descending limb, there are interdigitations of the cellular lining membranes, while, in the ascending limb, cellular borders are smooth and straight. Variations in the degree of cellular interdigitation and in the distribution of intramembranous particles, which are also more prominent in the descending limb, are considered to be important in the differential permeabilities of these limbs and in the function of the countercurrent mechanism (27—29).

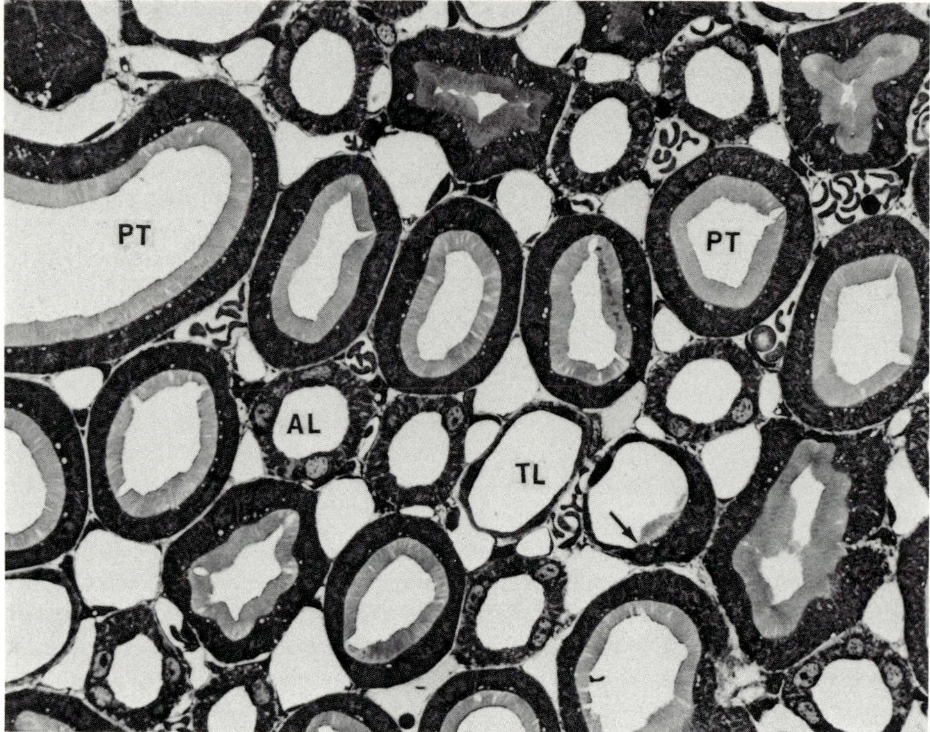

Figure 2-10. Outer renal medulla of an epoxy resin section showing proximal tubules (PT), thin loop of Henle (TL), and ascending thick loops (AL). The capillaries appear filled with red blood cells. Notice the abrupt transition of proximal tubule to thin loop of Henle (arrow). Toluidine blue stain (×550).

DISTAL TUBULE

The distal tubule has three segments. The ascending limb joins the loop of Henle to the macula densa, which is continuous with the convoluted portion. The thick ascending limb is located in the medullary ray of the cortex or in the inner stripe of the medulla (30). The cells in this region are cuboidal, with large and round central nuclei (Fig. 2-10). Basal infoldings are conspicuous and enclose very long mitochondria, which lie perpendicular to the basement membrane. Microvilli are present in variable numbers on the cell surface and are especially concentrated at cell borders (Fig. 2-15). The macula densa is considered with the other portions of the juxtaglomerular apparatus later in the chapter. The distal convoluted tubule is the terminal portion of the nephron, emptying into the collecting tubule, and is both shorter and less complex than its proximal counterpart. In paraffin sections, the cells are shorter and smaller than those of the proximal tubule, so the nuclei appear more crowded, and have clear cytoplasm. Although microvilli are well developed on the luminal surface, there is no glycocalyx and a brush border cannot be identified. There are extensive basal infoldings, with

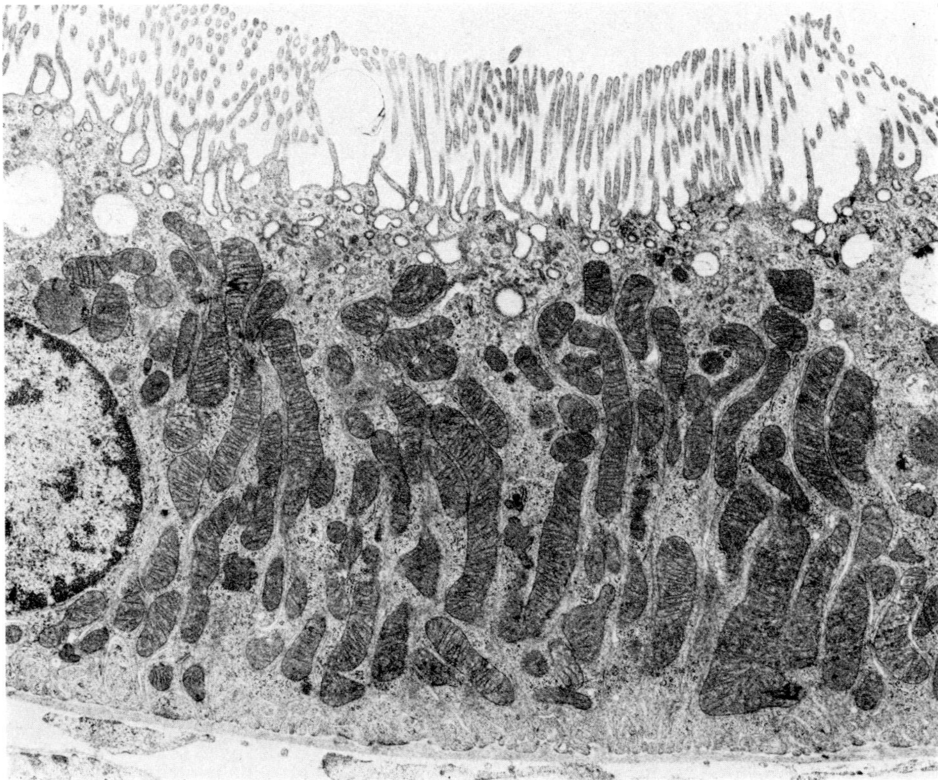

Figure 2-11. Transmission electron micrograph of a normal proximal tubule showing the brush border, numerous apical pinocytotic vesicles, and elongated mitochondria oriented perpendicular to the basement membrane ($\times$5,000).

adjacent elongate mitrochondria and complex lateral processes, which interdigitate with those from adjacent cells (Fig. 2-16). Tamm-Horsfall mucoprotein is secreted by the distal convoluted tubule and may be prominent as basophilic casts in biopsy specimens from dehydrated patients (31). Occasionally, these casts become extruded into the interstitium to provoke a mononuclear or granulomatous reaction (32,33).

COLLECTING DUCT SYSTEM

The renal collecting ducts transport urine from the nephrons to the papillae. The lining cells are clear and cuboidal through most of their length, becoming columnar in the ducts of Bellini near the papillary tip. Ultrastructurally, the lining cells are of two types (34). The predominant (principal) cells are of low electron density, contain few organelles, and have simple luminal surfaces with sparse microvilli and scattered cilia. The dark (intercalated) cells, which decrease

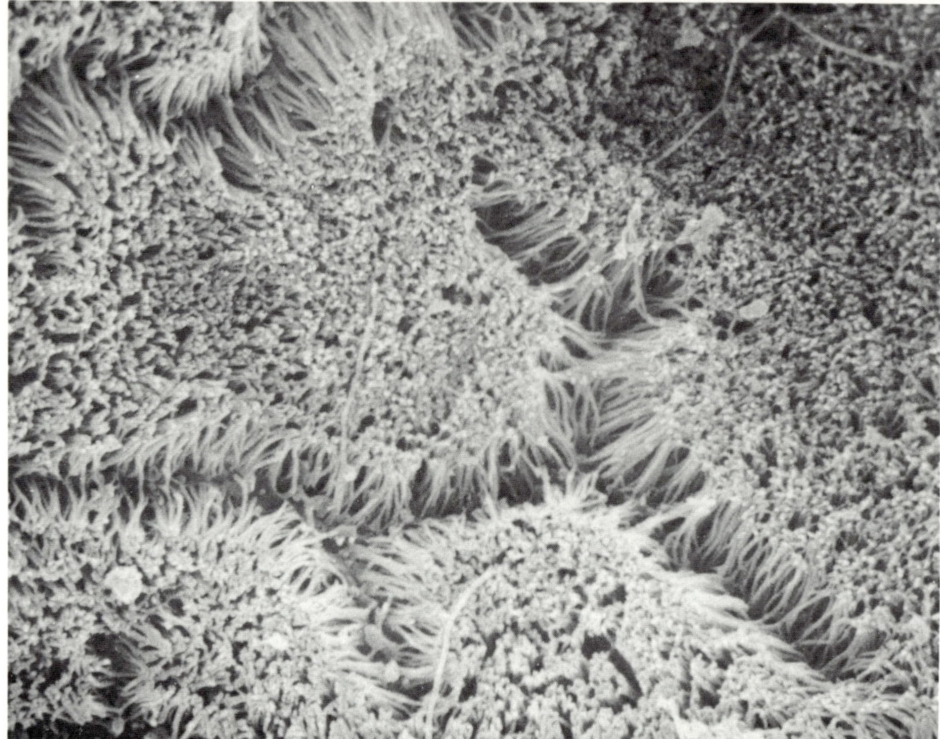

Figure 2-12. Scanning electron micrograph of the proximal tubule showing, in addition to the brush border, occasional cilia. Notice the separation between cells (×5,000).

in number from the cortex to the medulla, appear more electron-dense and are filled with oval mitochondria, free ribosomes, and rough endoplasmic reticulum (Figs. 2-14, 2-17). The luminal surfaces of these dark cells have complex and highly convoluted microplicae (Fig. 2-18). Cells with morphologic characteristics intermediate between the light and dark patterns have been recognized, suggesting that these patterns represent varied differentiation of one cell type under different metabolic or pathologic conditions (34).

INTERSTITIAL CELLS

The interstitial cells are most frequent in the renal papilla. They tend to be stellate in form and contain characteristic lipid droplets (Fig. 2-19). Because of their close relationship to the thin loops of Henle, these cells were considered to be concerned with the countercurrent mechanism, but recent evidence indicates that they are the major source of prostaglandin synthesis (35,36). Interstitial cells are the origin of medullary fibromata, the most common benign renal neoplasm (37).

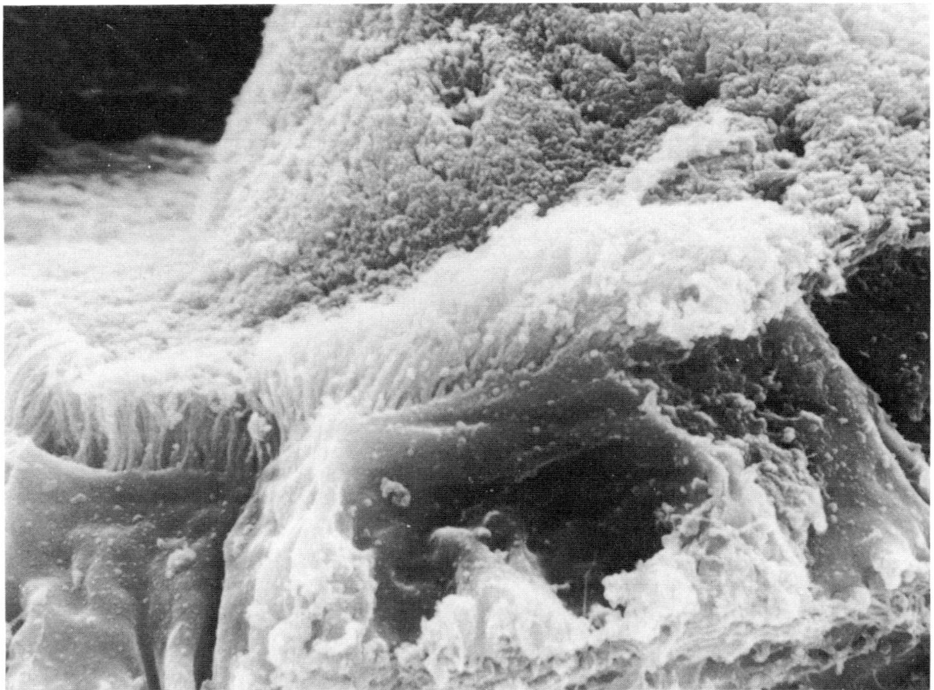

Figure 2-13. Scanning electron micrograph of proximal tubule demonstrating elaborate lateral projections of cytoplasm (×9,000).

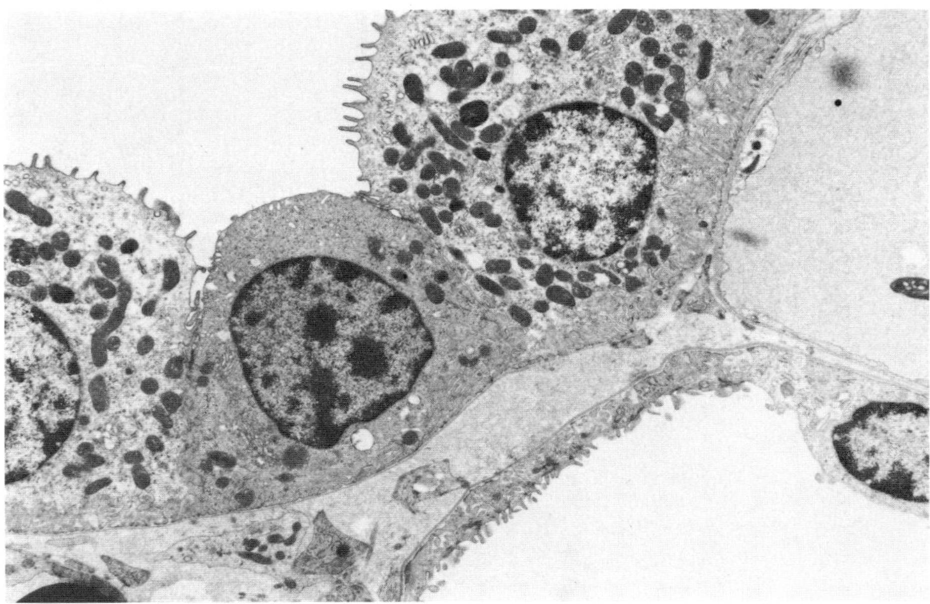

Figure 2-14. Electron micrograph of collecting tubule, thin loop of Henle (right lower corner), and capillary (right upper corner). A principal collection tubular cell is located between two dark cells (×7,500).

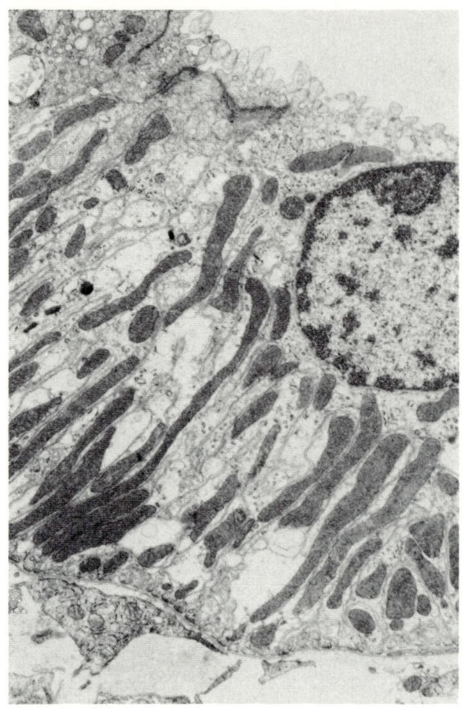

Figure 2-15. Electron micrograph of the ascending thick loop of a normal rat (×5,000).

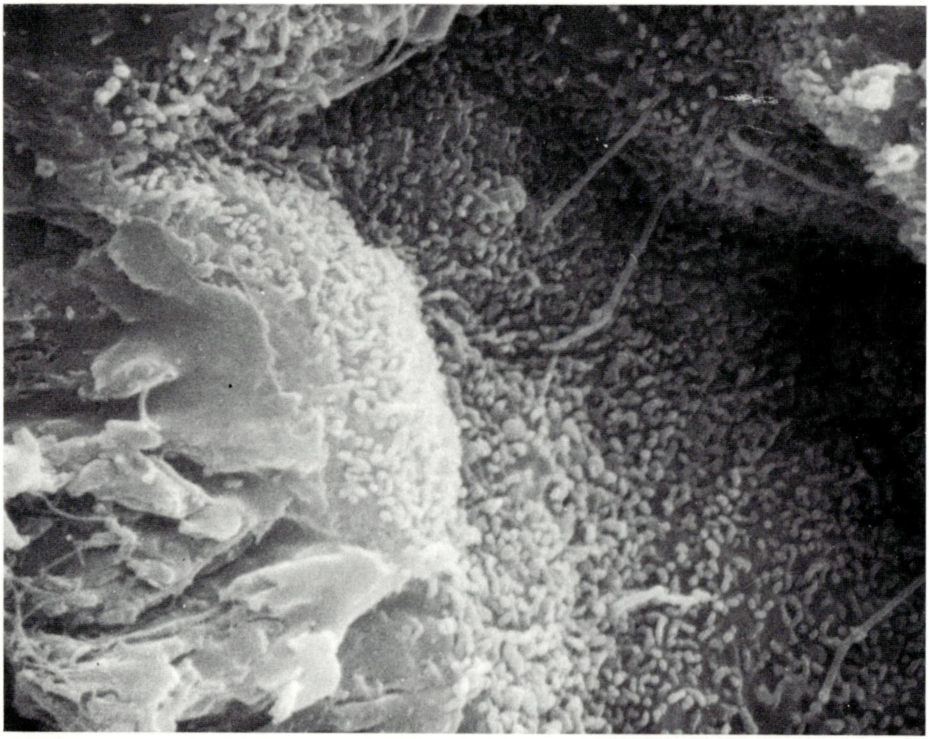

Figure 2-16. Scanning electron micrograph of the distal convoluted tubule of a normal rat showing prominent lateral folding of the cell membrane. The cell surface is covered by microvilli with a single cilium (×15,000).

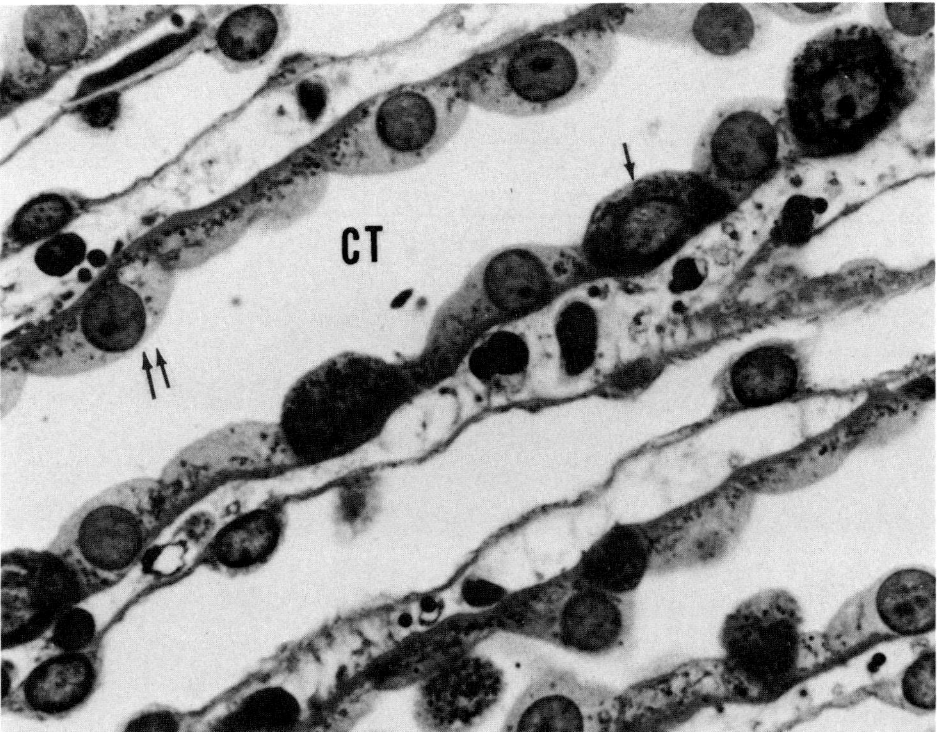

Figure 2-17. Collecting tubule (CT) showing light (double arrow) and dark (single arrow) cells (plastic embedded toluidine blue stain, ×600).

JUXTAGLOMERULAR APPARATUS

The juxtaglomerular apparatus is located at the glomerular hilus where the macula densa lies between the afferent and efferent arterioles. This orientation provides intimate contact between the fluid in the distal tubule, the granular cells of the arterioles, and the lacis cells at the base of the glomerulus. The arteriolar granular cells, which are most common in the afferent arteriole but are only rarely seen in the efferent arteriole, are arranged on the outer aspect of the muscular layer (38,39). These cells contain rhomboidal granules, which have been identified as renin and are the origin of rare renin-secreting tumors causing hypertension (40,41). The cells of the macula densa are narrower and taller than those elsewhere in the distal tubule and show few basal infoldings or mitochondria. The tubular basement membrane is attenuated and irregular between these cells and the lacis, which is continuous with the mesangium. The lacis cells contain microfilaments and may have contractile functions. In addition to a role in the control of blood pressure and sodium conservation, via renin secretion, the juxtaglomerular apparatus is involved in the tubuloglomerular feedback regulation of nephron filtration (42). The apparatus is unusually prominent in juxtamedullary glomeruli and knowledge of the region from which the biopsy specimen was taken is important when considering the possibility of juxtamedullary hypertrophy.

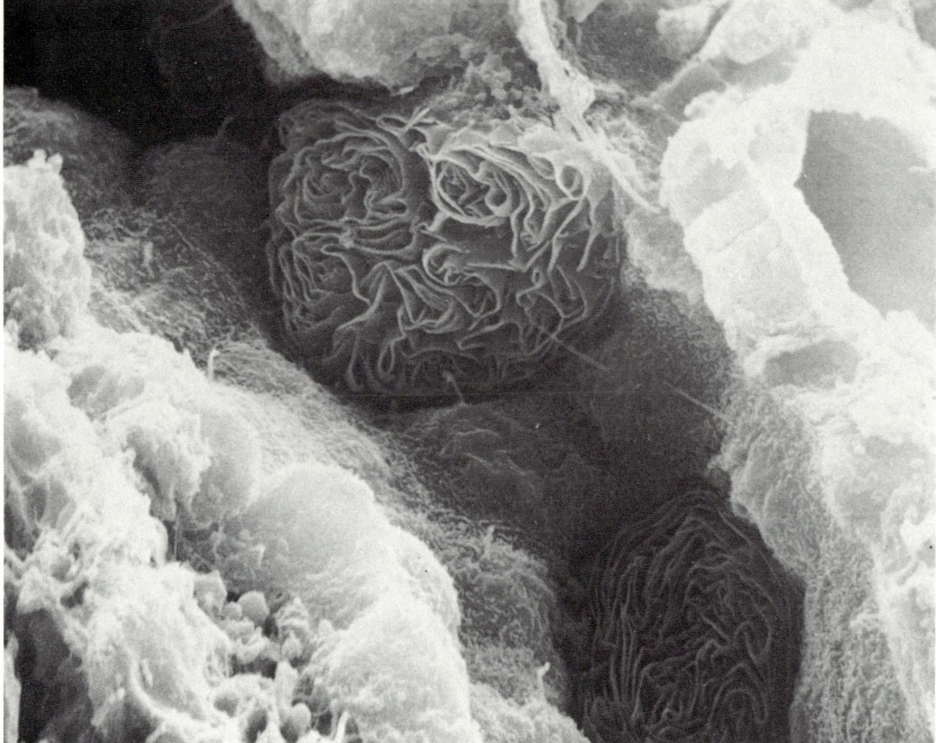

Figure 2-18. Scanning electron micrograph of collecting tubule. The dark cells appear covered by microplicae and light cells by microvilli (×2,025).

VASCULATURE

The kidneys receive approximately 25% of the cardiac output, and blood is transported to the glomeruli at high pressure via a series of wide and relatively straight vessels (43). The renal arteries arise from the abdominal aorta and branch to form segmental vessels that are effectively end arteries. At the corticomedullary junction, the segmental arteries lead into arcuate arteries, which form a series of arcades from whose convex surfaces arise the intralobular arteries. The interlobular arteries delineate cortical lobules and branch to form afferent arterioles, which drain into the glomerular capillaries and thence to the efferent arterioles. The glomerular capillary circulation is unique in the body because of its maintenance of a continuously high and controlled pressure by both proximal and distal arteriolar sphincters. The efferent arterioles of the outer cortex branch to form complex capillary networks which extend among proximal and distal convoluted tubules. From the larger juxtamedullary glomeruli, the efferent arterioles give off the arteriole rectae spuriae network, which supplies the medulla and is intimately involved with urinary concentration. Aside from the arteriolar epitheloid cells, the structure of the renal vasculature differs little from that elsewhere in the body. With advancing age, larger arteries show varying degrees of intimal fibrosis and elastica duplication, which

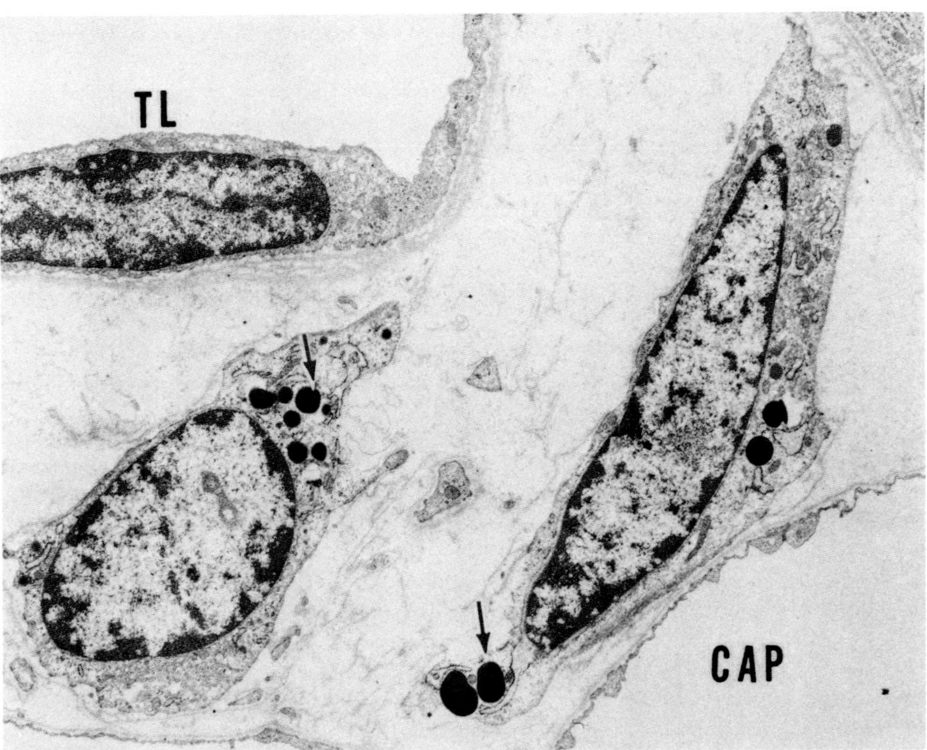

Figure 2-19. Electron micrograph of two interstitial cells between capillaries (CAP) and thin loop of Henle (TL). Note the intracytoplasmic lipid droplets (arrows) (×6,500).

need to be distinguished from the predominantly arteriolar changes occurring in hypertension. The capillary circulation lies in intimate contact with surrounding tubules and has an attenuated epithelium punctuated by fenestrations, 600 Å in diameter (Fig. 2-19).

REFERENCES

1. Van Damme B, Koudstaal J: Measuring glomerular diameters in tissue sections. *Virchows Arch* [*Pathol Anat*] 369:293, 1976.

2. Osterby R: Quantitative electron microscopy of the glomerular basement membrane: a methodological study. *Lab Invest* 25:15, 1971.

3. Nash DA, Rogers PW, Langlinais PC, et al: Diabetic glomerulosclerosis without glucose intolerance. *Am J Med* 59:191, 1975.

4. Tallquist G, Pasternack A, Tornroth T: Indentations of the glomerular basement membrane in renal diseases: a light and electron microscopic study on ultra-thin serial sections. *Lab Invest* 32:636, 1975.

5. Bariety J, Callard P: Striated membranous structures in renal glomerular tufts: an electron microscopic study of 340 human renal biopsies. *Lab Invest* 32:636, 1975.

6. Bariety J, Callard P: Round "virus-like" extracellular particles in glomerular tufts: an electron microscopic study of 190 human renal biopsies. *Virchows Arch* [*Pathol Anat*] 357:125, 1972.

7. Brenner BM, Hostetter TH, Humes HD: Molecular basis of proteinuria of glomerular origin. *N Engl J Med* 298:826, 1978.

8. Jones DB: Correlative scanning and transmission electron microscopy of glomeruli. *Lab Invest* 37:569, 1977.

9. Andrews PM: A scanning and transmission electron microscopic comparison of puromycin aminonucleoside-induced nephrosis to hyperalbuminemia-induced proteinuria with emphasis on kidney podocyte pedicel loss. *Lab Invest* 36:183, 1977.

10. Walker F: The origin, turnover and removal of glomerular basement-membrane. *J Pathol* 110:233, 1973.

11. Karnovsky MJ, Ainsworth SK: The ultrastructural basis of glomerular filtration. *Adv Nephrol* 2:35, 1973.

12. Heinemann HO, Maack TM, Sherman RL: Proteinuria. *Am J Med* 56:71, 1974.

13. Schneeberger EE, Levey RH, McCluskey RT, et al: The isoporous substructure of the human glomerular slit diaphragm. *Kidney Int* 8:48, 1975.

14. Farquhar MG: The primary glomerular filtration barrier—basement membrane or epithelial slits? *Kidney Int* 8:197, 1975.

15. Misra RP: The glomerular basement membranes in Black DAK (ed): *Renal Diseases,* 3rd ed. Oxford, Blackwell Scientific Publications, 1972, p 187.

16. Bradfield JWB, Cattell V, Smith J: The mesangial cell in glomerulonephritis. II. Mesangial proliferation caused by Habu snake venom in the rat. *Lab Invest* 36:487, 1977.

17. Vernier RL, Mauer SM, Fish AJ, et al: The mesangial cell in glomerulonephritis. *Adv Nephrol* 1:31, 1971.

18. Leiper JM, Thomson D, McDonald MK: Uptake and transport of Imposil by the glomerular mesangium in the mouse. *Lab Invest* 37:526, 1977.

19. Becker CG: Demonstration of actomyosin in mesangial cells of the renal glomerulus. *Am J Pathol* 66:97, 1972.

20. Scheinman JI, Fish AJ, Matas AJ, et al: The immunohistopathology of glomerular antigens. II. The glomerular basement membrane, actomyosin and fibroblast surface antigens in normal, diseased and transplanted human kidneys. *Am J Pathol* 90:71, 1978.

21. Bernik MB: Contractile activity of human glomeruli in culture. *Nephron* 6:1, 1969.

22. Tisher CC, Bulger RE, Trump BF: Human renal ultrastructure. I. Proximal tubule of healthy individuals. *Lab Invest* 15:1357, 1966.

23. O'Regan S; Smith M, Drummond KN: Antigens in human immune complex nephritis. *Clin Nephrol* 6:417, 1976.

24. Bourdeau JE, Carone FA: Protein handling by the renal tubule. *Nephron* 13:22, 1974.

25. Kretchmer N, Bernstein J: The dynamic morphology of the nephron: morphogenesis of the "protein droplet." *Kidney Int* 5:96, 1974.

26. Wallace AC, Nairn RC: Renal tubular antigens in kidney tumors. *Cancer* 29:977, 1972.

27. Humbert F, Pricam C, Pirrelet A, et al: Freeze-fracture differences between plasma membranes of descending and ascending branches of the rat Henle's thin loop. *Lab Invest* 33:470, 1975.

28. Schwartz MM, Venkatachalam MA: Structural differences in thin limbs of Henle: physiological implications. *Kidney Int* 6:103, 1974.

29. Jamison RL, Maffly RH: The urinary concentrating mechanism. *N Engl J Med* 295:1059, 1976.

30. Allen F, Tisher CC: Morphology of the ascending thick limb of Henle. *Kidney Int* 9:8, 1976.

31. Schenk EA, Schwartz RH, Lewis RA: Tamm-Horsfall mucoprotein. I. Localization in the kidney. *Lab Invest* 25:92, 1971.

32. Resnick JS, Sisson S, Vernier RL: Tamm-Horsfall protein: abnormal localization in renal disease. *Lab Invest* 38:550, 1978.

33. Zager RA, Cotran RS, Hoyer JR: Pathologic localization of Tamm-Horsfall protein in interstitial deposits in renal disease. *Lab Invest* 38:52, 1978.

34. Ordóñez NG, Spargo BH: The morpholgic relationship of light and dark cells of the collecting tubule in potassium-depleted rats. *Am J Pathol* 84:317, 1976.

35. Osvaldo L, Latta H: Interstitial cells of the renal medulla. *J Ultrastruct Res* 15:589, 1966.

36. Muirhead EE, Germain G, Leach BE, et al: Production of renomedullary prostaglandins by renomedullary interstitial cells grown in tissue culture. *Circ Res* 30 (suppl 2):161, 1972.

37. Lerman RJ, Pitcock JA, Stephenson P, et al: Renomedullary interstitial cell tumor (formerly fibroma of the renal medulla). *Human Pathol* 3:559, 1972.

38. Barajas L: The ultrastructure of the juxtaglomerular apparatus as disclosed by three-dimensional reconstructions from serial sections. *J Ultrastruct Res* 33:116, 1970.

39. Christensen JA, Meyer DS, Bohle A: The structure of the human juxtaglomerular apparatus: a morphometric, light microscopic study on serial sections. *Virchows Arch (A) Path Anat Histol* 367:83, 1975.

40. Oparil S, Haber E: The renin-angiotensin system. *N Engl J Med* 291:389,446, 1974.

41. Bonnin JM, Cain MD, Jose JS et al: Hypertension due to a renin-secreting tumor localized by segmental renal vein sampling. *Aust NZ J Med* 7:630, 1977.

42. Heirholzer K, Wiederholt M: Some aspects of distal tubular solute and water transport. *Kidney Int* 9:198, 1976.

43. Barger AC, Herd JA: The renal circulation. *N Engl J Med* 284:482, 1971.

3
Epithelial Cell Disease

The appearance of "normal" or "minimally changed" glomeruli in the majority of children with the nephrotic syndrome puzzled early students of renal disease. Ultrastructural studies, showing diffuse obliteration of epithelial foot processes, ended speculation about a nonglomerular origin of proteinuria in such patients, but they provided no clear solution to the mechanism of increased glomerular permeability. Whether the epithelial lesion is the primary abnormality or merely a secondary reaction still excites controversy. In fact, the epithelial cell and the glomerular basement membrane are functionally so closely interrelated that it is difficult to conceive of primary damage to either component of the putative filter mechanisms without significant alteration to the other. This theoretical argument has often obscured the diagnostic significance of isolated foot process obliteration. The demonstration of this appearance, with the concomitant exclusion of other abnormalities, remains one of the major contributions of electron microscopy to routine renal diagnosis. In the vast majority of patients with epithelial foot process obliteration, corticosteroid therapy will produce complete remission of the nephrotic syndrome, and this ultrastructural appearance is, therefore, an important diagnostic and prognostic finding.

ETIOLOGY AND PATHOGENESIS

Neither the causes nor the pathogenesis of epithelial cell disease are known. Experimental administration of the aminonucleoside of puromycin to rats produces proteinuria with an identical ultrastructural appearance (1). There is, however, little evidence of exposure to toxic chemicals in patients with epithelial cell disease, and the precise site of damage in this experimental model is still obscure. Changes in the carbohydrate content of the glomerular basement membrane have been demonstrated in aminonucleoside nephrotic rats, suggesting that reorientation of the fibrillar membrane components might allow increased passage of protein molecules by increasing "pore" size (2). These changes in the carbohydrate moieties are partially preventable by concomitant treatment of the experimental animals with corticosteroids (2), indicating one possible mechanism for the action of these agents in epithelial cell disease. There is, however, some evidence of direct action of aminonucleoside on the epithelial cell (3), so the site of steroid action remains uncertain.

In the human disease, there is a significant association with an atopic history (4), and the onset of nephrotic syndrome may follow infection or exposure to

34

allergens (5,6). Involvement of the immune system has, therefore, been pursued. One report of the immunofluorescent demonstration of IgE in the glomeruli of epithelial cell disease (7) was received with great interest, but this finding has not been confirmed in subsequent immunofluorescence studies (8). The apparent absence of humoral mechanisms, coupled with the occasional association of a similar morphologic lesion with Hodgkin's disease, led Shalhoub (9) to postulate a disorder of T cells in these patients. Numerous studies have since disclosed several alterations of the T-lymphocyte function in patients with epithelial cell disease, but clear evidence of lymphocytic mediation is not yet available (10). The recent detection of circulating immune complexes in both children (11) and adults (12) with epithelial cell disease has revived interest in humoral immune mechanisms. These complexes, which were present only during relapse, did not bind complement and have not been detected by assays requiring complement fixation (13). Lack of complement binding might explain the typically negative or minimal immunofluorescence findings (8), but the significance of these complexes and the mechanisms by which they might cause proteinuria are presently unknown. Clearly, the morphologic lesion may represent the endpoint of several pathogenetic pathways. The occurrence of familial epithelial disease (14,15,16), however, and the suggestion of an excess of some HLA antigens in these patients (4) lend some support to a uniform mechanism.

CLINICAL MANIFESTATIONS AND COURSE

Epithelial cell disease is predominantly a disorder of children, in whom it is the major cause of nephrotic syndrome (5,17,18), but this disease also occurs in adults with significant frequency (18,19,20). In the pediatric age group when first seen, most patients are younger than 6 years of age, the majority being 3 or 4 years old, and there is a clear male predominance (5,17). No clear sex difference is seen in adults, and all ages are affected (20). The initial manifestation does not differ significantly from that of the nephrotic syndrome caused by other disorders, although an atopic history of recent antigen exposure may point to the diagnosis of epithelial cell disease. Microscopic hematuria is uncommon and the proteinuria is often of selective type (5,17). A few patients, usually those with the most intense nephrotic syndrome, develop transitory renal dysfunction due to oligemia (5), and, very occasionally, irreversible renal failure has been reported (21). Reversible acute renal failure may also be caused by diuretic-induced acute interstitial nephritis (22). Progression into renal failure is usual in the congenital nephrotic syndromes, but these conditions differ in several aspects from epithelial cell disease and are discussed in Chapter 21.

Most adults and children with epithelial cell disease show complete remission of proteinuria within eight weeks after starting corticosteroid therapy (5,19,20,23). After withdrawal of steroids, however, approximately half the patients enter a period of intermittent relapse, which may last up to 10 years. Each relapse is steroid-responsive, and there is no tendency for the disease to progress to chronic renal failure. Relapse is rare after a disease-free interval of two years. A subgroup of patients shows only partial remission with corticosteroid therapy. Immunosuppressive drugs, especially cyclophosphamide, have achieved remission in a significant proportion of these steroid-dependent and steroid-resistant patients (20,24), although infertility has occurred in some children (25). Finally, a small group of patients achieves complete remission without any therapy. Few patients now remain untreated, but figures from the precorticosteroid era suggested that approximately half the patients eventually gained complete remission (26). In one large recent series, 10 of 181 patients entered permanent remission without any therapy (5).

Death from infection was frequent before the ready availability of antibiotics and corticosteroids (26) and still occurs occasionally. Progression to renal failure is, however, exceptional. The development of azotemia should always suggest an incorrect diagnosis, most often focal glomerulosclerosis, or a superadded complication such as interstitial nephritis (22) or renal vein thrombosis (27,28). The original diagnosis is especially likely to be incorrect if the nephrotic syndrome is corticosteroid resistant. In the absence of complications or severe infection, the eventual outlook for patients with epithelial cell disease is probably no different from that of the general population (29).

PATHOLOGIC CHARACTERISTICS

Light Microscopy

By definition, the glomeruli in epithelial cell disease appear entirely normal (Fig. 3-1). Actually, there is often some irregular prominence of epithelial cells, and

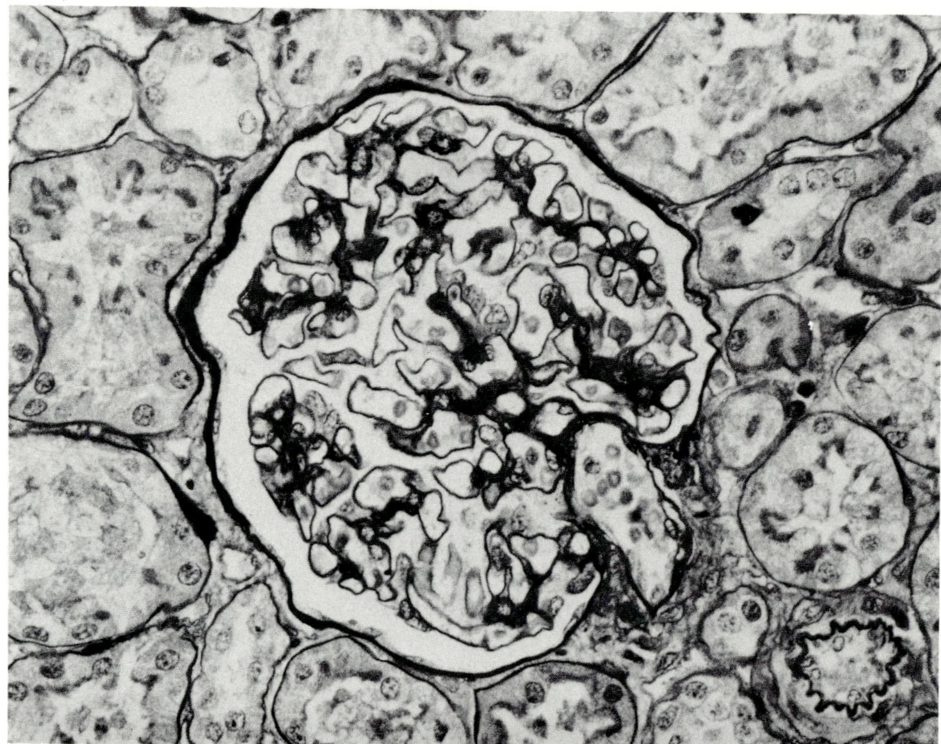

Figure 3-1. Glomerulus from a patient with epithelial cell disease. There is no increase in cellularity and the capillary loops appear normal in thickness (PAS stain, ×480).

minor degrees of mesangial enlargement are common (Fig. 3-2). Quantitative studies of the glomeruli in epithelial cell disease suggest a significant, although slight, increase in the numbers of intracapillary cells, but this increase is rarely detectable by qualitative assessment of an individual biopsy specimen (30). The presence of any glomerular abnormality is always an indication to search carefully for segmental lesions. Definite and diffuse mesangial enlargement is a disturbing finding since relentless progression to renal failure from focal glomerulosclerosis has been seen with this appearance, even when no segmental lesions could be demonstrated in the original biopsy specimen (31). In other studies, the behavior was more variable (5,32,33). There may be patchy interstitial edema and tubular vacuolation, the "lipoid nephrosis" described originally by Munk (34), but any interstitial scarring or inflammation is an inducement to consider other diseases in the differential diagnosis. Similarly, while occasional globally sclerotic glomeruli are ubiquitous at all ages, more than one or two sclerotic glomeruli must raise a suspicion of potentially progressive disease. However, focal global sclerosis with interstitial scarring does not appear to imply as aggressive a course as is seen with focal segmental sclerosis (see p. 53, Chap, 4).

Electron Microscopy

The characteristic ultrastructural appearance of the glomeruli is of total foot process obliteration, the basement membrane being covered by sheets of cyto-

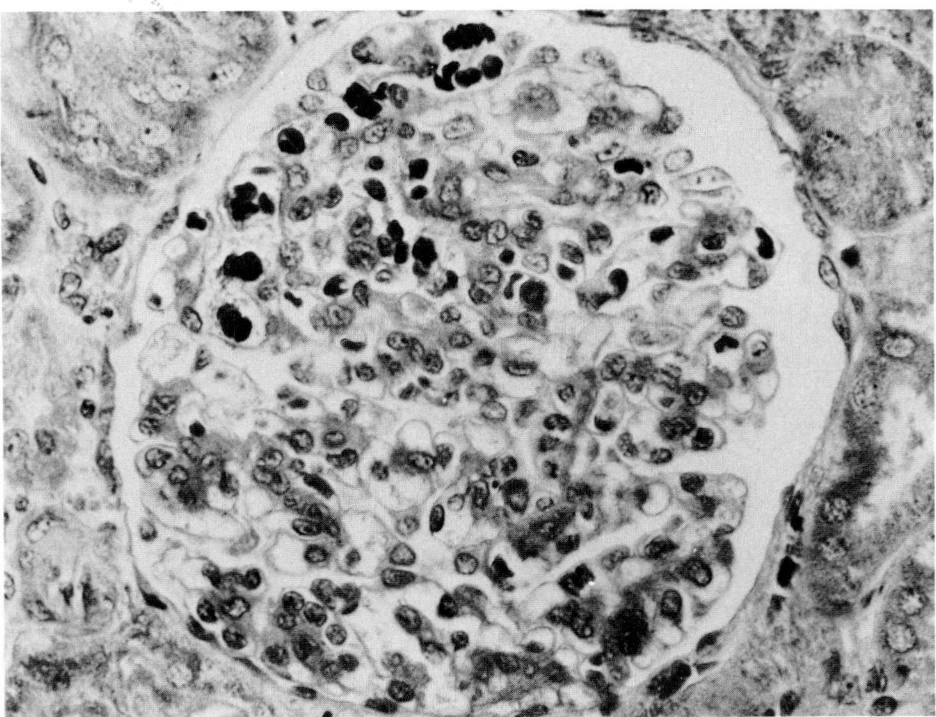

Figure 3-2. Mild diffuse hypercellularity in a biopsy speciman from a patient with epithelial cell disease (H&E stain, ×500).

plasm. There is frequently a zone of increased electron density, which may simulate deposit, within the epithelial cytoplasm adjacent to the membrane, but no deposits can be seen. Visceral epithelial cells show prominent intracytoplasmic organelles, suggesting increased cytoplasmic activity, and frequently contain cysts. Numerous microvilli usually protrude from the surface of the cells, but focal epithelial disruption (35,36) is rarely seen (Fig. 3-3). Scanning electron microscopic studies of both human epithelial cell disease (37) and of aminonucleoside nephrosis (3) have demonstrated that the loss of foot processes is due to their retraction into the parent cell bodies rather than to actual fusion. This retraction is presumably the result of extensive cell swelling.

All these changes are completely reversible, biopsy specimens taken during remission being indistinguishable from normal (Fig. 3-4). Confirmation of the diagnosis of epithelial cell disease, therefore, can only be obtained if the biopsy is taken during a proteinuric episode. Biopsy specimens examined during corticosteroid-induced remission show partial resolution of the normal foot process structure with irregular smudging of processes alternating with areas of normal morphology or total obliteration (Fig. 3-5). Endothelial and mesangial cells may show patchy hypertrophy but usually appear normal. Microthrombi were demonstrated in one exhaustive ultrastructural study (38) but are rarely

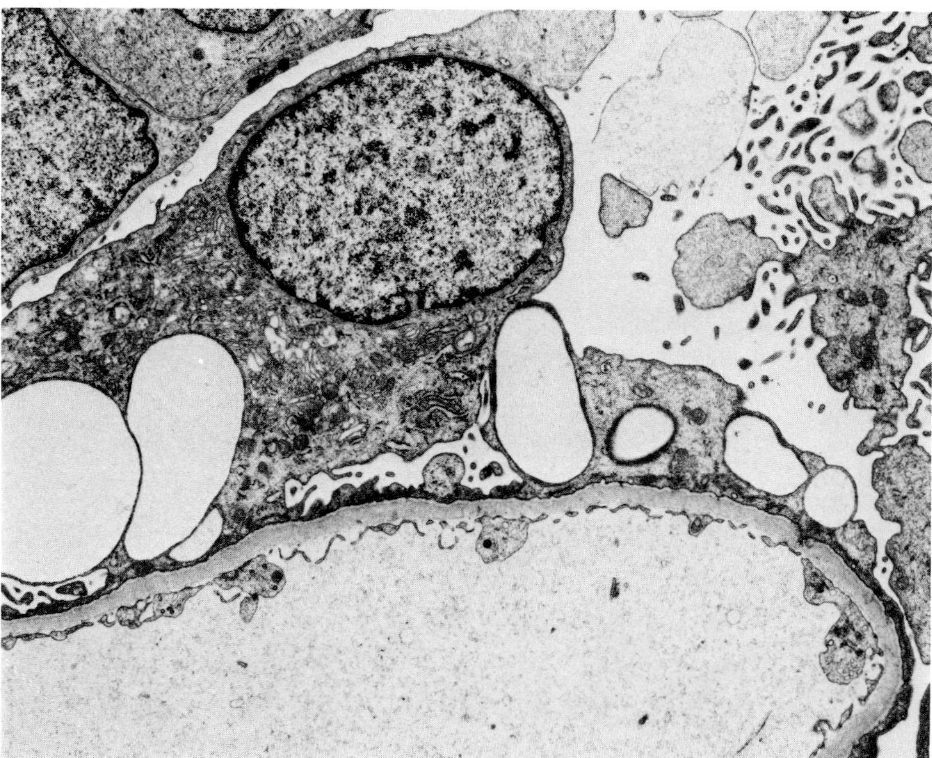

Figure 3-3. Complete obliteration of the foot processes is shown. The epithelial cell cytoplasm is hyperactive and shows prominent cyst formation and "villous" hyperplasia (×7,100).

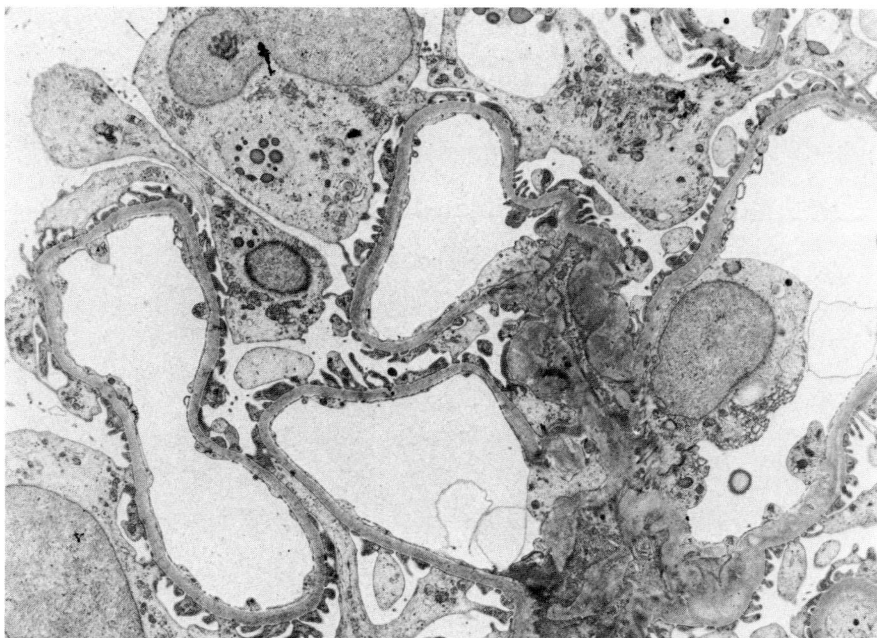

Figure 3-4. Glomerulus from a biopsy of a patient with epithelial cell disease taken during remission. The capillary loops are normal and the foot processes intact ($\times 4{,}000$).

encountered in routine practice, although clumps of interluminal platelets may be seen.

Immunofluorescence Microscopy

The results of most immunofluorescence studies of epithelial cell disease have been negative (5), but weak mesangial reactions for IgM and C3 have been described (8). The significance of these reactions is uncertain, but they are probably not immunologically specific and may merely reflect increased mesangial uptake of macromolecules like that demonstrated in the experimental nephrotic syndrome (39). Careful examination for segmental reactions, especially for IgM and C3, is advisable since these may be the first indication of segmental sclerosis, even when sclerotic lesions are not demonstrable by light microscopy. There is now general agreement that IgE cannot be demonstrated in the glomeruli of epithelial cell disease.

DIFFERENTIAL DIAGNOSIS

In the majority of biopsy specimens showing epithelial cell disease, the diagnostic findings are clear-cut. The major problems are in the assessment of mesangial increase and in the exclusion of segmental disease. There is considerable evidence that the presence of significant mesangial enlargement may be a poor prognostic sign (5,31), but the criteria for defining this enlargement are variable.

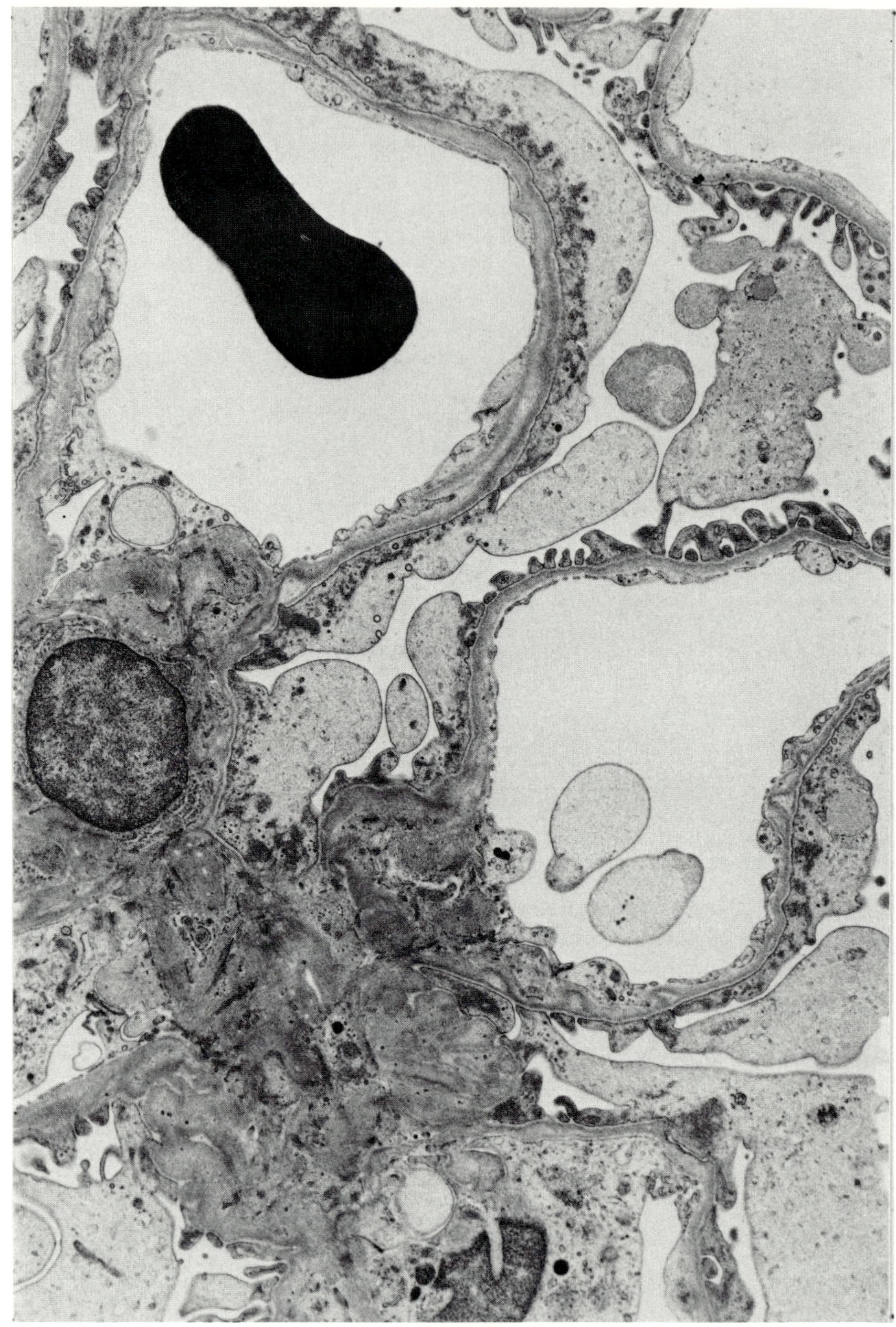

Figure 3-5. Glomerulus from a patient during steroid-induced remission. In some areas the foot processes are intact, while in others they remain obliterated (×7,000).

Probably the most reliable criterion is the presence of three or more nuclei in all or most mesangial areas (40). Segmental disease often accompanies such mesangial excess, either in the first or subsequent biopsies, and may be very sparse, sometimes occurring in only a few of many serial sections. There is, therefore, good reason for examining many levels of biopsy specimens from cases of epithelial cell disease, especially if mesangial enlargement, interstitial scarring, frequent sclerotic glomeruli, or segmental immunofluorescent reactions are present. Occasionally segmental capillary collapse is found by electron microscopy when light microscopy is within normal limits. While this appearance must raise the suspicion of evolving focal glomerulosclerosis, especially if there is widespread subendothelial irregularity of the basement membrane (41), it is not well enough correlated with a progressive course to be diagnostically useful (42).

Segmental glomerulosclerosis may be seen in some patients after repeated relapses of epithelial disease without carrying a grim prognosis (5,42,43). Only when seen in the initial episode of nephrotic syndrome can the presence of segmental sclerosis be regarded as a reliable sign of progressive disease. Definitive diagnosis of epithelial cell disease can only be achieved by the electron microscopic demonstration of foot process obliteration in the absence of other lesions. The presence of light microscopically normal glomeruli cannot, therefore, be taken as a reliable criterion for the diagnosis. Even the most careful light microscopic examination will miss some cases of amyloidosis and early membranous nephropathy (44). Furthermore, occasional patients may have proteinuria caused by the presence of large amounts of abnormal proteins, such as Bence-Jones proteins, and only the recognition of completely normal epithelial structure in the face of heavy proteinuria is likely to raise this diagnostic possibility.

ASSOCIATED CONDITIONS

In the vast majority of patients, epithelial cell disease occurs as an isolated phenomenon, without identifiable precipitating factors. Occasionally, the disease has been associated with gold (45,46) or heroin (47) administration or has manifested soon after the onset of diabetes mellitus (48,49). These occurrences are rare and of questionable significance, but there is a definite association with Hodgkin's disease. A number of patients with Hodgkin's disease have developed the nephrotic syndrome early in their course with only epithelial changes visible on biopsy specimens (50,51). In each of these patients, the nephrotic syndrome has responded completely to appropriate antitumor therapy and, in several, exacerbations have occurred in parallel with the reemergence of nodal or extranodal disease. The relationship appears to be specific since remissions have occurred with both cytotoxic therapy and local irradiation, and there has been no tendency toward the development of progressive renal disease. Rarely, a similar clinicopathologic syndrome has been associated with non-Hodgkin's lymphoma, of various patterns (50,51) and with benign lymphoid masses (52). Occasional examples of "minimal lesion" nephrotic syndrome have been described in association with epithelial malignancy, but adequate electron microscopic data for the diagnosis of epithelial cell disease have not been included in these reports (50).

There is a single report of acute nephrotic syndrome, with the morphologic features of epithelial cell disease, occurring soon after transplanation and remitting with corticosteroid and immunosuppressive therapy (53).

SUMMARY

Epithelial cell disease is a reversible cause of the nephrotic syndrome that occurs most frequently, though not invariably, in children. The diagnosis requires electron microscopic examination and is achieved by the demonstration of complete obliteration of epithelial foot processes in the absence of other abnormalities. This obliteration has been shown in scanning electron microscopy to be produced by swelling of the epithelial cell body with retraction of the foot processes rather than by fusion of adjacent processes, as was previously thought. There are rare systemic associations of epithelial cell disease. However,in most patients this disease has no identifiable causes, although an atopic history is common. Corticosteroid therapy produces complete remission in the majority of patients, but relapses are frequent and some patients remain resistant to or dependent on the continuation of corticosteroids. In some of the latter group, cyclophosphamide and other immunosuppressive agents have produced complete remission. Progression to renal failure does not occur in uncomplicated epithelial cell disease. However, the diagnosis may be simulated by focal glomerulosclerosis, in which segmental lesions are sometimes difficult to find and foot-process obliteration also occurs. Examination of serial- or step- sections, is therefore, recommended, especially if interstitial scarring, frequent sclerotic glomeruli, or segmental immunofluorescent reactions are discovered. Diffuse enlargement of the mesangium is a common accompaniment of focal glomerulosclerosis and is a potent stimulus to search for segmental disease. Even if segmental lesions cannot be discovered, however, the presence of excess diffuse mesangium is a disturbing prognostic sign.

REFERENCES

1. Caulfield JP, Reid JJ, Fraquhar MG: Alterations of the glomerular epithelium in acute animonucleoside nephrosis. Evidence for formation of occluding junctions and epithelial cell detachment. *Lab Invest* 34:43, 1976.

2. Misra RP: The glomerular basement membrane, in Black DAK (ed): *Renal Disease*, ed 3. Oxford, Blackwell Scientific Publications, p 187.

3. Andrews PM: A scanning and transmission electron microscopic comparison of puromycin aminonucleoside-induced nephrosis to hyperalbuminemia-induced proteinuria with emphasis on kidney podocyte pedicel loss. *Lab Invest* 36:183, 1977.

4. Thompson PD, Barratt TM, Stokes CR, et al: HLA antigens and atopic features in steroid-responsive nephrotic syndrome of childhood. *Lancet* 2:765, 1976.

5. Habib R, Kleinknecht C: The primary nephrotic syndrome of childhood: classification and clinicopathologic study of 406 cases. *Pathol Annu* 6:417, 1971.

6. Wittig HJ, Goldman AS: Nephrotic syndrome associated with inhaled allergens. *Lancet* 1:542, 1970.

7. Gerber MA, Paronetto F: IgE in glomeruli of patients with nephrotic syndrome. *Lancet* 1:1097, 1971.

8. Roy LP, Westberg NG, Michael AF: Nephrotic syndrome—no evidence for a role of IgE. *Clin Exp Immunol* 13:553, 1973.

9. Shalhoub RJ: Pathogenesis of lipoid nephrosis: a disorder of T-cell function. *Lancet* 2:556, 1974.

10. Mallick NP: The pathogenesis of minimal change nephropathy. *Clin Nephrol* 7:87, 1977.

11. Levinsky RK, Malleson PN, Barratt TM, et al: Circulating immune complexes in steroid-responsive nephrotic syndrome. *N Engl J Med* 298:126, 1978.

12. Poston RN, Cerio R, Cameron JS: Circulating immune complexes in minimal change nephritis. *N Engl J Med* 298:1089, 1978.

13. Woodroffe AJ, Foldes M, McKenzie PE, et al: Serum immune complexes and disease. *Aust NZ J Med* 9:129, 1979.

14. Bader PI, Grove J, Trygstad CW, et al: Familial nephrotic syndrome. *Am J Med* 56:34, 1974.

15. White RHR: The familial nephrotic syndrome. I. A European Survey. *Clin Nephrol* 1:215, 1973.

16. Moncrief MW, White RHR, Glasgow EF, et al: The familial nephrotic syndrome. II. A Clinicopathological study. *Clin Nephrol* 1:220, 1973.

17. Nephrotic syndrome in children: prediction of histopathology from clinical and laboratory characteristics at the time of diagnosis. A Report of the International Study of Kidney Disease in Children. *Kidney Int* 13:159, 1978.

18. Seymour AE, Spargo BH, Penska R: Contributions of renal biopsy studies to the understanding of disease. *Am J Pathol* 65:550, 1971.

19. Hayslett JP, Kashgarian M, Bensch KC, et al: Clinicopathological correlations in the nephrotic syndrome due to primary renal disease. *Medicine (Balt)* 52:93, 1973.

20. Cameron JS, Turner DR, Ogg CS, et al: The nephrotic syndrome in adults with "minimal change" glomerular lesions. *Quart J Med* 43:461, 1974.

21. Raij L, Keane WF, Leonard A, et al: Irreversible acute renal failure in idiopathic nephrotic syndrome. *Am J Med* 61:207, 1976.

22. Lyons H, Pinn VW, Cortell S, et al: Allergic interstitial nephritis causing reversible renal failure in four patients with idiopathic nephrotic syndrome. *N Engl J Med* 288:124, 1973.

23. Makker SP, Heymann W: The idiopathic nephrotic syndrome of childhood. A clinical reevaluation of 148 cases. *Am J Dis Child* 127:830, 1974.

24. Chin J, McLaine PM, Drummond KN: A controlled prospective study of cyclophosphamide in relapsing, corticosteroid responsive, minimal-lesion nephrotic syndrome in childhood. *J Pediat* 82:607, 1973.

25. Fairley KF, Barrie JU, Johnson W: Sterility and testicular atrophy related to cyclophosphamide therapy. *Lancet* 1:568, 1972.

26. Arneil GC: The nephrotic syndrome. *Pediat Clin NA* 18:547, 1971.

27. Duffy JL, Letteri J, Cinque T, et al: Renal vein thrombosis and the nephrotic syndrome: report of two cases with successful treatment of one. *Am J Med* 54:663, 1973.

28. Lewy PR, Jao W: Nephrotic syndrome in association with renal vein thrombosis in infancy. *J Pediat* 85:359, 1974.

29. Siegel NK, Goldberg B, Krassner LS, et al: Long-term follow-up of children with steroid-responsive nephrotic syndrome. *J Pediat* 81:251, 1972.

30. Ludwigsen E, Sorensen FH, Olsen S: A quantitative study of glomeruli in idiopathic nephrosis with minimal or no glomerular lesions. *Acta Pathol Microbiol Scand* (A) 85:911, 1977.

31. Schoeneman MJ, Bennett B, Greifer I: The natural history of focal segmental glomerulosclerosis with and without mesangial hypercellularity in children. *Clin Nephrol* 9:45, 1978.

32. Churg J, Habib R, White RHR: Pathology of the nephrotic syndrome in children: a report for the International Study of Kidney Disease in Children. *Lancet* 1:1299, 1970.

33. White RHR, Glasgow EF, Mills RJ: Clinicopathological study of nephrotic syndrome in childhood. *Lancet* 1:1353, 1970.

34. Munk F: (1913) Cited by Leiter, L: Nephrosis. *Medicine* 10:135, 1931.

35. Ryan GB, Karnovsky MJ: An ultrastructural study of the mechanisms of proteinuria in aminonucleoside nephrosis. *Kidney Int* 8:219, 1975.

36. Grishman E, Churg J: Focal glomerular sclerosis in nephrotic patients: an electron microscopic study of glomerular podocytes. *Kidney Int* 7:111, 1975.

37. Arakawa M: A scanning electron microscope study of the human glomerulus. *Am J Pathol* 64:457, 1971.

38. Duffy JL, Cinque T, Grishman E, et al: Intraglomerular fibrin, platelet aggregation, and subendothelial deposits in lipoid nephrosis. *J Clin Invest* 49:251, 1970.

39. Hoyer JR, Mauer SM, Michael AF: Unilateral renal disease in the rat. I. Clinical, morphologic and glomerular mesangial functional features of the experimental model produced by renal perfusion with the aminonucleoside of puromycin. *J Lab Clin Med* 85:756, 1975.

40. Sinniah R, Pwee HS, Lim CH: Glomerular lesions in asymptomatic microscopic hematuria discovered on routine medical examination. *Clin Nephrol* 5:216, 1976.

41. Kincaid-Smith P: *The Kidney: A Clinicopathological Study.* Oxford, Blackwell Scientific Publications, 1975, p 93.

42. Siegel NJ, Kashgarian M, Spargo BH, et al: Minimal change and focal sclerotic lesions in lipoid nephrosis. *Nephron* 13:125, 1974.

43. Habib R: Focal glomerular sclerosis. *Kidney Int* 4:355, 1973.

44. Jao W, Pollak VE, Norris SH, et al: Lipoid nephrosis: an approach to the clinicopathologic analysis and dismemberment of idiopathic nephrotic syndrome with minimal glomerular changes. *Medicine (Balt)* 52:445, 1973.

45. Lee JC, Dushkin M, Eyring EJ, et al: Renal lesions associated with gold therapy: light and electron microscopic studies. *Arthritis Rheum* 8:1, 1965.

46. Watanabe I, Whittier FC, Moore J, et al: Gold nephropathy: ultrastructural, fluorescence and microanalytic studies of two patients. *Arch Pathol Lab Med* 100:632, 1976.

47. Grishman E, Churg J, Porush JG: Glomerular morphology in heroin addicts. *Lab Invest* 35:415, 1976.

48. Urizar RE, Schwartz A, Top F Jr, et al: The nephrotic syndrome in children with diabetes mellitus of recent onset. *N Engl J Med* 281:173, 1969.

49. Brulles A, Caralps A, Vilardell M: Nephrotic syndrome with minimal glomerular lesions (lipoid nephrosis) in an adult diabetic patient. *Arch Pathol Lab Med* 101:270, 1977.

50. Eagen JW, Lewis EJ: Glomerulopathies of neoplasia. *Kidney Int* 11:297, 1977.

51. Galiano RG, Costanzi JJ, Beathard GA, et al: The nephrotic syndrome associated with neoplasia: an unusual paraneoplastic syndrome. Report of a case and review of the literature. *Am J Med* 60:1026, 1976.

52. Humphreys SR, Holley KE, Smith LH, et al: Mesenteric angiofollicular lymph node hyperplasia (lymphoid hamartoma) with nephrotic syndrome. *Mayo Clin Proc* 50:317, 1975.

53. Shapiro RS, Desmukh A, and Kropp K: Massive post-transplant proteinuria: biopsy proven nil disease. *Transplantation* 22:489, 1976.

4
Focal Glomerulosclerosis

In 1957, Rich described focal and segmental sclerosing lesions in the juxtamedullary glomeruli of 19 patients with "lipoid nephrosis" studied at autopsy (1). Noting that the frequency and severity of these lesions directly correlated with the duration of clinical disease, Rich suggested that the "uremia" present in several of these patients had resulted from progressive glomerular obliteration. The conclusions reached from these static observations were apparently supported by several biopsy studies of similar lesions in nephrotic patients with progressive renal disease (2). These anecdotal studies found that focal glomerulosclerosis could be present at the clinical onset of the disease but, in some patients, had apparently supervened on "minimal lesion" nephrotic syndrome. In 1970, two large biopsy studies of nephrotic children characterized the glomerular lesions and confirmed the previously noted resistance to corticosteroid therapy (3,4). The pessimistic outlook was apparently confirmed by a report of three patients with focal glomerulosclerosis and chronic renal failure, who developed proteinuria soon after renal transplantation and were found to have similar lesions in the transplanted kidneys (5). All these observations seemed to characterize a relatively specific glomerular lesion, which either occurred as a primary lesion or supervened upon epithelial cell disease. The lesion progressed relentlessly into chronic renal failure with no response to any therapy and recurred in the transplanted kidney. This well-defined clinicopathologic picture was soon challenged and has been the subject of continuing controversy. It has now become clear that the lesion of focal glomerulosclerosis is neither specific nor necessarily progressive. This chapter attempts to provide a summary of the present attitudes to focal glomerulosclerosis and to provide some guidelines to its recognition and interpretation.

PATHOGENESIS

The elucidation of all human glomerular diseases requires examination of the clinical circumstances in which they arise. Much of the misunderstanding of focal glomerulosclerosis probably arose from a failure to appreciate the ubiquity of this morphologic pattern in almost all types of glomerular disease. Careful examination of any large biopsy series demonstrates that the focal sclerosing pattern has no constant correlation with either the nephrotic syndrome or a progressive course. This clearly implies that the lesion is simply a pattern of reaction that may result from a wide variety of pathogenetic mechanisms. There is, nonetheless, a distinct association with proteinuria and/or the nephrotic syndrome in many patients; and most of the experimental models of focal glomerulosclerosis have, therefore, used animal systems in which proteinuria is the predominant component.

Early studies of aminonucleoside-induced proteinuria showed that repeated administration of the drug caused segmental glomerular lesions and an apparently self-perpetuating progressive course after its withdrawal (6). These observations suggested that chronic proteinuria alone might cause focal glomerulosclerosis rather than the reverse. Aging rats of several species develop increasing proteinuria with the progressive development of glomerular lesions identical to focal glomerulosclerosis (7), and similar lesions develop after uninephrectomy with protein overload (8). The aminonucleoside-induced disease also shows an increasing incidence and severity of sclerotic lesions after uninephrectomy and a threshold value of proteinuria is apparently required before glomerulosclerosis occurs (9). The development of glomerulosclerosis may correlate with epithelial cell damage demonstrated both by examination of polyanion, an epithelial sialoprotein whose function in glomerular permeability is attracting increasing interest (10), and by electron microscopy. A single dose of aminonucleoside causes diffuse loss of polyanion but, after repeated administration, its disappearance is segmental and occurs in the same segments as the sclerosis (11). Ultrastructurally, segmental epithelial disruption occurs in both aminonucleoside-treated rats (12) and in human focal glomerulosclerosis (13).

There is, therefore, considerable experimental evidence of an association between chronic proteinuria and focal glomerulosclerosis, although the precise mechanism of glomerular damage remains uncertain. The possibility that the association is indirect cannot, of course, be discounted. Hyperlipidemia, for example, is common with prolonged proteinuria and may lead to the accumulation of intraglomerular foam cells, which under certain experimental circumstances have been shown to precede the development of segmental glomerulosclerosis (14). Similarly, local coagulation may be implicated since fibrin-related antigens occur in the aminonucleoside-induced segmental lesions (11), and fibrin has been demonstrated ultrastructurally in one human study (15). None of these experimental models shares the juxtamedullary location of the human disease. The juxtamedullary glomeruli in humans are, however, larger than those in other species; they have a higher filtration rate (16) and are the oldest in the kidney (17), so that relative "overload," with or without other noxious stimuli, could preferentially localize injury in this region.

CLINICAL MANIFESTATIONS AND COURSE

This section reviews the clinical features of only those patients in whom idiopathic focal glomerulosclerosis is identified in the initial renal biopsy specimen, taken at or shortly after the onset of nephrotic syndrome. This restriction is based on three conclusions, which seem inescapable from personal experience and examination of the literature. First, lesions identical to focal glomerulosclerosis can develop in patients with relapsing corticosteroid-sensitive or corticosteroid-dependent epithelial cell disease without prejudicing the prognosis (18,18a). Second, the presence of focal glomerulosclerosis in a biopsy specimen taken at the onset of the nephrotic syndrome is very likely to indicate corticosteroid-resistant and progressive disease (18, 18a, 19). Third, the demonstration of focal glomerulosclerosis in patients with a nonnephrotic presentation is of uncertain prognostic significance. Focal glomerulosclerosis with nonnnephrotic proteinuria or other urinary abnormalities has been nonprogressive or minimally progressive in some series (19), but renal failure has developed in a significant number of patients in other studies (18a, 18b). While this restricted approach is not universally accepted, we consider that a relatively rigid series of clinical and pathologic criteria are required if the pathologist is to provide useful information to the physician performing renal biopsies.

In both adults (20–23) and children (24,25), the onset is typically insidious, with no systemic signs or identifiable precipitating events, although in a few patients this disease manifests after immunization or an infectious illness (24,25). Examination of the urinary sediment frequently reveals microscopic hematuria, and the proteinuria is usually nonselective (25). Although these features are suggestive of serious glomerular disease, there are no specific clinical features that allow diagnosis without renal biopsy. All ages may be affected and most studies report a predominance among males which is more pronounced in adults. There are sporadic reports of a familial tendency (26).

Therapy with corticosteroids and a variety of immunosuppressives is almost always fruitless in adults, but the pattern in children varies in individual reports. From the available literature, it is unfortunately difficult to be certain whether this variation represents included instances of late developing glomerulosclerosis in patients with relapsing epithelial cell disease or indicates a real heterogeneity in prognosis. Although adequate data are not provided in many reports, it is probable that typical focal glomerulosclerosis occurring soon after the onset of the nephrotic syndrome is an indication of a progressive course at all ages (18,18a). The nephrotic syndrome may pass through a series of remissions and relapses or be intractable to all therapy, and proteinuria may similarly remain fixed or show wide variation. The decline in renal function is progressive over a period of up to 10 years, although a substantial number of patients, usually those presenting with severe nephrotic features, progress rapidly to renal failure within two to three years, a condition known as "malignant" focal glomerulosclerosis (18b,18c). As with other progressive renal diseases, hypertension is a usual complication and may lead to further renal damage in addition to causing systemic vascular complications.

PATHOLOGIC CHARACTERISTICS

Light Microscopy

The characteristic fully developed lesion is a solidified area within the glomerular tuft which is adherent to Bowman's capsule and has a "hard," glossy character in H&E and PAS-stained sections because of accumulated "hyalin" (Figs. 4-1,4-

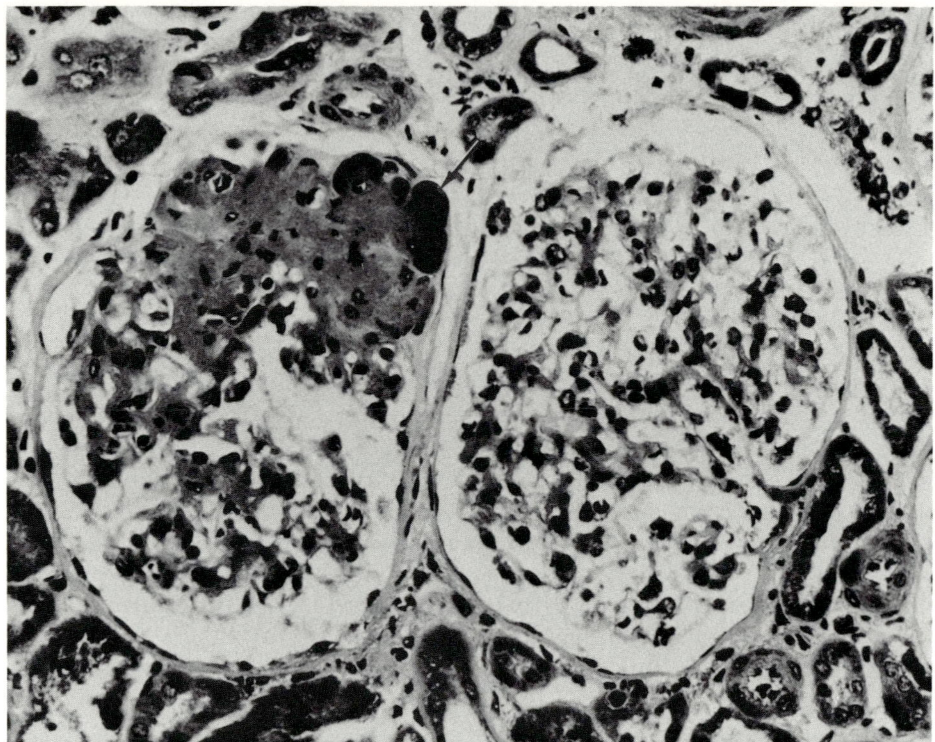

Figure 4-1. Biopsy from a patient with epithelial cell disease and nonprogressive focal glomerulosclerosis. The glomerulus on the left shows segmental sclerosis with conspicuous insudate (arrow), while the glomerulus on the right appears normal (Masson trichrome stain, ×325).

2). In contrast to the segmental lesions produced by inflammatory glomerular disease, there is no excess of cells in the affected area, which appears collapsed and consolidated rather than expanded by a true increase in matrix. The coalescence of mesangial and endothelial nuclei may, initially, give an impression of proliferation but can usually be distinguished from proliferative glomerulonephritis by either the lack of other segmental proliferation or the tangled, irregular appearance of the membrane. Later, accumulating "hyalin" may obscure the collapse pattern by expanding the affected area and may contain included vacuoles and/or foam cells. Overlying early lesions, there is often epithelial swelling with minor proliferation, but true crescents do not occur. Frequently, these epithelial cells contain large proteinaceous, PAS-positive droplets with, in some biopsy specimens, prominent intracytoplasmic cysts (27) (Fig. 4-3). In deep cortical biopsy specimens, preferential involvement of juxtamedullary glomeruli may be seen. There is often a tendency for the sclerotic lesions to occur adjacent to the glomerular hilum.

Early lesions may be very sparse, requiring diligent search of serial sections, and may consist only of segmental deposits of subendothelial "hyalin" or collections of intracapillary foam cells. Foam cells occur at all stages of focal glomerulosclerosis, both in the glomeruli and in the interstitium (Fig. 4-4). Me-

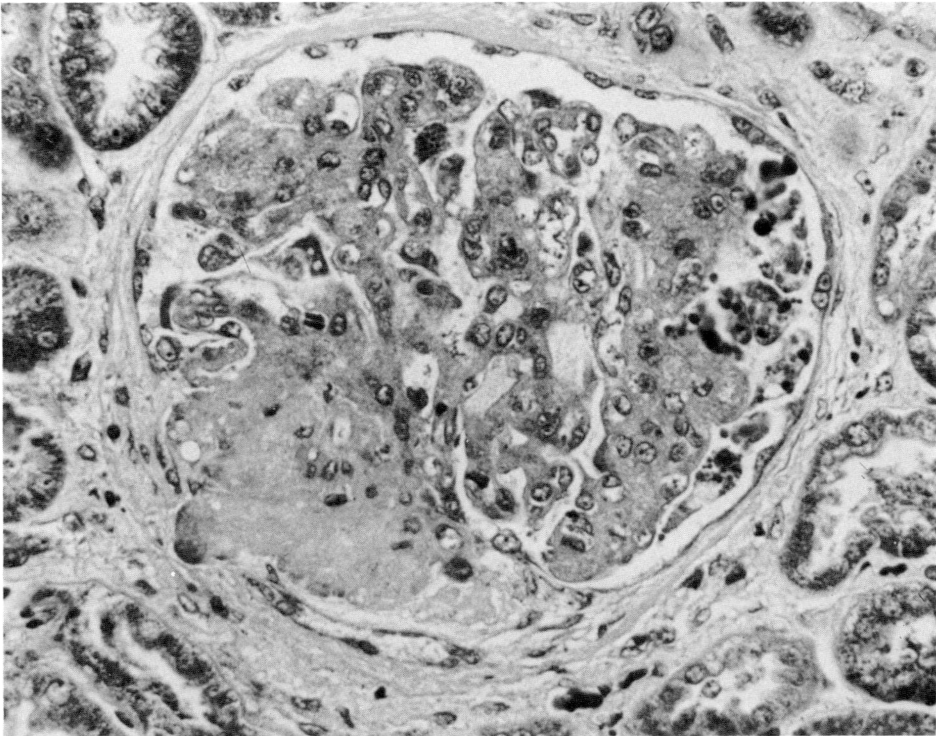

Figure 4-2. Advanced focal glomerulosclerosis. There is an area of consolidation adherent to the Bowman's capsule at the glomerular stalk (H&E stain, ×490).

sangial proliferation is a frequent accompanying feature and indicates a particular potential for progressive disease (28,29). The presence of mesangial proliferation in biopsy specimens from patients with the nephrotic syndrome is, therefore, a signal to search carefully for segmental disease and to express some reservations about the prognosis. Similarly, the presence of global glomerulosclerosis, with irregular glomerular and/or tubulointerstitial scarring, in biopsy specimens from patients with nephrotic syndrome is an inducement to search carefully for segmental disease and to be cautious in prognostic evaluation (18,30). Careful examination of PAS-stained sections may provide a clue to the diagnosis by showing irregular capillary condensation within globally sclerotic glomeruli, in contrast to the usual shrinkage pattern. In children, vascular changes are uncommon, but biopsy specimens from adults frequently show arteriolar hyalinosis, whether or not hypertension is present. Serial biopsy specimens in patients with progressive disease reveal increasing degrees of glomerular and tubulointerstitial damage, usually with preservation of the diagnostic glomerular pattern.

Electron Microscopy

There is complete obliteration of epithelial foot processes present in glomeruli with or without segmental disease. The diagnosis of focal glomerulosclerosis is,

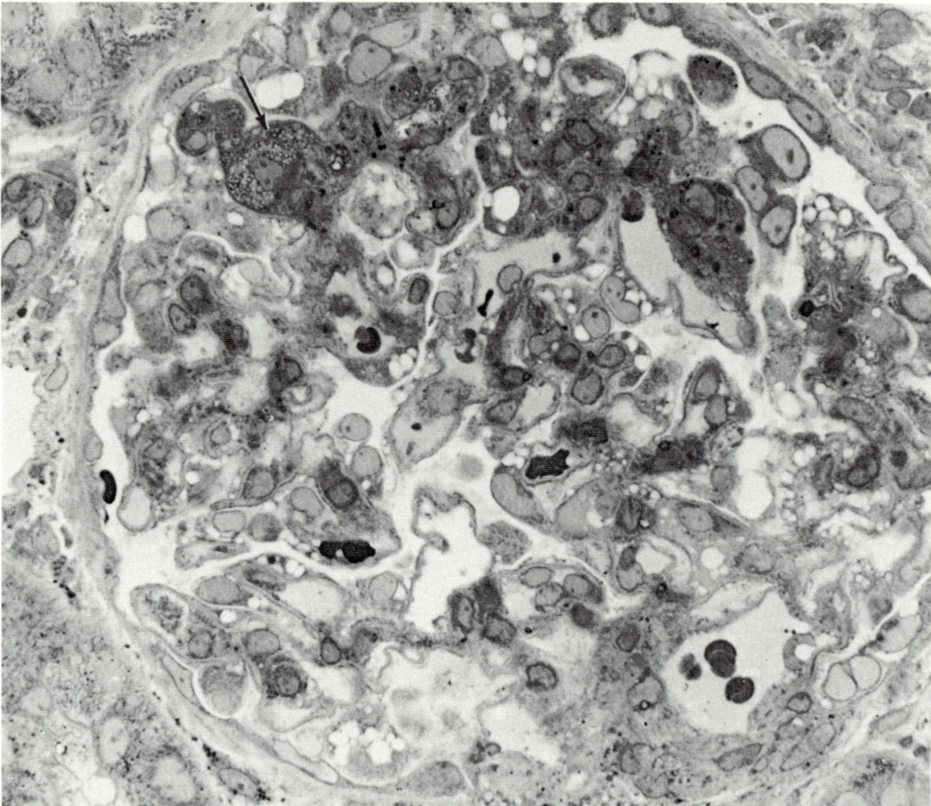

Figure 4-3. Early focal glomerulosclerosis. There is mild segmental prominence of the mesangium (upper third) with swelling and marked vacuolization of the epithelial cell cytoplasm. In addition, there is one intracapillary foam cell (arrow) (plastic embedded toluidine blue stain, ×625).

in fact, very unwise in the absence of such epithelial change. Sclerotic areas are characterized in the early stages by irregular capillary collapse, often with apparent hypertrophy of the included cells and increase in mesangial matrix (Figs. 4-5, 4-6). More advanced lesions show an extensive accumulation of granular, electron-dense material throughout the affected segments. This is typically seen as a nodular mass, correlating with the light microscopic hyalin deposits, expanding the distorted segment that is usually adherent to Bowman's capsule. Frequently, these masses contain lipid vacuoles, distorted membrane fragments, and abundant collagen (22) (Fig. 4-7). In some biopsy specimens, more discrete deposits may be visible in various locations but, if numerous, these suggest the possibility of glomerulosclerosis complicating other patterns of glomerular disease. In relation to the evolving sclerotic lesions, there is often epithelial cell detachment (13,27). This appears as areas of denuded basement membrane caused by epithelial degeneration with breakdown of cell membranes (Fig. 4-8). The space between the abnormal epithelial cell and the naked membrane may appear empty or may be filled with layers of membranous material, often admixed with degenerate cytoplasmic organelles (Fig. 4-9). Later stages of this epithelial disruption pattern may be recognizable only as collections of mi-

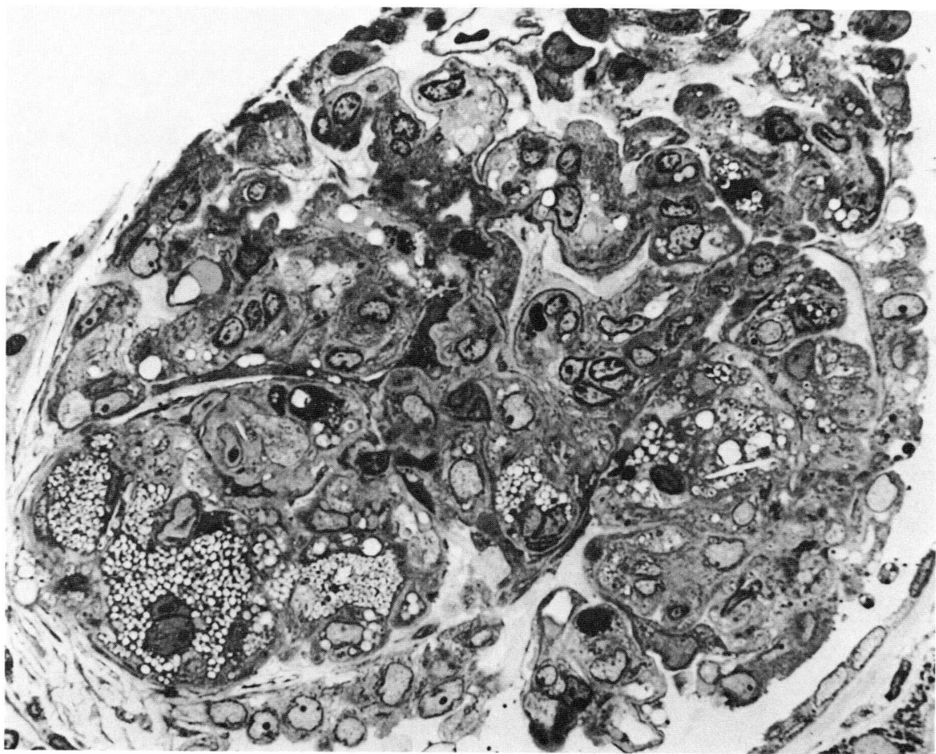

Figure 4-4. Glomerulus from a patient with focal glomerulosclerosis showing numerous lipid-containing foam cells (plastic embedded toluidine blue stain, × 725).

crovesicular bodies. These bodies, which are seen in a wide range of glomerular disorders (31), probably result from remodeling of intercellular junctions (32) and have no relationship to viral infection. Platelet clumps may be seen and actual microthrombi are occasionally found (15) (Fig. 4-8).

Immunofluorescence Microscopy

Bright, segmental reactions occur in sclerotic lesions as either granular, capillary wall patterns or irregular and ill-defined masses corresponding to the hyalin deposits (20,22,25). The reactions are usually for IgM and/or C3, but may include IgG, C1, C4, and such nonspecific reagents as albumin and α_2-macroglobulin (Figs. 4-10, 4-11). While light microscopic sclerosis and the segmental immunofluorescence deposits usually occur in parallel, the fluorescent reactions may precede recognizable light microscopic damage. This dichotomy, which also occurs in the experimental aminonucleoside model (11), is unexplained, but indicates the need to search carefully for segmental disease in paraffin sections if segmental immunofluorescence is seen. Reactions for IgA are rare and, especially if diffuse, are strong evidence against a diagnosis of focal glomerulosclerosis (33). Diffuse weak mesangial reactions for IgM may occur, as in epithelial cell disease (34), and a weak linear pattern of reaction for IgG, not associated with circulating antiglomerular basement membrane antibodies, has occasionally been described (34,35).

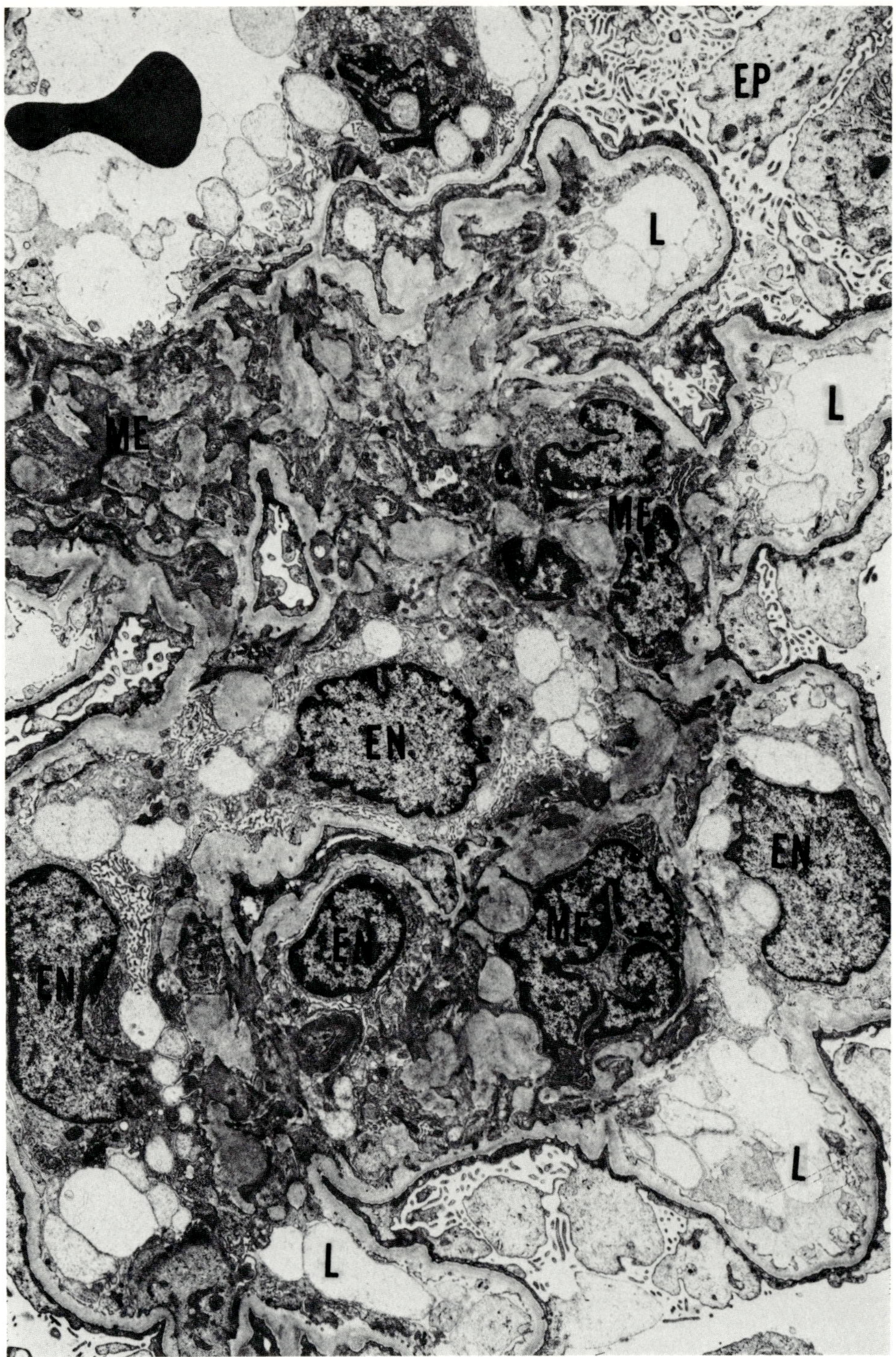

Figure 4-5. Electron micrograph from a biopsy of a patient with focal glomerulosclerosis. There is an increase in the mesangial matrix. The basement membrane is folded, and the epithelial foot processes are obliterated. Note the condensation of the epithelial cell cytoplasm along the basement membrane and the prominent epithelial villous hyperplasia. EN, endothelial cell; ME, mesangium; EP, epithelial cell; L, capillary lumen (×3,400).

52

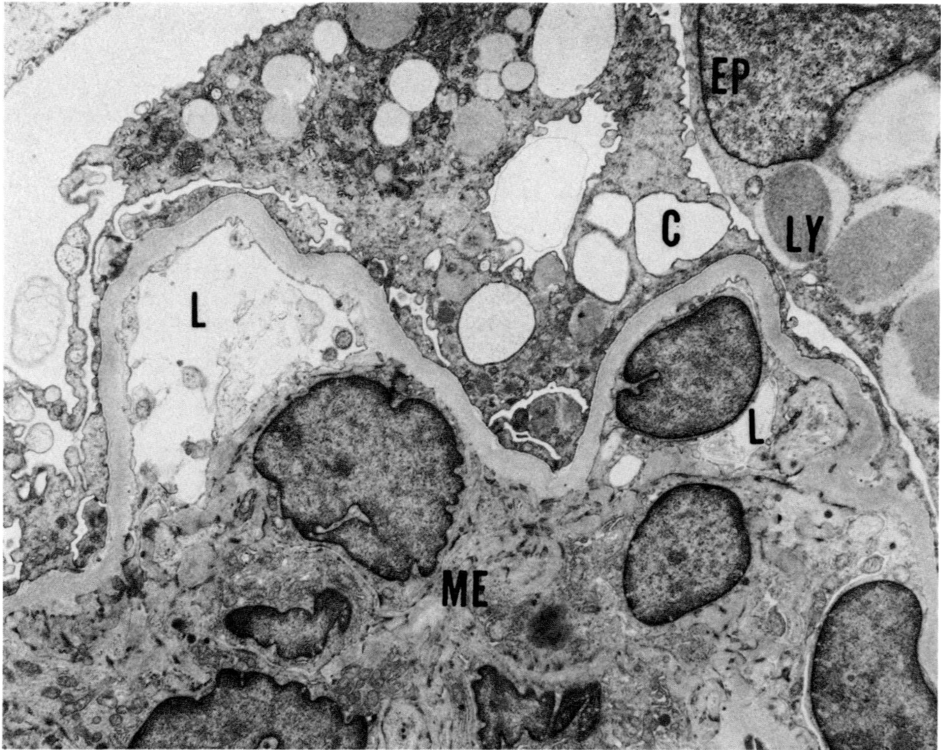

Figure 4-6. Focal glomerulosclerosis. The foot processes are obliterated and the epithelial cell (EP) is hypertrophied with prominent pseudocysts (C) and numerous lysosomes (LY), which probably represent protein transport droplets. The capillary lumina (L) are greatly reduced by enlargement of the mesangium (ME) (×5,400).

DIFFERENTIAL DIAGNOSIS

Focal Global Sclerosis

Habib (18,25) includes in her series of focal glomeruloscerosis patients a group in whom globally sclerotic glomeruli coexist with others showing no segmental or other abnormality. The nephrotic syndrome in this group of patients may be resistant to corticosteroid and immunosuppressive therapy, although rather less frequently than with typical segmental disease, and some patients show a slowly progressive course. This intermediate position between relapsing epithelial cell disease and focal glomerulosclerosis suggests an admixture of patients from each group rather than a separate disease entity. The presence of frequent globally sclerotic glomeruli is, however, a disturbing prognostic sign and an indication to search carefully for segmental lesions. A study of kidneys taken from autopsied patients without evidence of renal disease suggests that sclerosis of more than 10% of glomeruli in patients less than 40 years of age can be regarded as evidence of significant glomerular disease (36). Habib proposes, however, that sclerosis of 15 to 20% of the available glomeruli is required for inclusion in this group and recommends that, in children, only those whose biopsy specimens show tubulointerstitial scarring be considered to avoid confusion with congenital

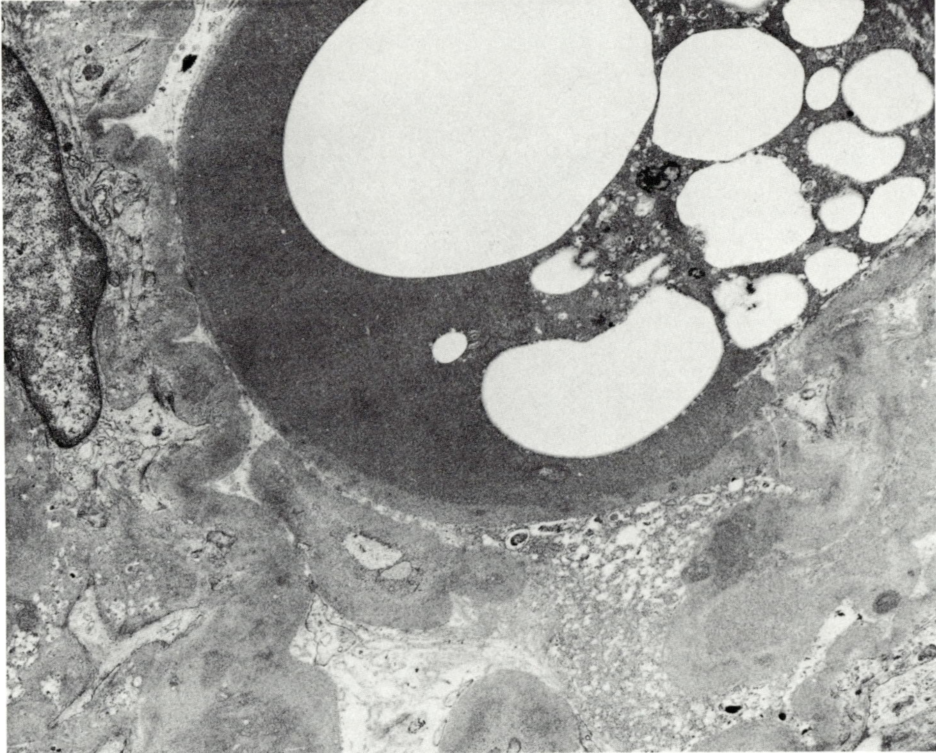

Figure 4-7. Sclerotic glomerular segment with electron-dense material and lipid vacuoles (×9,300).

glomerulosclerosis (18). The significance and pathogenesis of focal global glomerulosclerosis, without segmental lesions, remains uncertain. Some doubt about the prognostic reliability of global glomerulosclerosis has been recently introduced by a report showing no difference in outcome between patients with global sclerosis and those showing typical epithelial cell disease (37).

Focal Glomerulosclerosis in Other Glomerular Disorders

Lesions indistinguishable from the focal glomerulosclerosis associated with the nephrotic syndrome may be superimposed upon a wide range of glomerular disorders. These include diffuse glomerulonephritis, scarred focal and segmental glomerulonephritis, membranous nephropathy, hereditary glomerulonephritis (Alport and other types), and diabetic glomerulosclerosis (38,39). Segmental glomerulosclerosis is especially prone to complicate mesangial proliferative glomerulonephritis, particularly that associated with IgA deposition (33) and the glomerulomegaly associated with chronic lung and heart disease (40), obesity (41), and hepatic cirrhosis (42). There is clearly a need, therefore, to carefully review the clinical and pathologic features when these lesions are encountered before a diagnosis of focal glomerulosclerosis is applied. In most of these "secondary" forms of glomerulosclerosis, the lesions appear to represent only a

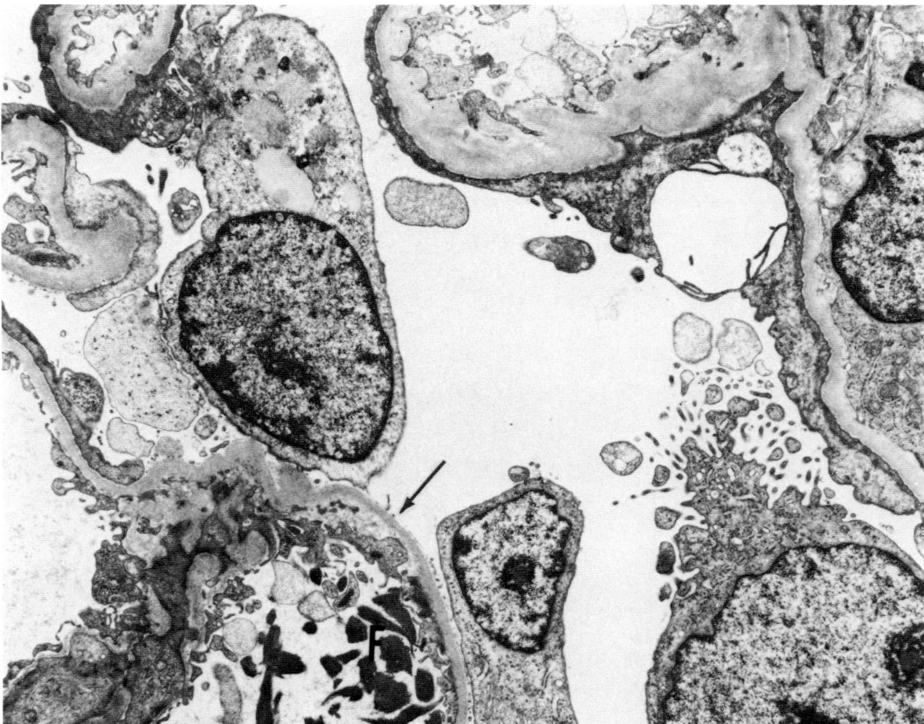

Figure 4-8. In addition to foot process obliteration, microvillous hyperplasia, and cyst formation, denudation of the outer aspect of the basement membrane (arrow) and fibrin thrombosis (F) are shown (×5,900).

nonspecific pattern of glomerular scarring that has complicated the basic disease. While their presence is suggestive of ongoing glomerular damage, the sclerotic lesions probably have no diagnostic or prognostic significance in the majority of patients. There is, however, some evidence that patients with segmental hyalinosis superimposed on membranous nephropathy progress more quickly into chronic renal failure than those without segmental disease (43), and that segmental sclerosis may represent one pathway for progressive glomerular damage in reflux nephropathy (44).

Focal Glomerulosclerosis with Proteinuria and the Nephrotic Syndrome

Clearly, any of the associated disorders described above may present with proteinuria. A diagnosis of isolated focal glomerulosclerosis implies, therefore, exclusion of other glomerular disease. As a corollary, the morphologic lesion of focal glomerulosclerosis occurring in patients with other clinical manifestations need have none of the dire prognostic implications discussed elsewhere in this chapter. Morphologic diagnosis in nephrotic patients is straightforward when there is complete obliteration of epithelial foot processes and the segmental lesions are typical and numerous. This situation is usually encountered in pa-

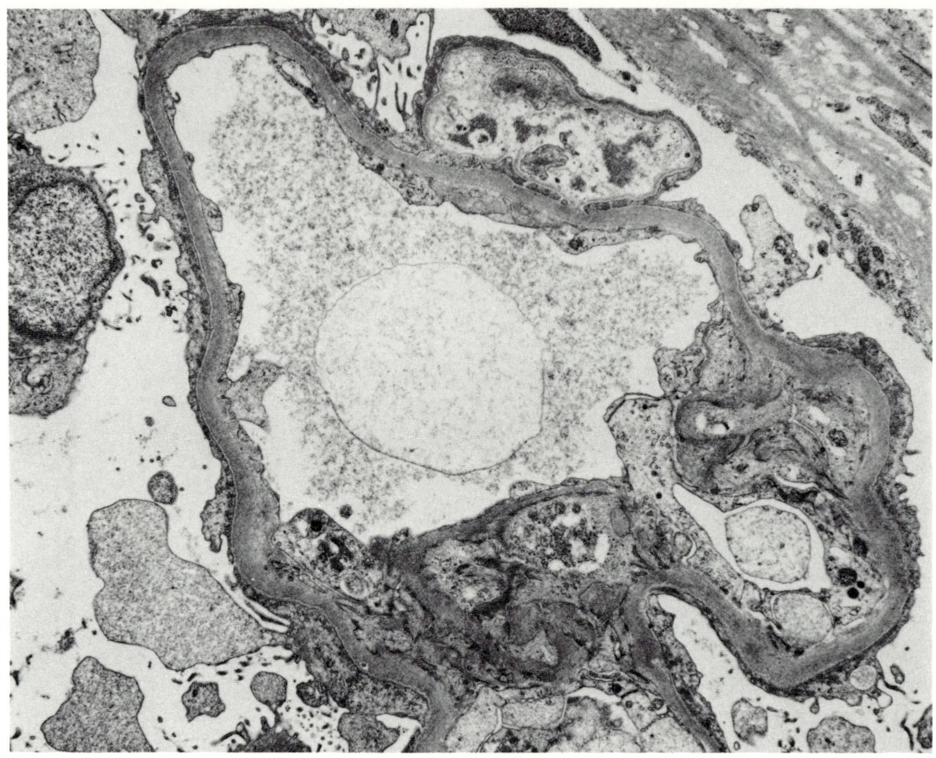

Figure 4-9. Focal lifting of the epithelial cell cytoplasm is shown, with reticulation and rarefaction between the epithelial cell and lamina densa (×6,300).

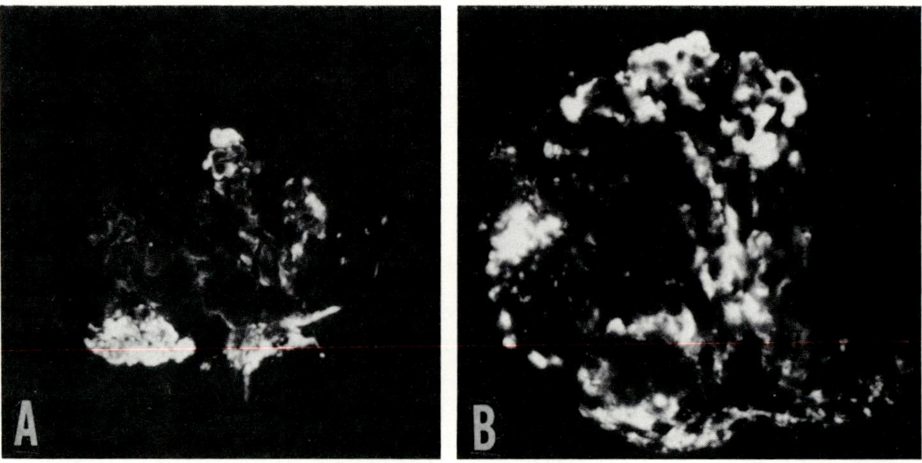

Figure 4-10. Immunofluorescence microscopy demonstrating segmental deposition of IgM (A) and C3 (B) in a biopsy specimen of a patient with focal glomerulosclerosis (×313).

56

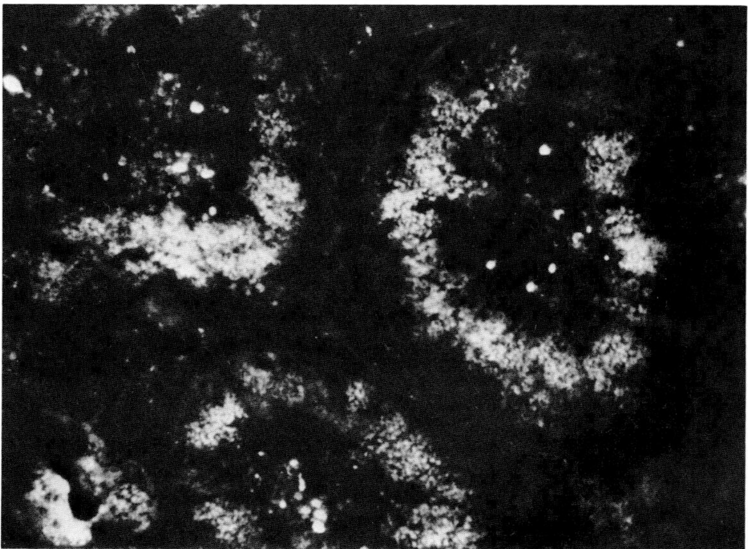

Figure 4-11. Numerous protein transport droplets in proximal tubules in a biopsy specimen from a patient with focal glomerulosclerosis and heavy proteinuria (antialbumin, ×350).

tients with recent onset of severe nephrotic syndrome that proves intractable to therapy. Diagnosis is more difficult when lesions are few or when they are found only in biopsy specimens taken after some months or years of constant or intermittent nephrotic syndrome. There is ample evidence that typical segmental glomerulosclerosis may occur during the course of otherwise uncomplicated, relapsing, and corticosteroid-sensitive epithelial cell disease without affecting the long-term prognosis (18,18b). The lesions in these patients are usually sparse, probably explaining the reported relationship between the frequency of glomerular lesions and subsequent clinical course (45). Isolated sclerotic lesions can, however, be found in biopsy specimens taken early in the clinical course and, especially if they are not typical, can be difficult to interpret. In these situations, the diagnosis can only be suspected morphologically and firm prognostic conclusions must await analysis of the patient's response to therapy. Similarly, disturbing clues are the presence of interstitial scarring, global glomerulosclerosis, ultrastructural capillary collapse or irregularity (46), and segmental immunofluorescence, stimulating careful search for characteristic lesions; however, these have undetermined prognostic significance as isolated phenomena. When unequivocal segmental glomerulosclerosis and hyalinosis is discovered, analysis of the mesangium may be important, since there is evidence that the combination of focal glomerulosclerosis and mesangial proliferation is particularly prone to relentless progression (28).

GLOMERULAR DISEASE AND HEROIN ABUSE (HEROIN NEPHROPATHY)

There has been increasing recent awareness of an association between chronic heroin abuse, proteinuria, and progressive renal disease. The first, anecdotal, reports concerned drug addicts with severe proteinuria, but more recent studies have examined the frequency and patterns of glomerular disease in unselected populations of addicts. These systematic studies have shown that the prevalence of glomerular disease is very low and have cast some doubt on the existence of a statistical relationship (47). However, the close similarity between the anecdotally reported clinical and pathologic features and the reduction in proteinuria occurring after cessation of the habit argue strongly for a real association (48,49). The most commonly described glomerular lesion in heroin addicts with proteinuria or the nephrotic syndrome is focal glomerulosclerosis (Figs. 4-12, 4-13), usually with mesangial proliferation (48,50). Focal epithelial disruption appears to be characteristic of the heroin-associated lesion, suggesting the possibility of a direct toxic effect (50). Immunofluorescence microscopy typically reveals diffuse mesangial reactions for IgM and C3 (51), although IgG may be the predominant immunoglobulin (49), and a change from IgG to IgM has been noted with increasing duration of heroin exposure (52). Linear IgG reactions, without circulating antiglomerular basement membrane antibodies, have also been described (32,52). Renal failure has developed in the majority of heroin addicts with focal glomerulosclerosis, and has occurred over periods of one to four years, but progression may be delayed or halted by cessation of heroin abuse (48,49). The pathogenesis of the glomerular changes is unknown, but elevated serum concentrations of IgM have been found in heroin addicts, and the possi-

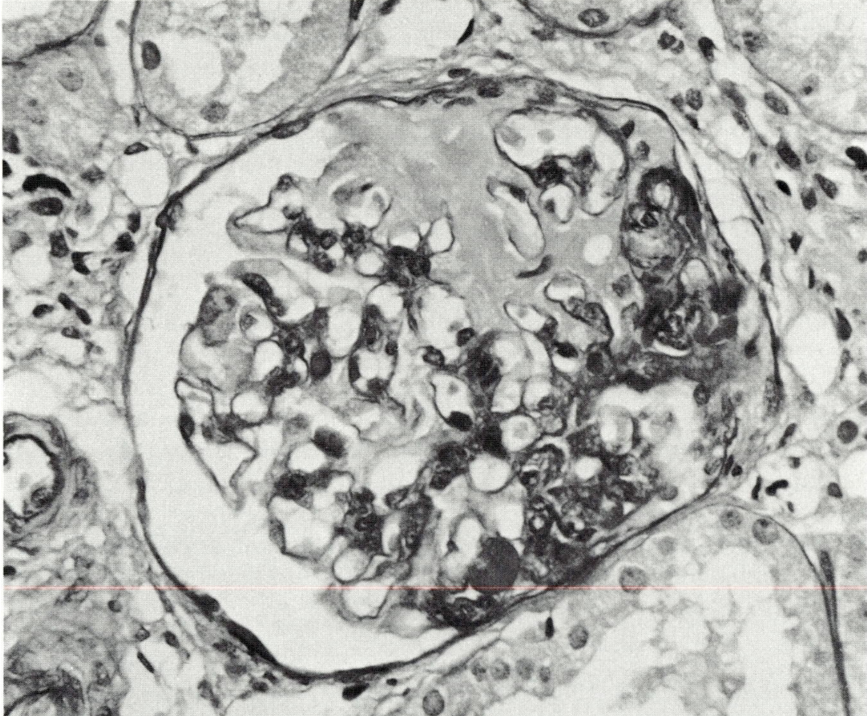

Figure 4-12. Glomerulus from a heroin addict showing segmental sclerosis and insudate (lower portion) (H&E stain, ×450).

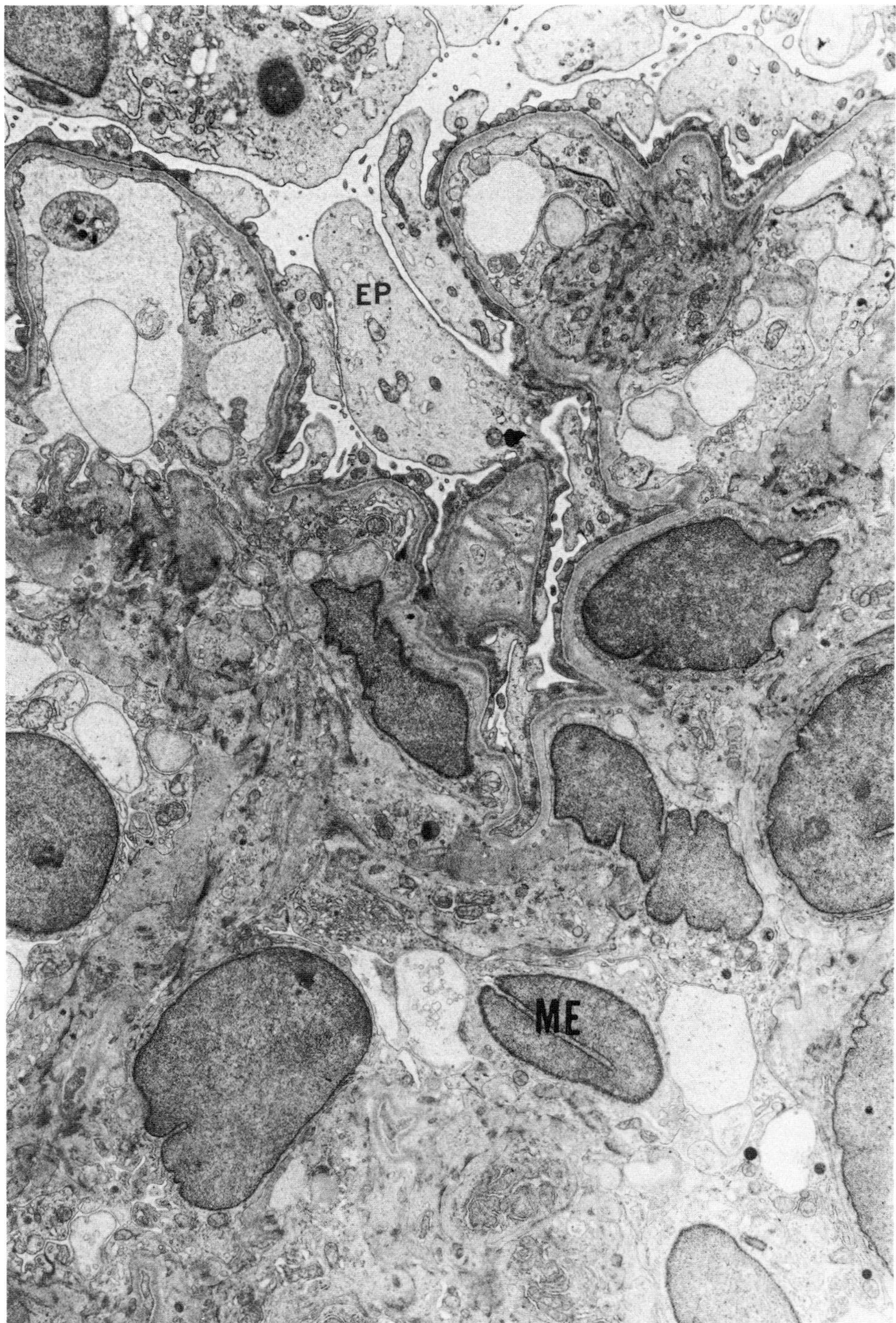

Figure 4-13. Electron micrograph of a portion of a glomerulus from a 28-year-old heroin addict showing mesangial proliferation, increase of mesangial matrix, and epithelial foot process obliteration. EP, epithelial cell; ME, mesangium (×6,000).

bility of IgM-containing immune complexes requires examination (48). Focal glomerulosclerosis is by no means the only renal lesion complicating heroin abuse. There is also a clear association with membranous nephropathy (47,49,50) and mesangiocapillary glomerulonephritis (49,50), and isolated examples of amyloidosis have been reported (53). Acute renal failure in heroin addicts may be caused by acute glomerulonephritis complicating septicemia (with or without endocarditis), rhabdomyolysis, and systemic arteritis (46).

FOCAL GLOMERULOSCLEROSIS AND TRANSPLANTATION

The recurrence of nephrotic syndrome soon after transplantation was reported soon after the characterization of the glomerular disease (5). A number of similar recurrences have since been described (54), but the behavioral patterns have been variable. Proteinuria may appear almost immediately (55) or at various stages up to two years (56) after transplantation. Biopsy specimens taken at the onset of proteinuria have usually shown only obliteration of epithelial foot processes, but typical glomerulosclerosis has developed over months or years, often in the juxtamedullary glomeruli (5). While graft failure from progressive glomerolsclerosis has been reported (55,56), gradual disappearance of the proteinuria with maintenance of graft function is more common. There is one report of the immediate recurrence of proteinuria in a second graft, with juxtamedullary sclerosis already present by 20 days after transplantation (55). The situation is, however, complicated by the occurrence of focal glomerulosclerosis in patients whose original disease was either nonglomerular (57) or some other form of glomerulonephritis (56). The frequency of recurrence has been reported as up to 60% in patients who have had transplants for focal glomerulosclerosis and renal failure (56), but it is generally thought to be less than 30% (54). Strangely, although there is a strong association between vesicoureteric reflux and focal glomerulosclerosis in the patient's own kidneys (44) and with glomerular lesions in transplanted kidneys (58), only rarely do the lesions in grafts affected by reflux resemble focal glomerulosclerosis. Whatever the frequency of recurrent focal glomerulosclerosis, its development in the grafts of patients with similar disease in their own kidneys suggests the presence of a circulating toxic factor. No such factor has as yet been demonstrated.

SUMMARY

Focal, segmental glomerulosclerosis is a common and nonspecific morphologic lesion occurring in a wide variety of glomerular diseases. When it occurs with severe proteinuria and the nephrotic syndrome, this pattern of glomerular disease has been associated with progressive glomerular obliteration leading eventually to chronic renal failure. Segmental glomerulosclerosis may, however, develop in patients after years of relapsing epithelial cell disease and, in this situation, appears not to affect the long-term prognosis. A gloomy prognosis is warranted, therefore, only when segmental sclerosis and diffuse obliteration of epithelial foot processes coexist in a biopsy specimen taken soon after the onset of the nephrotic syndrome—especially with associated mesangial proliferation—and if there is no response to corticosteroid therapy. In patients with severe proteinuria, this pattern may be associated with heroin abuse (usually with mesangial immunofluoresence for IgM) or reflux nephropathy, each of which may cause chronic renal failure. There is less evidence for progression into renal failure with the many other clinical and pathologic associations and specific diagnosis is important.

The pathogenesis of the glomerular lesions is unknown and probably variable according to the associated clinical and pathological features. There is, however, some experimental evidence to suggest that epithelial damage, similar to that seen in some human biopsy specimens from nephrotic patients, may lead to similar lesions. The lesions developing in chronic, relapsing epithelial cell disease may be related to the sclerosis developing in aging and protein overloaded rats. The possibility of direct epithelial damage, perhaps by a circulating factor, in nephrotic patients is supported by recurrence of proteinuria in a number of patients who have had transplants for focal glomerulosclerosis. The effect of such a toxin would, however, appear to be transient, for graft failure seldom occurs and recurrence in a second transplant has been recorded only once. The diagnosis of focal glomerulosclerosis may be obvious but, in some biopsy specimens, the lesions are sparse. Suggestive associated findings, stimulating more careful search for typical lesions, include focal interstitial scarring, focal global sclerosis, mesangial proliferation, segmental immunofluorescence for IgM and/or C3, and segmental capillary collapse on electron microscopy. Although the lesion of focal segmental glomerulsclerosis is a frequent finding in renal biopsy specimens, it is advisable for the pathologist to emphasize the presence of the lesions only in patients with severe proteinuria or the nephrotic syndrome.

REFERENCES

1. Rich AR: A hitherto undescribed vulnerability of the juxtamedullary glomeruli in lipoid nephrosis. *Bull Johns Hopkins Hosp* 100:173, 1957.

2. Hayslett JP, Krassner LS, Bensch KG, et al: Progression of "lipoid nephrosis" to renal insufficiency. *N Engl J Med* 281:181, 1969.

3. Churg J, Habib R, White RHR: Pathology of the nephrotic syndrome in children: A Report for the International Study of Kidney Disease in Children. *Lancet* 1:1299, 1970.

4. White RHR, Glasgow EF, Mills RJ: Clinicopathological study of nephrotic syndrome in childhood. *Lancet* 1:1353, 1970.

5. Hoyer, JR, Vernier RL, Najarian JS, et al: Recurrence of idiopathic nephrotic syndrome after renal transplantation. *Lancet* 2:343, 1972.

6. Borowsky BA, Kessner DM, Hartcroft WS, et al: Aminonucleoside-induced chronic glomerulonephritis in rats. *J Lab Clin Med* 57:512, 1961.

7. Bolton WK, Benton FR, Maclay JG, et al: Spontaneous glomerular sclerosis in aging Sprague-Dawley rats. I. Lesions associated with mesangial IgM deposits. *Am J Pathol* 85:277, 1976.

8. Lalich JJ, Burkholder PM, Paik WC: Protein overload nephropathy in rats with unilateral nephrectomy. A correlative light immunofluorescence and electron microscopial analysis. *Arch Pathol* 99:72, 1975.

9. Glasser RJ, Velosa JA, Michael AF: Experimental model of focal sclerosis. I. Relationship to protein excretion in aminonucleoside nephrosis. *Lab Invest* 36:519, 1977.

10. Seiler MW, Rennke HG, Venkatachalam MA, et al: Pathogenesis of polycation-induced alterations ("fusion") of glomerular epithelium. *Lab Invest* 36:48, 1977.

11. Velosa JA, Glasser RJ, Nevins TE, et al: Experimental model of focal sclerosis. II. Correlation with immunopathologic changes, macromolecular kinetics and polyanion loss. *Lab Invest* 36:527, 1977.

12. Ryan GB, Karnovsky MJ: An ultrastructural study of the mechanisms of proteinuria in aminonucleoside nephrosis. *Kidney Int* 8:219, 1975.

13. Cohen AH, Mampaso F, Zamboni L: Glomerular podocyte degeneration in human renal disease: an ultrastructural study. *Lab Invest* 37:30, 1977.

14. Wellman KF, Volk BW: Renal changes in experimental hypercholesterolemia in normal and in subdiabetic rabbits. II. Long term studies. *Lab Invest* 24:144, 1971.

15. Duffy JL, Cinque T, Grishman E, Churg J: Intraglomerular fibrin, platelet aggregation, and subendothelial deposits in lipoid nephrosis. *J Clin Invest* 49:251, 1970.

16. Cannon PJ: The kidney in heart failure. *N Engl J Med* 296:26, 1977.

17. McCrory WW: Normal staging of renal development during fetal life, in Strauss J (ed): *Pediatric Nephrology* New York, Stratton, 1976, Vol 2, p 279.

18. Habib R: Focal glomerular sclerosis. *Kidney Int* 4:355, 1973.

18a. Cameron JS, Turner DR, Ogg CS, et al: The long-term prognosis of patients with focal glomerulosclerosis. *Clin Nephrol* 10:213, 1978.

18b. Saint-Hillier Y, Morel-Maroger L, Woodrow D, et al: Focal and segmental hyalinosis. *Adv Nephrol* 5:67, 1975.

18c. Brown CB, Cameron JS, Turner DR, et al: Focal segmental glomerulosclerosis with rapid decline in renal function ("malignant FSGS"). *Clin Nephrol* 10:51, 1978.

19. Beaufils H, Alphonse JC, Guedon J, et al: Focal glomerulosclerosis: natural history and treatment. A report of 70 cases. *Nephron* 21:75, 1978.

20. Hyman LR, Burkholder PM: Focal sclerosing glomerulonephropathy with segmental hyalinosis: A clinicopathologic analysis. *Lab Invest* 28:533, 1973.

21. Velosa JA, Donadio JV Jr, Holley KE: Focal sclerosing glomerulonephropathy: a clinicopathologic study. *Mayo Clin Proc* 50:121, 1975.

22. Jenis EH, Teichman S, Briggs WA, et al: Focal segmental glomerulosclerosis. *Am J Med* 57:695, 1974.

23. Lim VS, Sibley R, Spargo B: Adult lipoid nephrosis: clinicopathological correlations. *Ann Intern Med* 81:314, 1974.

24. Newman WJ, Tisher CC, McCoy RC, et al: Focal glomerular sclerosis: contrasting clinical patterns in children and adults. *Medicine (Balt)* 55:67, 1976.

25. Habib R, Kleinknecht C: The primary nephrotic syndrome of childhood: classification and clinicopathologic study of 406 cases. *Pathol Annu* 6:417, 1971.

26. Moncrieff MW, White RHR, Glasgow EF, et al: The familial nephrotic syndrome. II. A clinicopathological study. *Clin Nephrol* 1:220, 1973.

27. Grishman E, Churg J: Focal glomerular sclerosis in nephrotic patients: an electron microscopic study of glomerular podocytes. *Kidney Int* 7:111, 1975.

28. Schoeneman MJ, Bennett B, Griefer I: The natural history of focal segmental glomerulosclerosis with and without mesangial hypercellularity in children. *Clin Nephrol* 9:45, 1978.

29. Grund K-E, Hara M, Bohle A: Diffuse mesangial cell proliferation in focal sclerosing glomerulonephritis. *Virchows Arch (A) Path Anat Histol* 370:297, 1976.

30. Jao W, Pollak VE, Norris SH, et al: Lipoid nephrosis: an approach to the clinicopathologic analysis and dismemberment of idiopathic nephrotic syndrome with minimal glomerular changes. *Medicine (Balt)* 52:445, 1973.

31. Bariety J, Callard P: Round "virus-like" extracellular particles in glomerular tufts: an electron microscopic study of 190 human renal biopsies. *Virchows Arch Abt (A) Path Anat* 357:125, 1972.

32. Ferrans VJ, Thiedemann KU, Maron BJ, et al: Spherical microparticles in human myocardium: an ultrastructural study. *Lab Invest* 35:349, 1976.

33. Clarkson AR, Seymour AE, Thompson AJ, et al: IgA nephropathy: a syndrome of uniform morphology, diverse clinical features and uncertain prognosis. *Clin Nephrol* 8:459, 1977.

34. Roy LP, Westberg NG, Michael AF: Nephrotic syndrome: no evidence for a role for IgE. *Clin Exp Immunol* 13:553, 1973.

35. Matalon R, Katz L, Gallo G, et al: Glomerular sclerosis in adults with nephrotic syndrome. *Ann Intern Med* 80:488, 1974.

36. Kaplan C, Pasternack B, Shah H, et al: Age-related incidence of sclerotic glomeruli in human kidneys. *Am J Pathol* 80:227, 1975.

37. Nash MA, Greifer I, Olbing H, et al: The significance of focal sclerotic lesions of glomeruli in children. *J Pediat* 88:806, 1976.

38. Kincaid-Smith P: *The Kidney: A Clinicopathological Study.* Oxford, Blackwell Scientific Publications, 1975, p 129.

39. Whitworth JA, Turner DR, Leibowitz S, et al: Focal segmental sclerosis or scarred focal proliferative glomerulonephritis? *Clin Nephrol* 9:229, 1978.

40. Rosenmann E, Dwarka L, Boss JH: Proliferative glomerulopathy in rheumatic heart disease and chronic lung disease. *Am J Med Sci* 264:213, 1972.

41. Weisenger JR, Kempson RL, Eldridge FL, et al: The nephrotic syndrome: a complication of massive obesity. *Ann Intern Med* 81:440, 1974.

42. Nochy D, Callard P, Bellon B, et al: Association of overt glomerulonephritis and liver disease: a study of 34 patients. *Clin Nephrol* 6:422, 1976.

43. Ehrenreich T, Churg J: Focal glomerulosclerosis in membranous nephropathy. *Am J Pathol* 87:37a, 1977.

44. Kincaid-Smith P: Glomerular and vascular lesions in chronic atrophic pyelonephritis and reflux nephropathy. *Adv Nephrol* 5:3, 1975.

45. Kohaut EC, Singer DB, Hill LL: The significance of focal glomerular sclerosis in children who have nephrotic syndrome. *Am J Clin Pathol* 66:545, 1976.

46. Siegel NJ, Kashgarian M, Spargo BH, et al: Minimal change and focal sclerotic lesions in lipoid nephrosis. *Nephron* 13:125, 1974.

47. Arruda JA, Kurtzman NA, Pillay, VK: Prevalence of renal disease in asymptomatic heroin addicts. *Arch Intern Med* 135:535, 1975.

48. Rao TKS, Nicastri AD, Friedman EA: Renal consequences of narcotic abuse. *Adv Nephrol* 7:261, 1977.

49. Llach F, Descouedres C, Massry SG: Heroin associated nephropathy: clinical and histological studies in 19 patients. *Clin Nephrol* 11:7, 1979.

50. Grishman E, Churg J, Porush JG: Glomerular morphology in nephrotic heroin addicts. *Lab Invest* 35:415, 1976.

51. Salomon MI, Poon TP, Goldblatt M, et al: Renal lesions in heroin addicts: a study based on kidney biopsies. *Nephron* 9:356, 1972.

52. Eknoyan G, Gyorkey F, Dichoso C, et al: Nephropathy in patients with drug addiction: evolution of pathological and clinical features. *Virchows Arch (A) Path Anat Histol* 365:1, 1975.

53. Derosena R, Koss MN, Pirani CL: Demonstration of amyloid fibrils in urinary sediment. *N Engl J Med* 293:1131, 1975.

54. Cameron JS, Turner DR: Recurrent glomerulonephritis in allografted kidneys. *Clin Nephrol* 7:47, 1977.

55. Case records of the Massachusetts General Hospital. *N Engl J Med* 294:1108, 1976.

56. Mathew TH, Mathews DC, Hobbs JB, et al: Glomerular lesions after renal transplantation. *Am J Med* 59:177, 1975.

57. Ettenger RB, Heuser ET, Malekzadeh MH, et al: Focal glomerulosclerosis in renal allografts. *Am J Dis Child* 131:1347, 1977.

58. Mathew TH, Kincaid-Smith P, Vikraman P: Role of vesicoureteric reflux in the transplanted kidneys. *N Engl J Med* 297:414, 1977.

5
Focal Glomerulonephritis

Focal glomerulonephritis is a morphologic term for irregular glomerular proliferation, which may be produced by a variety of diseases. Descriptively, the term indicates lesions in only some of the glomeruli in the biopsy specimen (focal), these lesions frequently involving only a portion of each involved glomerulus (segmental). As a primary diagnosis, focal glomerulonephritis is about as useful to the physician as an unqualified designation of anemia. The popularity of the term arose from early morphologic studies on autopsy material, in which the more obvious focal glomerular lesions, such as crescents, were emphasized at the expense of more subtle diffuse changes. This emphasis was maintained in the early phase of renal biopsy diagnosis, before immunofluorescence and electron microscopy became routine. Experience with these techniques has clearly demonstrated that the vast majority of apparently focal diseases are, in fact, merely the irregular expressions of more diffuse glomerular injury.

Recognition of the dichotomy between the focal light microscopic expression of a disease and its diffuse pathogenesis has produced a minor crisis in nomenclature. Pathologists have become uncertain whether they should adhere to conventional histopathologic criteria or rather strive to establish etiologic diagnoses and ignore the light microscopic changes. Several considerations indicate that a compromise between these extremes is appropriate. First, careful examination of a significant number of apparently focal disorders by light microscopy discloses clear evidence of diffuse glomerular disease. Second, experience in other areas of surgical pathology has shown that close attention to morphologic parameters, in conjunction with clinical investigation, frequently leads to the identification of significant clinicopathologic syndromes. Finally, light microscopic patterns of glomerular reaction may well express the response of the host to the injurious stimulus, and codification of the reaction patterns to apparently identical stimuli may provide, as in systemic lupus, crude guidelines for therapy and prognosis.

The essential approach to a biopsy specimen showing focal and/or segmental changes is, therefore, to establish the presence or absence of diffuse disease. In some biopsy specimens only immunofluorescence or electron microscopy will establish the diagnosis. Frequently, however, careful light microscopic examination will disclose deposits, diffuse mesangial proliferation, or other changes. By these means, specific clinicopathologic diagnoses can be made for most patients whose biopsies show irregular glomerular disease (Table 5-1). Inevitably, there

Table 5–1. Differential Diagnosis of Focal Glomerulonephritis

	Light Microscopy[a]	Immunofluorescence	Electron Microscopy	Other
Anti-GBM glomerulonephritis	FS	Linear IgG	—	± Pulmonary hemorrhage
IgA nephropathy	M and FS or FS	Mesangial IgA, C3, etc.	Mesangial deposits	± Synpharyngitic hematuria
Henoch-Schönlein glomerulonephritis	M and FS or FS	Mesangial IgA, C3, etc.	Mesangial deposits	Skin rash ± arthritis, abdominal pain
Lupus glomerulonephritis	M and FS or FS	Various glomerular and TBM patterns	Various deposits, tubulovesicular bodies	± Systemic syndrome, antinuclear factor, etc.
Hereditary glomerulonephritis	FS or M and FS		Splitting GBM	± Family history, etc.
Bacterial endocarditis	M and FS or FS	Various patterns	Various deposits	Cardiac disease
Resolving postinfectious glomerulonephritis	M and FS	Mesangial ± capillary wall C3	Mesangial ± capillary wall deposits	Recent acute nephritis
Hypertension (alterative glomerulitis)	FS	Negative	—	Vascular changes
Vasculitis	FS	Negative	—	± Systemic disease
Wegener's granulomatosis	FS	Negative	—	Pulmonary and upper respiratory tract disease
Idiopathic focal glomerulonephritis	FS	Negative	—	

[a] M = mesangial proliferation; FS = focal and/or segmental proliferation.

remains a minority of cases that cannot presently be allocated to a particular syndrome. Continued clinicopathologic examination of these cases will almost certainly identify new syndromes but, at present, little is known about their pathogenesis and behavior. The possibility of systemic vasculitis must always be considered when apparently idiopathic focal glomerulonephritis is discovered, and this subject, like the other entities mentioned in Table 5-1, is discussed elsewhere in this book (see Chapter 12).

IDIOPATHIC FOCAL GLOMERULONEPHRITIS

Most published studies of focal glomerulonephritis describe its occurrence in association with isolated or recurrent hematuria (1–4). Indeed, the term *focal nephritis* was for many years used almost routinely by physicians to describe this clinical manifestation (5,6). Few of these studies provide sufficient immunofluorescence or ultrastructural data for retrospective evaluation, but it is probably significant that no similar reports have appeared since IgA antisera have been widely used. Indeed, two substantial studies specifically state that focal glomerulonephritis is either absent (7) or invariably associated with mesangial disease (8) in patients with this syndrome. Careful ultrastructural studies of the biopsy specimens from these patients sometimes reveal irregular changes that may be indicative of focal disease, but light microscopic evidence of focal glomerulonephritis is, in our experience, extremely rare.

Occasional examples of focal glomerulonephritis, without ultrastructural or immunofluorescent deposits, are encountered in patients with the nephrotic syndrome (9) and in elderly patients with either an acute systemic illness or severe nephritic features (10) (Fig. 5-1). In each of these situations, the glomeruli show irregular areas of intracapillary proliferation, frequently with areas of necrosis and scattered crescents (Figs. 5-2–5-4). The pathogenesis in each of these clinical situations is unknown, but renal expression of a systemic vasculitis (see Chapter 12) is a strong possibility, and the lesions usually respond rapidly to corticosteroid therapy or removal of associated infection.

SUMMARY

Focal glomerulonephritis is a morphologic lesion, not a diagnosis. In almost all cases in which biopsy specimens show irregular inflammatory involvement of glomeruli, a specific diagnosis will be possible with careful study by light, electron, or immunofluorescence microscopy. The irregularity of glomerular reaction in the face of apparently diffuse injurious stimuli is not understood, but may provide an index of the host response to these stimuli. The pathologist provides the physician with little useful diagnostic information by making an unqualified

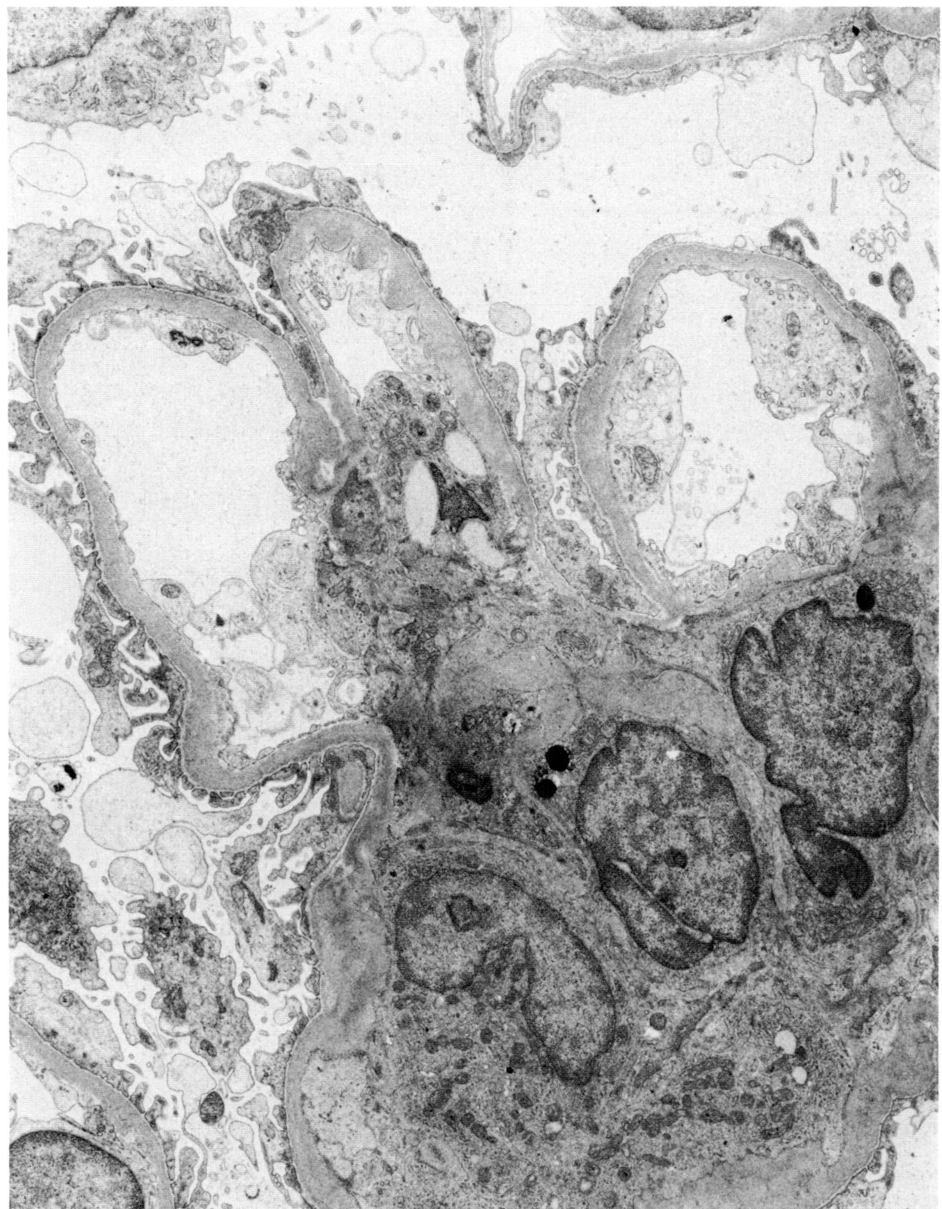

Figure 5-1. Electron micrograph from a biopsy specimen of a patient with idiopathic focal glomerulonephritis. There is mesangial hypercellularity and focal foot process obliteration. Prominent subendothelial irregularities are present in the middle loop. No significant glomerular lesions were seen by light microscopy (×6,700).

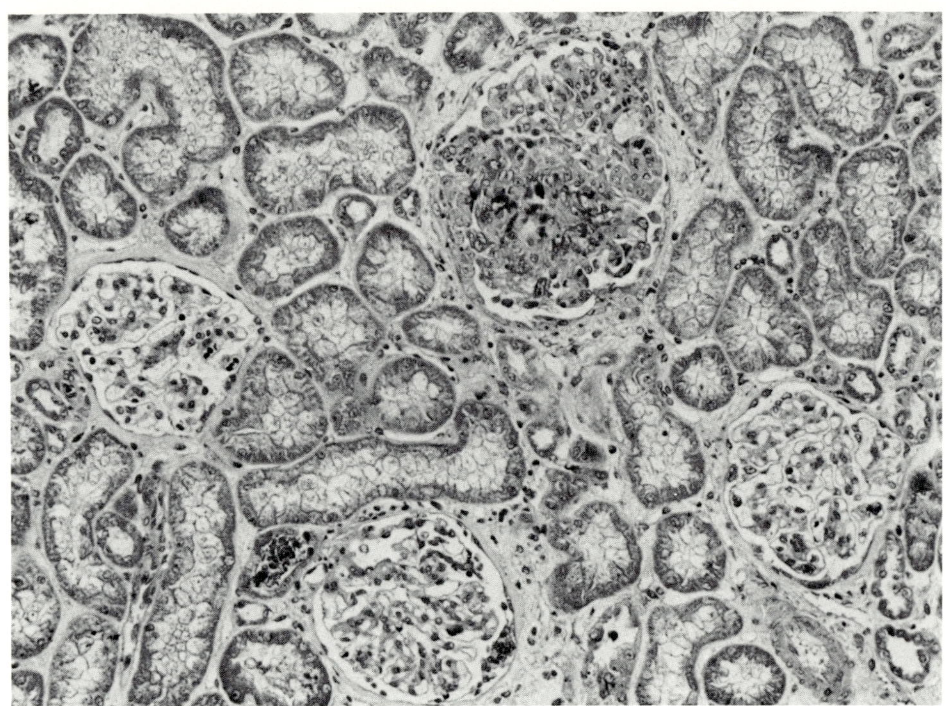

Figure 5-2. Renal biopsy specimen from a patient with idiopathic focal glomerulonephritis showing intra- and extracapillary lesions in one of four glomeruli (H&E stain, ×180).

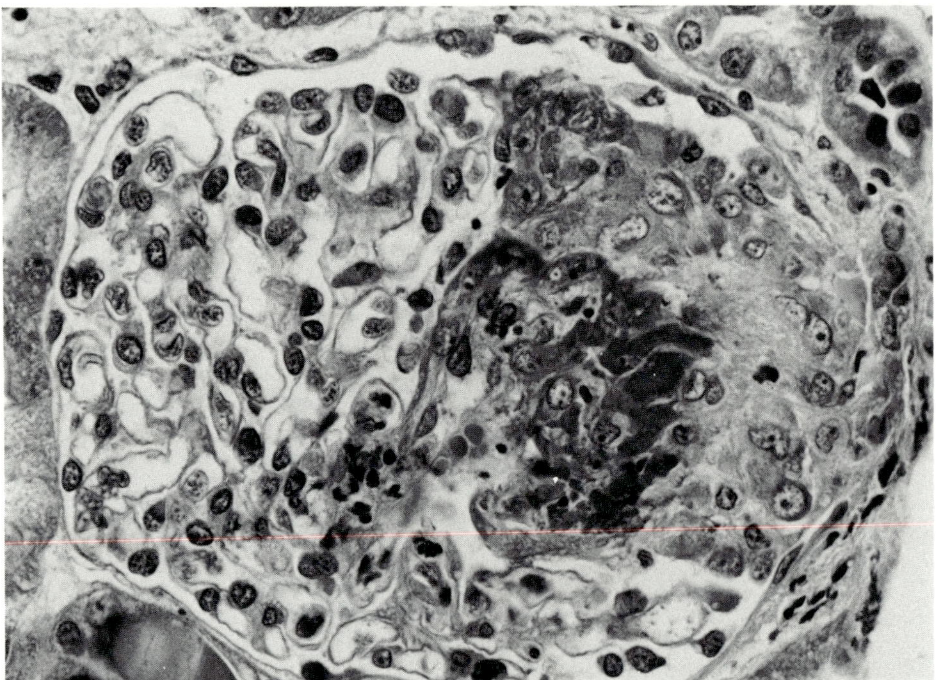

Figure 5-3. Higher magnification of another glomerulus of the same biopsy specimen as Figure 5-2, demonstrating localized area of segmental proliferation with necrosis adherent to Bowman's capsule (H&E stain, ×640).

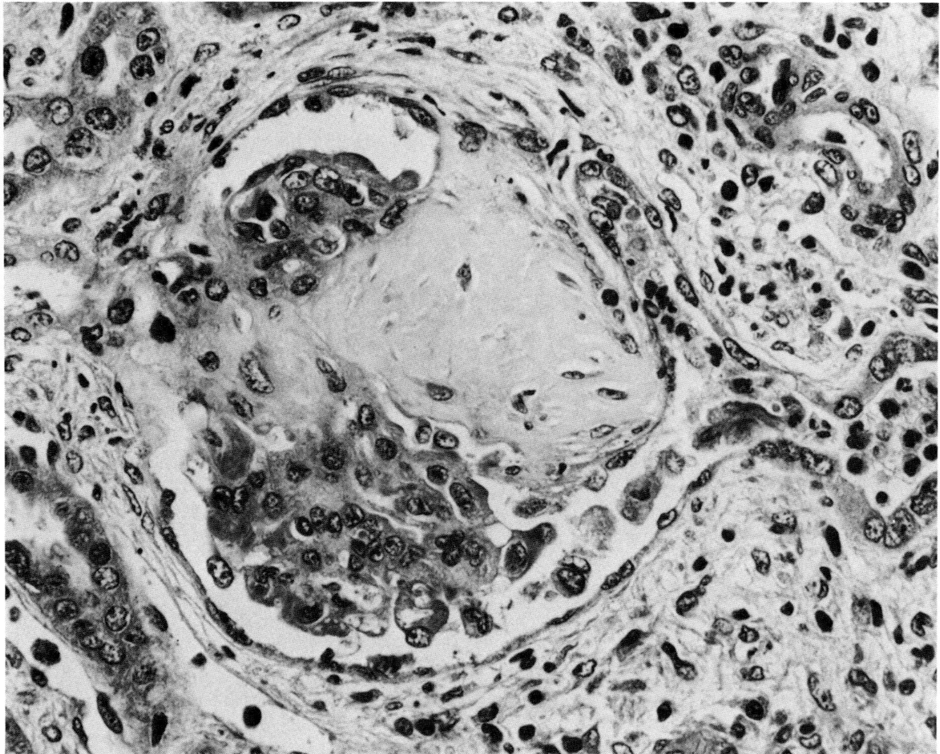

Figure 5-4. Biopsy specimen from the same patient as Figure 5-3 six months later, showing a healed segmental lesion (H&E stain, ×480).

diagnosis of focal glomerulonephritis, and strenuous efforts are recommended to allocate biopsy specimens showing this pattern to specific clinicopathologic groupings.

REFERENCES

1. Bates RB, Jennings RB, Earle DP: Acute nephritis related to group A hemolytic streptococcus infection. *Am J Med* 23:510, 1957.

2. Alexander F, Lannigan R, Bull R: Clinical, light, and electron microscopy findings in idiopathic hematuria. *J Clin Pathol* 26:750, 1973.

3. Singer DB, Hill LL, Rosenberg HS, et al: Recurrent hematuria in childhood. *N Engl J Med* 279:7, 1968.

4. Bodian M, Black JA, Kobayashi N, et al: Recurrent hematuria in childhood. *Quart J Med* 34:359, 1965.

5. Baehr G: Benign and curable form of hemorrhagic nephritis. *JAMA* 86:1001, 1926.

6. Ellis A: Natural history of Bright's disease: clinical, histological and experimental observations. *Lancet* 1:1, 1942.

7. Glasgow EF, Moncrieff MW, White RHR: Symptomless hematuria in childhood. *Br Med J* 2:687, 1970.

8. Sinniah R, Pwee HS, Lim CH: Glomerular lesions in asymptomatic microscopic hematuria discovered on routine medical examination. *Clin Nephrol* 5:216, 1976.

9. Heptinstall RH, Joekes AM: Focal glomerulonephritis: a study based on renal biopsies. *Quart J Med* 28:329, 1959.

10. Beaufils M, Morel-Maroger L, Srear JD, et al: Acute renal failure of glomerular origin during visceral abscesses. *N Engl J Med* 295:185, 1976.

6
Mesangial Proliferative Glomerulonephritis

Diffuse mesangial proliferation is the sole or predominant abnormality in a significant number of renal biopsy specimens. Until recently, this appearance was either attributed to previous poststreptococcal glomerulonephritis or, apparently, ignored. Appreciation of the significance of mesangial disease was precipitated by the recognition of mesangiopathic immunofluorescence patterns (1) and by the demonstration of prognostic differences between nephrotic children with mesangial proliferative and other forms of glomerular disease (2). In focusing attention on the mesangium by disparate techniques, these observations created problems of nomenclature that have not yet been fully resolved. First, the light microscopic expressions of mesangiopathic immunofluorescent disease tend to be spotty and were previously designated as focal glomerulonephritis. Second, the light microscopic pattern of mesangial proliferation occurs in a number of conditions with established designations, and conflicts have arisen over the choice of morphologic, immunopathologic, or clinical criteria as determinants of nomenclature. This chapter concentrates particularly on those diseases that are characterized by mesangiopathic immunofluorescence and frequently show mesangial proliferation by light microscopy.

The recognition of mesangial proliferation requires experience and good quality sections. Perhaps because of the variety of insults to which the mesangium is subjected, there is a wide range of "normal" mesangial volume, the upper limit to this range varying among different observers. Careful quantitative studies have demonstrated increased mesangial volume in a number of diseases, but these techniques are impracticable for routine application. The most satisfactory criterion for the diagnosis of mesangial proliferation is probably the presence of three or more nuclei per mesangial area (3). Diagnosis is straightforward in biopsy specimens showing diffuse mesangial proliferation but may be complicated by either irregular distribution of this proliferation or by the superimposition of true segmental lesions. The mesangial proliferative diseases are peculiarly prone to such segmental changes, and there is little doubt that the results of many biopsies previously categorized as focal and segmental glomerulonephritis would now be included in the mesangial category. By emphasizing the mesangial changes in this way, there is, of course, a danger that the mesangiopathic and mesangial proliferation diseases may become "wastebaskets" of heterogeneous and disparate conditions. Only by concentrating on basic patterns of reaction, however, can the pathologist begin to dissect discrete clinicopathologic groups from apparently amorphous morphologic conditions.

PATHOGENESIS

The mesangium is the major focus of glomerular reaction to a wide variety of stimuli (4). The mesangial cells are critically situated in intimate relationship with both capillary lumina and the juxtaglomerular apparatus. Circulating macromolecular substances are held up by the glomerular basement membrane and move along the subendothelial space to the mesangium, where they can be either phagocytosed or transported to the distal tubule (5). Mesangial cells, therefore, act as the glomerular representatives of the reticuloendothelial system, although they are of different origin (6). The mesangial accumulation of macromolecular substances is enhanced by alterations of glomerular permeability produced in animals by either aminonucleoside or nephrotoxic serum (7). The frequency of mesangial changes in human glomerulonephritis is, therefore, not surprising, even if the nature of the damaging effects is not always known.

The most cogent studies of mesangial function have examined the deposition of immune complexes. In experimental animals, the primary determinant of the site of immune complex deposition is the size of the complex (1). Small complexes (300,000−500,000 daltons) deposit along capillary walls while larger complexes (1×10^6 daltons) accumulate in the mesangium. The pattern of glomerular reaction is, however, related more to the site of complex deposition than to size, since the acute diffuse glomerulonephritis caused by capillary wall deposition is altered to a mesangial proliferative pattern when small complexes are redirected to the mesangium by corticosteroid administration. As in the human diseases, experimental mesangial proliferative glomerulonephritis caused by immune complex deposition is frequently complicated by segmental lesions. This mixed pattern has been attributed to spillage of complexes onto capillary walls after mesangial capacity is overloaded. Thus, a continuous low burden of large immune complexes might evoke a "pure" mesangial proliferative pattern, while either an intermittently or constantly higher burden could be expected to evoke superadded segmental disease. Large mesangial complexes of this type are produced by formation in antibody excess or, possibly, by the participation of IgM immunoglobulins (1). An alternative mechanism for the production of immune complex mesangial proliferation glomerulonephritis is the reaction of antigens previously deposited in the mesangium with circulating antibodies to form complexes in situ (8).

Most studies of human mesangial disease have concentrated on the mechanisms of IgA deposition. Circulating immune complexes and cryoglobulins have been demonstrated in a number of the conditions associated with IgA deposits, suggesting analogy with the experimental models of immune complex mesangial disease (9−11). In many of these conditions, the serum concentrations of IgA are often increased, but the causes for this increase are unknown and the mesangial deposits do not appear to represent either aggregated IgA alone or reaction with fixed mesangial antigen. The frequent correlation of respiratory infections and renal disease suggests reaction of infectious antigens with preformed IgA antibody to form antibody excess complexes. Showers of such complexes could exacerbate underlying mesangial disease to produce acute damage and episodes of macroscopic hematuria. The clinicopathologic differences between IgA nephropathy and the Henoch-Schönlein syndrome could represent differences in the method of antigen presentation or in immune complex load rather than basically distinct pathogenetic pathways.

The relationship of mesangial IgA disease and mucosal infection is supported by the excessive frequency of this form of nephritis in patients with cirrhosis (11). In this situation, gut-derived antigens or complexes could reach the circulation in excessive quantities by either deficient hepatic reticuloendothelial activity or portal-systemic shunts. Similarly, the occurrence of transitory IgA nephropathy in association with untreated celiac disease suggests that defects in mucosal integrity could predispose to unrestricted entry of antigens from the gut (11a). While the precise mechanism of the IgA mesangial diseases are, therefore, unknown, there is good evidence that they are expressions of immune complex disease. The complexes are likely to be formed of IgA antibody and antigens entering via mucosae in various sites although, with few exceptions (12), the IgA secretory component can be demonstrated in neither the serum nor the deposits (13). The varying clinical manifestations of the IgA mesangial diseases could result from differences in antigen presentation or from either hereditary or acquired abnormalities of antibody formation.

GLOMERULONEPHRITIS WITH MESANGIAL IgA

Immunofluorescent reactions for IgA are relatively common in a variety of glomerular diseases (14,15). Usually, these are relatively minor components of more typical reactions with other immunoglobulins. Berger's description (16) of diffuse mesangial IgA was used to categorize a syndrome of benign recurrent hematuria occurring in young men. As Berger noted, however, the syndrome is neither benign nor restricted by a hematuric presentation. Subsequent studies of patients with this immunofluorescence in their biopsies have disclosed a number of subgroups, and it is likely that further subdivisions will be created. At present the major clinical associations with mesangial IgA reactions are the Henoch-Schönlein syndrome, cirrhotic glomerulonephritis, some cases of lupus glomerulonephritis, and the cases of apparently isolated disease described by Berger.

IgA NEPHROPATHY (BERGER'S DISEASE)

Incidence and Clinical Manifestations

IgA nephropathy is very common in France (16,17), Singapore (3), and Australia (15), but occurs less frequently in Britain (18), Holland (19), and North America (20–22). In areas of high incidence, 18–22% of patients with apparently primary glomerulonephritis show diffuse mesangial IgA, whereas elsewhere the incidence is only 2–5%. The disease occurs at all ages, but is most common in the second and third decades, and affects males up to five times more frequently than females (14,17). Familial disease is rare, and an association with the HLA-Bw 35 has been claimed by some workers but has not been substantiated by other studies, including our own (23,23a,23b). Serum concentrations of polymeric IgA are persistently increased in approximately half the patients, but complement studies are usually normal (13,14). Circulating immune complexes have been demonstrated in a small proportion of patients but may be found more frequently if assays with specific IgA endpoints can be developed (9).

The most characteristic clinical manifestation of IgA nephropathy is with macroscopic hematuria, often recurrent, which usually follows an episode of pharyngitis and may be associated with fever and loin pain (14). The hematuric syndrome is typically closely associated with the pharyngitis ("synpharyngitic") rather than delayed for one to two weeks as in postinfectious glomerulonephritis. In a minority of patients, the onset is with an acute nephritic episode, clinically distinguishable from poststreptococcal glomerulonephritis only by the close association of the nephritis and pharyngitis. Between hematuric episodes, there is usually persistent proteinuria and microscopic hematuria, but the sediment may return to normal. A significant number of patients are referred for the investigation of proteinuria, usually associated with microscopic hematuria, and occasionally, the proteinuria may be sufficient to cause the nephrotic syndrome (14,17). Hypertension is common in patients with IgA nephropathy, and a few patients may first have malignant hypertension or chronic renal failure. There is an unexplained tendency for patients with the disease to develop acute renal failure, from a variety of causes, and a biopsy specimen taken during an acute azotemic episode may be the first indication of IgA nephropathy.

Pathologic Characteristics

Light Microscopy
The glomeruli in IgA nephropathy may appear normal but usually show varying degrees of mesangial proliferation and sclerosis (Figs 6-1, 6-2). Careful examination of mesangial areas often reveals small hyaline nodules protruding toward Bowman's space. The mesangial proliferative changes are least prominent in children (25) and tend to increase in severity with prolonged disease. Irregularity in the distribution of mesangial proliferation may produce an apparent segmental pattern, and true segmental lesions occur in approximately two-thirds of the cases (15) (Fig. 6-3). These lesions may be intense and necrotizing, with fibrin exudation, disruption of loops, and crescents, or they may be sclerotic. Sclerotic lesions appear as either segmental masses of excessive membrane, indicating previous proliferation, or areas of capillary collapse and hyalinosis (24,25) (Fig. 6-4). These hyalinotic areas are indistinguishable from the pattern of focal glomerulosclerosis occurring in the nephrotic syndrome. In some biopsy specimens, the segmental lesions are predominant and mesangial disease may be minimal, but careful examination usually discloses some areas of mesangial proliferation or deposit. Rarely, varying degrees of mesangial interposition are seen in individual glomeruli, especially adjacent to segmental lesions, but diffuse mesangiocapillary glomerulonephritis has not been reported with isolated IgA nephropathy. In adults, areas of tubulointerstitial scarring are common. Arterio-

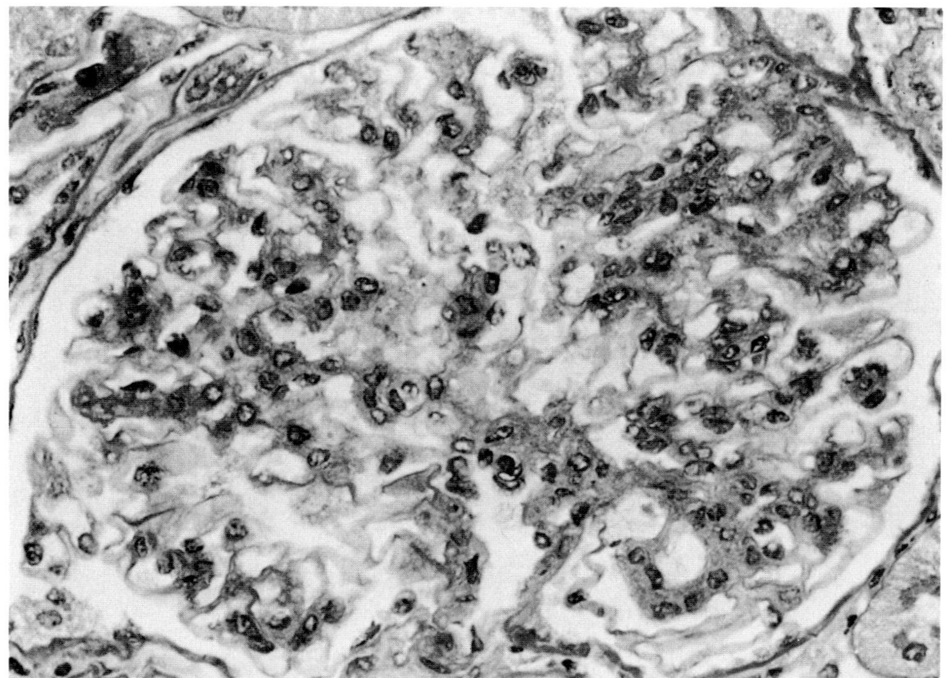

Figure 6-1. IgA nephropathy. There is diffuse mesangial hypercellularity and adhesion to Bowman's capsule (H&E stain, ×550).

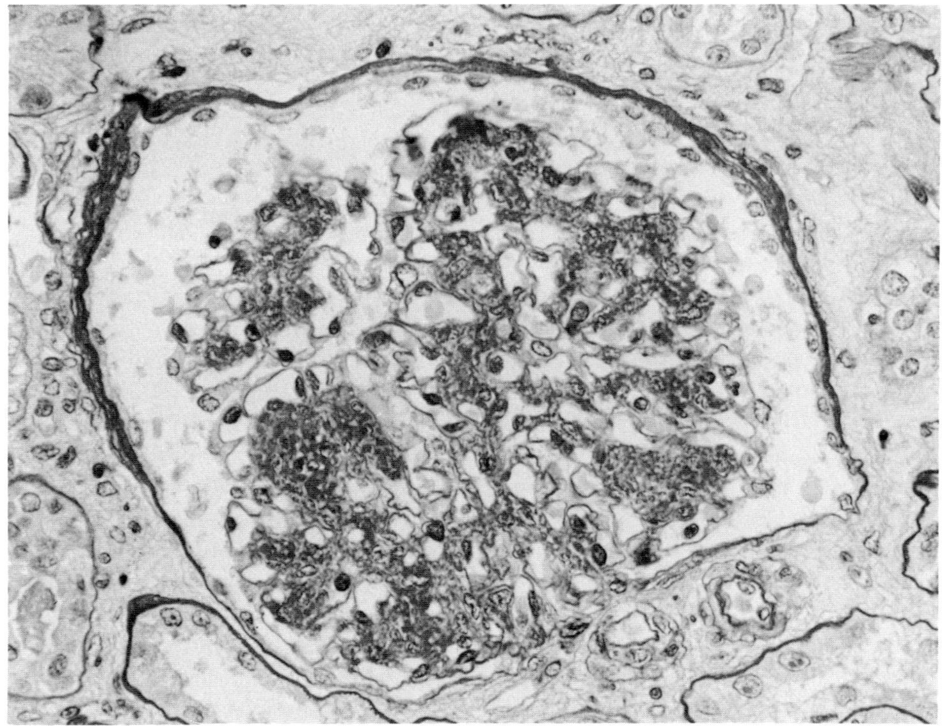

Figure 6-2. IgA nephropathy. Diffuse mesangial enlargement with accumulation of hyaline material indicating mesangial deposits (H&E stain, ×480).

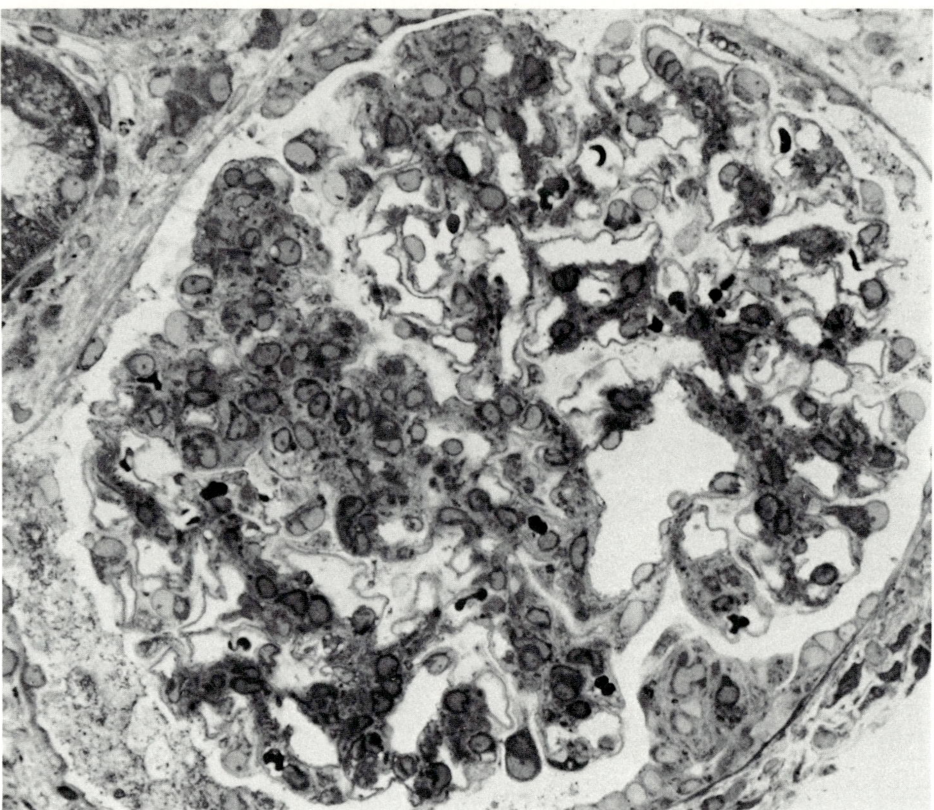

Figure 6-3. IgA nephropathy. Mesangial proliferation with segmental accentuation (plastic embedded toluidine blue stain, ×750).

lar hyalinosis, correlating poorly with hypertension, is present in a high proportion of cases and often has a nodular pattern.

Immunofluorescence Microscopy
The IgA reactions occur either as confluent masses or as discrete granules and outline the mesangia in a pattern resembling a deciduous tree in winter (Fig. 6-5). While these reactions are typically diffuse, individual mesangial areas and even occasional glomeruli may be spared. Extension of the reactions onto capillary walls is frequent and is roughly correlated with the severity of segmental disease (Fig. 6-6). The staining pattern for IgA is followed by immunoglobulins G and M in many, but not all, biopsy specimens, although these reactions are usually of lesser intensity. Fibrin is present in the mesangium in about half the cases and may also be seen in crescents. In the majority of biopsy specimens, C3 is distributed in a similar pattern to IgA, often with extension into arterioles in parallel with light microscopic hyalinosis (Fig. 6-7). The early acting complement components are, however, invariably absent, indicating, in conjunction with the presence of properdin (26), complement activation by the alternate pathway (27). IgA deposits can also be demonstrated in the superficial dermal capillaries, supporting a systemic immune complex disease (28).

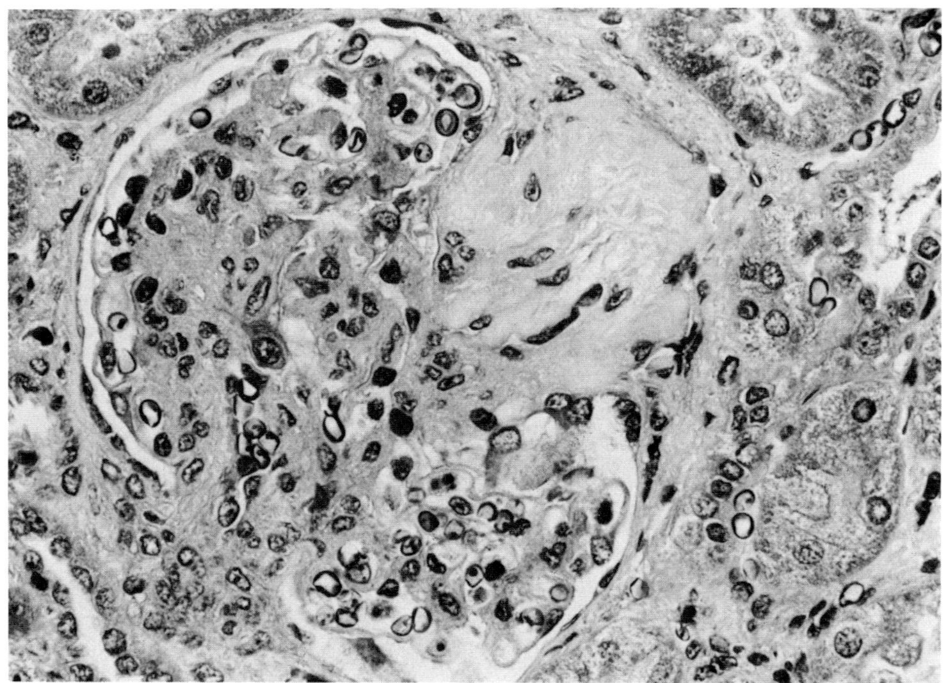

Figure 6-4. IgA nephropathy. Mesangial hypercellularity and segmental sclerosis adherent to Bowman's capsule, indicating healed segmental necrosis (H&E stain, ×500).

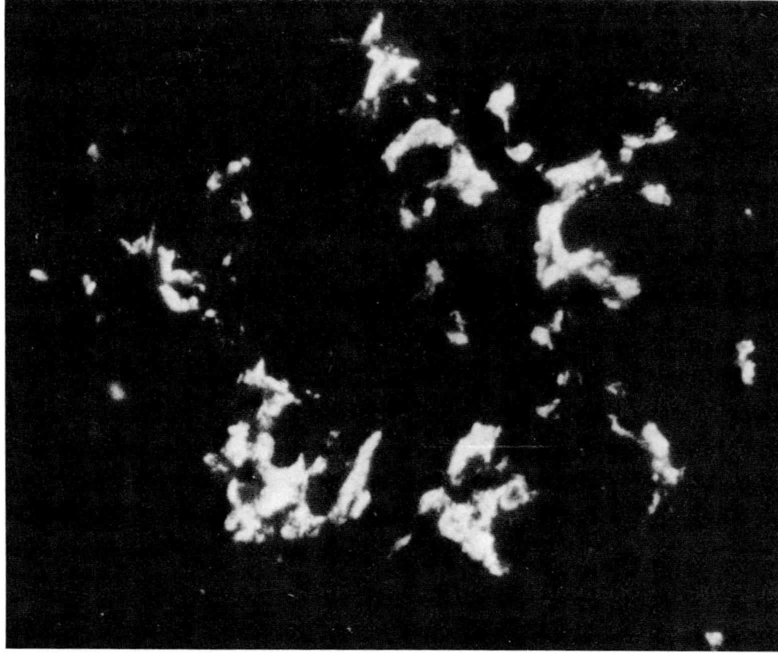

Figure 6-5. IgA nephropathy. The deposits are essentially confined to the mesangium (antihuman IgA, ×450).

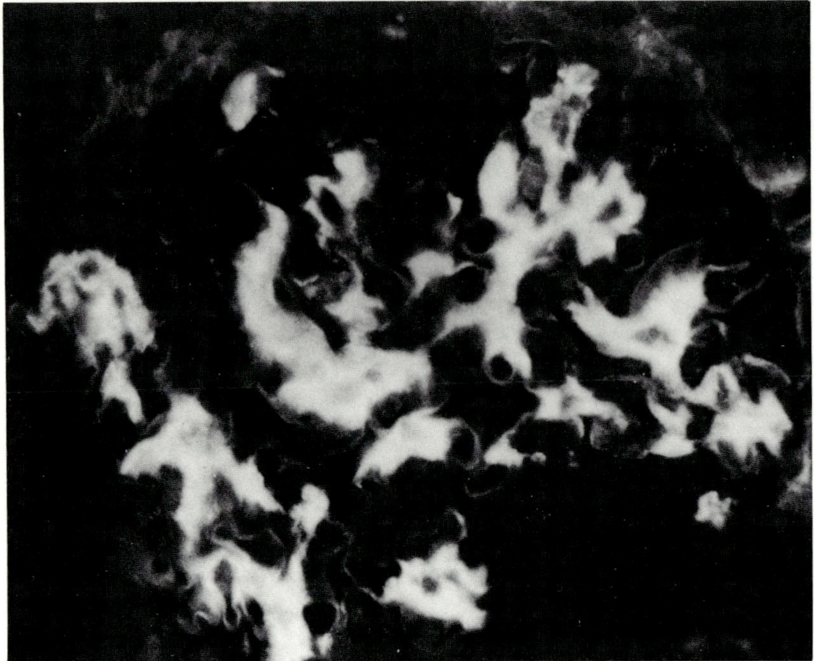

Figure 6-6. IgA nephropathy. Large clumps of fluorescent deposits involving the mesangium and continuous loops (antihuman IgA, ×500).

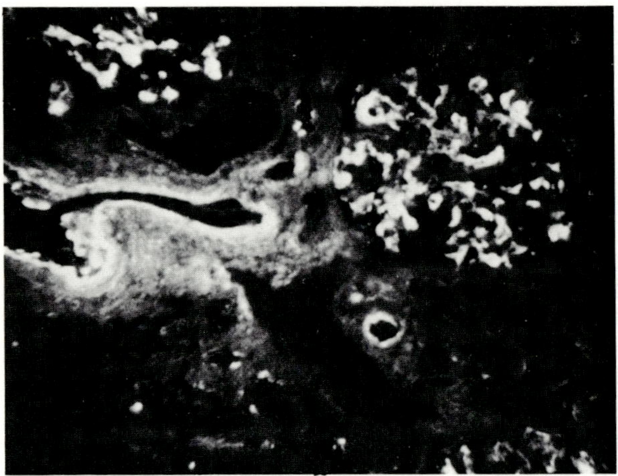

Figure 6-7. IgA nephropathy. Fluorescent deposits of C3 involving mesangium and arteriolar walls (×130).

Electron Microscopy

The mesangia are variably enlarged by combinations of increased cytoplasm and matrix. There is progressive increase in matrix with disease duration, and the mesangia are finally composed almost entirely of matrix, which may contain frequent collagen fibers. Deposits are usually restricted to mesangia although capillary wall deposits in various locations are seen in some biopsy specimens, especially in those with extensive segmental disease (Figs. 6-8, 6-9). In those biopsy specimens with minimal mesangial sclerosis, the deposits are nodular and are located beneath the overlying basement membrane. This nodular pattern is lost with progressive mesangial sclerosis, and the deposits in more advanced disease are diffused among the matrix. There is often considerable variation in the distribution of deposit, some mesangial areas being apparently uninvolved. A characteristic, although not specific, pattern of subepithelial irregularity or etching is found in the majority of cases (14).

Natural History

The prevailing belief that IgA nephropathy is benign is not supported by long-term studies. Instead, there is accumulating evidence for relentless progression into chronic renal failure in a number of patients, especially if hypertension is not controlled. Progression appears to be more likely in patients presenting with nonhematuric manifestations (14,17,19) and is, therefore, more common in adults, since children generally present with macroscopic hematuria (24). The rapidity of progression into renal failure varies, but the average is six years (17).

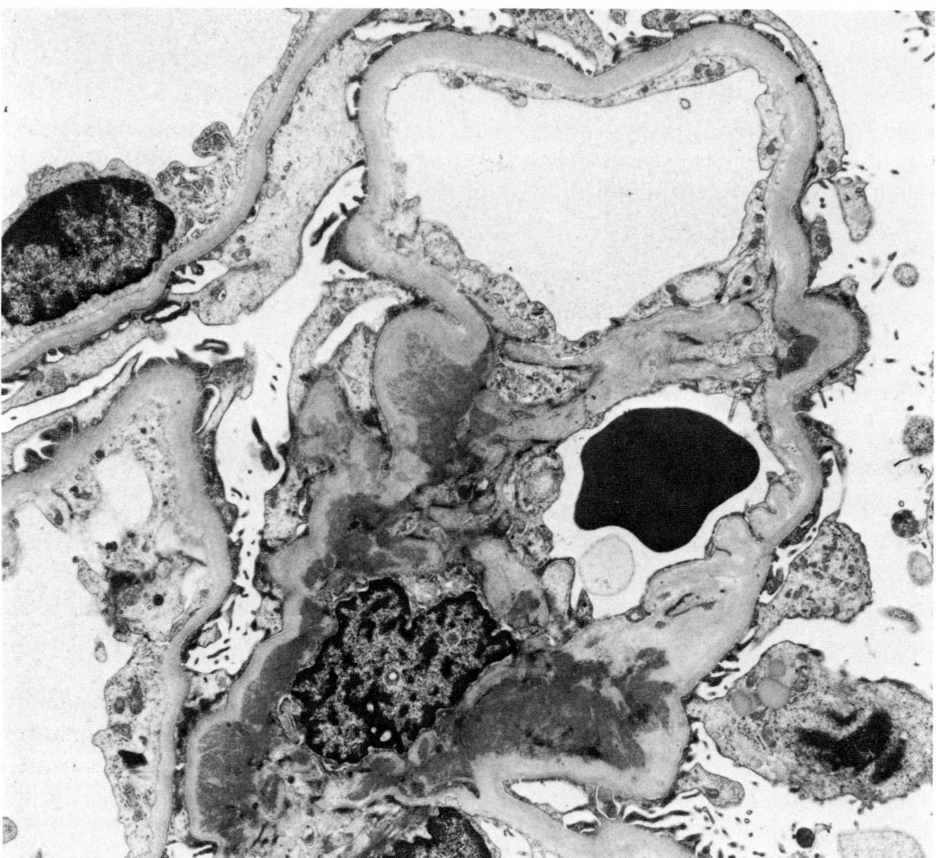

Figure 6-8. IgA nephropathy. The mesangium is enlarged by matrix and abundant deposit (×7,000).

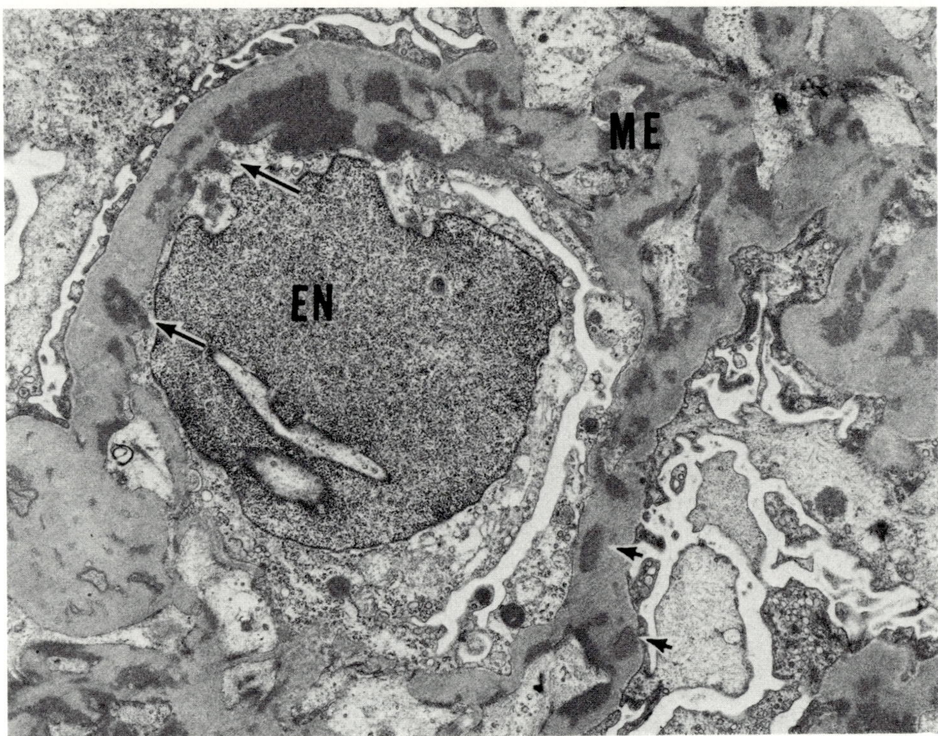

Figure 6-9. IgA nephropathy. The mesangium (ME) is enlarged by matrix and deposits, which are extending into the subendothelial area (arrows). Small deposits are also present within the basement (arrow heads). EN, endothelial cell (×9,000).

Whether a similar but less rapid tendency toward advancing renal destruction occurs in patients with hematuric presentations is not yet clear. There is no proven therapy for IgA nephropathy and transplantation remains the last resort for patients with renal failure. Recurrent mesangial IgA reactions occur in the grafts of approximately half the transplanted patients within one to four years (17,29,30). Progressive glomerular damage in affected grafts is, however, minimal and microscopic hematuria is usually the sole expression of recurrent IgA deposition.

HENOCH-SCHÖNLEIN (ANAPHYLACTOID) PURPURA (HSP)

Clinical Manifestations

The HSP syndrome affects children predominantly but also occurs occasionally in adults up to an advanced age (31–33). There is a slight male predominance, with occasional familial cases, and an increased incidence in the winter months. The syndrome often follows an upper respiratory infection but is not specifically associated with any particular organism. The clinical features are produced by a systemic vasculitis of leukocytoclastic type, which predominantly affects the skin, gut, joints, and kidneys (34). The presence of cryoglobulins (10) and circulating immune complexes in many patients with HSP suggests that this vasculitis is produced by immune complex deposition, although hypocomplementemia is unusual (32). As in IgA nephropathy, serum IgA concentrations are often raised, but these tend to return to normal with subsidence of the disease (32). The skin lesions are the most typical manifestations of the syndrome, consisting of palpable, purpuric areas distributed over the lower extremities, buttocks, and elbows. Typically these appear in crops during the acute illness and then disappear, but recurrent episodes of skin and other manifestations may continue for months or years (32).

Renal involvement is probably invariable in the HSP syndrome, but the incidence of significant renal disease is uncertain, estimates ranging from 20 to 100% of patients, depending on diagnostic criteria (35). Probably, about half of both children (36) and adults (33) develop appreciable renal damage, usually within the first month after onset, but occasionally not for months or years (31,32). The first notice of renal disease is generally macroscopic hematuria (32). There is, however, a wide range of renal manifestations, extending from microscopic hematuria to oliguric acute renal failure. Proteinuria usually accompanies the hematuria and is of sufficient severity to cause the nephrotic syndrome in some patients. The nephrotic syndrome typically is admixed with features of acute nephritis and may be associated with renal dysfunction. The severity of clinical presentation is closely correlated with the light microscopic appearances on renal biopsy and with the long-term prognosis.

Pathologic Characteristics

Light Microscopy

The principal glomerular changes of HSP are mesangial proliferation and epithelial crescents, these occurring either separately or in various combinations (Figs. 6-10–6-14). The crescents range in extent from small foci of epithelial proliferation to complete encirclement of the tuft, and the proportion of glomeruli involved by crescents, whatever their extent, is the major morphologic factor determining prognosis (32,37). The lobules underlying crescents show intracapillary swelling that may be associated with fibrin exudation, polymorph accumulation, and disruption of the capillary wall. Mesangial proliferation may be absent but can usually be detected in at least a segmental pattern, and in some biopsy specimens it is the major feature. Occasionally, proliferation is extensive and is associated with widespread mesangial interposition to produce the pattern of mesangiocapillary glomerulonephritis. In lesser affected biopsy specimens, extraglomerular changes are minimal, but interstitial inflammatory aggregates and tubular damage may be seen with severe crescentic disease (Fig. 6-13). Only very rarely is evidence of vasculitis found in renal biopsies (32). Serial renal biopsy specimens usually show diminution of both crescentic and mesangial proliferation, but mesangial changes may remain visible for some years and some patients show progressive glomerular damage (32).

Immunofluorescence Microscopy

A small number of patients with clinically typical HSP show no immunofluorescent reactions (32,38). These patients presumably are affected by a closely similar disease of different pathogenesis, and whether their prognosis differs from that of HSP is presently unknown. The vast majority of biopsy specimens, how-

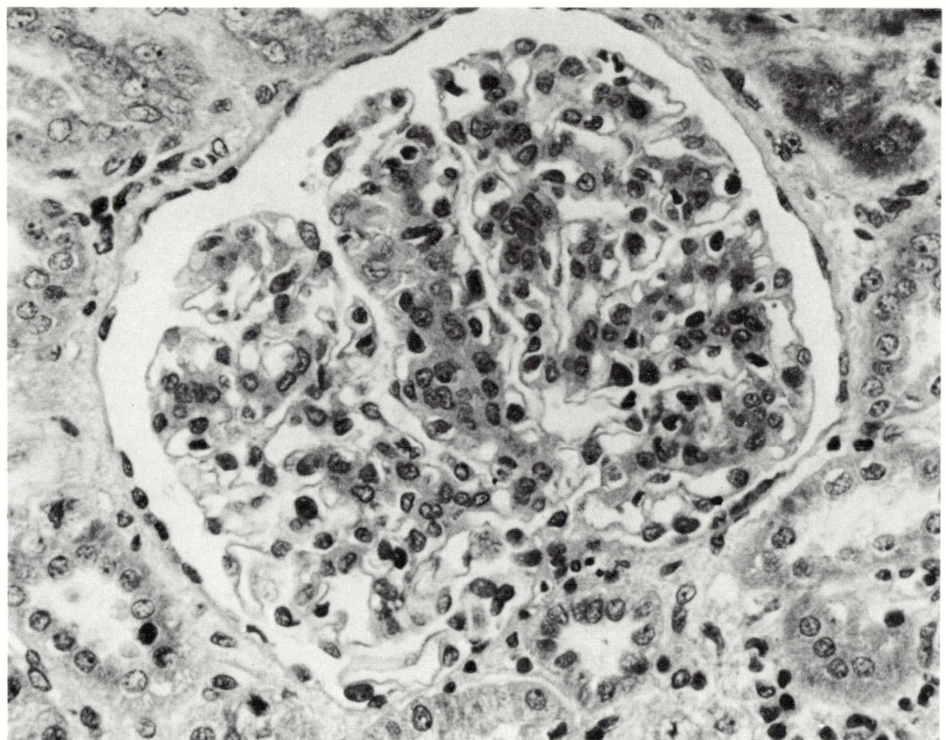

Figure 6-10. Glomerulus from a biopsy specimen of a patient with Henoch-Schönlein purpura, showing mesangial hypercellularity (H&E stain, ×550).

ever, show diffuse reactions for IgA that are predominantly mesangial, but show varying involvement of capillary walls (Fig. 6-15a). There is some correlation tween the extent of capillary wall involvement and the severity of light microscopic disease (32). Reactions for IgG, IgM, and fibrin frequently accompany those for IgA but are usually less intense. Staining for C3 is present in the majority of biopsy specimens, either in a similar distribution to that for IgA or in a distinct pattern of irregularly distributed granules (32,38) (Fig. 6-15b). As in IgA nephropathy, properdin can be demonstrated (27), and the early acting complement components are absent. Biopsies of both normal and abnormal skin show IgA reactions in dermal capillaries (28,39).

Electron Microscopy
Mesangial deposits, correlating with those seen by immunofluorescence, are distributed either through mesangial matrix or beneath the overlying basement membrane (40) (Fig. 6-16). These rarely have the nodular character seen in IgA nephropathy but, in some biopsy specimens, mesangial matrix may be increased beyond the amount expected for the duration of clinical disease. The proportion of biopsy specimens showing extramesangial deposits is uncertain but is probably quite high (38). Subendothelial extensions of the mesangial deposits are frequent and subepithelial deposits may be seen (41) (Fig. 6-17). These may resemble the pattern of membranous nephropathy, which has occasionally been associated with HSP (32), or be indistinguishable from the humps of postinfectious glomerulonephritis (38). A pattern of subepithelial etching, similar to that seen

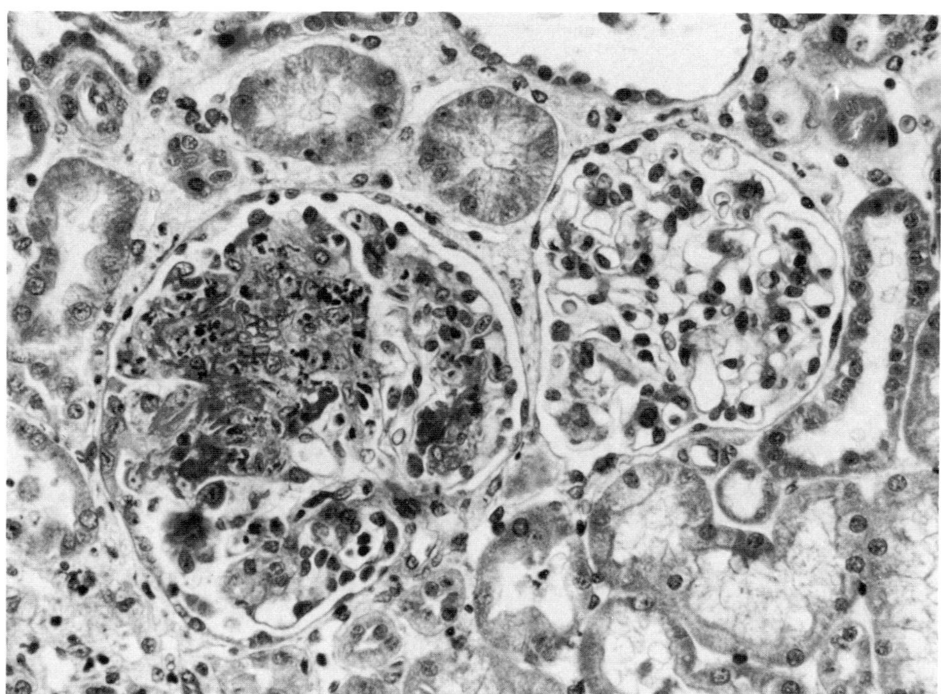

Figure 6-11. Focal necrotizing glomerulonephritis in a case of Henoch-Schönlein purpura. The glomerulus on the left shows segmental cell proliferation with inflammatory exudate and fibrin deposition with necrosis (×375).

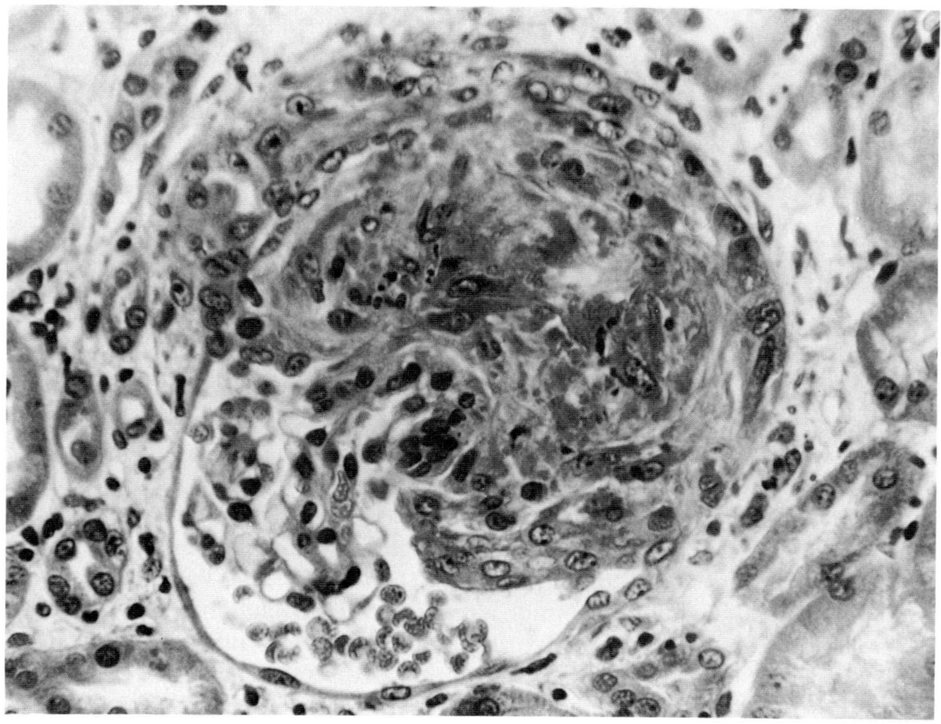

Figure 6-12. The same biopsy specimen as Figure 5-11, showing a glomerulus invaded by a large epithelial crescent (H&E, ×438).

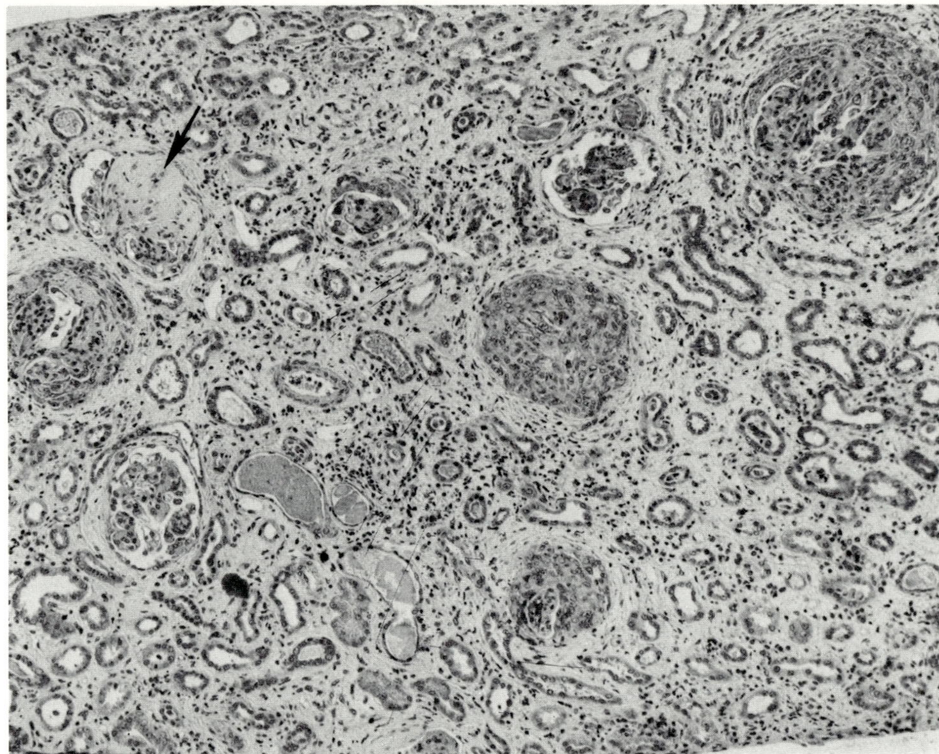

Figure 6-13. The same case as in Figure 5-11, seen two months later. In addition to the marked crescentic proliferation involving most glomeruli, there is focal segmental sclerosis (arrow) and marked tubular atrophy. The interstitium is scarred and infiltrated by moderate numbers of mononuclear inflammatory cells (H&E stain, ×120).

in IgA nephropathy, is occasionally seen, and there may be considerable basement membrane irregularity (42).

Natural History

The manifestations of renal disease decrease in intensity over a variable period and are usually stable after two years, when an assessment of the long-term prognosis can reasonably be made (35). Recrudescence of glomerulonephritis often accompanies recurrent systemic disease, but the number of recurrences does not appreciably affect prognosis (35). In a large series of patients with HSP glomerulonephritis followed for several years, 14 to 22% developed chronic renal failure (32,37), but these figures are not necessarily applicable to all patients with HSP. The severity of the initial clinical and morphologic features provide an accurate guide to the eventual prognosis (32,37). Patients with only microscopic hematuria and/or minor glomerular abnormalities on biopsy specimens seldom develop progressive disease. Conversely, those with a mixed nephritic/nephrotic presentation or with more than 50% crescentic involvement have a high risk of chronic renal failure. In an intermediate position are patients with macroscopic hematuria, in whom the severity of associated proteinuria

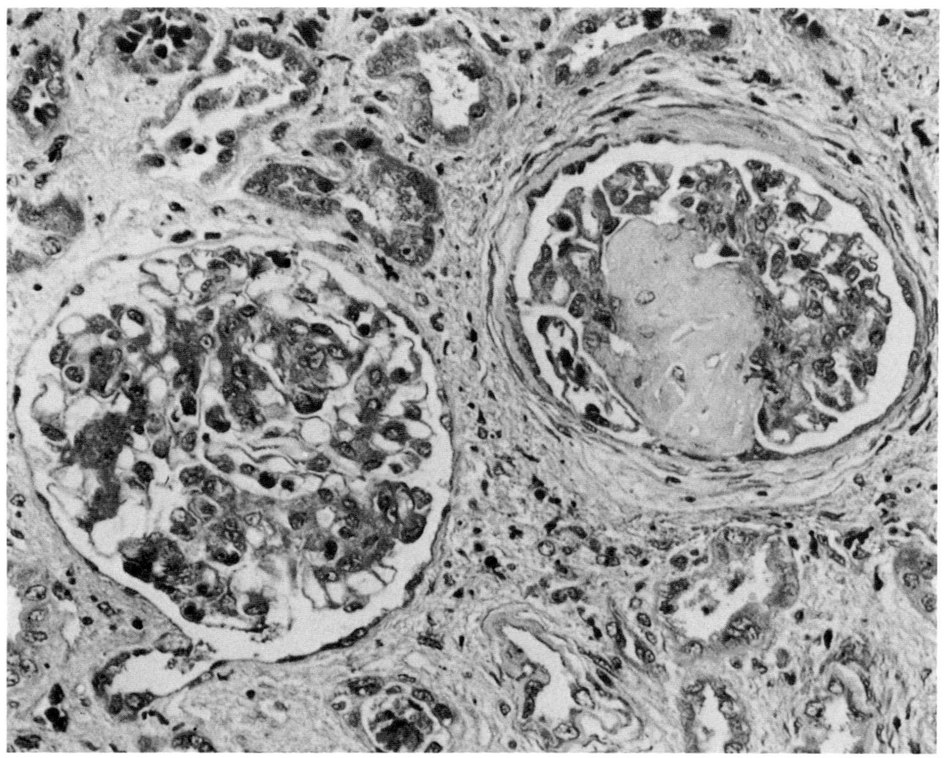

Figure 6-14. The same biopsy specimen as in Figure 6-13. One glomerulus shows segmental sclerosis, probably the result of previous necrosis, while the other has significant enlargement of the mesangium (H&E stain, ×400).

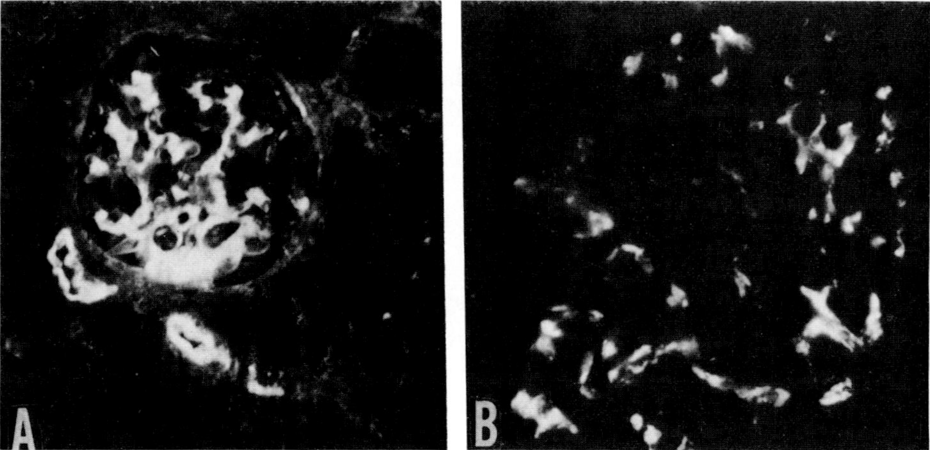

Figure 6-15. Henoch-Schönlein purpura. (*a*) Heavy mesangial deposition of IgA in the mesangium and glomerular arterioles. (*b*) Another glomerulus from the same biopsy specimen, demonstrating irregular granular mesangial deposits of C3 (*a*, ×110; *b*, ×313).

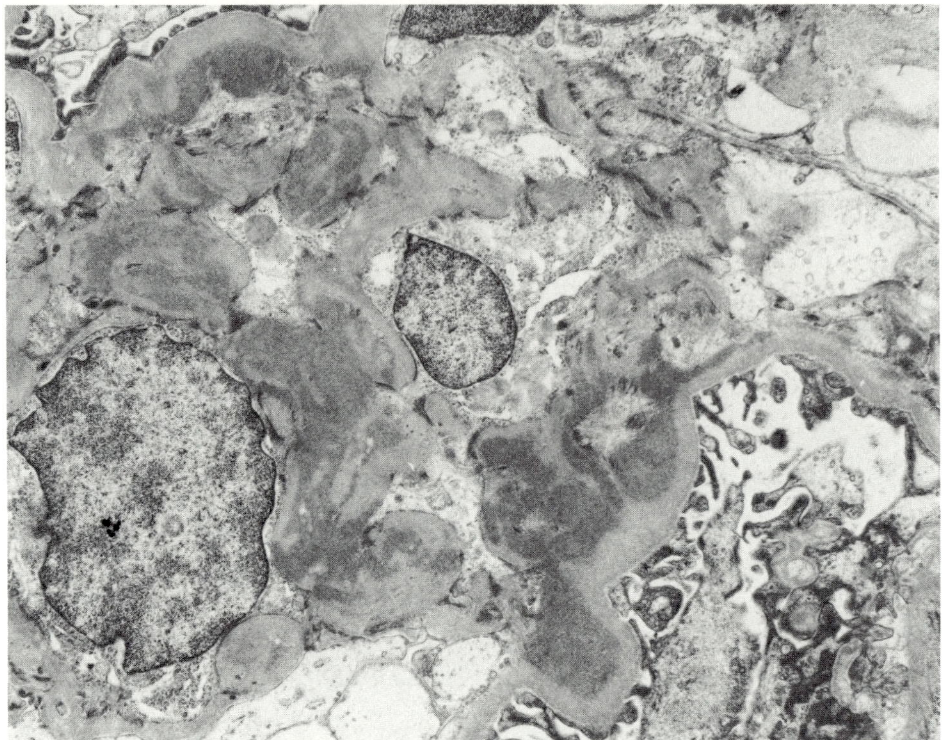

Figure 6-16. Henoch-Schönlein purpura. The mesangium is enlarged by increased in cellularity, mesangial matrix, and dense deposits (×8,100).

appears to be the major prognostic factor. Morphologically, the extent of intracapillary proliferation is not well correlated with the eventual outcome, even the mesangiocapillary pattern showing resolution in about half of those affected. Corticosteroid and immunosuppressive therapy is widely used and has been claimed to offer some protection from progression (32), although no significant differences have been shown between treated and untreated groups (35,37). Renal transplantation has occasionally been complicated by recurrent disease (41a) but has generally been successful (32), although the frequency of recurrent IgA reactions has not yet been assessed.

CIRRHOTIC GLOMERULONEPHRITIS

Although there has been prolonged debate over the glomerular changes in hepatic cirrhosis, a fairly characteristic pattern of glomerulosclerosis is now well recognized. This is characterized by glomerular enlargement with mesangial expansion, widening of the glomerular basement membrane and a characteristic pattern of irregular membrane lucency (42,43) (Figs. 6-18, 6-19). Recent prospective studies have demonstrated a high prevalence of glomerulonephritis in patients with chronic liver disease, most often related to abuse of alcohol (43,43a).

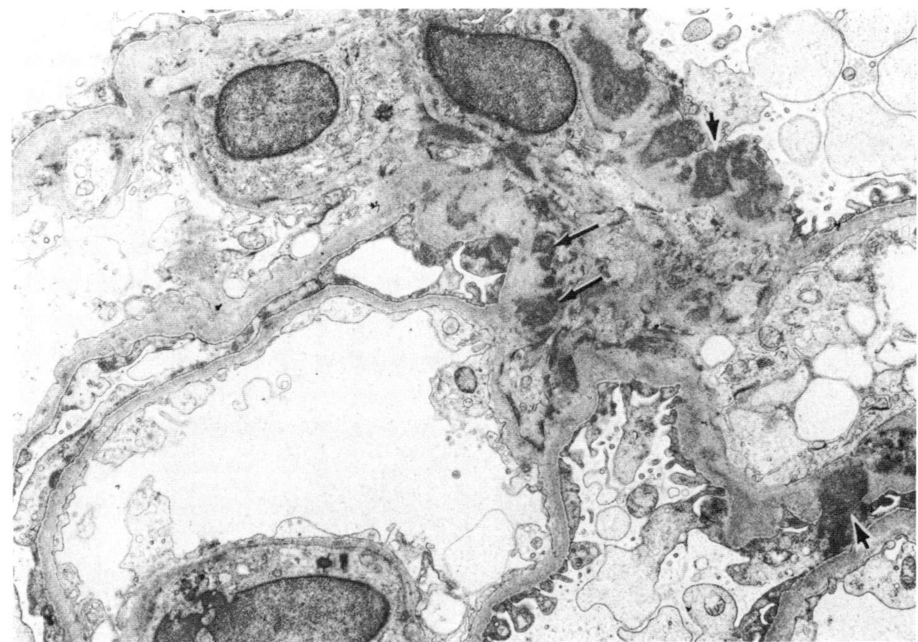

Figure 6-17. Mesangial (arrows) and subepithelial (arrow heads) deposits in a case of Henoch-Schönlein purpura. ME, mesangium (×6,600).

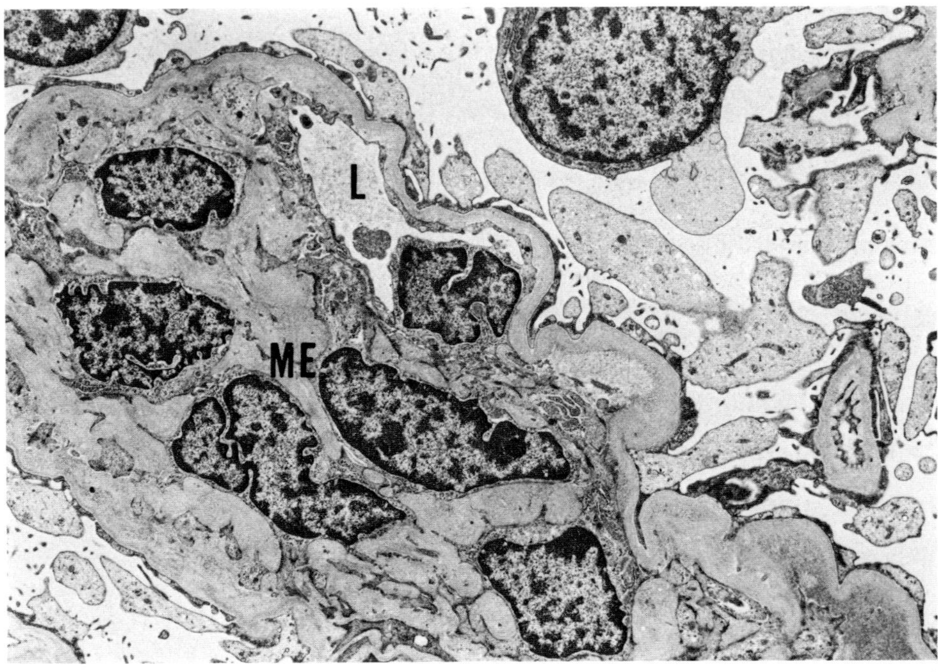

Figure 6-18. Renal biopsy specimen from a patient with cirrhosis, showing mesangial hypercellularity and mesangial dense deposits (lower right corner), which stained with antiserum from IgA. L, capillary lumen; ME, mesangium (×3,875).

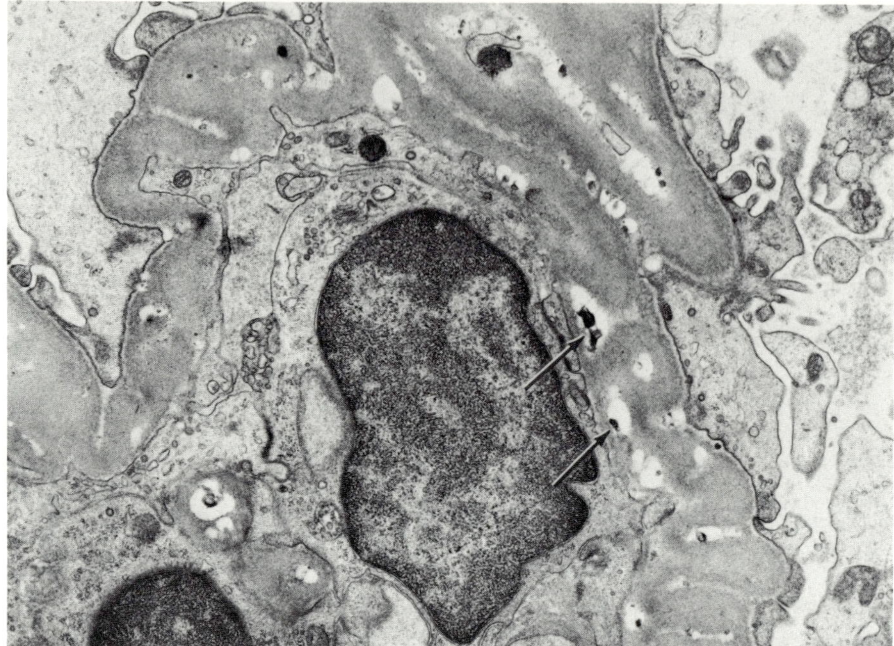

Figure 6-19. Electron micrograph of portion of a glomerulus from a patient with cirrhosis. There are irregular, lucent areas, some of which appear empty, while others contain small dark particles (arrows) (×9,500).

Glomerular changes may be present in up to three-quarters of cirrhotic patients and need not be manifest by urinary abnormalities (11). The most characteristic component of this glomerulonephritis has been the presence of mesangial IgA. Reactions for IgA may be found in glomeruli showing only glomerulosclerosis, but varying degrees of mesangial proliferation are common and may extend to the pattern of mesangiocapillary glomerulonephritis (11). As in IgA nephropathy and HSP, serum IgA concentrations are increased and IgA-containing cryoglobulins, presumably representing immune complexes, have been detected (11). The secretory component has been reported to circulate in increased concentration (12) but is not present in the glomeruli (11). Cirrhotic glomerulonephritis may be expressed as microscopic hematuria, proteinuria, or the nephrotic syndrome, and has progressed in some patients to chronic renal failure (11).

GLOMERULONEPHRITIS WITH MESANGIAL IgM

Recently, there have been several reports of mesangial proliferative glomerulonephritis occurring in association with either macroscopic hematuria (44,45) or nephrotic proteinuria (45,46). In these reports, IgM was the major immunoglobulin demonstrated by immunofluorescence, IgA was usually absent, and there were variable reactions for complement. Mesangial deposits were found by electron microscopy in some, but not all, of the biopsy specimens. The clinical features varied considerably, especially in the response of the patients with nephrotic syndrome to corticosteroid therapy, and more experience is necessary to determine whether these cases represent distinctive clinicopathologic groups.

DIFFERENTIAL DIAGNOSIS

Each of the syndromes described is characterized by typical immunofluorescence or clinical features. Differentiation between these syndromes is, therefore, usually not difficult if clinical data are considered. There are, however, cases that fall between the well-defined groups as well as a number of other conditions with similar light and immunofluorescent microscopic features. The only disease, aside from those so far discussed, in which IgA reactions are common is lupus glomerulonephritis. Generally, other immunoglobulins occur in lupus renal involvement, but occasional examples of mesangial lupus disease exhibit only IgA reactions. Confusion with the other IgA diseases is not likely since the early acting complement components are invariably present in lupus.

Mesangial proliferation is typically seen in the resolving phase of acute postinfectious glomerulonephritis, and there has almost certainly been confusion in the past between this condition and IgA nephropathy. Careful separation of the two conditions is important if valid prognostic data are to be obtained, and reports of long-term studies of postinfectious glomerulonephritis may be viewed with some suspicion if immunofluorescent data are not provided. Similarly, segmental disease identical to focal glomerulosclerosis occurs in IgA nephropathy, and these conditions may well have been confused. Mesangial proliferation is common in focal glomerulosclerosis associated with the nephrotic syndrome (47) and may also occur, in the same clinical context, in some cases of membranous nephropathy. Finally, there are sporadic cases in which no cause for mesangial proliferation can be determined. Most often, biopsies are performed in these cases for the investigation of proteinuria and/or hematuria, and immunofluorescent studies are completely negative. There is, as yet, insufficient information about the natural history of these lesions for definite comment, but the possibility that they represent the residua of IgA nephropathy after resolution of the deposits does not appear likely.

SUMMARY

Mesangial disease may be discovered by either light or immunofluorescence microscopy. Mesangial proliferative glomerulonephritis, on the one hand, may be unassociated with immunofluorescent reactions while, on the other, mesangiopathic immunofluorescence may occur with minimal mesangial change detectable by light microscopy. Nonetheless, the various diseases associated with mesangial changes probably indicate glomerular damage by broadly similar mechanisms. The mesangium is a major mechanism for the disposal of circulating macromolecular substances but may, under some circumstances, be unable to dispose of deposited materials. In these situations, which are assumed to be produced by immune complex deposition, mesangial proliferation occurs and may be accompanied by an assortment of segmental lesions. The best studied examples of this pattern of disease are those associated with IgA reactions. Whether the IgA in these apparently disparate diseases is a uniting feature indicating a common pathogenesis is not yet certain, but all are associated with mucosal abnormalities in the respiratory or gastrointestinal systems. There is considerable variation in both the morphologic patterns and clinical expressions of most of these diseases, and more intensive study will be required before definite prognostic data are available. In Henoch-Schönlein purpura, however, a series of well-defined prognostic guidelines have been isolated, these depending largely on the number of glomeruli involved by crescents.

There are many morphologic expressions of the IgA diseases, and they closely resemble a number of other conditions. Since immunofluorescence studies for IgA have been done routinely for only about 10 years, it is likely that examples of IgA nephropathy were included in reviews of other conditions with similar clinical and morphologic features. Thus, especially in those parts of the world where the IgA diseases are common, early clinicopathologic reviews of diseases associated with mesangial proliferation may now be invalid.

REFERENCES

1. Germuth FG Jr, Rodriguez E: Focal mesangiopathic glomerulonephritis: prevalence and pathogenesis. *Kidney Int* 7:216, 1975.

2. Churg J, Habib R, White RHR: Pathology of the nephrotic syndrome in children: a report for the International Study of Kidney Disease in children. *Lancet* 1:1299, 1970.

3. Sinniah R, Pwee HS, Lim CH: Glomerular lesions in asymptomatic microscopic hematuria discovered on routine medical examination. *Clin Nephrol* 5:216, 1976.

4. Vernier RL, Mauer SM, Fish AJ, et al: The mesangial cell in glomerulonephritis. *Adv Nephrol* 1:31, 1971.

5. Leiper JM, Thomson D, McDonald MK: Uptake and transport of Imposil by the glomerular mesangium in the mouse. *Lab Invest* 37:526, 1977.

6. Bradfield JWB, Catell V, Smith J: The mesangial cell in glomerulonephritis: II. Mesangial proliferation caused by habu snake venom in the rat. *Lab Invest* 36:487, 1977.

7. Mauer SM, Fish AJ, Day NK, et al: The glomerular mesangium: II. Studies of macromolecular uptake in nephrotoxic nephritis in rats. *J Clin Invest* 53:531, 1974.

8. Mauer SM, Sutherland DER, Howard RJ, et al: The glomerular mesangium: III. Acute immune mesangial injury: a new model of glomerulonephritis. *J Exp Med* 137:553, 1973.

9. Woodroffe AJ, Foldes M, McKenzie PE, et al: Serum immune complexes and disease. *Aust NZ J Med* 9:129, 1979.

10. Garcia-Fuentes M, Chantler C, Williams DG: Cryoglobulinemia in Henoch-Schönlein purpura. *Br Med J* 2:163, 1977.

11. Berger RJ, Yaneva H, Nabarra B: Glomerular changes in patients with cirrhosis of the liver. *Adv Nephrol* 7:3, 1978.

11a. Katz A, Dyck RF, Bear RA: Celiac disease associated with immune complex glomerulonephritis. *Clin Nephrol* 11:39, 1979.

12. André F, André C: Cirrhotic glomerulonephritis and secretory immunoglobulin A. *Lancet* 1:197, 1976.

13. Witworth JA, Liebowitz S, Kennedy MC, et al: IgA and glomerular disease. *Clin Nephrol* 5:33, 1975.

14. Clarkson AR, Seymour AE, Thompson AJ, et al: IgA nephropathy: a syndrome of uniform morphology, diverse clinical features and uncertain prognosis. *Clin Nephrol* 8:459, 1977.

15. Hyman LR, Wagnild JP, Beirne GJ, et al: Immunoglobulin-A distribution in glomerular disease: analysis of immunofluorescence localization and pathogenetic significance. *Kidney Int* 3:397, 1973.

16. Berger J: IgA glomerular deposits in renal disease. *Transplant Proc* 1:939, 1969.

17. Droz D: Natural history of primary glomerulonephritis with mesangial deposits of IgA. *Contr Nephrol* 2:150, 1976.

18. Sissons JGP, Woodrow DR, Curtis JR, et al: Isolated glomerulonephritis with mesangial IgA deposits. *Br Med J* 2:611, 1975.

19. Van Der Peet J, Arisz L, Brentjens JRH, et al: The clinical course of IgA nephropathy in adults. *Clin Nephrol* 8:335, 1977.

20. Zimmerman SW, Burkholder PM: Immunoglobulin A nephropathy. *Arch Intern Med* 135:1217, 1975.

21. McCoy RC, Abramowsky CR, Tisher CC: IgA nephropathy. *Am J Pathol* 76:123, 1974.

22. Alexander F, Barabas AZ, Jack RGJ: IgA nephropathy. *Human Pathol* 8:173, 1977.

23. Sabatier JC, Genin C, Assenat H, et al: Mesangial IgA glomerulonephritis in HLA-identical brothers. *Clin Nephrol* 11:35, 1979.

23a. Brettle R, Peters DK, Batchelor JR: Mesangial IgA glomerulonephritis and HLA antigens. *N Engl J Med* 299:200, 1978.

23b. Nagy J, Hámori A, Ambrus M, et al: More on IgA glomerulonephritis and HLA antigens. *N Engl J Med* 300:92, 1979.

24. Levy M, Beaufils H, Gubler MC, et al: Idiopathic recurrent macroscopic hematuria and mesangial IgA-IgG deposits in children (Berger's disease). *Clin Nephrol* 1:63, 1973.

25. Lawler W, Williams G, Tarpey P, et al: IgA localization in glomerular diseases. *J Clin Pathol* 30:914, 1977.

26. Evans DJ, Williams DG, Peters DK, et al: Glomerular deposition of properdin in Henoch-Schönlein syndrome and focal nephritis. *Br Med J* 2:326, 1973.

27. Gotze O, Muller-Eberhard HJ: The C3 activator system: an alternate pathway of complement activation. *J Exp Med* 134:905, 1971.

28. Baarte de La Faille-Kuyper EH, Kater L, Huijten RH, et al: Occurrence of vascular IgA deposits in clinically normal skin of patients with renal disease. *Kidney Int* 9:424, 1976.

29. Berger J, Yaneva H, Nabarra B, et al: Recurrence of mesangial deposition of IgA after renal transplantation. *Kidney Int* 7:232, 1975.

30. Mathew TH, Mathews DC, Hobbs JB, et al: Glomerular lesions after renal transplantation. *Am J Med* 59:177, 1975.

31. Meadow SR, Glasgow EF, White RHR et al: Schönlein-Henoch nephritis. *Quart J Med* 41:241, 1972.

32. Levy M, Broyer M, Arsan A, et al: Anaphylactoid purpura nephritis in childhood: natural history and immunopathology. *Adv Nephrol* 6:183, 1976.

33. Bar-on H, Rosenmann E: Schönlein-Henoch syndrome in adults: a clinical and histological study of renal involvement. *Israel J Med Sci* 8:1702, 1972.

34. Sams WM, Thorne EG, Small P, et al: Leukocytoclastic vasculitis. *Arch Dermatol* 112:219, 1976.

35. Meadow SR: The prognosis of Henoch-Schönlein nephritis. *Clin Nephrol* 9:87, 1978.

36. Hurley RM, Drummond KN: Anaphylactoid purpura nephritis: clinicopathological correlations. *J Pediat* 81:904, 1972.

37. Counahan R, Winterborn MH, White RHR, et al: Prognosis of Henoch-Schönlein nephritis in children. *Br Med J* 2:11, 1977.

38. Heaton JM, Turner DR, Cameron JS: Localization of glomerular 'deposits' in Henoch-Schönlein nephritis. *Histopathol* 1:93, 1977.

39. Tsai CC, Giangiacomo J, Zuckner J: Dermal IgA deposits in Henoch-Schönlein purpura and Berger's nephritis. *Lancet* 1:342, 1975.

40. Sinniah R, Feng PH, Chem BTM: Henoch-Schönlein syndrome: a clinical and morphologic study of renal biopsies. *Clin Nephrol* 9:219, 1978.

41. Brun C, Bryld C, Fenger L, et al: Glomerular lesions in adults with the Schönlein-Henoch syndrome. *Acta Pathol Microbiol Scand (A),* 79:569, 1971.

41a. Weiss JH, Bhathena DB, Curtis JJ, et al: A possible relationship between Henoch-Schönlein syndrome and IgA nephropathy (Berger's disease): an illustrative case. *Nephron* 22:582, 1978.

42. Olsen S: Mesangial thickening and nodular glomerular sclerosis in diabetes mellitus and other diseases. *Acta Pathol Microbiol Scand (A) 80* (Suppl 233):203, 1972.

43. Callard P, Feldmann G, Prandi D, et al: Immune complex type glomerulonephritis in cirrhosis of the liver. *Am J Pathol* 80:329, 1975.

43a. Nochy D, Callard P, Bellon B, et al: Association of overt glomerulonephritis and liver disease: a study of 34 patients. *Clin Nephrol* 6:422, 1976.

44. Van De Putte LBA, De La Riviere GB, Van Breda Vreisman PJC: Recurrent or persistent hematuria: sign of mesangial immune complex deposition. *N Engl J Med* 290:1165, 1974.

45. Cohen AH, Border WA, Glassock RJ: Nephrotic syndrome with glomerular mesangial IgM deposits. *Lab Invest* 38:610, 1978.

46. Bhasin HK, Abuelo JG, Nayak R, et al: Mesangial proliferative glomerulonephritis. *Lab Invest* 39:21, 1978.

47. Waldherr R, Gubler MC, Levy M, et al: The significance of pure diffuse mesangial proliferation in idiopathic nephrotic syndrome. *Clin Nephrol* 10:171, 1978.

7
Postinfectious Glomerulonephritis

Glomerulonephritis associated with infectious agents may take many forms. There is increasing evidence that viruses are implicated in the pathogenesis of systemic lupus erythematosus, and infectious antigens have been identified in the deposits of membranous nephropathy (1,2). The best known association is, however, the acute nephritic syndrome following infection with group A streptococci. Recently, the definition of this apparently discrete disease has become blurred. Organisms other than streptococci have been implicated in its pathogenesis, and biopsy studies of patients with typical clinical features have demonstrated a variety of morphologic patterns. Furthermore, glomerulonephritis has been recognized with increasing frequency in association with persistent internal infections. Accordingly, the concept of postinfectious glomerulonephritis has broadened to include two distinct but interlinked patterns of disease: acute and transitory glomerulonephritis following superficial infection and persistent glomerular inflammation complicating prolonged deep infections. In each disease pattern, the continued activity of glomerulonephritis is dependent on the presence of infectious antigens, and removal of these antigens causes resolution of the glomerular lesions.

PATHOGENESIS

The various forms of human postinfectious glomerulonephritis closely resemble the morphologic lesions occurring in experimental serum sickness. These lesions follow either single or multiple injections of foreign, soluble protein, usually bovine serum albumin (BSA), and are produced by the deposition of circulating immune complexes (3,4).

Acute Serum Sickness

After a single injection of BSA, the serum concentration falls gradually because of equilibration and catabolism for about 10 days, when there is an abrupt decline produced by immune elimination. Elimination occurs by complexing of the BSA with circulating antibody at a critical concentration and is accompanied by hypocomplementemia, acute glomerulonephritis, vasculitis, and other inflammatory lesions. The glomerulonephritis is characterized by diffuse intracapillary swelling with polymorph infiltration and subepithelial humps. Antibody immunoglobulin and complement can be demonstrated by immunofluorescence microscopy; the antigen may be masked, although its presence can be proven by other techniques. The morphologic and immunopathologic changes are evanescent and there are no long-term sequelae. The latent period, glomerular changes, and reversibility of this model are very similar to human acute postinfectious glomerulonephritis in which circulating immune complexes are well documented (5). The particular association of this form of disease with streptococci is not yet explained, and injections of streptococci into experimental animals have not reproduced the typical glomerular changes (6). The disease in man is, however, restricted to a limited number of "nephritogenic" streptococcal serotypes, and these share antigenic characteristics with the glomerular basement membrane (3). Cross reactivity of antibodies within immune complexes could, therefore, favor localization within the glomerulus. Streptococcal antigens have only occasionally been identified in the glomerular lesions (7,8), and they are presumably masked by overlying antibody and complement as in the acute serum sickness model. Not all animals challenged with a bolus of BSA develop glomerulonephritis, probably because of differences in the rapidity and type of antibody formation, and similar differences may explain the relative rarity of acute postinfectious glomerulonephritis in man.

Chronic Serum Sickness

Repeated BSA injections produce a variety of glomerular disease patterns, the character of the glomerular lesion depending on the size of the immune complexes. Thus, differences in the type and quantity of antibody produced and in the dose of administered antigen may vary the size or antigen/antibody ratio of the complexes formed by individual animals. Generally, small complexes deposit along capillary walls and cause diffuse glomerulonephritis, while larger complexes localize in the mesangium to produce a mesangial pattern, with or without the superimposition of segmental features produced by the spillage of complexes onto capillary walls. Almost any pattern of glomerular change may be induced by varying the conditions of the model, but antigen, antibody, and complement can be demonstrated by immunofluorescence regardless of the morphologic lesion. The prolonged antigenemia occurring in this model is analogous to that occurring in chronic septicemic conditions in man. As in the experimental system, not all patients with chronic septicemic conditions can be expected to develop glomerulonephritis, since the conditions for production of phlogistic complexes depend on critical concentrations of antigen and antibody. When glomerulonephritis occurs, it is likely to have a mesangial pattern because the release of small quantities of infectious antigen tend to form large complexes in antibody excess. Infectious antigens have been demonstrated in the glomerular lesions of a variety of glomerular diseases associated with chronic infection, and eradication of these antigens from the circulation has, as expected, been followed by resolution (9,10).

ACUTE POSTINFECTIOUS GLOMERULONEPHRITIS

The acute nephritic syndrome following streptococcal infection is one of the most common renal diseases in childhood. The disease is less common in adults, in whom its manifestations and clinical course may be atypical. While the majority of patients with this clinical syndrome undoubtedly have acute postinfectious glomerulonephritis, biopsy studies show other, more ominous, glomerular lesions in a significant minority (11). Thus, the diagnosis of acute postinfectious glomerulonephritis cannot be proven by clinical criteria alone, even if rising titers of antibodies to streptococcal products can be demonstrated. Recognition of this fact is crucial to an analysis of the literature since a number of the major prognostic studies have not required typical biopsy features at onset for inclusion. That the prognosis of patients selected by clinical criteria alone should be heterogenous is, therefore, not surprising. The major controversy at present is whether patients with typical biopsy changes of acute postinfectious glomerulonephritis are prone to the later development of chronic renal disease.

Clinical Manifestations and Course

Acute glomerulonephritis typically occurs one to two weeks after infection with group A streptococci of a restricted number of "nephritogenic" serotypes. The principal serotypes implicated have been 1, 2, 12, 49, 55, 57, and 60 (12,13). Primary infection may be either of the pharynx or, especially in hot and humid environments, the skin and there may be seasonal variation in the site of precipitating infection. Cutaneous infections are usually persistent but pharyngitis is self-limiting, and the organisms may not be recoverable when nephritis occurs. Diagnosis of streptococcal infection is then dependent on the serologic evidence of a rise in titers to streptococcal products. The most commonly used tests are antistreptolysin-0 for pharyngeal infections and antihyaluronidase for pyoderma, but neither may be elevated if the original infection was treated with penicillin, and an increased titer does not prove that nephritis is related to infection (12). The frequency of glomerulonephritis after streptococcal infection probably varies in different populations but has been estimated at up to 24% in epidemic situations (14). Acute glomerulonephritis may be produced by organisms other than streptococci more commonly than is generally appreciated (15). Acceptable evidence for such an association has been reported for staphylococci, meningococci, pneumococci, mycoplasmas, and leprosy, with less certain instances complicating *Salmonella, Varicella, Toxoplasma,* mumps, and hepatitis B infections, and Guillain-Barré syndrome (16−25). A variety of other organisms have been associated with other types of glomerulonephritis (9,10).

The disease may occur at any age, although children are most commonly affected, and shows no consistent predilection for either sex. Typically, nephritis begins abruptly with oliguria, hematuria, which may be either macroscopic or a dull brownish color, and facial edema. Some degree of hypertension is usual during the acute phase, and there is proteinuria of varying degree with an active urinary sediment. There is a range of severity in each of these features so that several may be absent while one may dominate the clinical picture. Thus, in adults the initial manifestations may be the nephrotic syndrome, acute pulmonary edema or acute hypertension, while morphologically typical disease may occur in children with no overt clinical features (26,27). A morphologic picture similar to acute postinfectious glomerulonephritis has rarely been reported in transplanted kidneys (27a, 27b), but the etiology and significance of these occurrences is unclear. The acute syndrome is accompanied by profound depressions of serum C3 and properdin, the early-acting complement components usually remaining within normal limits, these changes returning to normal over three to six weeks (28). The clinical and urinary expressions of the disease are evanescent and generally disappear within one to two weeks. Both proteinuria and hematuria wane rapidly, and the majority of patients are clinically cured within a few months (27,28). An abnormal urinary sediment may, however, persist for five or more years after the acute episode, and occasional patients in this persistent group may suffer exacerbations of the disease upon reinfection with another nephritogenic organism (27,28,30).

PATHOLOGIC CHARACTERISTICS

Acute Glomerulonephritis

Light Microscopy

The glomeruli are diffusely enlarged, hypercellular, and appear bloodless, with exaggeration of the normal lobular pattern (27,31,32). The hypercellularity is caused by a variable admixture of intracapillary proliferation and granulocyte accumulation (Fig. 7-1). Thus, some biopsy specimens show massive infiltration of the glomeruli by granulocytes but only relatively minor mesangial proliferation, while others demonstrate almost total occlusion of capillary loops by cellular proliferation but only sparse granulocytes, and there are a number of intermediate patterns (Fig. 7-2). The granulocytes are usually predominantly neutrophilic, but eosinophils are prominent in some biopsy specimens. Cellular proliferation is principally mesangial, and there is generally no significant increase in matrix, although varying degrees of mesangial interposition may occur. Careful examination of capillary walls often reveals the characteristic humps (10,32,33). These are most easily recognized in sections stained with Masson trichrome or in plastic-embedded material but can often be recognized in routine H&E preparations (Fig. 7-3). While the process is diffuse, there may be some variation in the intensity of involvement between individual glomeruli and even between segments of the same glomerulus. Crescents are occasionally seen and may be diffuse, but are usually sporadic and segmental (27,32,34) (Fig. 7-4). Tubulointerstitial damage and inflammation occurs in parallel with the glomerular changes (32) (Fig. 7-4). Necrotizing arteritis has rarely been reported in association with acute postinfectious glomerulonephritis, but has apparently not been systemic, nor has it affected the prognosis (35).

Electron Microscopy

The characteristic ultrastructural feature of acute postinfectious glomerulonephritis is the subepithelial hump (Figs. 7-5, 7-6). While characteristic, however, humps are not peculiar to this disease and are always accompanied by deposits in

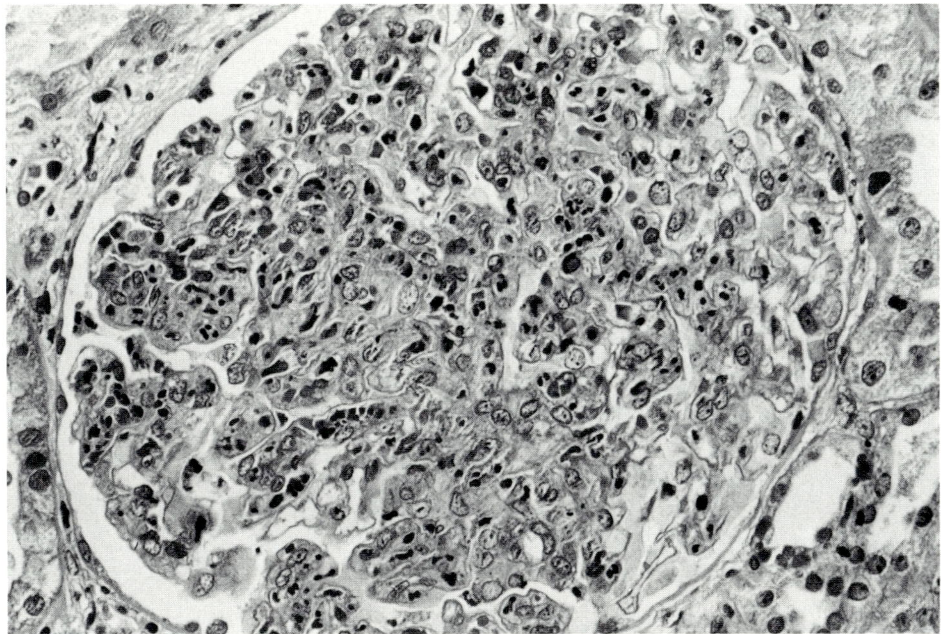

Figure 7-1. Acute poststreptococcal glomerulonephritis. The glomerular tufts are enlarged and show both proliferation and exudation (H&E stain, ×325).

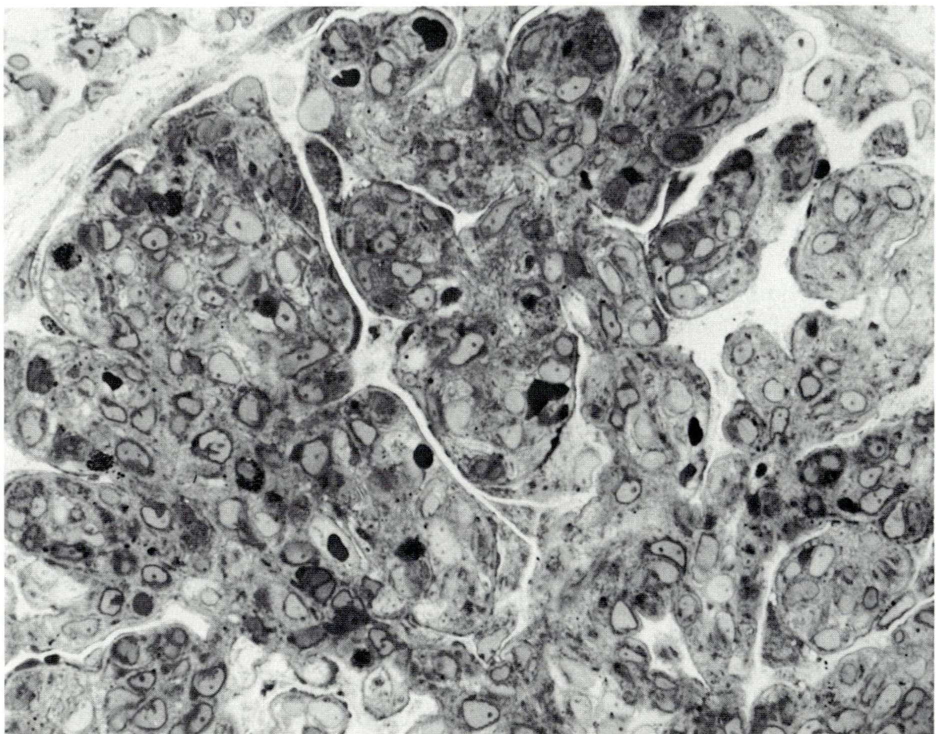

Figure 7-2. Acute poststreptococcal glomerulonephritis. Most of the capillary loops are obliterated by cell proliferation (plastic embedded toluidine blue stain, ×650).

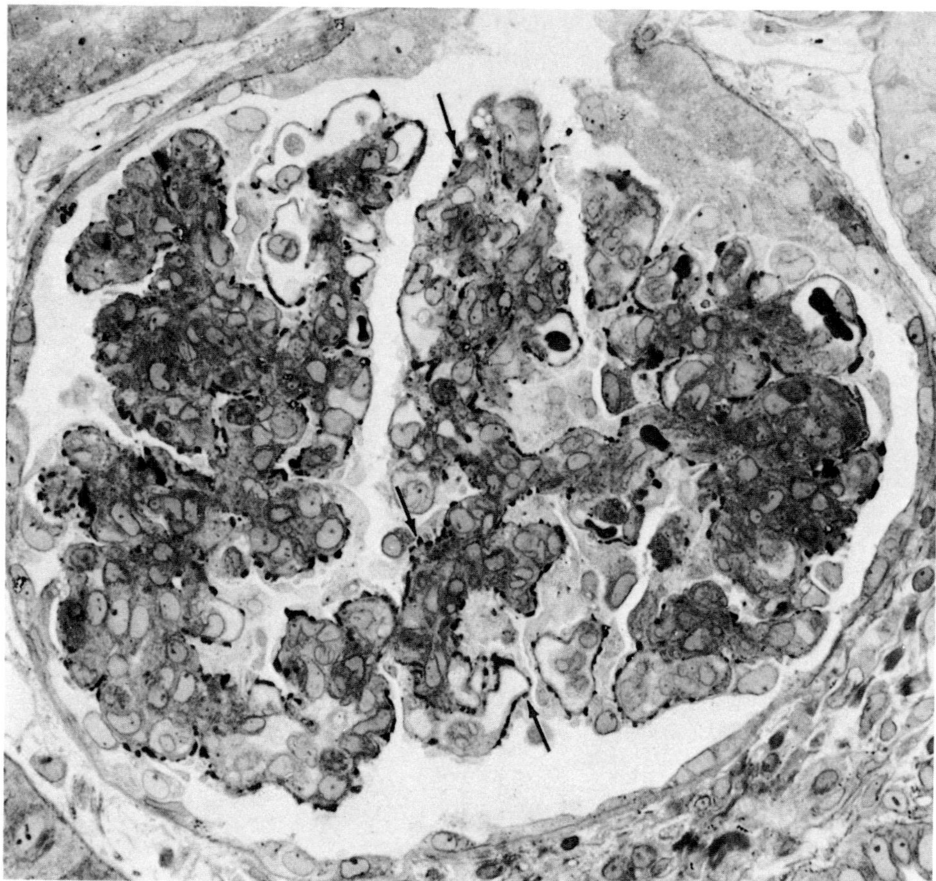

Figure 7-3. Acute poststreptococcal glomerulonephritis with numerous "humps" along the capillary walls (arrows) (plastic embedded toluidine blue stain, ×620).

other locations. Mesangial and subendothelial deposits are invariable and linear centrimembranous strips, sometimes continuous with humps, are common (32) (Figs. 7-7, 7-8). The humps are dome-shaped deposits of varying size, which are situated on the epithelial aspect of the basement membrane and are associated with obliteration of the overlying foot processes (27) (Fig. 7-9). They are often preferentially localized over mesangial regions (32), and careful examination of these areas is indicated when acute postinfectious glomerulonephritis is suspected. There is a rough correlation between the number of humps and the intensity of inflammation, although the individual deposits are not necessarily related to inflammation in the adjacent lobule (Fig. 7-10). Frequently, however, foci of endothelial ulceration with adhesion of polymorphs to the denuded basement membrane can be found beneath humps (36) (Fig. 7-11). The presence of very numerous humps, especially if they are atypical, is often correlated with unusually severe inflammation, with or without crescents, and delayed resolution (11). Within the lobules, mesangial and endothelial cells are hypertrophic and fibrin is often visible in subendothelial regions (Figs. 7-10, 7-12). Basement membrane irregularities, sometimes with actual perforation, are often seen overlying such fibrin deposits (32).

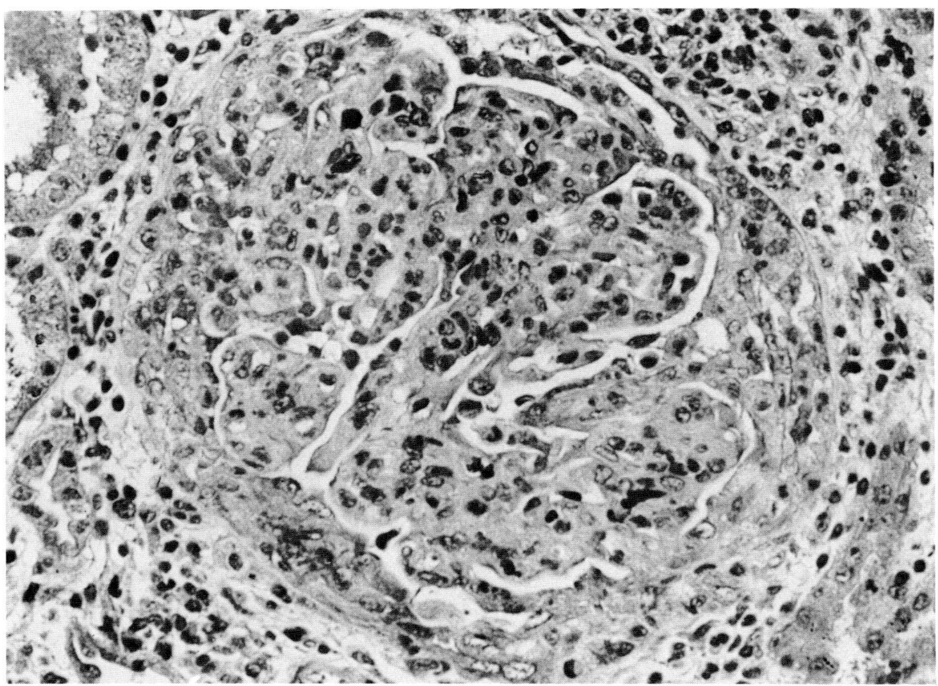

Figure 7-4. Acute postinfectious glomerulonephritis with intra- and extracapillary proliferation. The interstitium is heavily infiltrated by acute inflammatory cells (H&E stain,

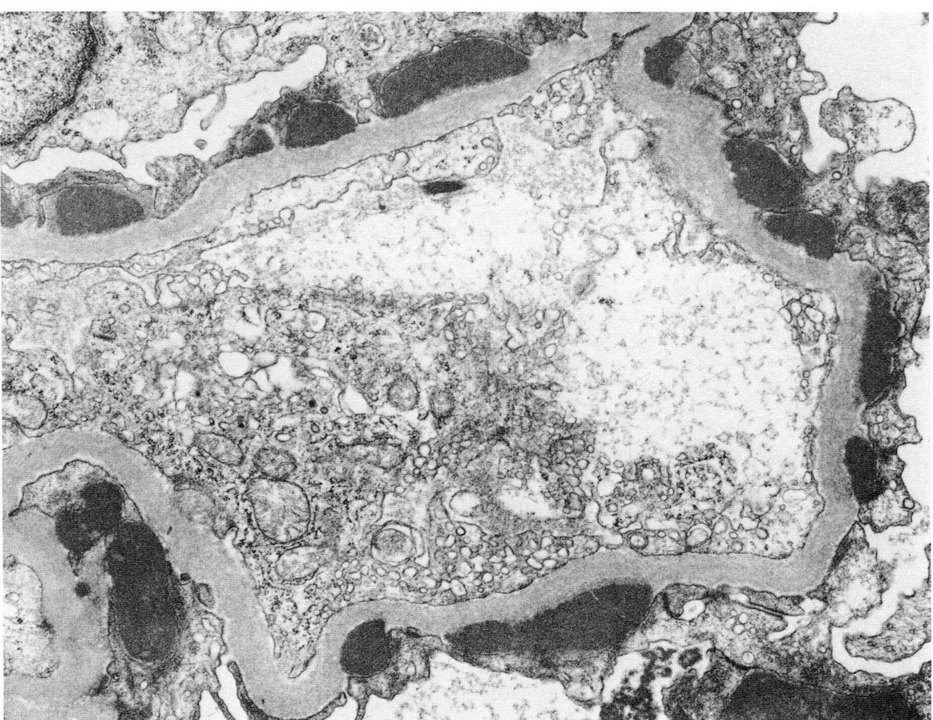

Figure 7-5. Numerous humps are present along the basement membrane. The capillary
loop is partially obstructed by hypertrophic endothelium (×12,800).

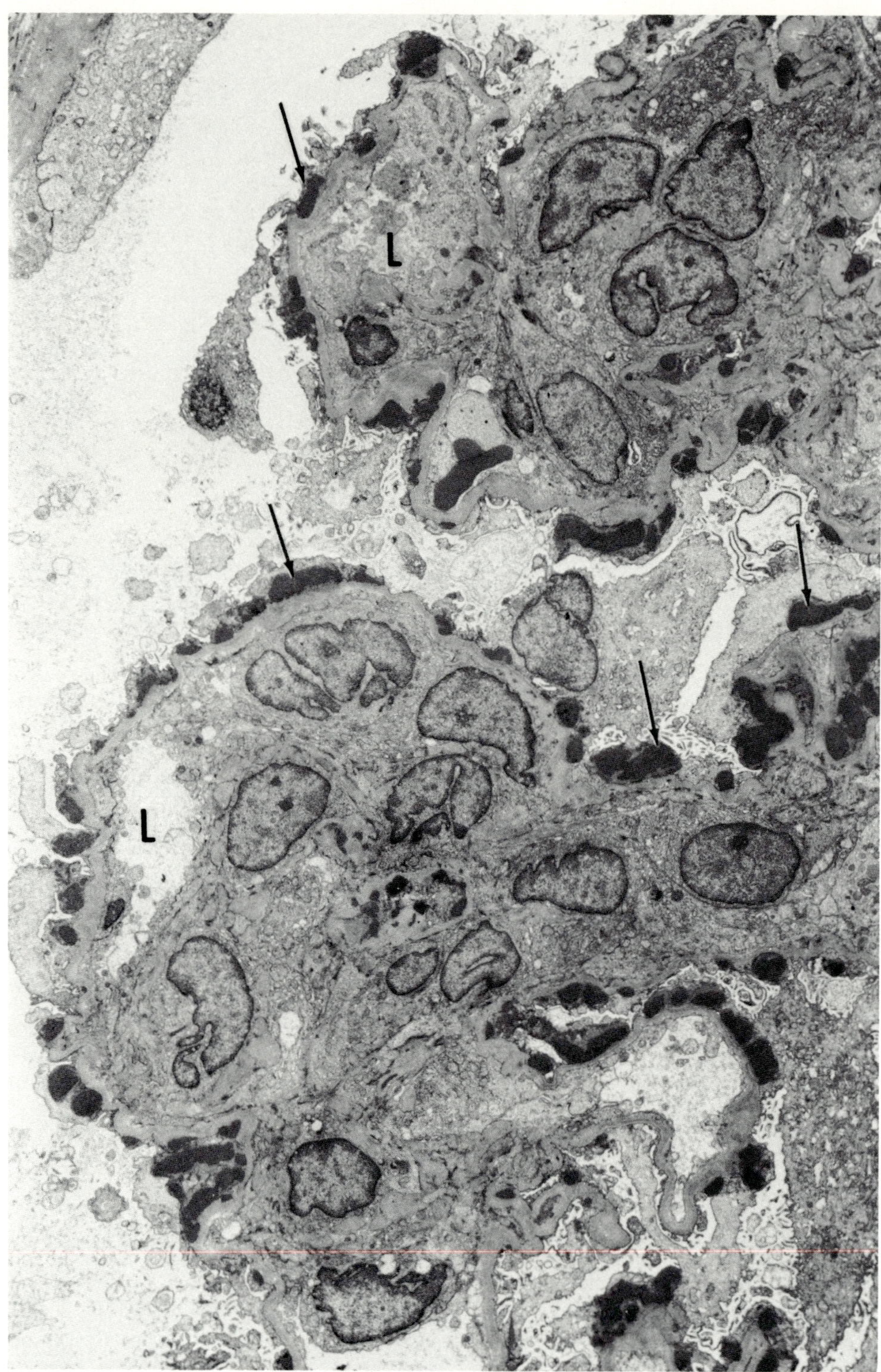

Figure 7-6. Numerous humps (arrows) and endocapillary cell proliferation with narrowing of the capillary lumen in acute poststreptococcal glomerulonephritis. Note the absence of inflammatory exudate. L, capillary lumen (×2,700).

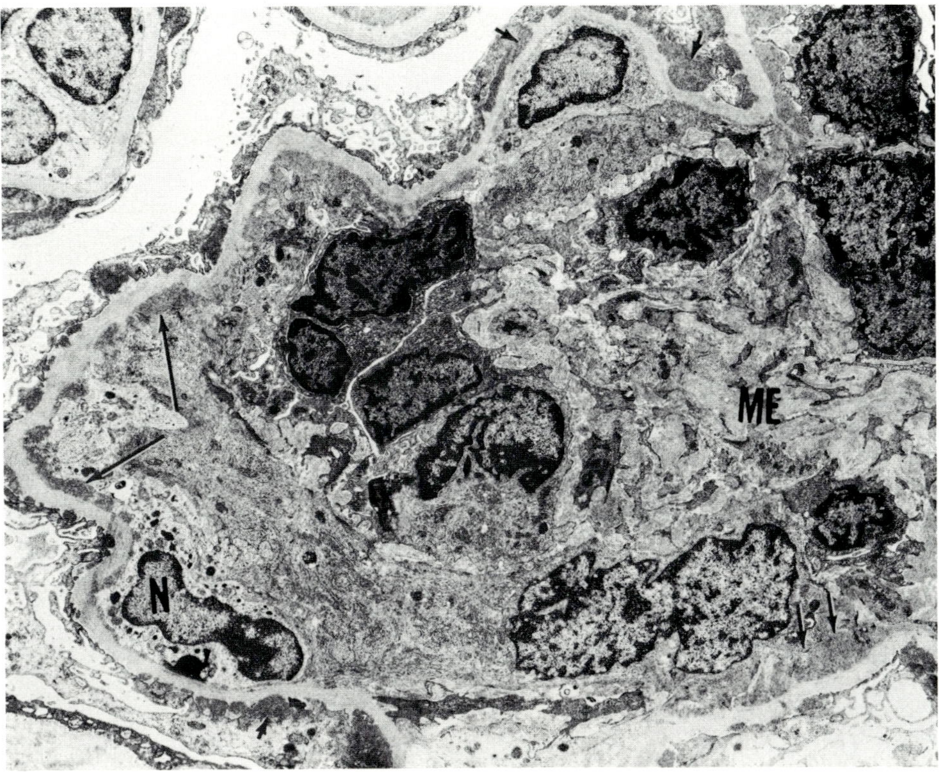

Figure 7-7. Portion of a glomerulus showing marked increase in mesangial matrix and endocapillary proliferation with large amounts of subepithelial (arrow heads), subendothelial (long arrows), and mesangial (short arrows) deposits. ME, mesangium; N, neutrophilic leukocyte (×6,200).

Immunofluorescence Microscopy

Intense, granular reactions for IgG and C3 are present along the basement membrane in locations corresponding to the humps (7,10,11,33) (Figs. 7-13, 7-14). The granules are typically coarse and irregular, often in continuity with similar reactions in adjacent arterioles. Mesangial reactions are sometimes present as well, and there may be interrupted strips of membrane reaction corresponding to the centrimembranous deposits. Reactions for IgG are most prominent in biopsy specimens taken very early in the course of the disease and may be absent later when the C3 reactions are predominant. Properdin usually accompanies the C3 reactions, but early-acting complement components are absent, and immunoglobulins other than IgG are either absent or present in only trace amounts. Fibrin may be seen in some biopsy specimens. A variety of streptococcal products have been identified in the glomeruli but appear not to be in the humps (7,8,10). One patient was reported to have developed linear reactions along tubular basement membranes during the course of acute postinfectious glomerulonephritis with an intense interstitial nephritis (37).

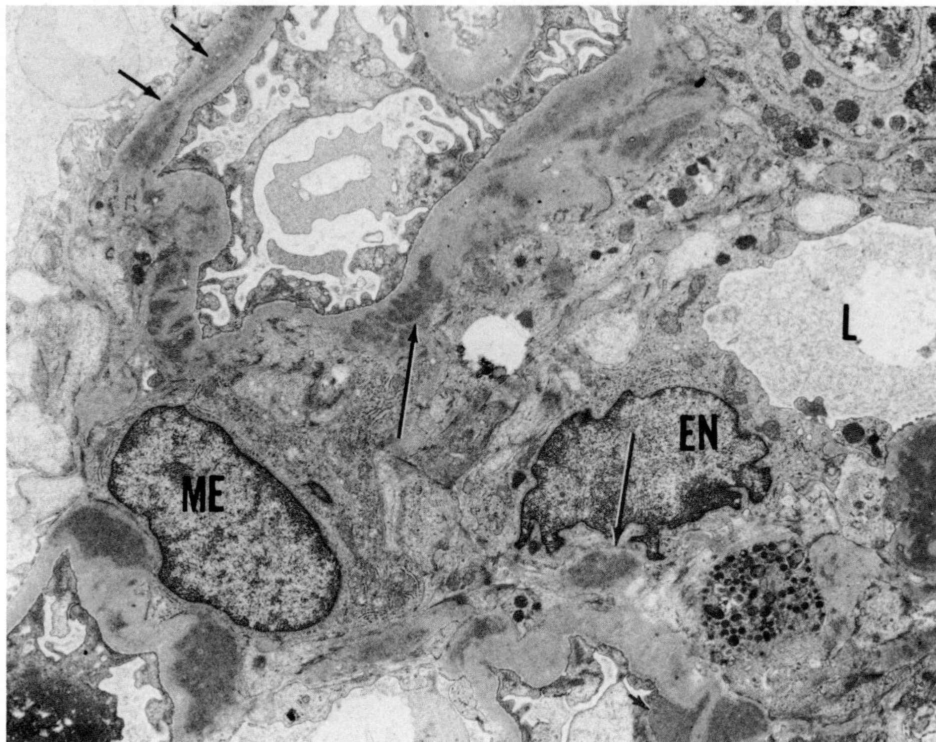

Figure 7-8. Portion of a glomerulus showing mesangial (long arrows), intramembranous (short arrows), and subepithelial (arrow head) deposits. ME, mesangium; EN, endothelial cell; L, capillary lumen (×7,100).

Resolving Glomerulonephritis

The intense inflammatory changes in this condition progressively resolve into a pattern of diffuse excess in mesangial matrix, with or without hypercellularity (27,28) (Fig. 7-15). The typical morphologic features of acute inflammation have usually disappeared by eight weeks from the onset of nephritis, and humps are rarely seen after this time. Resolution of the humps leaves irregularity of the subepithelial membrane contour and areas of lucency may be seen within the membrane (27,28) (Figs. 7-16−7-19). Resolution of the inflammatory changes may be irregular so that a pattern of focal glomerulonephritis may be simulated before inflammation completely subsides. The mesangial excess pattern may persist for up to 10 years after the acute syndrome, but usually returns toward the normal range within 3−4 years. In this phase, mesangial deposits or reactions for C3 may occur, but there is no evidence to suggest that these indicate a potential for progressive disease (Fig. 7-20). A patchy linear pattern of immunofluorescence for IgG has been reported in the resolving phase by one group, but this experience appears to be unique (30).

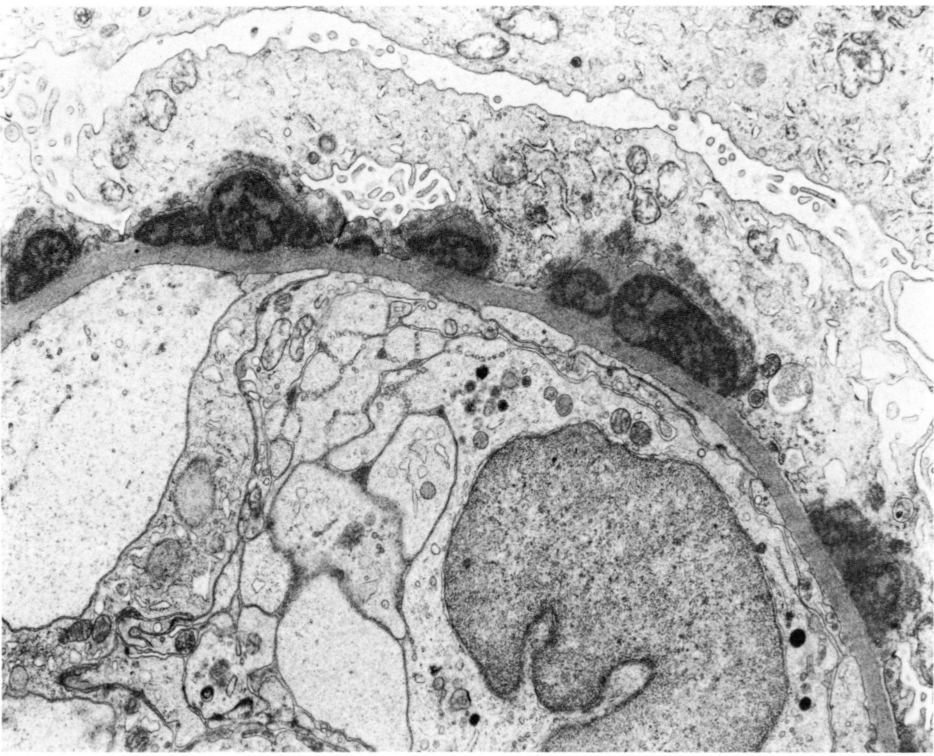

Figure 7-9. Part of a peripheral capillary loop showing numerous humps with irregular areas of decreased electron density. The epithelial cell is hyperactive and shows "villous" hyperplasia. The cytoplasm adjacent to the humps has increased electron density and the foot processes are obliterated (×9,500).

DIFFERENTIAL DIAGNOSIS

The typical pattern of acute postinfectious glomerulonephritis with humps is pathognomic and cannot easily be confused with other glomerular diseases. This specificity is not applicable to any individual feature but is rather an expression of the total clinical and morphologic pattern. In particular, humps occur in a variety of disorders and have no peculiar diagnostic significance. Mesangiocapillary glomerulonephritis has been alleged to develop from acute postinfectious glomerulonephritis, but we have not encountered this transition. An acute nephritic onset is common in the various forms of mesangiocapillary glomerulonephritis and clinical confusion is, therefore, possible, but differentiation between the diseases is almost always possible by careful examination of the initial biopsy specimen (11). Rarely, however, acute postinfectious glomerulonephritis has been reported to evolve into membranous nephropathy (39). In the resolving phase, the mesangial sclerotic pattern is, while characteristic, entirely nonspecific. Before immunofluorescence microscopy was routine, cases of IgA nephropathy were almost certainly diagnosed as resolving postinfectious

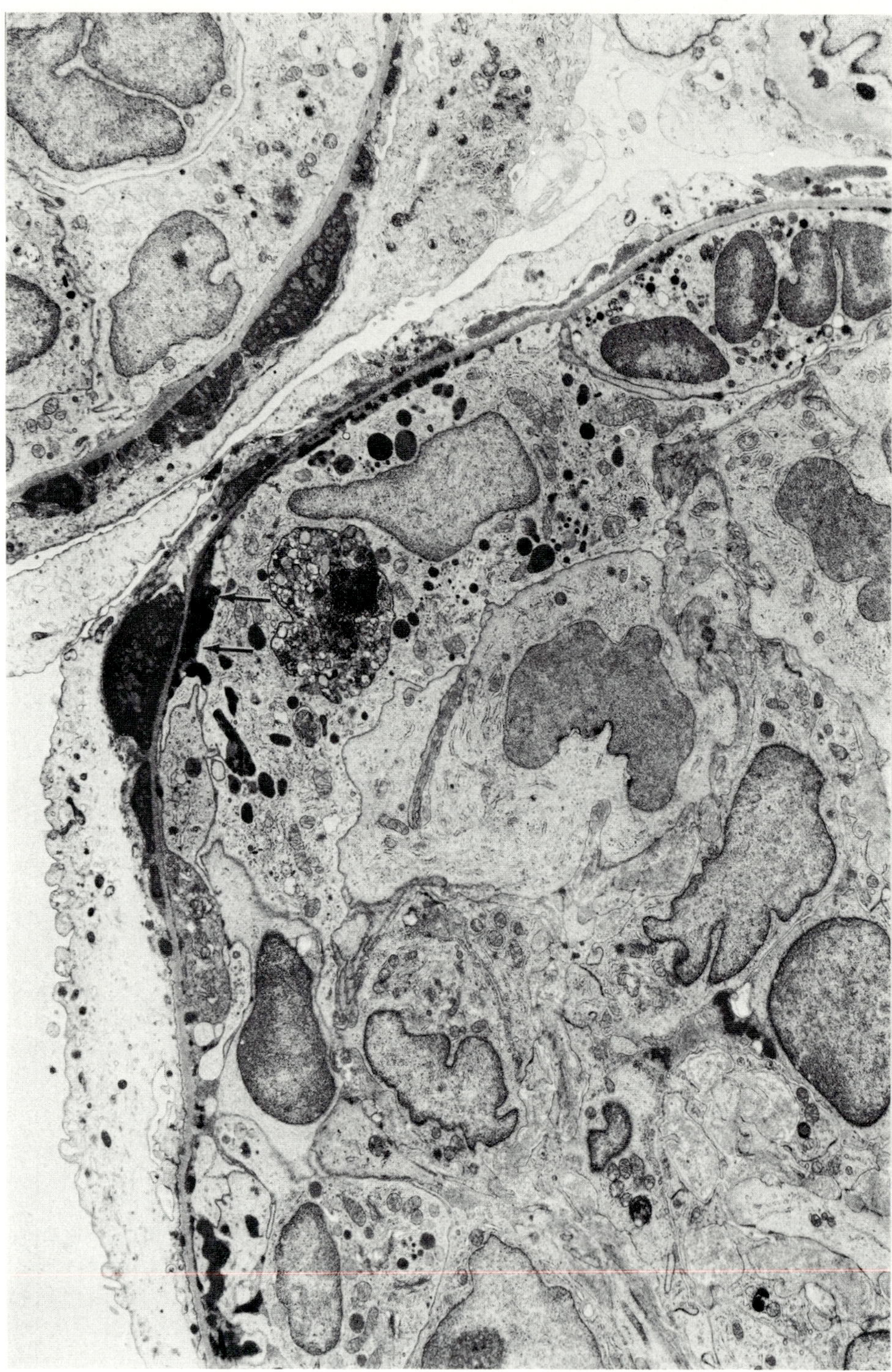

Figure 7-10. Acute poststreptococcal glomerulonephritis. There are numerous humps along the basement membrane. The capillary loops are obliterated by cell proliferation. Numerous polymorphs appear in direct contact with the basement membrane. Small amounts of fibrin are present in the subendothelial area (arrows) (×6,100).

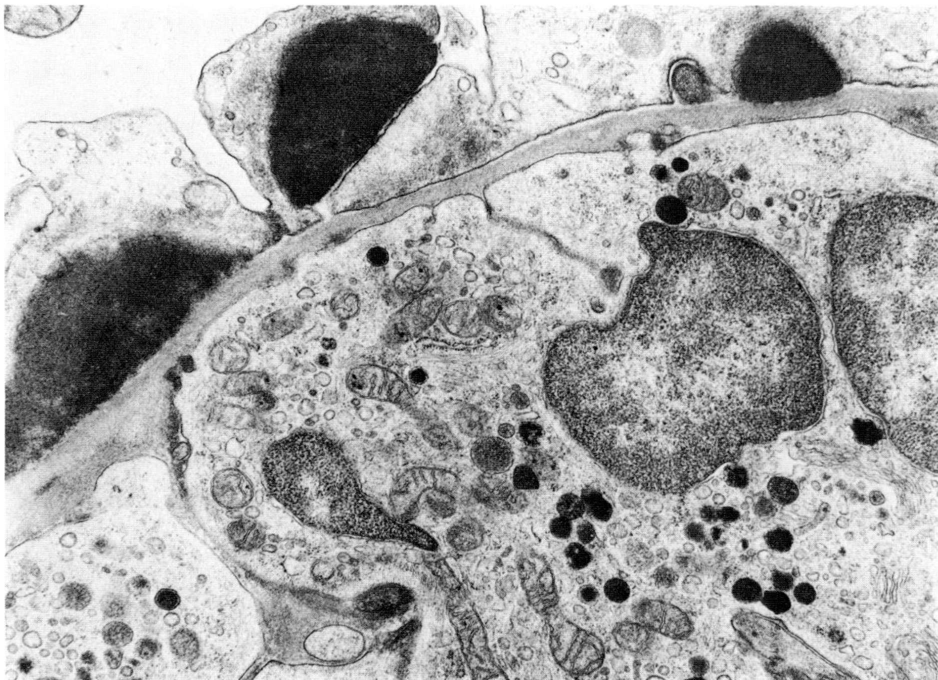

Figure 7-11. Acute poststreptococcal glomerulonephritis. Higher magnification showing humps and polymorphonuclear leukocytes in direct contact with the basement membrane, which has been denuded of its endothelial lining (×12,875).

glomerulonephritis, and this confusion may well have contributed to the controversy over prognosis. A mesangial proliferative or sclerotic pattern can only be confidently attributed to previous postinfectious glomerulonephritis when a previous biopsy specimen has demonstrated the characteristic features of the acute disease. In all other situations, even when a history of previous acute glomerulonephritis can be obtained, this pattern can do no more than raise a suspicion of previous postinfectious disease, and specific diagnosis relies on the electron and immunofluorescence microscopic findings.

PROGNOSIS

Considerable controversy continues over the sequelae of acute postinfectious glomerulonephritis, and the subject is best considered in the two following categories.

Short-Term Prognosis

The overwhelming majority of patients show a return to normal renal function and blood pressure within a year, although abnormalities in the sediment persist for several years (11,32,40,41). A small proportion, however, are left with permanent functional impairment. Progressive or irreversible renal damage is more

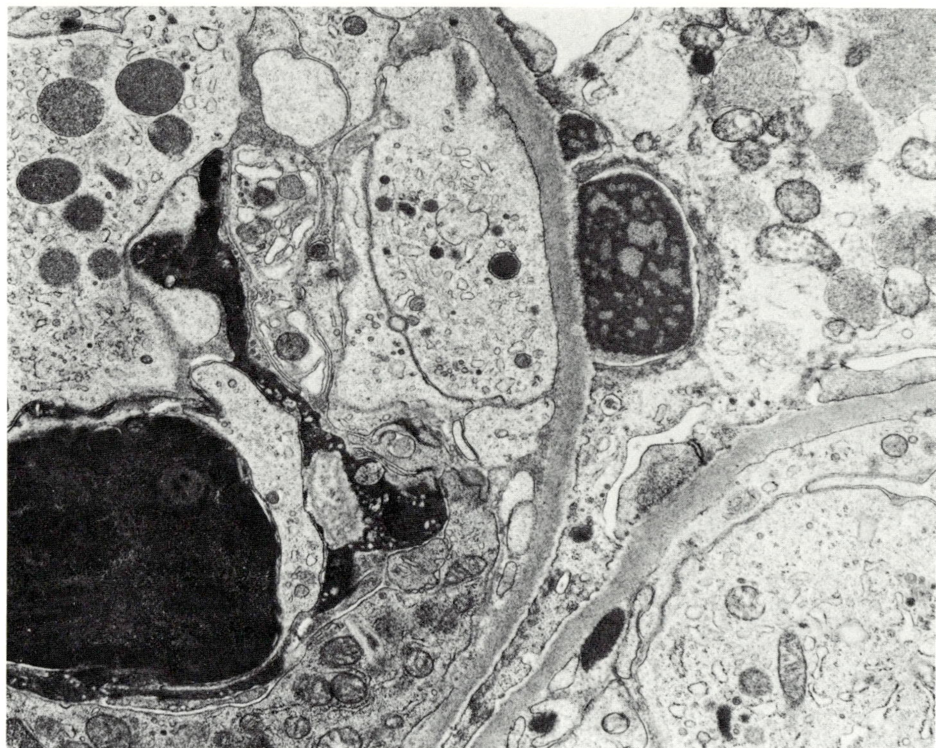

Figure 7-12. Acute poststreptococcal glomerulonephritis. The capillary loop is occluded by cell proliferation and a fibrin thrombus. The epithelial cytoplasm adjacent to the humps has an increased in electron density. Numerous protein transport droplets are also seen (×10,000).

likely, but not inevitable, in those patients with epithelial crescents. Extensive crescentic disease may produce chronic renal failure and/or death (27,32,42) or leave residual renal damage with persistent proteinuria and hypertension (11,30,32). There is some uncertainty whether a history suggesting postinfectious glomerulonephritis confers any prognostic benefit on patients with diffuse crescentic glomerulonephritis. Several studies have suggested a better prognosis in those patients with significant elevation of the antistreptolysin-0 titer, but the number of glomeruli involved by crescents was not always similar in this group and the group without such an elevation (43, 44). Valid comparative data to examine the problem is not available at present, but there is some evidence for an improved prognosis in those patients with significant endocapillary proliferation (45). Focal epithelial crescents are likely to leave residual scarring, but do not affect the normal pattern of resolution (11).

Long-Term Prognosis

Although urinary abnormalities may persist, most studies find no evidence for progressive renal disease after acute postinfectious glomerulonephritis

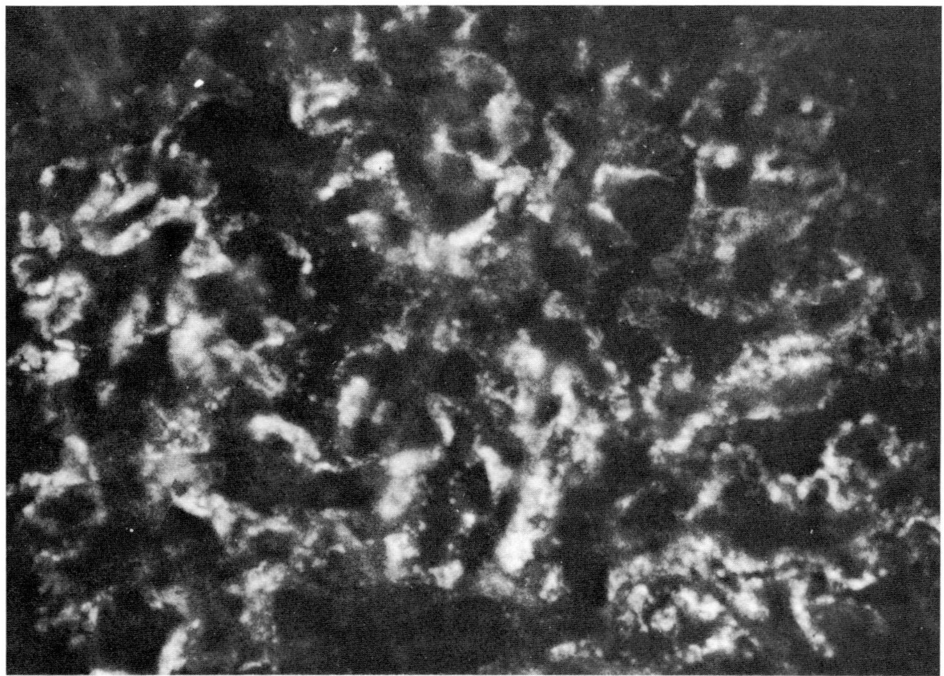

Figure 7-13. Coarse granular peripheral deposits of C3 along the capillary loops in acute poststreptococcal glomerulonephritis (×550).

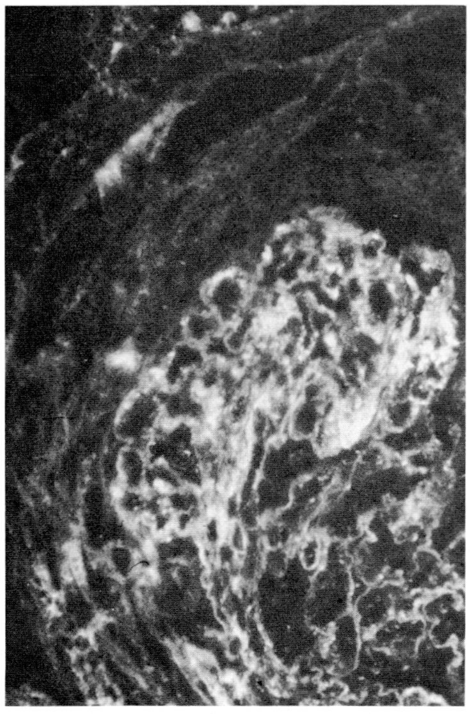

Figure 7-14. Acute poststreptococcal glomerulonephritis. The capillary tufts are compressed by an epithelial crescent. coarse granular deposits are prominent along the capillary walls (Antihuman IgG, × 500).

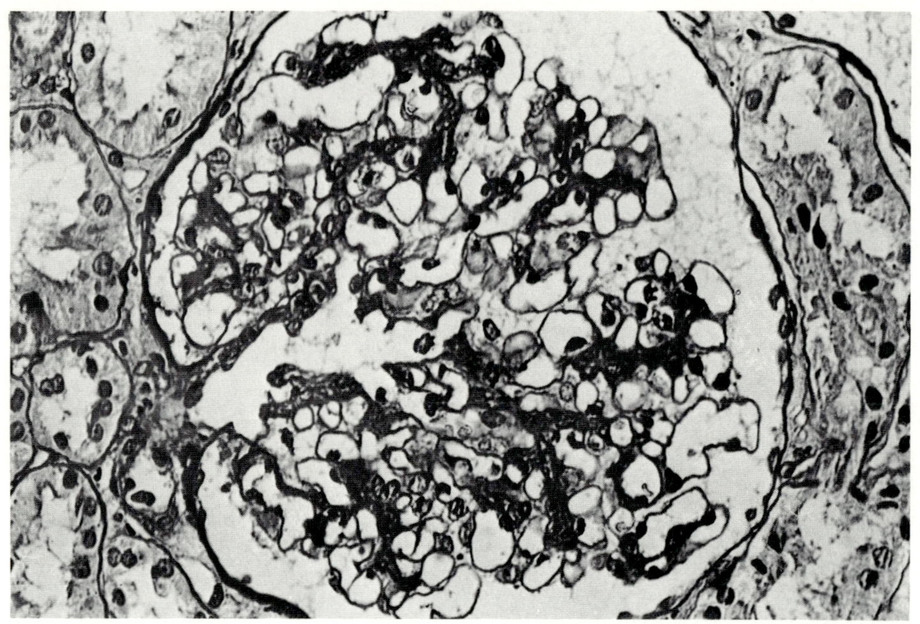

Figure 7-15. Resolving poststreptococcal glomerulonephritis. There is a moderate increase of mesangial matrix six months after the acute episode of glomerulonephritis (PAS stain, ×500).

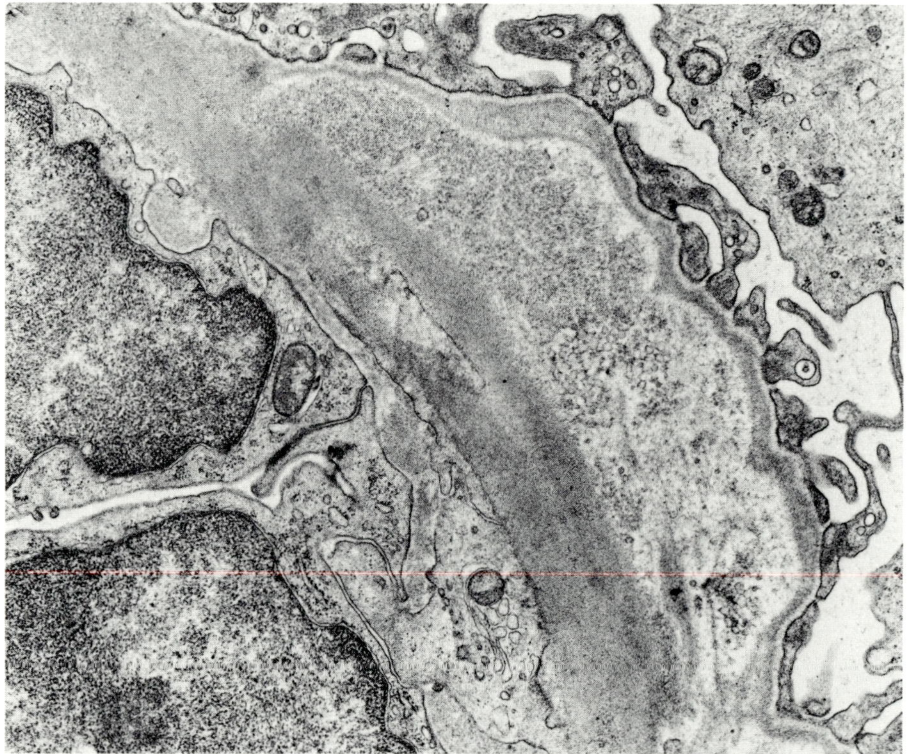

Figure 7-16. Partially reabsorbed deposits during the resolution phase of poststreptococcal glomerulonephritis (×15,200).

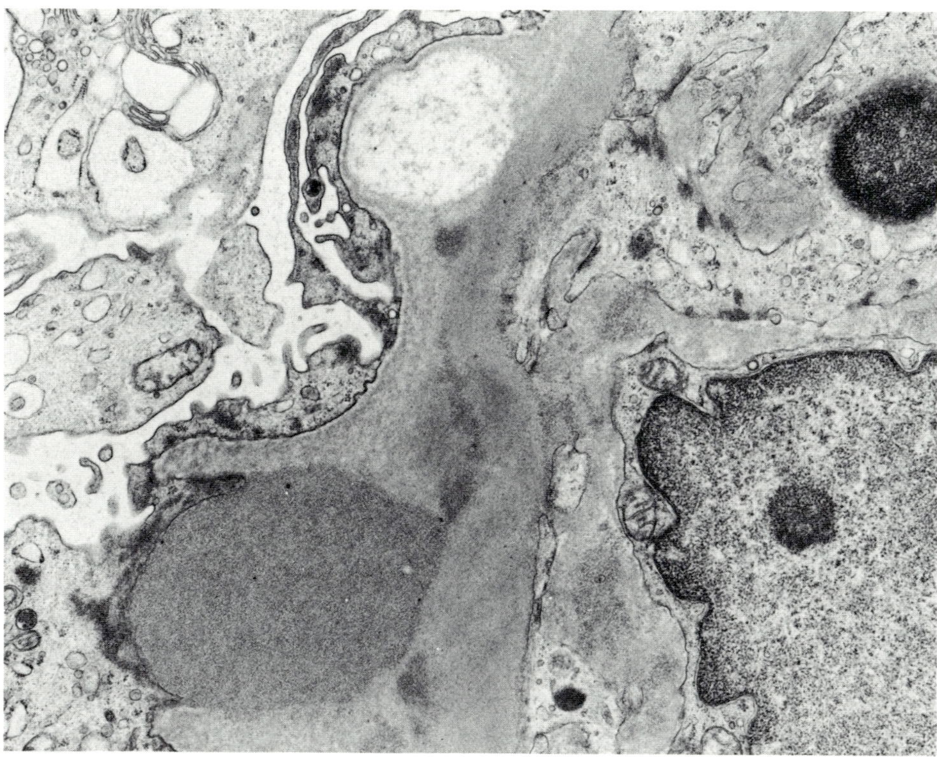

Figure 7-17. Resolving poststreptococcal glomerulonephritis eight weeks after the acute episode. A large subepithelial deposit appears partially surrounded by basement membrane, while the area of decreased electron density probably represents reabsorbed deposits (×13,300).

(11,32,40,41,46). One group, however, describes the development of chronic renal failure or hypertension and proteinuria in more than half of a large group of patients whose progress was followed for more than 10 years (47). These progressive features developed after an initial phase of apparent resolution and were accompanied by increasing tubulointerstitial scarring with glomerular obsolescence and vascular thickening. The reasons for these different prognostic experiences are not yet clear, but it may be significant that many of the group with progressive features were adults with severe disease at onset, since there is a general suspicion that adults are more prone to residual damage. Furthermore, not all the patients in this group were available for follow-up, and the criteria for initial diagnosis were not as stringent as in some of the other studies. The incidence of persistent disease is higher in patients with evidence of established glomerular disease at initial presentation and, as already discussed, clinical diagnosis of acute postinfectious glomerulonephritis is incorrect in a significant proportion of patients (11,27). Some degree of caution must, therefore, remain in the assessment of the long-term prognosis after acute postinfectious glomerulonephritis, but the evidence from most studies suggests that permanent cure is the rule.

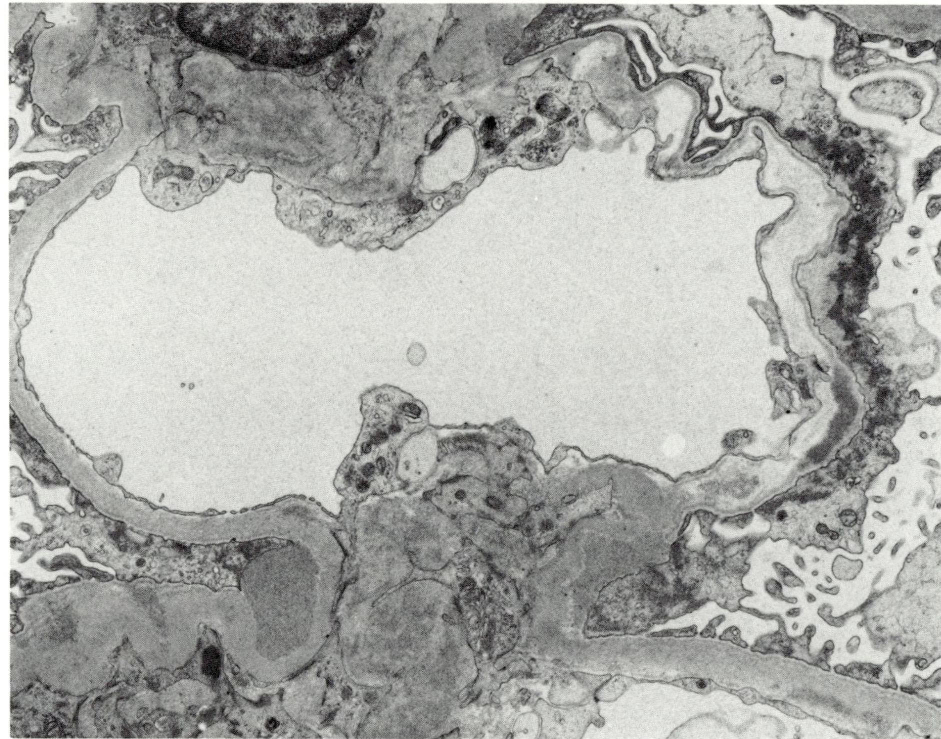

Figure 7-18. Electron micrograph of a capillary loop during the resolution phase of poststreptococcal glomerulonephritis, showing mesangial, subepithelial, and intramembranous deposits. The prominent focal clearing of the lamina densa (right) probably represents reabsorbed deposits ($\times 8,600$).

GLOMERULONEPHRITIS ASSOCIATED WITH INFECTIVE ENDOCARDITIS

Minor degrees of glomerular damage are probably very common in patients with infective endocarditis, and renal failure may be a major complication. There are two general patterns of glomerular damage: proliferative glomerulonephritis and segmental thrombosis (focal embolic glomerulonephritis) (48,49). Depending on the type of endocarditis, two forms of proliferative glomerulonephritis are described: acute, diffuse glomerulonephritis in association with acute endocarditis or septicemia, and progressive, irregular glomerular inflammation occurring with more prolonged inflammation (49,50). These forms correspond to those occurring with experimental acute and chronic serum sickness and probably reflect differences in the size and composition of immune complexes. There is little doubt that the proliferative glomerulonephritis of infective endocarditis, like the other vasculitic complications, is produced by the deposition of immune complexes. The development of these lesions is accompanied by hypocomplementemia with circulating immune complexes, and granular reactions for immunoglobulins and complement are present in the kidney, skin, and choroid plexus (51,52). The pathogenesis of the thrombotic lesions is less certain. Experimental induction of glomerulonephritis in animals with infective en-

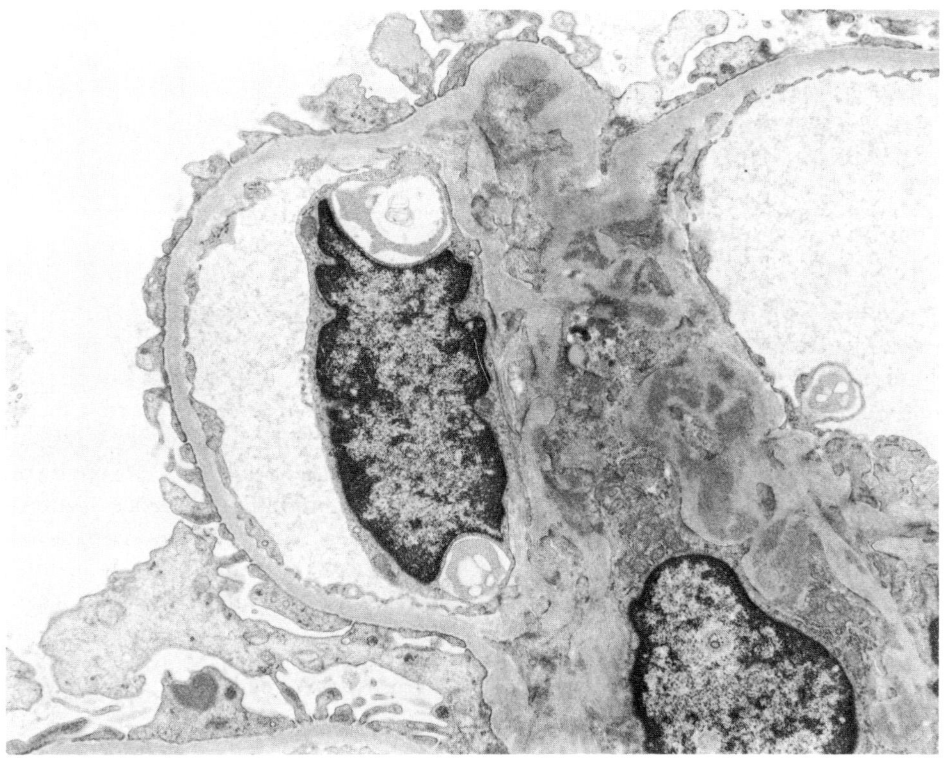

Figure 7-19. Resolving poststreptococcal glomerulonephritis. Electron micrograph of a renal biopsy specimen taken one year after an episode of acute glomerulonephritis, showing small mesangial deposits (×7,500).

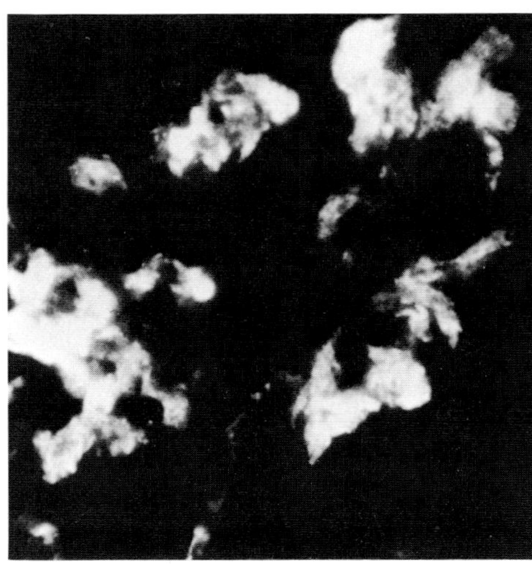

Figure 7-20. Resolving poststreptococcal glomerulonephritis. Immunofluorescent preparation six months after the acute episode. Most of the deposits are in the mesangium (Anti-C3, ×350).

docarditis has been achieved by prior immunization with the infecting organisms, but the thrombotic lesions occur even with sterile vegetations (53). Whether these thrombi are formed in situ or whether they represent emboli from valvular vegetations is uncertain, but there is little evidence at present for an immune pathogenesis.

Clinical Manifestations and Course

Renal involvement is usually indicated by microscopic hematuria with varying degrees of proteinuria, but some patients may have advancing renal failure. Some degree of renal failure occurred in 25 to 35% of patients with infective endocarditis before antibiotics became available, but the incidence is now in the region of 10% (54). Microscopic hematuria alone may occur with cortical infarcts and focal embolic lesions, but the presence of hypocomplementemia or circulating immune complexes suggests proliferative glomerulonephritis. The activity of the glomerulonephritis, whatever its type, is dependent on the presence of infectious antigen. Thus, control of the glomerular disease is achieved by sterilization of the valvular vegetations, and specific therapy for the renal lesion is usually unnecessary. Diminishing activity of the glomerular disease is reflected by a decline in the concentration of circulating immune complexes and normalization of serum complement (51). A wide variety of bacteria, viruses, and fungi have been implicated in the glomerulonephritis complicating infective endocarditis, and a number of the infectious antigens have been identified in the glomerular lesions (9,10).

Pathologic Characteristics

Proliferative Glomerulonephritis

The acute glomerulonephritis complicating acute endocarditis or septicemia, usually staphylococcal in type, is indistinguishable in all respects from acute postinfectious glomerulonephritis (49) (Fig. 7-21). Persistent glomerulonephritis, occurring with longstanding infections, usually has an irregular pattern. Segmental proliferation, with adhesions to Bowman's capsule, is the major feature and may be complicated by crescent formation (50,55) (Fig. 7-22). In many, but not all, of these persistent lesions there is underlying mesangial proliferation, and pure mesangial proliferative or mesangiocapillary patterns occasionally occur (50,55,56). Electron microscopy usually demonstrates mesangial and subendothelial deposits, and immunofluorescent reactions for IgG, IgM, C3, and occasionally, IgA, are present in mesangia and along capillary walls (49,50,55,56) (Figs. 7-23, 7-24). There is one report of anti-basement membrane activity in a glomerular eluate (57), which has not been confirmed elsewhere.

Focal Embolic Glomerulonephritis

The typical pattern here is of distension and occlusion of one or more capillary loops by thrombus. This process may progress to actual necrosis of a portion of the tuft with localized epithelial reaction (48). Immunofluorescence and electron microscopic studies of these lesions have not been reported.

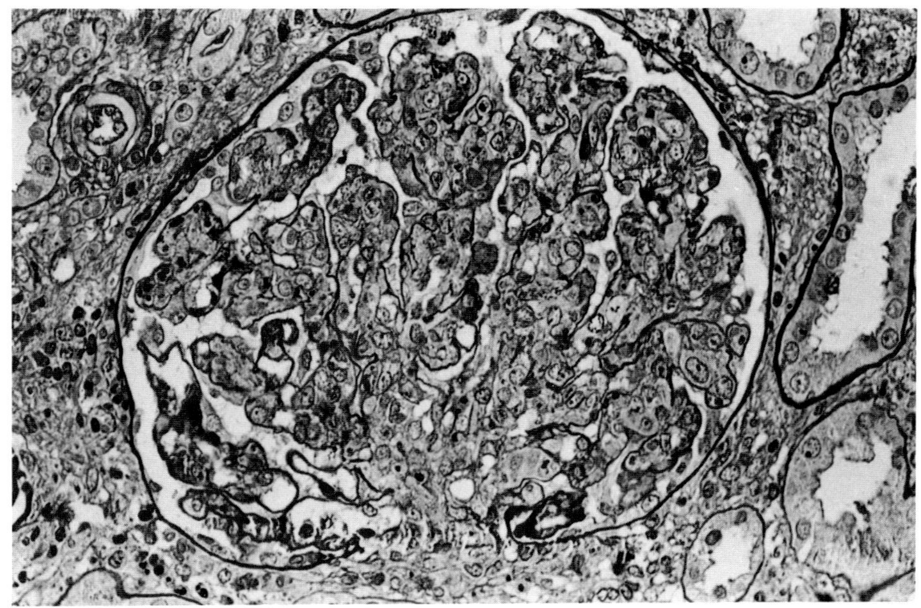

Figure 7-21. Diffuse proliferative glomerulonephritis in a patient with staphylococcal endocarditis (PAS stain, ×420).

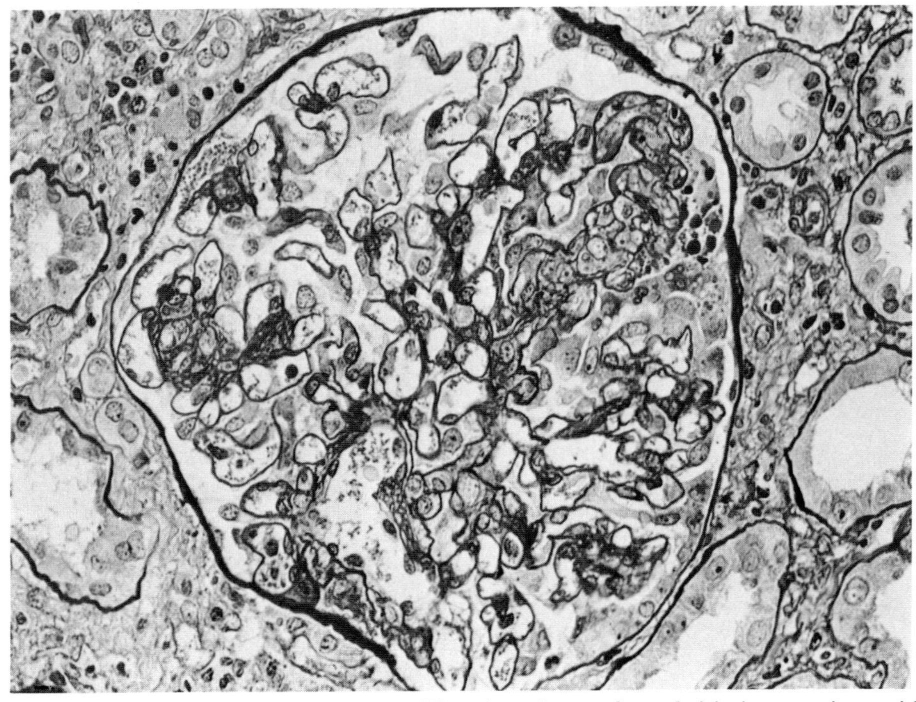

Figure 7-22. Focal and segmental proliferative glomerulonephritis in a patient with staphylococcal endocarditis (PAS stain, ×500).

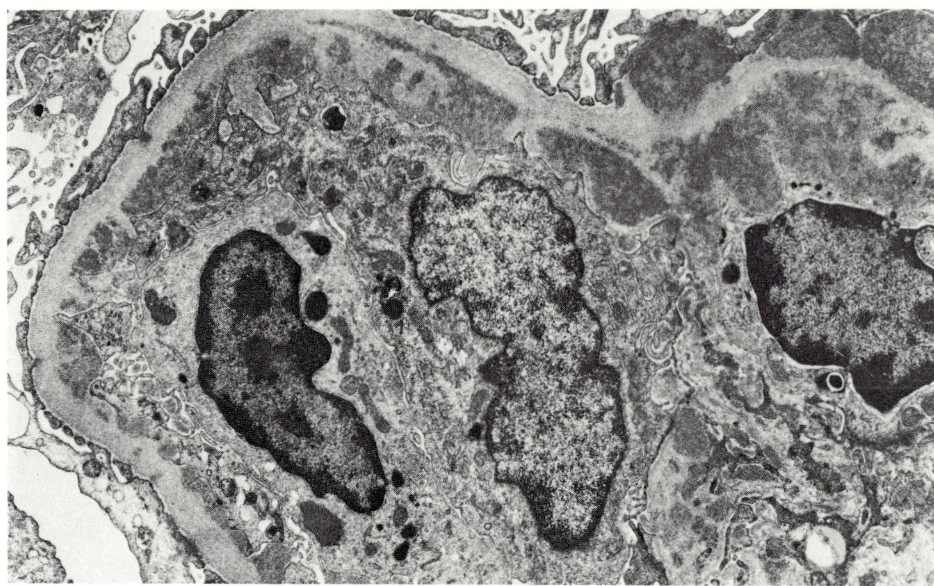

Figure 7-23. Biopsy specimen from a patient with staphylococcal bacterial endocarditis. The loop is obliterated by endocapillary proliferation. There are large amounts of subendothelial (left), mesangial (right), and subepithelial (right upper corner) deposits (×7,300).

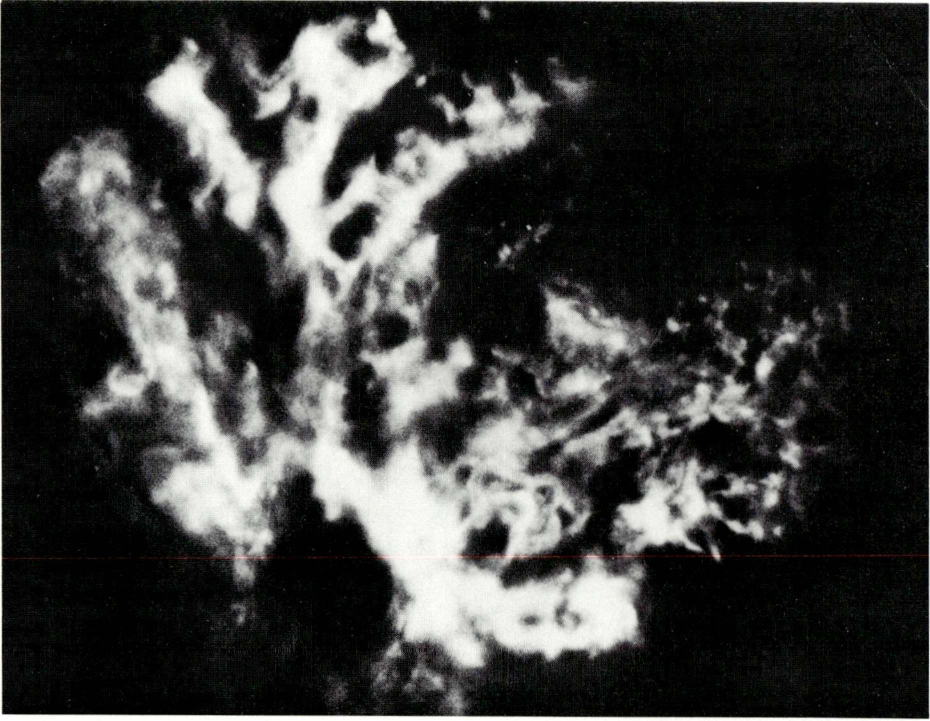

Figure 7-24. The same case as in Figure 7-23, showing mainly mesangial, but also peripheral, granular fluorescent deposits (Anti-human IgG, ×500).

114

Prognosis

Complete eradication of infectious antigen halts the progress of the glomerulonephritis with ensuing resolution (49,50). Renal dysfunction or abnormalities in the urinary sediment may remain if severe glomerular damage has occurred, but recovery is usually complete. Preexisting glomerular damage may be present in patients with endocarditis complicating narcotic addiction, and this possibility should be considered if significant proteinuria persists after the valvular disease is controlled (58). The incidence of focal embolic lesions is reduced, but not abolished, by antibiotic therapy (59), and it is doubtful whether these lesions are of major significance.

GLOMERULONEPHRITIS ASSOCIATED WITH INFECTED VENTRICULOATRIAL SHUNTS (SHUNT NEPHRITIS)

Chronic infection of ventriculoatrial or other shunts inserted for hydrocephalus occurs in 27% of patients and is complicated by glomerulonephritis in 4% (60). A wide variety of organisms have been implicated in these infections, but coagulase-negative staphylococci are the most commonly associated with glomerulonephritis (9,10). Persistent infection is associated with fever, general ill health, and a systemic syndrome of hepatosplenomegaly, anemia, and hypocomplementemia (61–63). Renal involvement may be detected by proteinuria or hematuria, either gross or microscopic, but is often not suspected until the onset of the nephrotic syndrome (62–64). The glomerular lesions are predominantly mesangial in type and range in severity from mild and irregular proliferation to the classic pattern of mesangiocapillary glomerulonephritis (61–66). Electron microscopy demonstrates deposits in subendothelial and mesangial regions, but humps do not occur. Granular mesangial and capillary-wall reactions for IgG, IgM, IgA, C3, C1, and properdin have been reported by immunofluorescence, with IgM and C3 being found most commonly (61,65,66). Bacterial antigens have been identified in the glomerular deposits in some cases (9,62,63,65), and cryoglobulins, presumably representing immune complexes, are usually present in the serum (62,63,66). Antibiotic therapy alone is usually ineffective in eradicating the organism, and excision of the infected shunt is usually required (60). After removal of the organism, there is complete resolution of all clinical, serologic, and urinary features of the glomerulonephritis.

SUMMARY

Glomerulonephritis following infection may be diffuse and evanescent when exposure to the organism is brief, or irregular and persistent when exposure is prolonged. Although either pattern may cause enough damage to leave residual renal dysfunction, resolution is usually complete once the organism is eradicated. The behavior and morphologic characteristics of these glomerular diseases are very similar to those of the experimental lesions produced by antigen injection, and there is no doubt that both the human and experimental diseases are caused by the deposition of immune complexes. Acute postinfectious glomerulonephritis is characterized by diffuse endocapillary proliferation, granular reactions for IgG and C3, and typical subepithelial deposits called humps. The humps are not specific for the disease but, in the context of an acute glomerulonephritis, suggest that rapid resolution is likely. There is controversy over the frequency of hypertension and progressive renal failure as late complications of acute postinfectious glomerulonephritis, but most studies show no significant long-term sequelae. Persistent glomerulonephritis complicating chronic internal infections is seen most commonly in association with infective endocarditis and infected ventriculoatrial shunts. The glomerular lesions in these conditions tend to be of mesangial proliferative type but often have an irregular character. Occasionally, glomerular damage may be sufficiently extensive to leave residual damage when the infection is eradicated, but complete resolution usually occurs. The ability of the glomerulus to recover after the extensive damage seen in these conditions indicates the importance of excluding underlying infection in cases of unexplained glomerulonephritis. Furthermore, this resilience suggests that complete recovery may be possible in a number of apparently primary glomerular diseases if an underlying cause can be identified and removed.

REFERENCES

1. Panem S, Ordóñez NG, Katz AI, et al: Viral immune complexes in systemic lupus erythematosus: specificity of C-type viral complexes. *Lab Invest* 39:413, 1978.

2. Gamble CN, Reardan JB: Immunopathogenesis of syphilitic glomerulonephritis: elution of antitreponemal antibody from glomerular immune-complex deposits. *N Engl J Med* 292:449, 1975.

3. Cochrane CG, Koffler D: Immune complex disease in experimental animals and man. *Adv Immunol* 16:185, 1973.

4. Germuth FG Jr, Rodriguez E: *Immunopathology of the renal glomerulus. Immune complex disease and antibasement membrane disease.* Boston, Little, Brown and Co, 1973, p. 15.

5. Woodroffe AJ, Border WA, Theofilopoulos AN, et al: Detection of circulating immune complexes in patients with glomerulonephritis. *Kidney Int* 12:268, 1977.

6. Michael AF, Hoyer JR, Westberg NG: Experimental models for the pathogenesis of acute poststreptococcal glomerulonephritis, in Wannamaker LW, Matsen JM (eds), *Streptococci and Streptococcal Diseases. Recognition, Understanding and Management,* New York, Academic Press, 1972, p 481.

7. Zabriskie JB, Utermohlen V, Read SE, et al: Streptococcus-related glomerulonephritis. *Kidney Int* 3:100, 1973.

8. Lange K, Ahmed U, Kleinberger H, et al: A hitherto unknown streptococcal antigen and its probable relation to acute poststreptococcal glomerulonephritis. *Clin Nephrol* 5:207, 1976.

9. O'Regan S, Smith M, Drummond KN: Antigens in human immune complex nephritis. *Clin Nephrol* 6:417, 1976.

10. Kim Y, Michael AF: Chronic bacteremia and nephritis. *Ann Rev Med* 29:315, 1978.

11. Hinglais N, Garcia-Torres R, Kleinknecht D: Long-term prognosis in acute glomerulonephritis. *Am J Med* 56:52, 1974.

12. Peter G, Smith AL: Group A streptococcal infections of the skin and pharynx (first of two parts). *N Engl J Med* 297:311, 1977.

13. Stollerman GH: Rheumatogenic and nephritogenic streptococci. *Circulation* 43:915, 1971.

14. Anthony BF, Kaplan EL, Wannamaker LW, et al: Attack rates of acute nephritis after type 49 streptococcal infection of the skin and respiratory tract. *J Clin Invest* 48:1697, 1969.

15. Meadow SR: Poststreptococcal glomerulonephritis—a rare disease? *Arch Dis Child* 50:379, 1975.

16. Rainford DJ, Woodrow DR, Sloper JC, et al: Postmeningococcal acute glomerular nephritis. *Clin Nephrol* 9:249, 1978.

16a. Sato M, Nakazora H, Ofuji T: The pathogenetic role of *Staphylococcus aureus* in primary human glomerulonephritis. *Clin Nephrol* 11:190, 1979.

17. Hyman LR, Jenis EH, Hill GS, et al: Alternate C3 pathway activation in pneumococcal glomerulonephritis. *Am J Med* 58:810, 1975.

18. Vitullo BB, O'Regan S, De Chadarevian JP, et al: Mycoplasma pneumonia associated with acute glomerulonephritis. *Nephron* 21: 284, 1978.

19. Date A, Thomas A, Mathai R, et al: Glomerular pathology in leprosy: an electron microscopic study. *Am J Trop Med Hyg* 26:266, 1977.

20. Sitprija V, Pipatanagul V, Boonpucknavig V, et al: Glomerulitis in typhoid fever. *Ann Intern Med* 81:210, 1974.

21. Yuceoglu AM, Berkovich S, Minkowitz S: Acute glomerulonephritis as a complication of Varicella. *J AMA* 202:113, 1967.

22. Ginsburg BE, Wasserman J, Huldt G, et al: Case of glomerulonephritis associated with acute toxoplasmosis. *Br Med J* 3:664, 1974.

23. Monteiro GE, Lillecrap CA: Case of mumps nephritis. *Br Med J* 4:721, 1967.

24. Brzosko WJ, Krawczynski K, Nazareqicz T, et al: Glomerulonephritis associated with hepatitis-B surface antigen immune complexes in children. *Lancet* 2:477, 1974.

25. Rodriguez-Iturbe B, Garcia R, Rubio L, et al: Acute glomerulonephritis in the Guillain-Barré-Strohl syndrome. *Ann Intern Med* 78:391, 1973.

26. Sagel I, Tresser G, Ty A, et al: Occurrence and nature of glomerular lesions after group A streptococci infections in children. *Ann Intern Med* 79:492, 1973.

27. Dodge WF, Spargo BH, Bass JA, et al: The relationship between the clinical and pathologic features of poststreptococcal glomerulonephritis. A study of the early natural history. *Medicine (Balt)* 47:227, 1968.

27a. Porter KA, Dossetor JB, Marchioro LT, et al: Human renal transplants: I. Glomerular changes. *Lab Invest* 16:153, 1967.

27b. Turner DR, Cameron JS, Bewick M, et al: Transplantation in mesangiocapillary glomerulonephritis with intramembranous dense "deposits": recurrence of disease. *Kidney Int* 9:439, 1976.

28. West CD, Ruley EF, Forristal J, et al: Mechanisms of hypocomplementemia in glomerulonephritis. *Kidney Int* 3:116, 1973.

29. Kaplan EL, Anthony BF, Chapman SS, et al: Epidemic acute glomerulonephritis associated with type 49 streptococcal pyoderma. I. Clinical and laboratory findings. *Am J Med* 48:9, 1970.

30. Baldwin DS, Gluck MC, Schacht RG, et al: The long-term course of poststreptococcal glomerulonephritis. *Ann Intern Med* 80:342, 1974.

31. Jennings RB, Earle DP: Post-streptococcal glomerulonephritis: histopathologic and clinical studies of the acute, subsiding acute and early chronic latent phrase. *J Clin Invest* 40:1525, 1961.

32. Lewy JE, Salinas-Madrigal L, Herdson PB, et al: Clinico-pathologic correlation between renal functions, morphologic damage and clinical course of 46 children with acute poststreptococcal glomerulonephritis. *Medicine (Balt)* 50:453, 1971.

33. Fish AJ, Herdman RC, Michael AF, et al: Epidemic acute glomerulonephritis associated with type 49 streptococcal pyoderma. I. Correlative study of light, immunofluorescent and electron microscopic findings. *Am J Med* 48:28, 1970.

34. Gill DG, Turner DR, Chantler C, et al: The progression of acute proliferative poststreptococcal glomerulonephritis to severe epithelial crescent formation. *Clin Nephrol* 8:449, 1977.

35. Ingelfinger JR, McCluskey RT, Schneeberger EE, et al: Necrotizing arteritis in acute poststreptococcal glomerulonephritis. *J Pediat* 91:228, 1977.

36. Morita T, Wenzl JE, Kimmelstiel P: The relationship of neutrophilic and eosinophilic leukocytes to the glomerular capillary basement membrane in acute proliferative glomerulonephritis. *Lab Invest* 25:445, 1971.

37. Morel-Maroger L, Kourilsky O, Mignon F, et al: Antitubular basement membrane antibodies in rapidly progressive poststreptococcal glomerulonephritis: report of a case. *Clin Immunol Immunopathol* 2:185, 1974.

38. Törnröth T: The fate of subepithelial deposits in acute poststreptococcal glomerulonephritis. *Lab Invest* 35:461, 1976.

39. Richet G, Fillastre JP, Morel-Maroger L, et al: Change from diffuse proliferative to membranous glomerulonephritis: serial biopsies in four cases. *Kidney Int* 5:57, 1974.

40. Dodge WF, Spargo BH, Travis LB, et al: Poststreptococal glomerulonephritis: a prospective study in children. *N Engl J Med* 286:273, 1972.

41. Potter EV, Abidh S, Sarrett AR, et al: Clinical healing two to six years after poststreptococcal glomerulonephritis in Trinidad. *N Engl J Med* 298:767, 1978.

42. McCluskey RT, Baldwin DS: Natural history of acute glomerulonephritis. *Am J Med* 35:213, 1963.

43. Leonard CD, Nagle RB, Striker GE, et al: Acute glomerulonephritis with prolonged oliguria: an analysis of 29 cases. *Ann Intern Med* 73:703, 1970.

44. Morrin PAF, Hinglais N, Nabarra B, et al: Rapidly progressive glomerulonephritis: a clinical and pathologic study. *Am J Med* 65:446, 1978.

45. Elfenbein IB, Baluarte JH, Cubillas-Rojas M, et al: Quantitative morphometry of glomerulonephritis with crescents: diagnostic and predictive value. *Lab Invest* 32:56, 1975.

46. Perlman LV, Herdman RC, Kleinman H, et al: Poststreptococcal glomerulonephritis: a ten year follow-up of an epidemic. *J Am Med Ass* 194:63, 1965.

47. Baldwin DS: Poststreptococcal glomerulonephritis: a progressive disease? *Am J Med* 62:1, 1977.

48. Bell ET: Glomerular lesions associated with endocarditis. *Am J Pathol* 8:639, 1932.

49. Gutman RA, Striker GE, Gillialand BC, et al: The immune complex glomerulonephritis of bacterial endocarditis. *Medicine (Balt)* 51:1, 1972.

50. Boulton-Jones JM, Sissons JGP, Evans DJ, et al: Renal lesions of subacute infective endocarditis. *Br Med J* 2:11, 1974.

51. Bayer AS, Theofilopoulos AN, Eisenberg R, et al: Circulating immune complexes in infective endocarditis. *N Engl J Med* 295:1500, 1976.

52. Davis JA, Weisman MH, Dail DH: Vascular disease in infective endocarditis: report of immune-mediated events in skin and brain. *Arch Intern Med* 138:480, 1978.

53. Arnold SB, Valone JA, Askenase, PW, et al: Diffuse glomerulonephritis in rabbits with streptococcus viridans endocarditis. *Lab Invest* 32:681, 1975.

54. Weinstein L, Schlesinger JJ: Pathoanatomic, pathophysiologic and clinical correlations in endocarditis (second of two parts). *N Engl J Med* 291:1122, 1974.

55. Morel-Maroger L, Sraer J-D, Herreman G, et al: Kidney in subacute endocarditis: pathological and immunofluorescence findings. *Arch Pathol* 94:205, 1972.

56. Uff JS, Evans DJ: Mesangio-capillary glomerulonephritis associated with Q-fever endocarditis. *Histopathol* 1:463, 1977.

57. Levy RL, Hong R: The immune nature of subacute bacterial endocarditis (SBE) nephritis. *Am J Med* 54:645, 1973.

58. Ayres BF, Bastian PD, Haines D, et al: Renal and cardiac complications of drug abuse. *Med J Aust* 2:489, 1976.

59. Spain DM, King DW: The effect of penicillin on the renal lesions of subacute bacterial endocarditis. *Ann Intern Med* 36:1086, 1952.

60. Schoenbaum SL, Gardner P, Shillito J: Infections of cerebrospinal fluid shunts: epidemiology, clinical manifestations and therapy. *J Infect Dis* 131:543, 1975.

61. Peeters W, Mussche M, Becaus I, et al: Shunt nephritis. *Clin Nephrol* 9:122, 1978.

62. Bolton WK, Sande MA, Normansell DE, et al: Ventriculojugular shunt nephritis with Corynebacterium bovis. *Am J Med* 59:417, 1975.

63. Kaufman DB, McIntosh R: The pathogenesis of the renal lesion in a patient with streptococcal disease, infected ventriculoatrial shunt, cryoglobulinemia and nephritis. *Am J Med* 50:262, 1971.

64. Moncrieff MW, Glasgow EF, Arthur LJH, et al: Glomerulonephritis associated with *Staphylococcus albus* in a Spitz Holter valve. *Arch Dis Child* 48:69, 1973.

65. Dobrin RS, Day NK, Quie PG, et al: The role of complement, immunoglobulin and bacterial antigen in coagulase-negative staphylococcal shunt nephritis. *Am J Med* 59:660, 1975.

66. Strife CF, McDonald BM, Ruley EJ, et al: Shunt nephritis: the nature of the serum cryoglobulins and their relation to the complement profile. *J Pediat* 88:403, 1976.

8
Mesangiocapillary Glomerulonephritis*

In 1965, West and Gotoff independently described the association of persistent hypocomplementemia and a morphologically characteristic form of chronic glomerulonephritis (1,2). Because of the combination of capillary-wall thickening and endocapillary proliferation, this morphologic pattern became known as membranoproliferative glomerulonephritis. In fact, neither the morphology nor the association with hypocomplementemia has proven to be a specific disease marker. The thickening of capillary walls may occur via a number of mechanisms, of which two are predominant (3). Most common is the subendothelial extension (interposition) of mesangial cytoplasm and matrix to produce apparent splitting of the basement membrane (4,5). There is rarely extensive true membranous change, and this mesangial interposition pattern is better described as mesangiocapillary than membranoproliferative glomerulonephritis. Extensive mesangial interposition is usually associated with subendothelial deposits, and this pattern of disease has been termed type I or subendothelial deposit mesangiocapillary glomerulonephritis (6). In contrast, the capillary wall may be thickened by a peculiar dense transformation of the basement membrane, with or without interposition, and this picture has been designated type II or dense intramembranous (DIM) mesangiocapillary glomerulonephritis (6). A number of other alterations of the membrane have been recognized and are sometimes described as type III variants. Any of these patterns may be associated with centrolobular sclerosis to produce the picture of lobular glomerulonephritis, which is no longer regarded as a discrete disease entity.

Although these subdivisions suggest varying patterns of a single clinicopathologic entity, the conditions share no pathologic or pathogenetic aspects and are linked only by a similar appearance in H&E-stained sections. There is, therefore, no longer any justification for the use of the term *mesangiocapillary* (or *membranoproliferative*) *glomerulonephritis* as a general diagnostic category for these disparate conditions. The subendothelial deposit pattern may be associated with a wide range of conditions, though most cases are idiopathic, and is almost certainly a chronic immune complex disease. In contrast, the dense intramembranous pattern marks a specific disease entity, albeit of unknown pathogenesis. To conform with general usage, both conditions are discussed in

*This category of renal disease includes membranoproliferative, lobular, mixed, membranous and proliferative, and chronic hypocomplementemic glomerulonephritis.

120

this chapter, but we recommend that the term *mesangiocapillary glomerulonephritis* be restricted to biopsies showing extensive mesangial interposition with subendothelial deposits. When the dense intramembranous lesion is detected, a primary diagnosis of dense deposit disease is indicated, with a supplementary description of the associated proliferative changes.

MESANGIOCAPILLARY GLOMERULONEPHRITIS (MCGN) WITH SUBENDOTHELIAL DEPOSITS (TYPE I)

This pattern of glomerular disease is, like membranous nephropathy, merely a morphologic endpoint with no etiologic specificity. While no cause can be found in the majority of patients with MCGN, a number of associations are well recognized, and effective therapy in some of these conditions may lead to resolution of the glomerular lesions. The idiopathic form, however, is usually relentlessly progressive to chronic renal failure.

Pathogenesis

Many of the conditions associated with MCGN are known to be immune complex disorders, and specific antigens have been detected in the glomerular deposits of a significant number of these conditions (Table 8-1). This implies that the idiopathic disease is likely to have a similar pathogenesis (30). Circulating immune complexes have, in fact, been demonstrated in some patients with this lesion, and chronic immune complex deposition probably accounts in part for the associated hypocomplementemia (31). The presence or absence of circulating complexes is not, however, clearly correlated with serum complement concentrations, and other mechanisms are probably implicated (32). In most biopsy specimens showing the changes of MCGN, both immunoglobulins and complement are found by immunofluorescence but, in some, only complement is detected. This may represent masking of reaction sites, as occurs in experimental serum sickness (33), and could prevent easy identification of antigens in the deposits. The majority of antigens identified in the secondary forms of MCGN have been exogenous, but DNA is present in the deposits associated with schistosomiasis, and renal tubular antigen has been identified in patients with sickle cell disease (10,25). Exhaustive examination with a panel of antigens of biopsies from patients with idiopathic disease may, therefore, provide etiologic information in the future. There are few reports of satisfactory experimental models, but spontaneous disease has occurred in one population of Scottish sheep (30).

Clinical Manifestations and Course

The disease usually affects children or young adults and is slightly more common in females (6,34–36). Onset before the age of 4 years is rare, and most patients are less than 30 years old at presentation, although occasional examples develop in middle age (6,36).

Mesangiocapillary glomerulonephritis occurs most frequently with the nephrotic syndrome, often with a mixed nephritic-nephrotic pattern, but some pa-

Table 8-1 Conditions associated with MCGN and Subendothelial Deposits

Clinical Condition	Reference Number
Chronic infection[a]	
Infected ventriculoatrial shunts	7
Infective endocarditis	8
Chronic suppuration	7,9
Schistosomiasis	10
Malaria	11,12
Hepatitis B	13
Neoplasms	
Epithelial tumors	14
Leukemia and malignant lymphoma	14
Macroglobulinemia	14
Cryoglobulinemia	15
Multiple myeloma	16
Systemic connective tissue disorders	
Systemic lupus [a]	17
Polyarteritis	6
Sjögren's syndrome	18
Henoch-Schönlein purpura	19
Complement deficiencies	
C1 esterase inhibitor (angioedema)	20
C2	21
Miscellaneous	
Hepatic cirrhosis	22
Toxic epidermal necrolysis	23
α_1-antitrypsin deficiency [a]	24
Sickle cell disease [a]	25
Kartagener's syndrome	26
Klinefelter's syndrome	6
Heroin abuse	27,27a
Partial lipodystrophy [b]	28,29

[a]Specific antigens have been identified in the deposits.
[b]Usually associated with dense deposit disease.

tients are referred for investigation of an abnormal urinary sediment and up to one-third have a typical acute nephritic syndrome (6,34). This nephritic onset and the frequent occurrence of upper respiratory tract infection before manifestation has suggested that the disease may develop from acute postinfectious glomerulonephritis. There is, however, no clear evidence for a specific association with streptococcal or other organisms in most cases, and the progression of well-documented acute postinfectious glomerulonephritis to MCGN has not been reported (30). Macroscopic hematuria may occur as part of a nephritic syndrome or as an isolated phenomenon, and microscopic hematuria is common (6). The clinical course is usually indolent and slowly progressive over 10 or more years. This progression may be punctuated by episodes of acute nephritis or nephrotic syndrome and rapidly progressive deterioration associated with crescentic disease occurs at onset or later in about 10% of the patients (6). Many patients are anemic and hypocomplementemia is present in about two-thirds, often with marked variation during the course (6,37–39). The predominant complement depletion is of C3, with associated C3 nephritic factor in about one-third of patients, but early acting components are also depressed and the complement profile usually suggests activation of the classical pathway (40).

Pathologic Characteristics

Light Microscopy

The glomeruli are diffusely enlarged with thickening of capillary walls and centrolobular proliferation producing a lobular pattern (4,6,35,41) (Fig. 8-1). Lobulation is more pronounced in this form of glomerulonephritis than in any other, and the lobules may appear to lie as discrete nodules in Bowman's space. Depending on the duration of the disease, there is progressive centrolobular accumulation of matrix, which may form central balls resembling the nodules of diabetic glomerulosclerosis (Fig. 8-2). This pattern was previously termed *lobular glomerulonephritis* but is now recognized as an integral part of the MCGN lesion (3,36,41). In sections stained with PAS or PASM, continuations of the mesangial matrix can be seen to surround capillary loops, producing a double-contour pattern, sometimes erroneously described as splitting of the basement membrane, and causing the thickening of capillary walls (5) (Fig. 8-3). Double contours vary in number between glomeruli, but a diagnosis of MCGN is unwise unless several loops in all or most glomeruli show this change. Within the double contours, "slugs" of hyaline material, corresponding to subendothelial deposits, are often prominent.

Cellular proliferation is always principally mesangial, but there may be a significant endothelial component, especially in patients with acute nephritis. Occasionally, the initial biopsy specimen has a light microscopic pattern very similar to acute postinfectious glomerulonephritis, and the characteristic features of MCGN can only be recognized in subsequent examinations. In such cases, the immunopathologic and ultrastructural features usually allow differentiation from postinfectious glomerulonephritis, even if specific diagnosis is not possible. Acute presentation or deterioration may also be caused by focal or diffuse crescentic disease, but the typical endocapillary changes can almost always be recognized beneath the crescents (Fig. 8-4). A few biopsy specimens have diagnostic changes of MCGN in only a proportion of the glomeruli, the remainder showing only mesangial proliferation. If the immunopathologic and ultrastructural features are diffuse, these biopsy specimens may be regarded as a developing stage of MCGN with a strong probability of relentless progression. Atypical findings on these special studies are, however, indications to consider associated conditions and to express caution about the long-term prognosis. In prolonged disease, glomerular foam cells may accumulate and segmental sclerosis may appear (Figs. 8-5, 8-6).

Electron Microscopy

Mesangial areas are strikingly enlarged by cellular proliferation and accumulated matrix. In advanced disease, this excessive matrix may contain collagen fibers and areas of calcification. The capillary lumina are reduced by a combina-

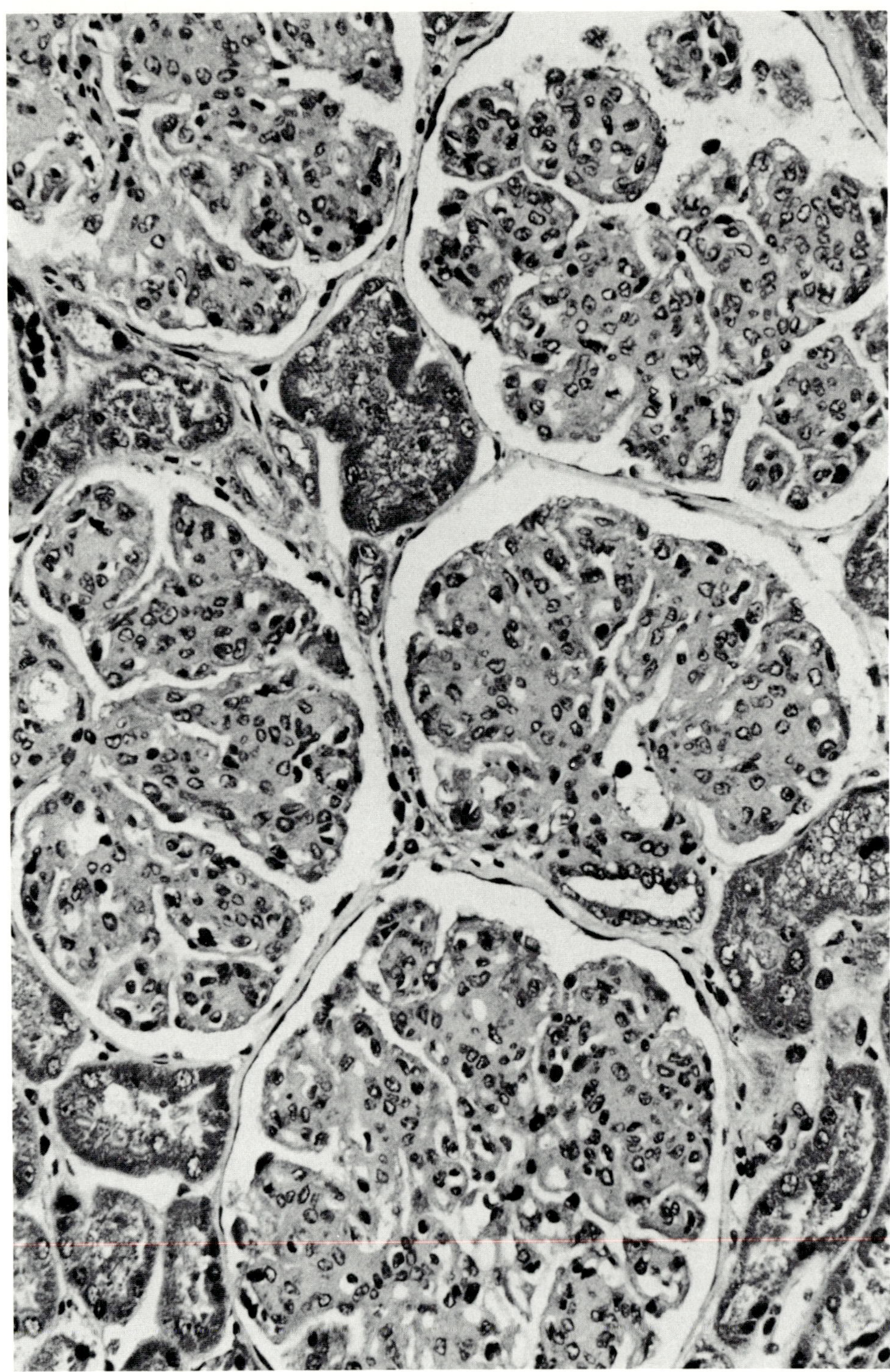

Figure 8-1. Biopsy specimen from a patient with MCGN with subendothelial deposits (type I). There is increased lobulation, diffuse mesangial hypercellularity, and thickening of the capillary walls (H&E stain, ×425).

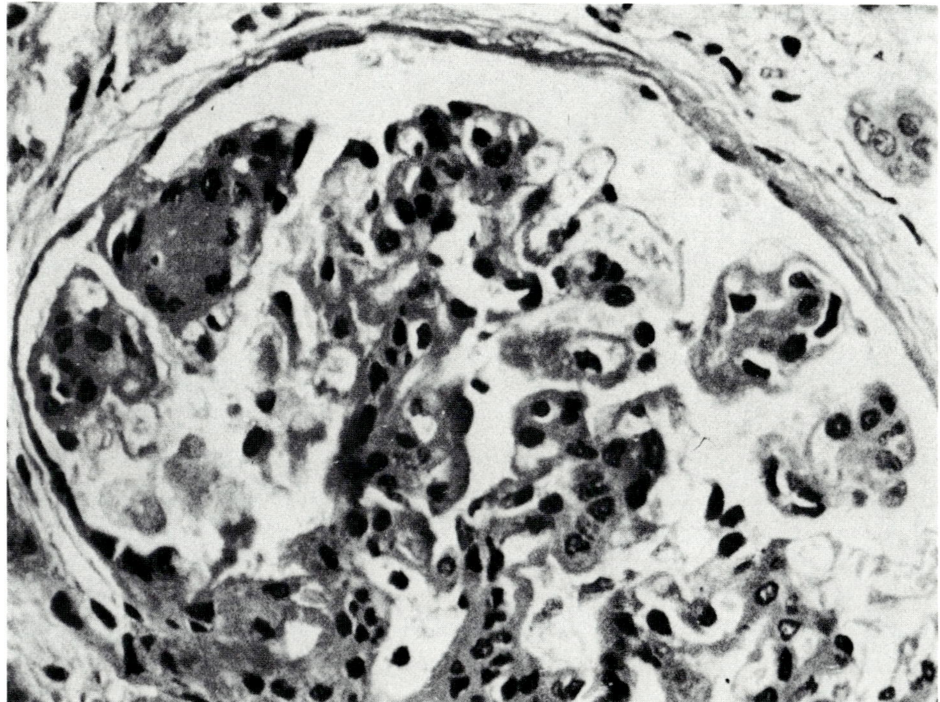

Figure 8-2. MCGN with subendothelial deposits (type I) and centrolobular sclerosis (PAS stain, ×800).

tion of peripheral mesangial expansion and the interposition of cells and matrix beneath the endothelium. Typically, there is a continuous layer of mesangial cytoplasm around the entire capillary with an irregular layer of new matrix underlying the intact basement membrane (5,20) (Figs. 8-7, 8-8, 8-9). Frequently, however, tangential sectioning demonstrates only part of this process, and a similar pattern may be produced by sections across the peripheral regions of mesangia. Dense deposits are present in mesangia and subendothelial regions, the latter sometimes forming large masses in a wire-loop configuration (Fig. 8-10). These deposits may extend into the membrane and often show irregularly lucent areas in advanced disease (Fig. 8-11). Subepithelial deposits, sometimes resembling humps, are present in a number of cases (3,6,41).

Immunofluorescence Microscopy
There are two general patterns of immunofluorescence in idiopathic MCGN (38,42). The majority of biopsy specimens show granular reactions for both immunoglobulins and complement along capillary walls (Fig. 8-12). In these cases the predominant immunoglobulin is IgG, and the early acting complement components C1 and C4 can be demonstrated as well as C3, although C3 may be present alone in the mesangium. The other pattern is of C3 reactions, without immunoglobulins or other complement components, distributed either in

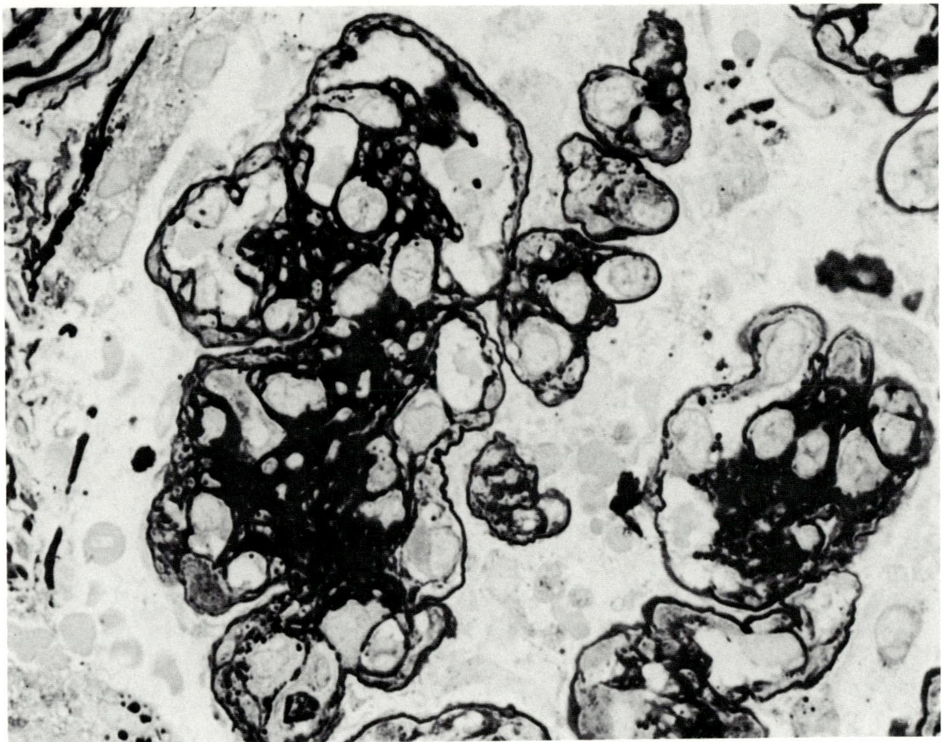

Figure 8-3. MCGN with subendothelial deposits (type I). Glomerulus showing marked increase in mesangial matrix in the centrolobular areas with peripheral extension of mesangium producing a double contour pattern in the loops (PASM stain, ×888).

mesangia or along capillary walls. Reactions for properdin may be found with either pattern but are more common in biopsy specimens showing only C3. In some cases staining with fibrinogen may reveal a prominent "train-track" pattern in the glomerular tufts (Fig. 8-13). The distribution and type of reactions in the "secondary" forms of MCGN may be distinct from these usual patterns, and the identification of atypical immunofluorescent reactions is an indication to search for associated disease.

Differential Diagnosis

The pathologic features of established MCGN are easily recognized, and diagnostic problems usually arise in cases of evolving disease or in other diseases showing lobular patterns or extensive interposition. Lobular changes occur in diabetic glomerulonephritis and multiple myeloma, but the electron and immunofluorescence microscopic features of these conditions are easily distinguished from MCGN. Mesangial interposition is common in many glomerular diseases characterized by mesangial proliferation, and occasional double contours, especially near the stalk or around segmental lesions, can be ignored.

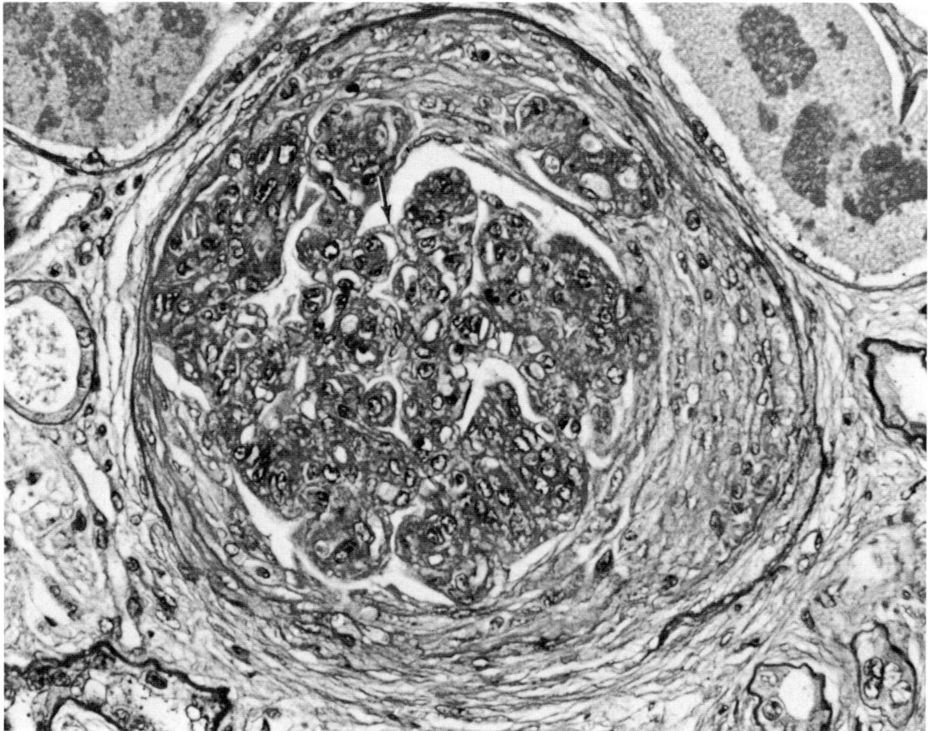

Figure 8-4. MCGN with subendothelial deposits (type I). The glomerular tuft is surrounded by an epithelial crescent. Some capillary loops have a double contour appearance (arrow) (PAS stain, ×450).

Double contours are sometimes very extensive in preeclampsia but, as in the other conditions causing interposition, consideration of the electron and immunofluorescence microscopic features should prevent diagnostic confusion.

Prognosis

The usual course for idiopathic MCGN is relentless progression to renal failure. The mean mortality in one large series was 6.4% over 10 years with 50% of the patients either dead or in renal failure 11 years after presentation (6). More rapid progression occurs in patients with azotemia or the nephrotic syndrome at presentation, but there is dispute over the prognostic significance of hypocomplementemia (6,38,43). Spontaneous remission occurs occasionally, and there is, therefore, dispute over the value of therapy (6,41). Most studies have found no improvement in prognosis with various forms of therapy (6,35), but partial or complete remissions have been reported with corticosteroid and immunosuppressive regimes (44,45). Recurrent glomerulonephritis occurs in transplanted kidneys and has occasionally developed de novo, but its frequency is difficult to establish because of the similar mesangiocapillary changes occurring in transplant glomerulopathy (46,46a). Diagnosis of recurrent or de novo

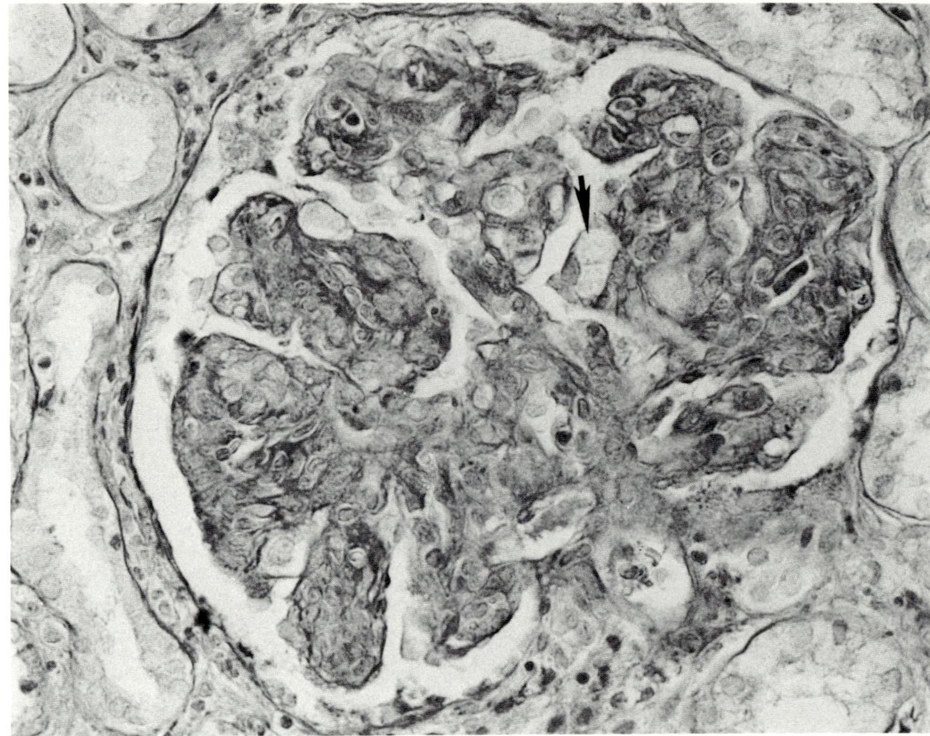

Figure 8-5. MCGN with subendothelial deposits (type I) and numerous foam cells (arrow) (PAS stain, ×550).

MCGN in transplanted kidneys is best restricted to those biopsy specimens showing subendothelial deposits and typical immunofluorescence findings (47).

DENSE DEPOSIT DISEASE (MESANGIOCAPILLARY GLOMERULONEPHRITIS, TYPE II)

Dense deposit disease (DDD) is a specific clinicopathologic entity with a unique morphologic appearance and a particular relationship to alternate pathway complement activation.

Pathogenesis

The morphologic feature peculiar to DDD is a unique dense transformation of renal basement membranes (48). Biochemical studies of the abnormal membranes demonstrate an excess of sialic acid and a deficiency in cystine but no immunoglobulin. Most interest in the investigation of the disease has centered on its characteristic complement abnormalities (30,32). With very few exceptions

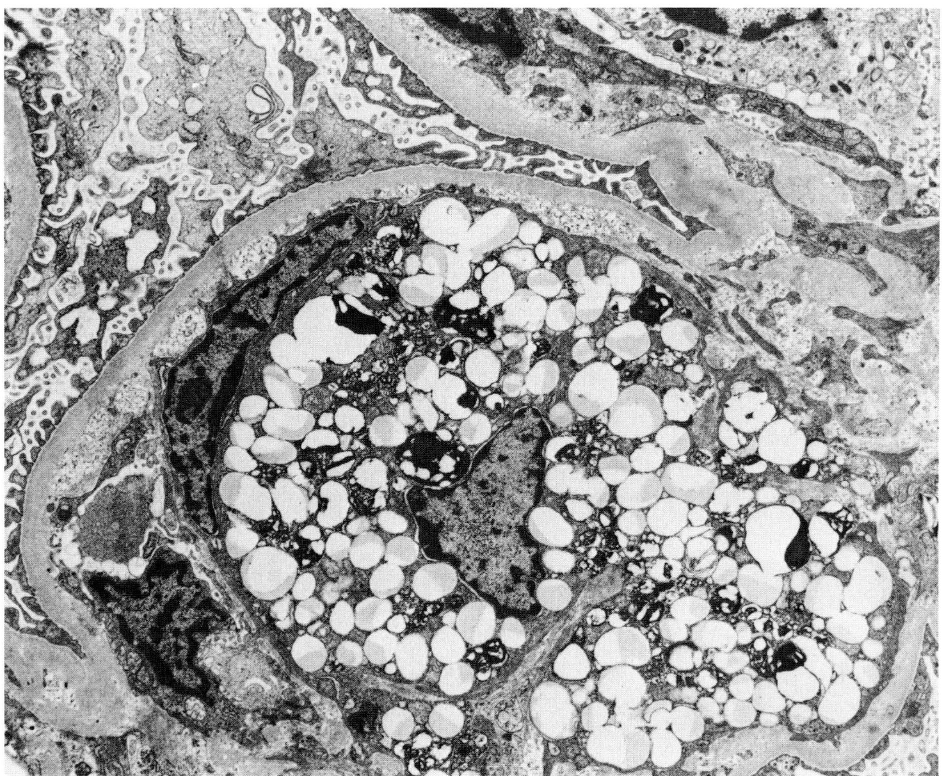

Figure 8-6. Electron micrograph of a mesangial foam cell from the same biopsy specimen as Figure 8-5 (×6,000).

(49), patients with DDD show persistent and profound depletion of serum C3, with normal values for the early acting components, and an abnormal circulating substance, C3 nephritic factor (C3NeF) (40). This factor causes continued activation of the alternate complement pathway by altering the delicate balance between activator and inactivator enzymes. Normally, activation of the alternate complement pathway is controlled by a variety of mechanisms, including spontaneous decay of the cleaving enzymes and a naturally occurring substance, C3b inactivator. This inactivator prevents C3b, a major cleavage product of C3, from interacting with C3 proactivator (factor B) and C3 proactivator convertase (factor D) to produce persistent C3 activation in a continuously reinforcing system. C3NeF increases the generation of C3b and destroys the normal balancing systems by promoting the stability of the converting enzymes and reducing their sensitivity to C3b inactivator (50). The nature of C3NeF is still uncertain, but it appears to be an auto-antibody immunoglobulin of IgG class acting against a component of the alternate complement system (51). The depressed C3 concentrations in patients with DDD are only partially caused by C3NeF, which may persist after nephrectomy, since there is also evidence for decreased C3 synthesis (30,32).

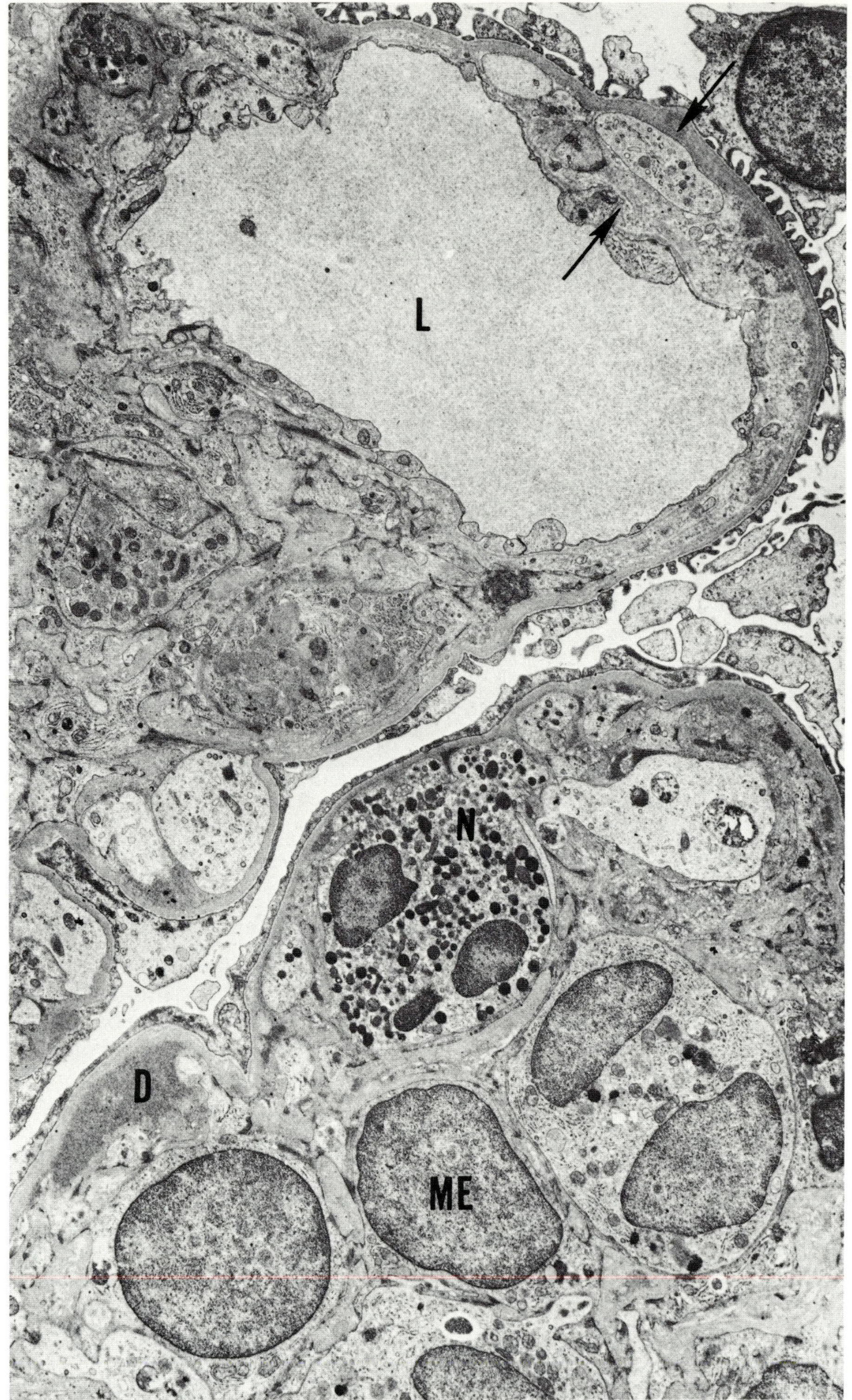

Figure 8-7. MCGN with subendothelial deposits (type I). There is proliferation of mesangium and peripheral extension of mesangial material in the periphery of the loop (arrows). In addition to the thickening of the capillary wall, there is prominent inflammatory cell infiltration and small amounts of mesangial deposits (D). L, capillary lumen; ME, mesangium; N, neutrophilic leukocyte (×6,400).

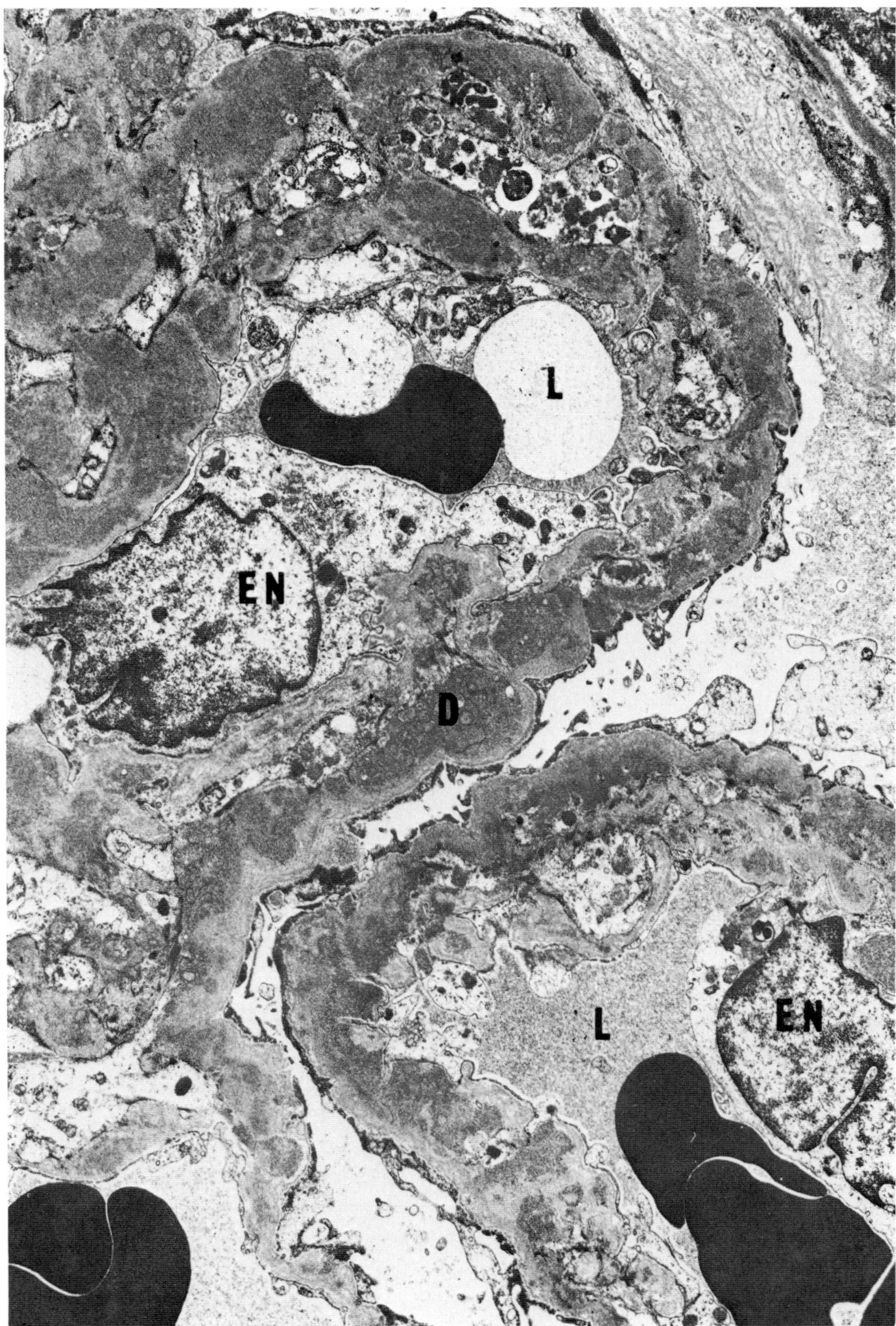

Figure 8-8. Electron micrograph illustrating "splitting" of the basement membrane by mesangial interposition in MCGN with subendothelial deposits (type I). Large subendothelial deposits (D) are present along the loops. L, capillary lumen; EN, endothelium (×6,100).

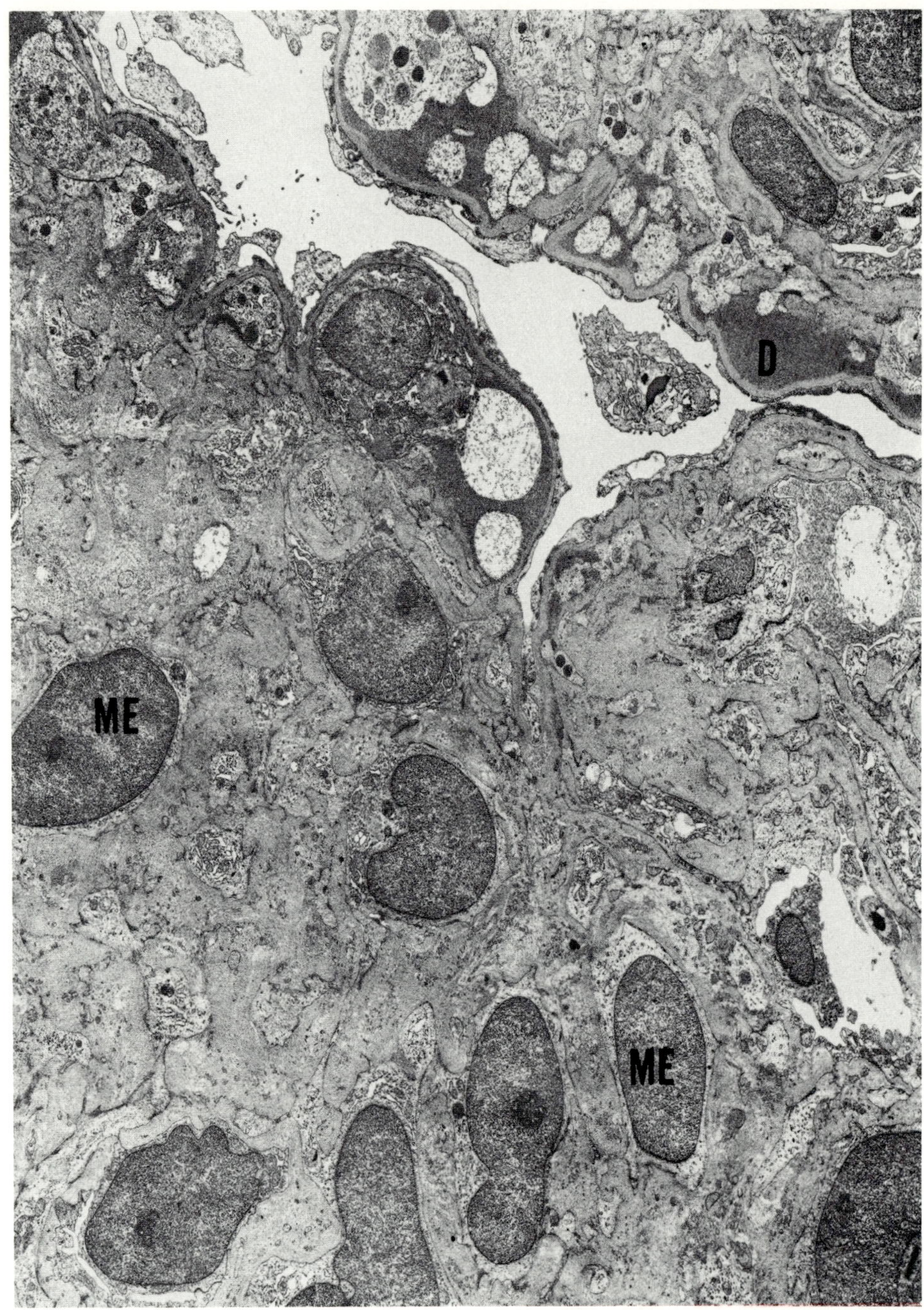

Figure 8-9. Advanced MCGN with subendothelial deposits (type I). There is marked proliferation of mesangial cells and increase in mesangial matrix in the central portions of the glomerular lobules. The capillary loops are narrowed and show subendothelial deposits (D). ME, mesangium (×5,750).

132

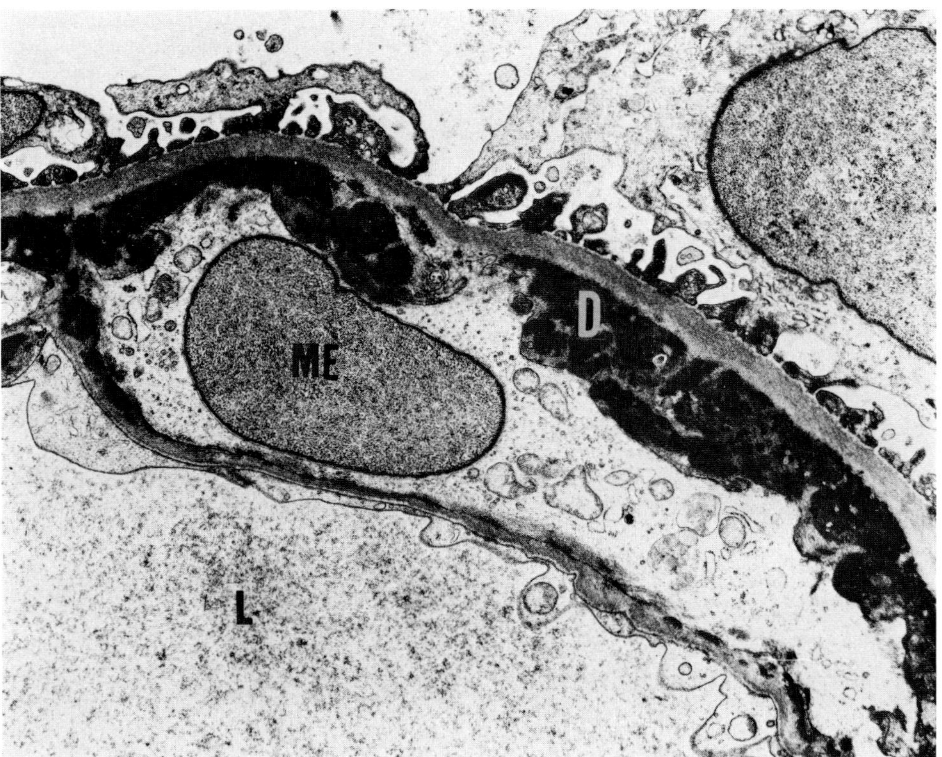

Figure 8-10. MCGN with subendothelial deposits (type I). Peripheral capillary loop showing large subendothelial deposits (D) and mesangial cell (ME) interposition. L, capillary lumen (×16,700).

Analysis of the role of these complement abnormalities in the pathogenesis of DDD has been aided by an association with partial lipodystrophy in about 10% of patients (52). Circulating C3NeF and profound depressions of serum C3 are common in patients with partial lipodystrophy, and may precede the development of renal disease by some years (28). The glomerular lesion in patients with partial lipodystrophy is almost always DDD, but MCGN of subendothelial deposit type has occasionally been reported (28,29). The observation of complement depletion preceding glomerulonephritis suggests that prolonged complement activation may contribute to the development of the membrane lesion. There is some experimental evidence to suggest the formation of dense deposits by alternate pathway complement cleavage, but prolonged systemic activation of complement in experimental animals has not produced glomerular disease (3,53). Aside from partial lipodystrophy, the only known association of complement abnormalities with DDD is in one patient with mucocutaneous candidiasis, in whom *Candida* antigens could be identified in the glomeruli (54). In general, the lack of immunoglobulins in the diseased basement membranes is against an immune complex pathogenesis. Circulating immune complexes have been iden-

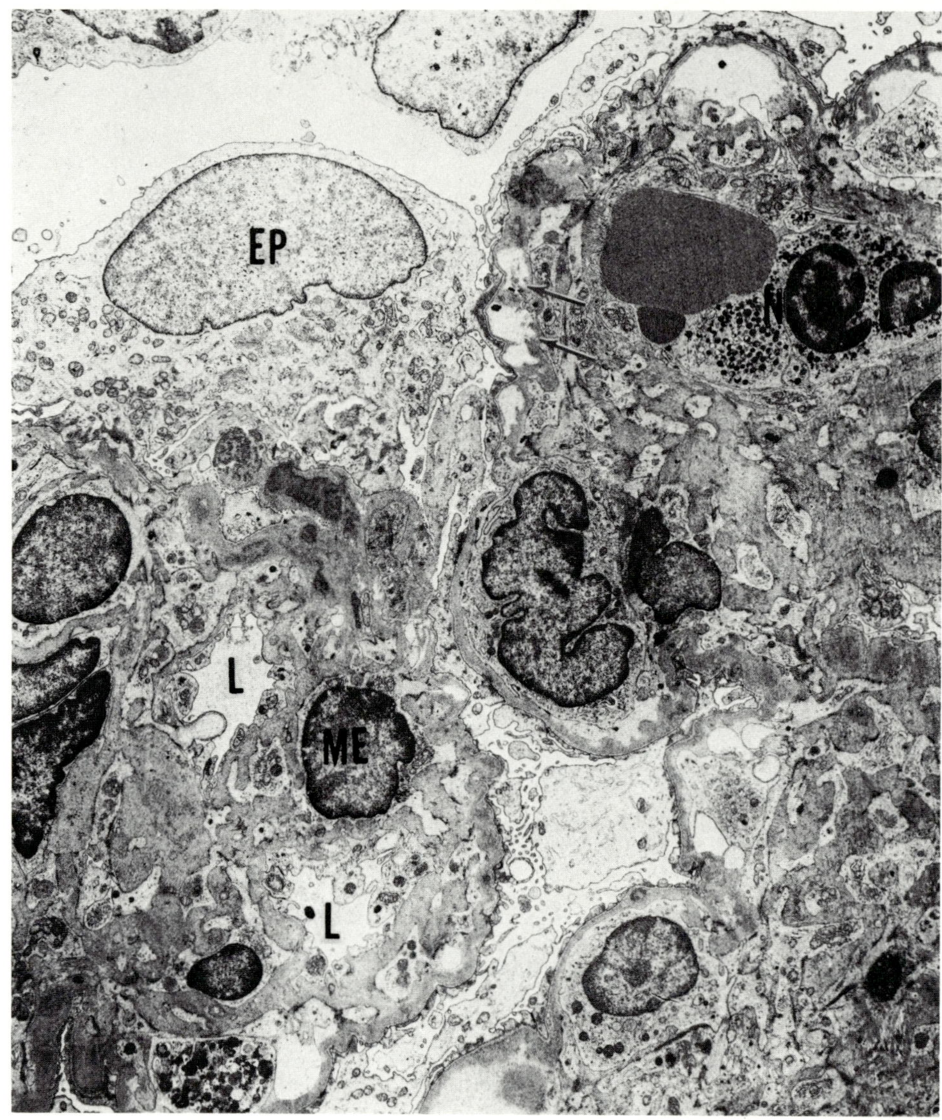

Figure 8-11. Advanced MCGN with subendothelial deposits (type I). There is peripheral mesangial interposition, marked increase in mesangial matrix, and prominent irregular intramembranous electron lucent areas (arrows). L, capillary lumen; EP, epithelial cell; EN, endothelial cell; ME, mesangium; N, neutrophilic leukocyte (×2,450).

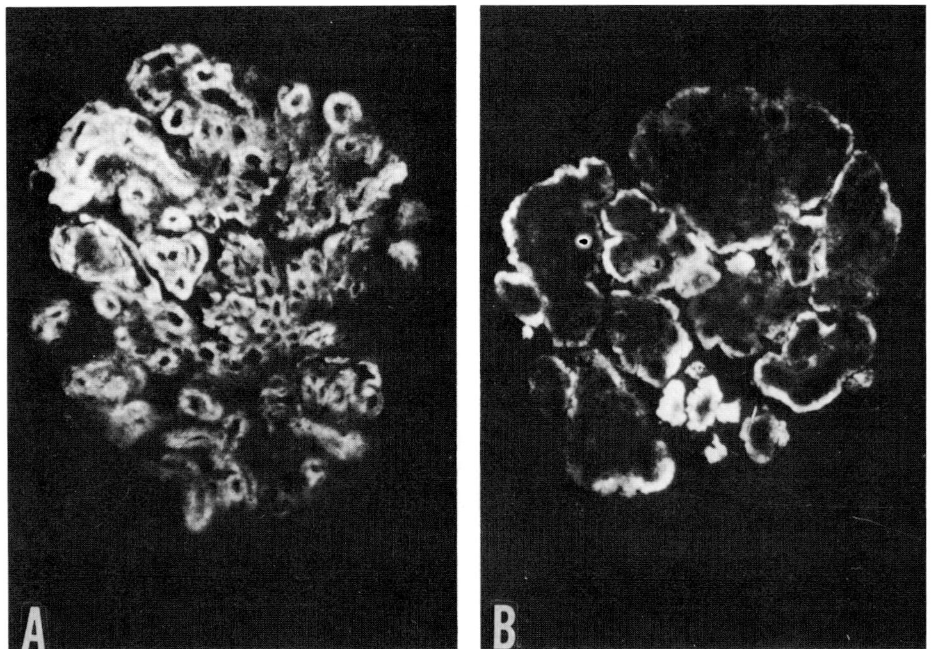

Figure 8-12. MCGN with subendothelial deposits (type I). (*a*) Granular peripheral and mesangial deposits of IgG. (*b*) Granular fluorescent deposits of C3 in capillary walls with lobular distribution (×250).

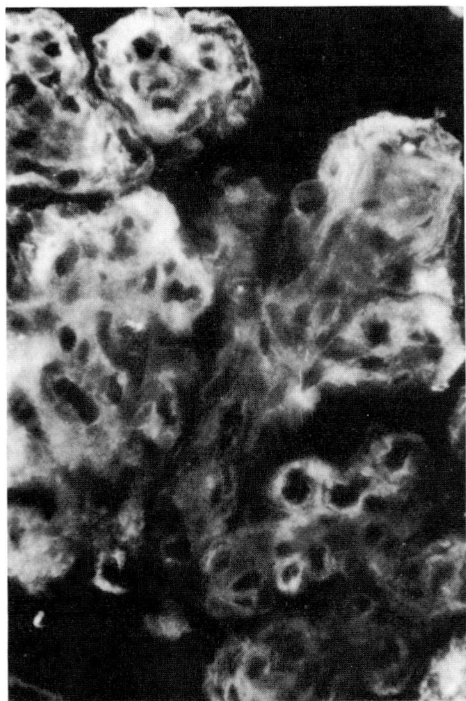

Figure 8-13. MCGN with subendothelial deposits (type I). Centrolobular mesangial deposits of fibrinogen with "train-track" features along capillary loops (×400).

tified in a few patients, but these may represent secondary developments, corresponding to the subepithelial humps (55). There may, in fact, be an increased tendency to superimposed immune complex disease because of immune deficiency secondary to complement depletion (32).

Clinical Manifestations and Course

The disease affects children and young adults exclusively, being rare in people over the age of 25 and never seen in children younger than 4 years (52). Most series report a slight male predominance (52,56,57). Clinical manifestation often follows an upper respiratory infection, often of streptococcal type (58). The infection may precede an acute nephritic syndrome or an episode of macroscopic hematuria, but up to a third of patients present with the nephrotic syndrome (56−59). A minority of patients are first seen with rapidly progressive renal failure secondary to crescentic disease, and there is a potent tendency for the development of crescents to cause an abrupt deterioration in renal function at any time during the course (56,58). The disease pursues a relentless course to renal failure, often with nephrotic, nephritic and hematuric episodes. As has already been discussed, profound and persistent depression of serum C3 is usual, often with circulating C3NeF (28,39,40,57). In some patients, however, the serum concentration of C3 is variable and C3NeF is absent (39,57). Concentrations of the early acting complement components are usually normal (40).

Pathologic Characteristics

Light Microscopy

The characteristic feature of established DDD is an eosinophilic, refractile, and ribbonlike thickening of basement membranes (Fig. 8-14). This is usually most pronounced in the glomeruli but can often be detected also in Bowman's capsules and tubular basement membranes. As expected from the excess of sialic acid residues, this thickening is brilliantly PAS-positive and has a very characteristic dark blue color in plastic-embedded sections stained with toluidine blue (Fig. 8-15). This membrane stains green with the Masson trichrome stain, reacts with thioflavin T to produce brilliant fluorescence, and has a quite typical light brown color in silver-stained sections, sometimes with thin peripheral bands of normal black staining (48,56,58, 59a). Although these membrane appearances are highly characteristic, they may be absent early in the disease, and extensive intramembranous deposits in other conditions may produce a similar appearance. Light microscopic diagnosis is, therefore, not always either possible or completely reliable, and electron microscopy is necessary for unequivocal identification of the membrane changes.

There is no constant relationship between the extent of the membrane lesion and the degree of cellular proliferation (48). Proliferation may be either segmental or completely absent, but there is usually diffuse mesangial enlargement caused by increases in both cells and matrix. Frequently, brightly eosinophilic and refractile granules can be detected in the mesangial areas (Fig. 8-14). Mesangial proliferation may be pronounced, and some biopsy specimens show a

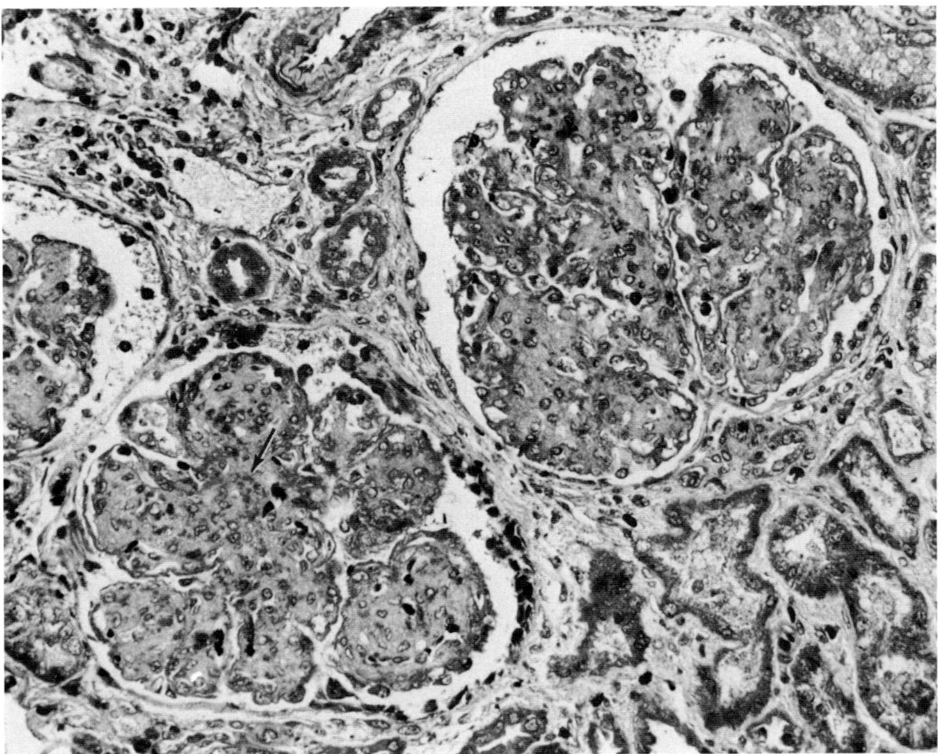

Figure 8-14. Dense deposit disease. There is mesangial hypercellularity with accentuation of the glomerular lobular architecture and thickening of the capillary walls. Granular eosinophilic deposits are present in the central portions of the lobules (arrow) (H&E stain, ×300).

lobular pattern with extensive interposition, which mimics Type I MCGN (Fig. 8-15). In such biopsy specimens, careful examination of the membrane is necessary to prevent the confusion of the two conditions that has occurred in the past. Polymorphs are often present in increased numbers within glomerular capillaries, and subepithelial "humps" can sometimes be recognized by light microscopy (58). The disease is frequently complicated by crescents and may present with a diffuse crescentic pattern that obscures the membrane lesions (Fig. 8-16).

Electron Microscopy

Dense deposit disease is characterized by the presence of a ribbonlike zone of increased density located centrally within the thickened basement membrane (48,58). This material lacks the granularity seen in conventional deposits and is often distributed in a segmental pattern, especially adjacent to mesangial areas (58). Similar dense transformation may occur in the mesangial matrix, in Bowman's capsule and in the basement membranes of the convoluted tubules (Figs. 8-17–8-22). Areas of density may also be found in the membranes of peritubular capillaries and in the elastic laminae of arterioles, but the collecting tubule mem-

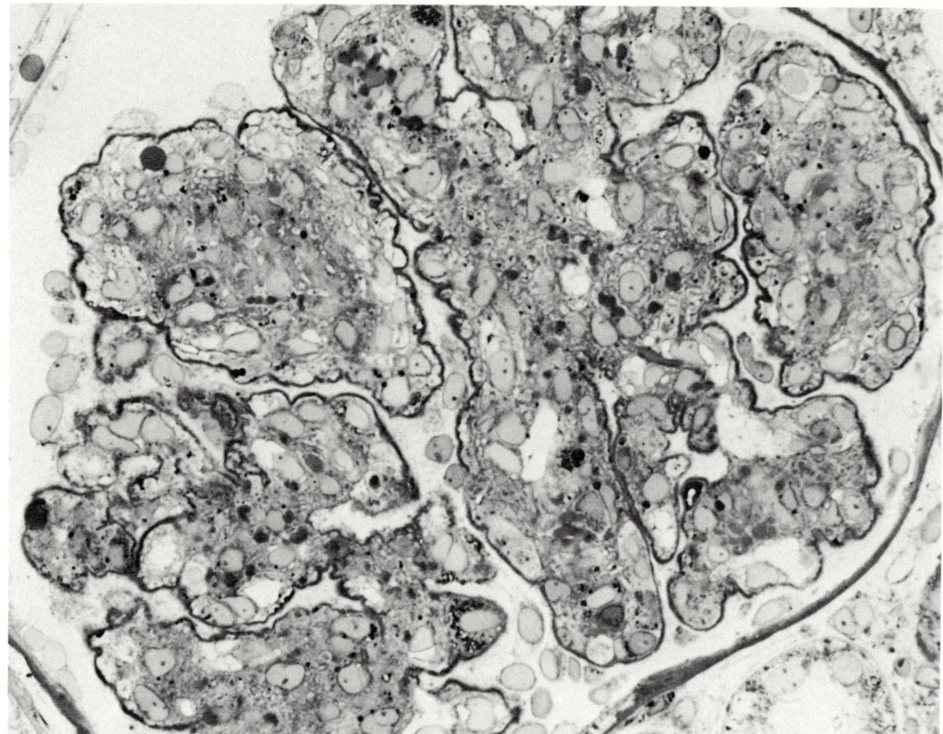

Figure 8-15. Dense deposit disease. There is hypercellularity and a continuous ribbonlike thickening of the glomerular basement membrane. Intramembranous dark material is also present in Bowman's capsule (plastic embedded toluidine blue stain, ×670).

branes are spared (52,58). In addition to the ribbonlike dense transformation, granular subepithelial deposits indistinguishable from "humps" are common, and there may also be flattened, irregular deposits associated with epimembranous spikes (58,60).

Immunofluorescence Microscopy

The typical pattern gives an accurate diagnosis and consists of weak and discontinuous reactions for C3 along capillary walls enclosing brightly staining granules and small masses in the mesangia (58) (Fig. 8-23). Reactions are usually limited to C3, although properdin has been demonstrated in some cases; the early acting complement components are usually absent (39,57–60a). Careful examination with high magnification demonstrates that the reactions are not homogeneous but appear to represent zones of staining around, rather than within, the dense material (60a). Thus, the membrane reactions are formed by parallel, thin strips of staining along either aspect of the dense material, while the mesangial granules are, in fact, rings with nonstaining centers (Fig. 8-23). Similar bilaminar patterns of reactions are commonly seen in Bowman's capsules and along tubular basement membranes. Granular capillary wall reactions for C3 and various

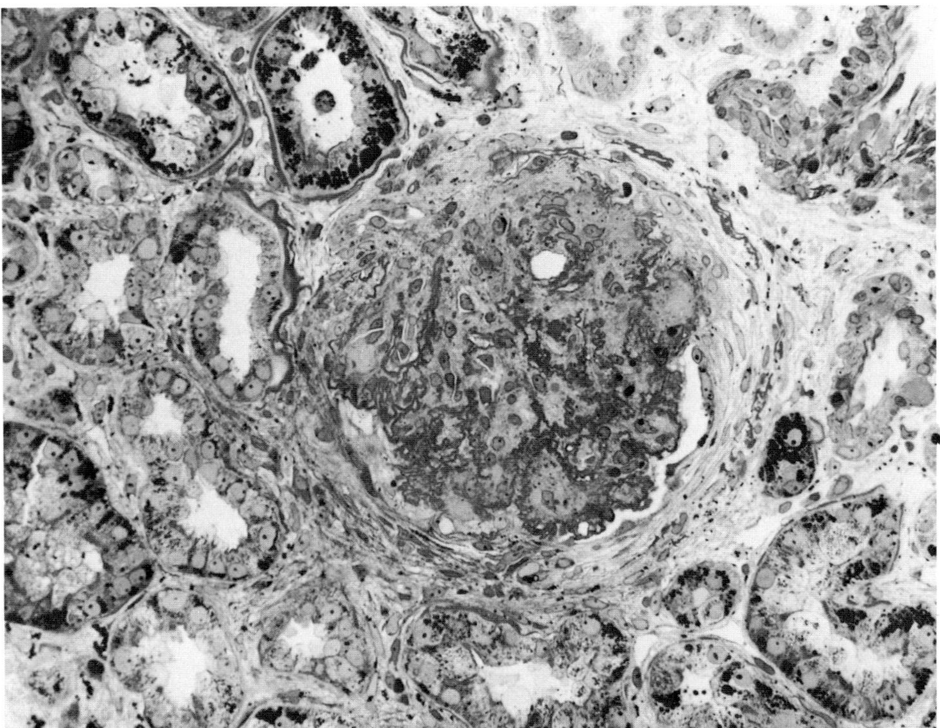

Figure 8-16. Advanced dense deposit disease with fibroepithelial crescent and central sclerosis of the glomerular lobules. Note the presence of intramembranous deposits in both glomerular and tubular basement membranes (left upper corner). In addition, numerous lipid and protein transport droplets are present in the proximal tubular epithelium (plastic embedded toluidine blue stain, ×310).

immunoglobulins may be superimposed upon this typical pattern, possibly corresponding to subepithelial humps.

Differential Diagnosis

There is little difficulty in the diagnosis of typical DDD, but extensive intramembranous deposits occurring in other diseases may produce a superficially similar light and electron microscopic appearance. Generally, careful ultrastructural examination, paying particular attention to the lack of granularity in DDD, and consideration of the immunopathologic findings will resolve the diagnosis. Occasionally, however, precise diagnosis may be extremely difficult and may require ultrastructural examination of silver-impregnated ultrathin sections (61,62). Dense transformation of basement membranes similar to DDD occur with systemic deposition of kappa light chains in myelomatosis but may be distinguished by the granular pattern of the dense material and the immunofluorescent demonstration of light chains in the dense deposits (16). A mesangial proliferative pattern of glomerulonephritis with deposits similar to those of DDD, but less

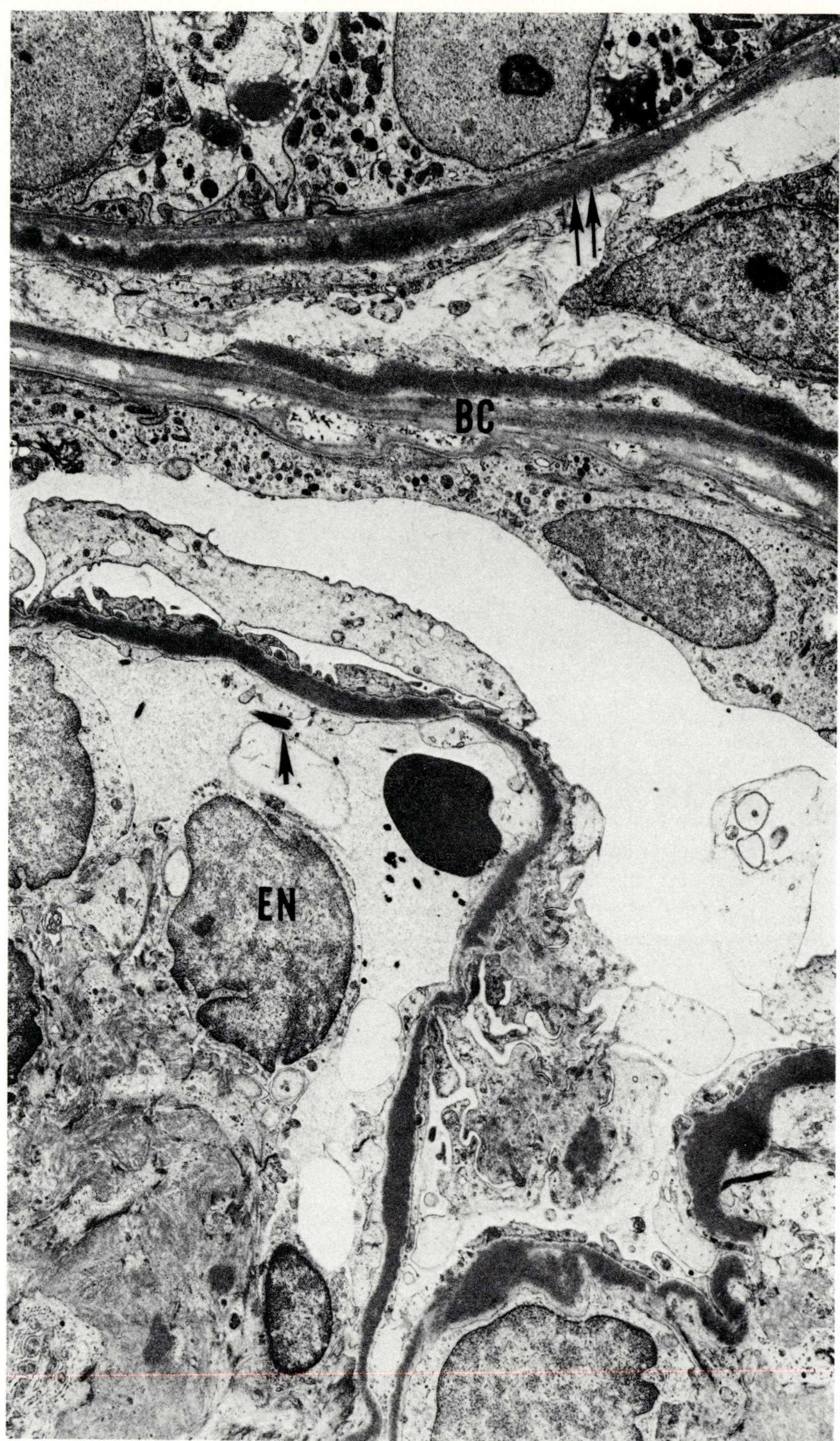

Figure 8-17. Electron micrograph from a biopsy specimen of a patient with dense deposit disease. There is homogenous dense material within the lamina densa of the glomerular basement membrane as well as in the outer aspect of Bowman's capsule (BC) and tubular basement membrane (double arrow). Small tactoids of fibrin are present in the capillary lumen (arrow). EN, endothelial cell (×5,600).

140

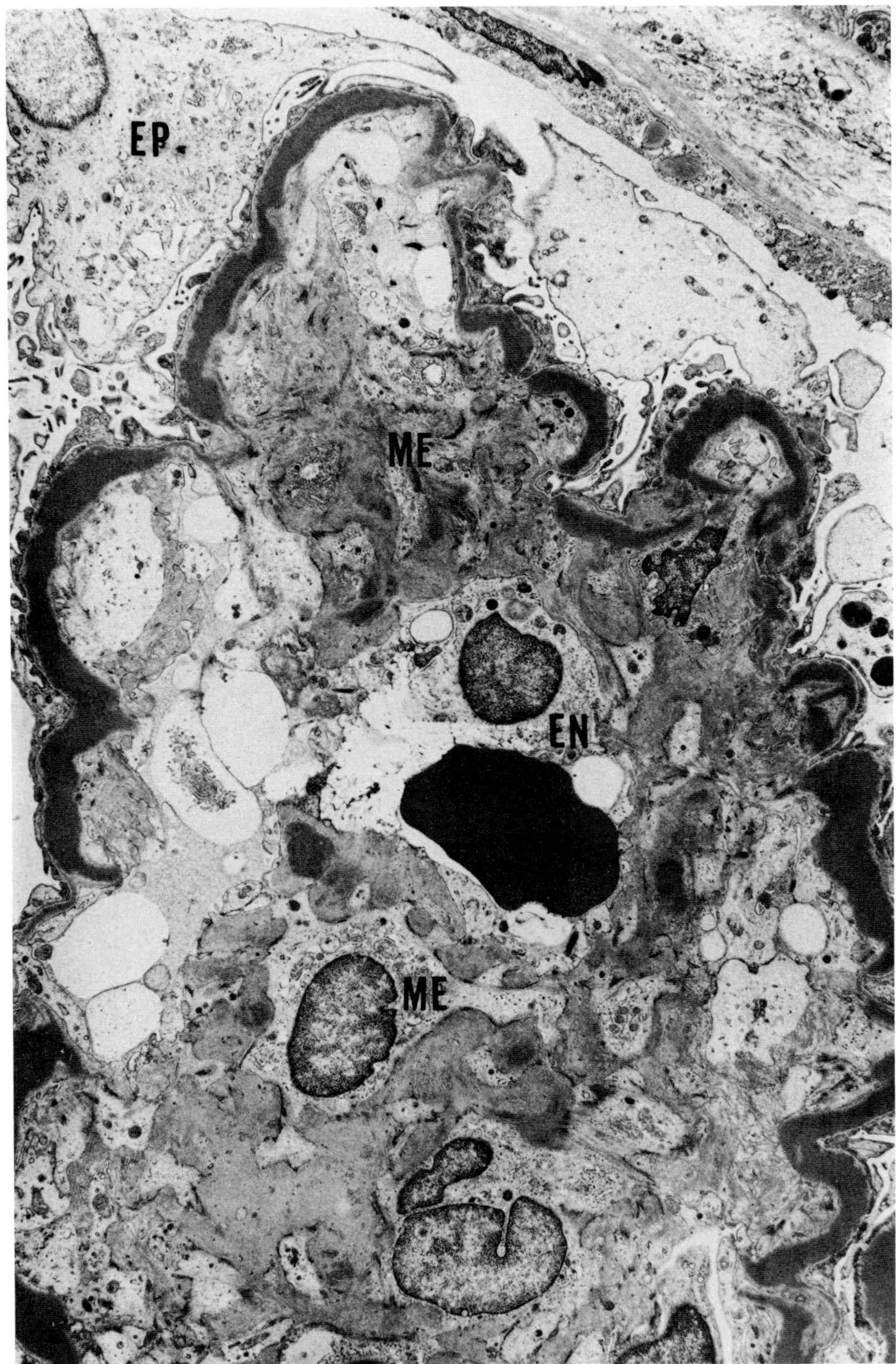

Figure 8-18. Dense deposit disease. Peripheral loop with segmental dense deposits within the lamina densa and peripheral mesangial extension. The capillary lumen is narrowed and contains a red blood cell. EN, endothelial cell; EP, epithelial cell; ME, mesangium (×4,850).

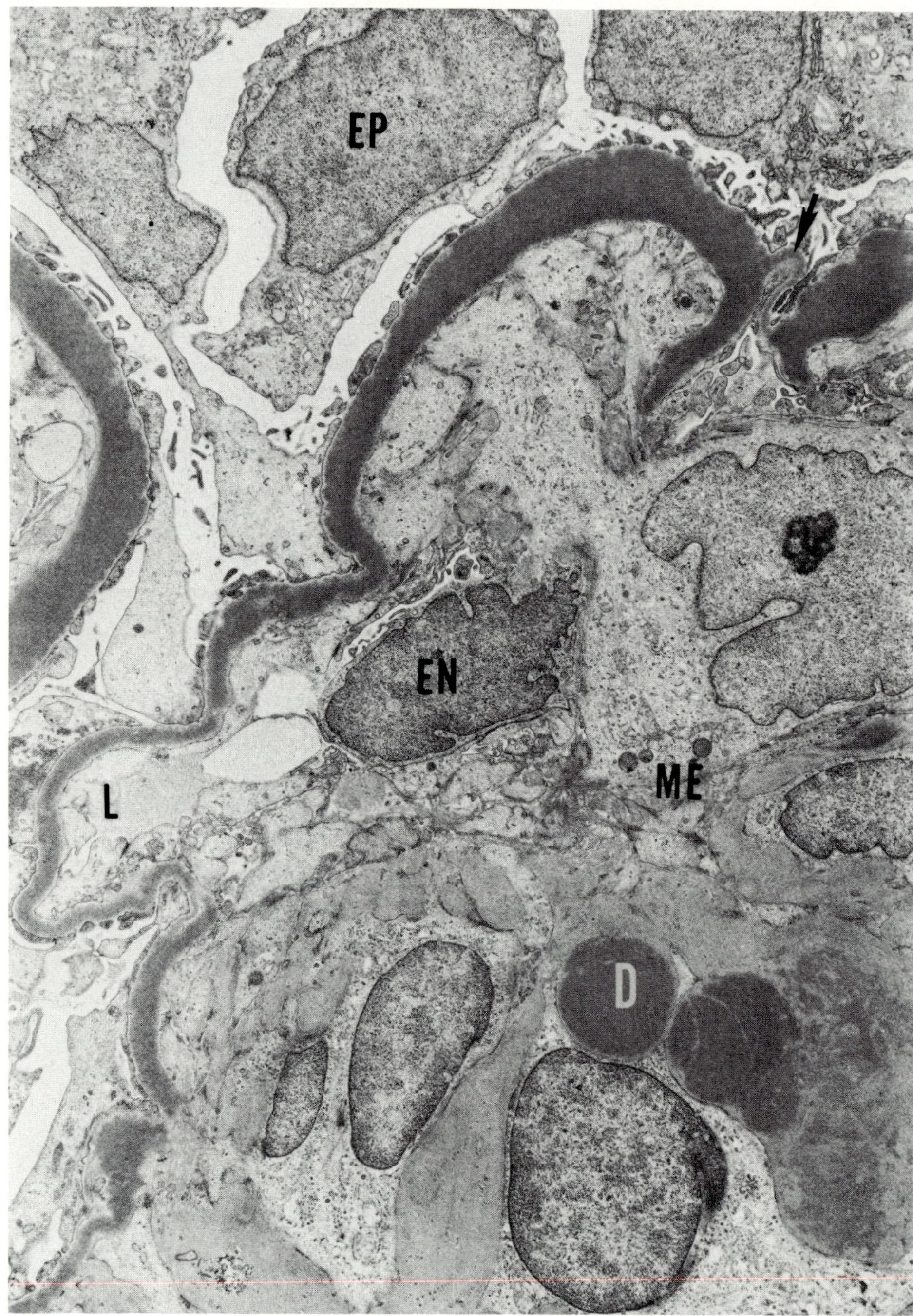

Figure 8-19. Dense deposit disease. Electron micrograph demonstrating irregular thickening of the capillary walls by dense intramembranous deposits. The capillary loops arc narrowed and there is focal attenuation of the basement membrane (arrow). Nodular electron dense deposits (D) are present in the mesangium. L, capillary lumen; EN, endothelial cell; EP, epithelial cell; ME, mesangium (×6,700).

142

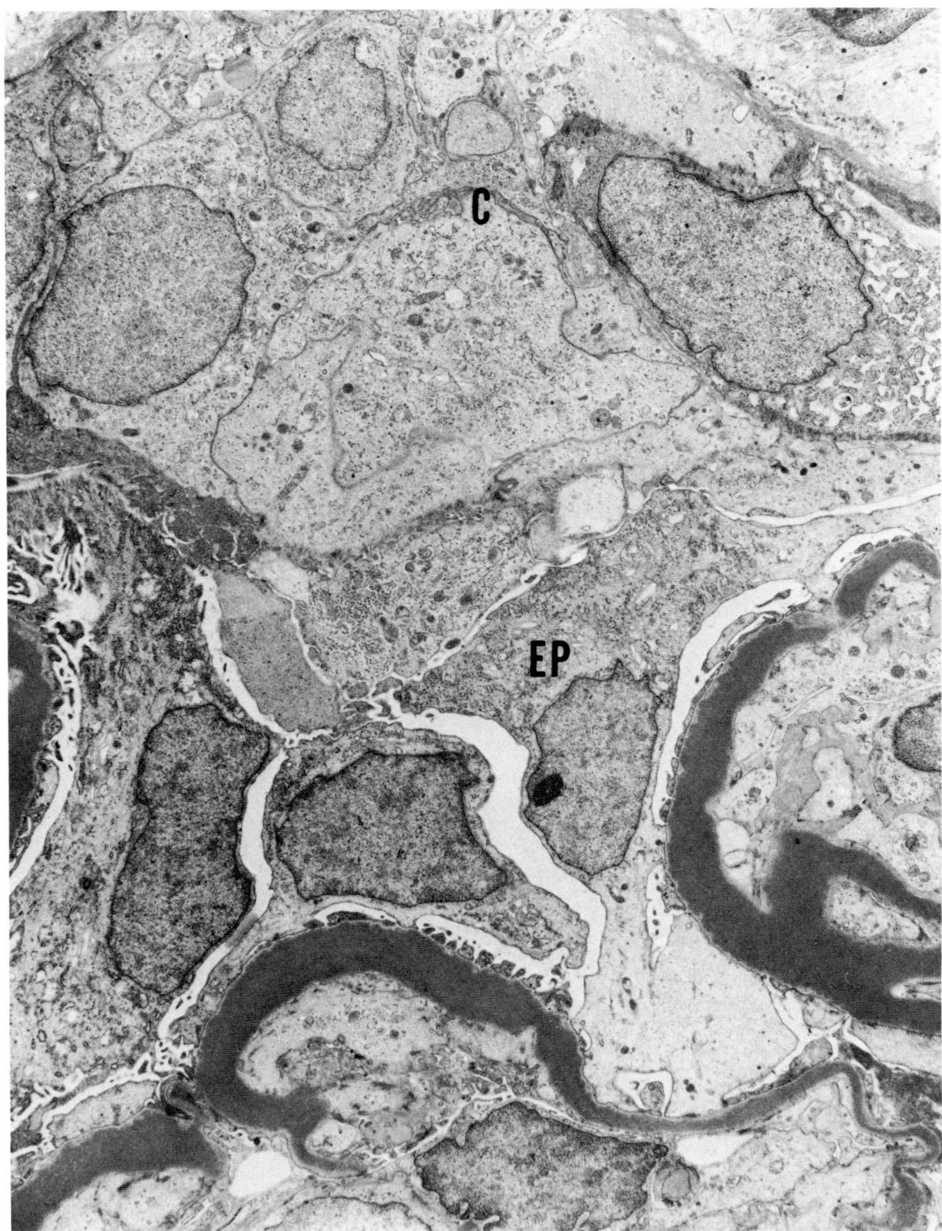

Figure 8-20. Dense deposit disease. Electron micrograph of the same case as in Figure 8-16. The glomerular basement membrane is irregularly thickened by intramembranous deposits with a much greater density than the lamina densa. The upper portion of the picture shows an epithelial crescent (C). EP, visceral epithelial cell (×5,350).

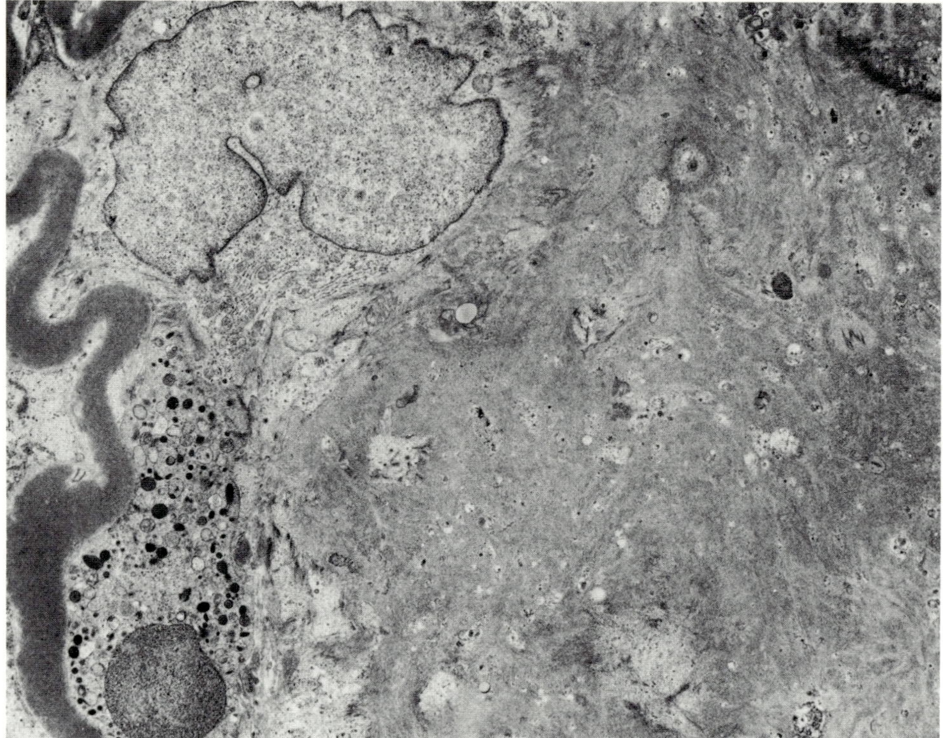

Figure 8-21. Dense deposit disease. Same case as in Figure 8-16, showing marked increase in mesangial matrix in the central areas of lobular sclerosis (right) and intramembranous dense deposits ($\times$5,400).

extensively distributed, has recently been described. Depression of serum C3 was present in these patients, but C3NeF could not be detected and the lesion was clinically indolent (63).

Prognosis

Progressive renal destruction is almost invariable, and only very rare examples of spontaneous remission have been recorded (58). The decline in renal function may be steady or abrupt with the development of crescentic disease. There is no evidence for any beneficial effect of therapy with either corticosteroids or immunosuppressive agents (52). In long-term studies, the mean annual mortality is 5%, and 50% of patients are either dead or in chronic renal failure by 9 to 11 years after presentation (56,58). Aside from the presence of crescents, no morphologic feature appears to be correlated with the rapidity of this progression but, clinically, the presence of hypergammaglobulinemia or the nephrotic syndrome are poor prognostic signs (56). Recurrence of the membrane abnormality is almost invariable in transplanted kidneys; it may occur as early as two months after transplantation and has affected two sequential grafts in the same patient (64,46a). There is no constant relationship between persistent or renewed

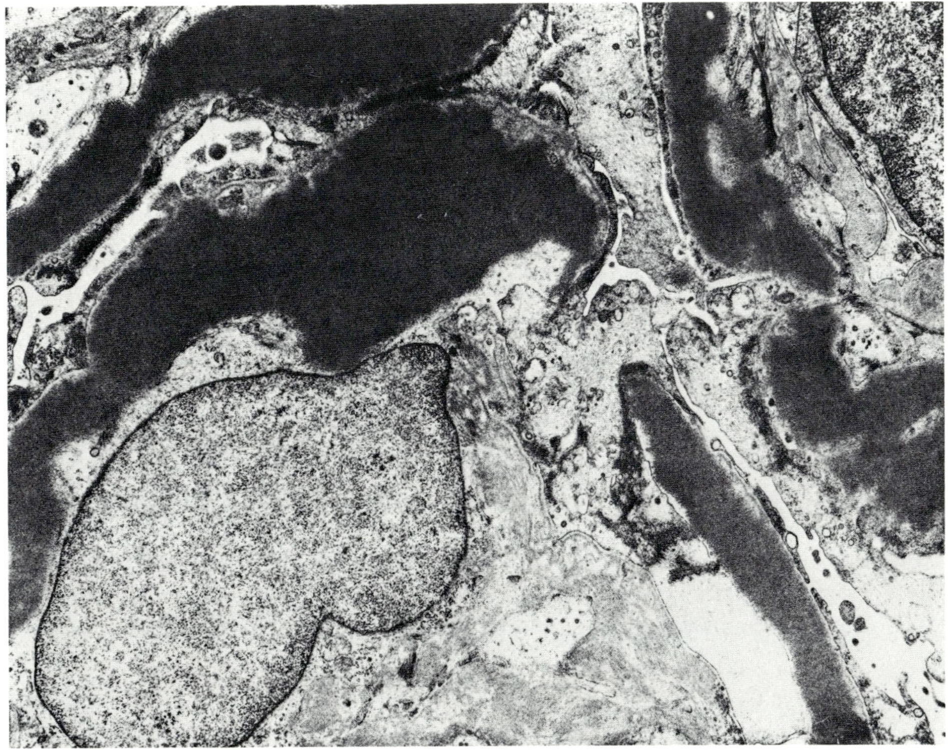

Figure 8-22. Electron micrograph from a biopsy specimen of a patient with crescentic dense deposit disease showing rupture of the basement membrane (×8,400).

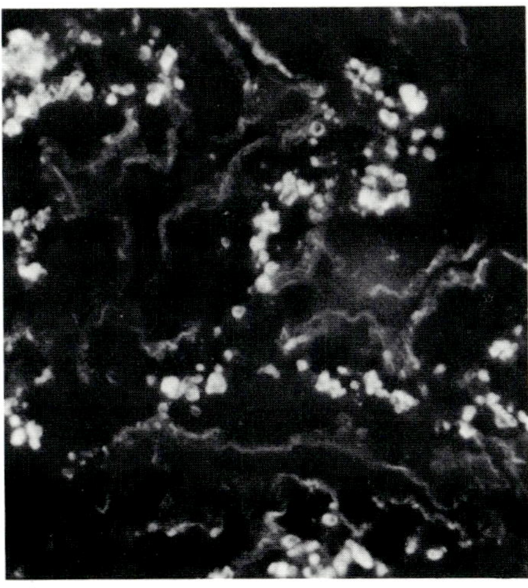

Figure 8-23. Dense deposit disease showing weak linear fluorescent staining along the capillary basement membranes and bright granular deposits in the mesangium. Note that some of the mesangial deposits have a ringlike appearance (antihuman C3, ×250).

145

hypocomplementemia after transplantation and the development of recurrent disease (64a). The abnormal density appears earliest near the vascular pole and adjacent to the mesangia (65,65a). Morphologic recurrence is usually not accompanied by cellular proliferation, and the clinical manifestations are usually minimal and nonprogressive (46,65a). There is one report of the unique association of DDD and de novo membranous nephropathy in a transplanted kidney (65).

VARIANTS OF MESANGIOCAPILLARY GLOMERULONEPHRITIS (TYPE III)

Recently, there have been reports of glomerular lesions, appearing under the light microscope, similar to MCGN or DDD but showing a characteristic ultrastructural pattern of membrane disruption (61,62). This disruption was produced by massive accumulation within the membrane, and on either side, of granular deposits, which often appeared refractile and eosinophilic on light microscopy (Figs. 8-24, 8-25). The extent of membrane disruption can be demonstrated best by silver impregnation of the ultrathin sections examined by electron microscopy, since this technique distinguishes the silver-negative deposits of the variant from the argyrophilic density of DDD. The clinical features and prognosis of these patients appear similar to those with MCGN or DDD. Another

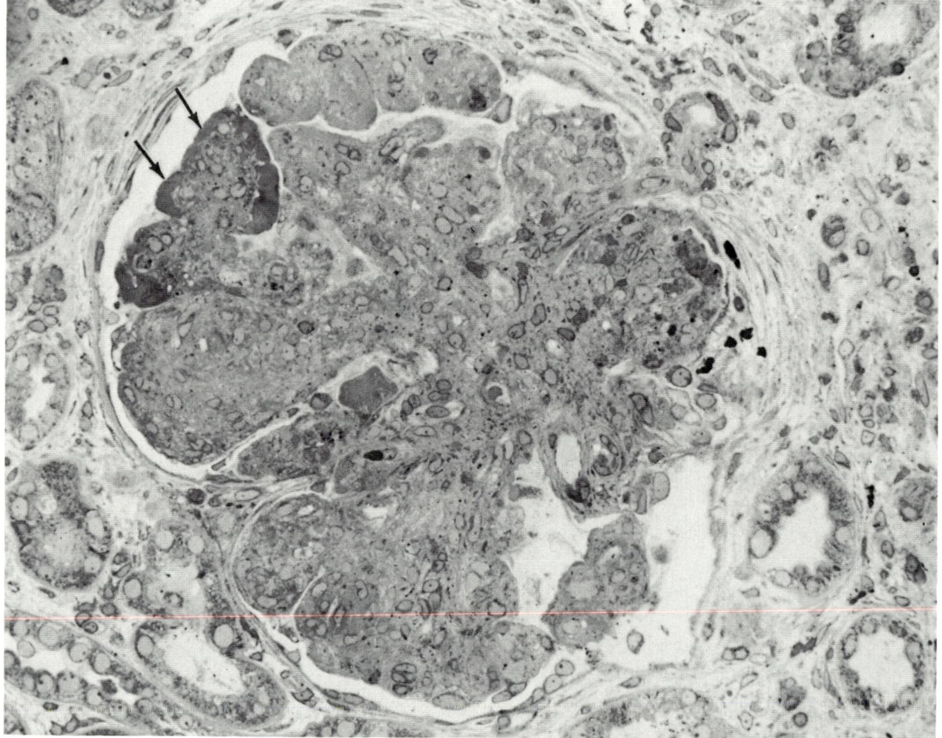

Figure 8-24. MCGN, type III. The glomerulus is enlarged, hypercellular, and shows accentuation of its lobular architecture. The basement membrane is irregularly thickened by large amounts of deposits (arrows) (plastic embedded toluidine blue stain, ×450).

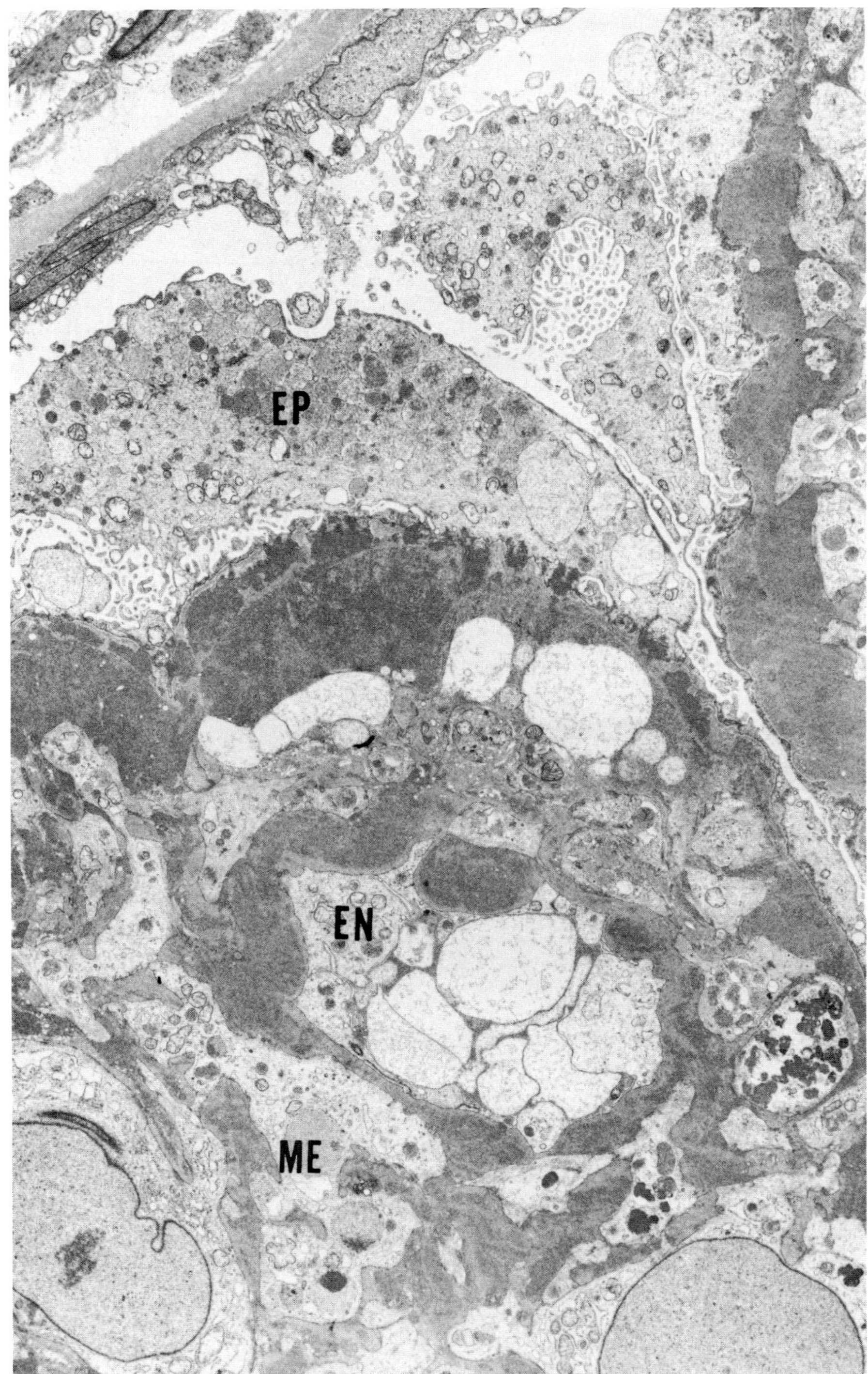

Figure 8-25. MCGN, type III. Glomerulus from the same patient as in Figure 8-24, showing diffuse, ill-defined basement membrane thickening due to medium dense, homogenous material associated with mesangial interposition. These deposits are difficult to distinguish from the lamina densa. Although they are mainly located within the basement membrane in some areas, they are in continuity with the subendothelial and supepithelial zones (middle portion of the picture). The outer aspect of the basement membrane is markedly irregular and the foot processes are obliterated. EP, epithelial cell; EN, endothelium; ME, mesangium (×5,000).

pattern of glomerulonephritis with features of both MCGN and membranous nephropathy has been described (66). Occasional biopsy specimens from patients with apparently primary glomerular disease may show this mixed pattern, but the possibility of lupus must always be seriously considered.

SUMMARY

The concept of mesangiocapillary glomerulonephritis has passed through a number of phases since its relationship to hypocomplementemia was recognized in 1965. Presently, many authors describe one clinicopathologic disease with two morphologic and serologic subgroups. The evidence presented in this chapter, however, indicates that these subgroups are, in reality, two quite distinct diseases. MCGN with subendothelial deposits is a chronic immune complex disease with a characteristic pattern of mesangial proliferation and circumferential interposition. DDD, on the other hand, is characterized by a unique dense transformation of basement membranes and may show little or no proliferation, although some cases evolve into an MCGN-like pattern. The clinical presentation and prognosis of these two diseases are similar and both show depression of serum C3, often with C3NeF. These changes in complement are almost invariable in DDD and are presently unexplained, although their occurrence in some patients before the onset of renal disease suggests that they may play a part in the development of the membrane lesion. Both hypocomplementemia and C3NeF are less constant in MCGN and are probably secondary to complement activation by prolonged immune complex deposition. The diseases should be considered and diagnosed as separate entities to allow more precise study of their pathogenesis and natural history.

REFERENCES

1. West CD, McAdams AJ, McConville JM, et al: Hypocomplementemic and normocomplementemic persistent (chronic) glomerulonephritis: clinical and pathological characteristics. *J Pediat* 67:1089, 1965.

2. Gotoff SP, Fellers FX, Vawter GF, et al: The beta 1C globulin in childhood nephrotic syndrome: laboratory diagnosis of progressive glomerulonephritis. *N Engl J Med* 273:524, 1965.

3. Jones DB: Membranoproliferative glomerulonephritis. One of many diseases? *Arch Pathol Lab Med* 101:457, 1977.

4. Jones DB: The nature of scar tissue in glomerulonephritis. *Am J Pathol* 42:185, 1963.

5. Arakawa M, Kimmelstiel P: Circumferential mesangial interposition. *Lab Invest* 21:276, 1969.

6. Habib R, Kleinknecht C, Gubler MC, et al: Idiopathic membranoproliferative glomerulonephritis in children. *Clin Nephrol* 1:194, 1973.

7. Kim Y, Michael AF: Chronic bacteremia and nephritis. *Ann Rev Med* 29:319, 1978.

8. Uff JS, Evans DJ: Mesangio-capillary glomerulonephritis associated with Q-fever endocarditis. *Histopathol* 1:463, 1977.

9. Pertschuk DO, Vuletin JC, Sutton AL, et al: Demonstration of antigen and immune complex in glomerulonephritis due to Staphylococcus aureus. *Am J Clin Pathol* 66:1027, 1976.

10. Rocha H, Cruz T, Brito E, et al: Renal involvement in patients with hepatosplenic Schistosomiasis mansoni. *Am J Trop Med Hyg* 25:108, 1976.

11. White RHR: Quartan malarial nephrotic syndrome. *Nephron* 11:147, 1977.

12. Bhamarapravati N, Boonpucknavig S, Boonpucknavig V, et al: Glomerular changes in acute Plasmodium falciparum infection: an immunopathologic study. *Arch Pathol* 96:289, 1973.

13. Brzosko WJ, Krawczynski K, Nazarewicz T, et al: Glomerulonephritis associated with hepatitis-B surface antigen immune complexes in children. *Lancet* 2:477, 1974.

14. Eagen JW, Lewis EJ: Glomerulonephritis of neoplasia. *Kidney Int* 11:297, 1977.

15. Feiner H, Gallo G: Ultrastructure in glomerulonephritis associated with cryoglobulinemia: a report of six cases and review of the literature. *Am J Pathol* 88:145, 1977.

16. Randall RE, Williamson WC Jr, Mullinax F, et al: Manifestations of systemic light chain deposition. *Am J Med* 60:293, 1976.

17. Hill GS, Hinglais N, Tron F, et al: Systemic lupus erythematosus: morphologic correlations with immunologic and clinical data at the time of biopsy. *Am J Med* 64:61, 1978.

18. Moutsopoulos HM, Balow JE, Lawley TJ, et al: Immune complex glomerulonephritis in Sicca syndrome. *Am J Med* 64:955, 1978.

19. Levy M, Broyer M, Arsan A, et al: Anaphylactoid purpura nephritis in childhood: natural history and immunopathology. *Adv Nephrol* 6:183, 1976.

20. Herdman RC, Pickering RC, Michael AF, et al: Chronic glomerulonephritis associated with low serum complement activity (chronic hypocomplementemic glomerulonephritis). *Medicine (Balt)* 49:207, 1970.

21. Kim Y, Friend PS, Dresner IG, et al: Inherited deficiency of the second component of complement with membranoproliferative glomerulonephritis. *Am J Med* 62:765, 1977.

22. Nochy D, Callard P, Bellon B, et al: Association of overt glomerulonephritis and liver disease: a study of 34 patients. *Clin Nephrol* 6:422, 1976.

23. Krumlovsky FA, Del Greco F, Herson PB, et al: Renal disease associated with toxic epidermal necrolysis (Lyell's disease). *Am J Med* 57:817, 1974.

24. Moroz SP, Cutz E, Balfe JW, et al: Membranoproliferative glomerulonephritis in childhood cirrhosis associated with alpha$_1$-antitrypsin deficiency. *Pediatrics* 57:232, 1976.

25. Pardo V, Strauss J, Kramer H, et al: Nephropathy associated with sickle cell anemia. An autologous immune complex nephritis. II. Clinicopathologic study of seven patients. *Am J Med* 59:650, 1975.

26. Egbert BM, Schwartz E, Kempson RL: Kartagener syndrome: report of a case with mesangiocapillary glomerulonephritis. *Arch Pathol Lab Med* 101:95, 1977.

27. Treser G, Cherubin C, Longergan ET, et al: Renal lesions in narcotic addicts *Am J Med* 57:687, 1974.

27a. Llach F, Descouedres C, Massry SG: Heroin associated nephropathy: clinical and histological studies in 19 patients. *Clin Nephrol* 11:7, 1979.

28. Sissons JGP, West RJ, Fallows J, et al: The complement abnormalities of lipodystrophy. *N Engl J Med* 294:461, 1976.

29. Bennett WM, Bardana EJ, Wuepper K, et al: Partial lipodystrophy, C3 nephritic factor and clinically inapparent mesangiocapillary glomerulonephritis. *Am J Med* 62:757, 1977.

30. West CD: Pathogenesis and approaches to therapy of membranoproliferative glomerulonephritis. *Kidney Int* 9:1, 1976.

31. Ooi YM, Vallota EH, West CD: Serum immune complexes in membranoproliferative and other glomerulonephritides. *Kidney Int* 11:275, 1977.

32. Peters DK, Williams DG: Complement and mesangiocapillary glomerulonephritis. Role of complement deficiency in the pathogenesis of nephritis. *Nephron* 13:188, 1974.

33. Wilson CB, Dixon FJ: Antigen quantitation in experimental immune complex glomerulonephritis. *J Immunol* 105:279, 1970.

34. West CD: Membranoproliferative hypocomplementemic glomerulonephritis. *Nephron* 11:134, 1973.

35. Cameron JS, Glasgow EF, Ogg CS, et al: Membranoproliferative glomerulonephritis and persistent hypocomplementaemia. *Br Med J* 4:7, 1970.

36. Mandalenakis N, Mendoza N, Pirani CL, et al: Lobular glomerulonephritis and membranoproliferative glomerulonephritis. *Medicine (Balt)* 50:319, 1971.

37. West CD, McAdams AJ: Serum β1c globulin levels in persistent glomerulonephritis with low serum complement: variability unrelated to clinical course. *Nephron* 7:193, 1970.

38. Zucchelli P, Sasdelli M, Cagnoli L, et al: Membranoproliferative glomerulonephritis: correlations between immunological and histological findings. *Nephron* 17:449, 1976.

39. Davis AE, Schneeberger EE, Grupe WE, et al: Membranoproliferative glomerulonephritis (MPGN type I) and dense deposit disease (DDD) in children. *Clin Nephrol* 9:184, 1978.

40. Ooi YM, Vallota E, West CD: Classical complement pathway activation in membranoproliferative glomerulonephritis. *Kidney Int* 9:46, 1976.

41. Bohle A, Gartner HV, Fischbach H, et al: The morphological and clinical features of membranoproliferative glomerulonephritis in adults. *Virchows Arch (A) Pathol Anat Histol* 363:213, 1974.

42. Levy M, Gubler M-C, Sich M, et al: Immunopathology of membranoproliferative glomerulonephritis with subendothelial deposits (Type I MPGN). *Clin Immunol Immunopathol* 10:477, 1978.

43. Cameron JS, Ogg CS, White RHR, et al: The clinical features and prognosis of patients with normocomplementemic mesangiocapillary glomerulonephritis. *Clin Nephrol* 1:8, 1973.

44. McAdams AJ, McEnery PT, West CD: Mesangiocapillary glomerulonephritis: changes in glomerular morphology with long-term alternate day prednisone therapy. *J Pediat* 86:23, 1975.

45. Kincaid-Smith P: The treatment of chronic mesangiocapillary (membrano-proliferative) glomerulonephritis with impaired renal function. *Med J Aust* 2:587, 1972.

46. Cameron JS, and Turner DR: Recurrent glomerulonephritis in allografted kidneys. *Clin Nephrol* 7:47, 1977.

46a. Curtis JJ, Wyatt RJ, Bhathena D, et al: Renal transplantation for patients with type I and type II membranoproliferative glomerulonephritis: serial complement and nephritic factor measurements and the problem of recurrent disease. *Am J Med* 66:216, 1979.

47. Mathew TH, Mathews DC, Hobbs JB, et al: Glomerular lesions after renal transplantation. *Am J Med* 59:177, 1975.

48. Galle P, Mahieu P: Electron dense alteration of the kidney basement membranes. A renal lesion specific of a systemic disease. *Am J Med* 58:749, 1975.

49. Méry JPh, Kourilsky O, Morel-Maroger L, et al: Partial lipodystrophy and glomerulonephritis without complement activation. *N Engl J Med* 298:1034, 1978.

50. Fearon DT: Glomerulonephritis, complement and C3NeF. *N Engl J Med* 294:495, 1976.

51. Williams DG, Bartlett A, Duffus P: Identification of nephritic factor as an immunoglobulin. *Clin Exp Immunol* 33:425, 1978.

52. Droz D, Zanetti M, Noël L-H, et al: Dense deposits disease *Nephron* 19:1, 1977.

53. Verroust PJ, Wilson CB, Dixon FJ: Lack of nephritogenicity of systemic activation of the alternate complement pathway. *Kidney Int* 6:157, 1974.

54. Chesney RW, O'Regan S, Guyda HJ, et al: Candida endocrinopathy syndrome with membranoproliferative glomerulonephritis: demonstration of glomerular Candida antigen. *Clin Nephrol* 5:232, 1976.

55. Case records of the Massachusetts General Hospital. *N Engl J Med* 296:160, 1977.

56. Antoine B, Faye C: The clinical course associated with dense deposits in the kidney basement membranes. *Kidney Int* 1:420, 1972.

57. Vargas R, Thompson KJ, Wilson D, et al: Mesangiocapillary glomerulonephritis with dense "deposits" in the basement membrane of the kidney. *Clin Nephrol* 5:73, 1976.

58. Habib R, Gubler MC, Loirat C, et al: Dense deposit disease: a variant of membranoproliferative glomerulonephritis. *Kidney Int* 7:204, 1975.

59. Lamb V, Tisher CC, McCoy RC, et al: Membranoproliferative glomerulonephritis with dense intramembranous alterations. A clinicopathologic study. *Lab Invest* 36:607, 1977.

59a. Churg J, Duff JL, Bernstein J: Identification of dense deposit disease. A report for the International Study of Kidney Diseases in Children. *Arch Pathol Lab Med* 103:67, 1979.

60. Jenis EH, Sandler P, Hill GS, et al: Glomerulonephritis with basement membrane dense deposits. *Arch Pathol* 97:84, 1974.

60a. Kim Y, Vernier RL, Fish AJ, et al: Immunofluorescence studies of dense deposit disease: the presence of railroad tracks and mesangial rings. *Lab Invest* 40:474, 1979.

61. Anders D, Agricola B, Sippel M: Basement membrane changes in membranoproliferative glomerulonephritis. II. Characterization of a third type by silver impregnation of ultrathin sections. *Virchows Arch (A) Pathol Anat Histol* 376:1, 1977.

62. Strife CF, McEnery PT, McAdams AJ, et al: Membranoproliferative glomerulonephritis with disruption of the glomerular basement membrane. *Clin Nephrol* 7:65, 1977.

63. Davis AE, Schneeberger EE, McCluskey RT, et al: Mesangial proliferative glomerulonephritis with irregular intramembranous deposits: another variant of hypocomplementemic glomerulonephritis. *Am J Med* 63:481, 1977.

64. Turner DR, Cameron JS, Bewick M, et al: Transplantation in mesangiocapillary glomrulonephritis with intramembranous dense "deposits": recurrence of disease. *Kidney Int* 9:439, 1976.

64a. Leibowitch J, Halbwachs L, Wattel S, et al: Recurrence of dense deposits in transplanted kidney: II. Serum complement and nephritic factor profiles. *Kidney Int* 15:396, 1979.

65. Beaufils H, Gubler MC, Karam J, et al: Dense deposit disease: long term follow-up of three cases of recurrence after transplantation. *Clin Nephrol* 7:31, 1977.

65a. Droz D, Nabarra B, Noel L-H, et al: Recurrence of dense deposits in transplanted kidneys: I. Sequential survey of the lesions. *Kidney Int* 15: 386, 1979.

66. Burkholder PM, Marchand A, Krueger P: Mixed membranous and proliferative glomerulonephritis: a correlative light, immunofluorescence and electron microscopic study. *Lab Invest* 23:459, 1970.

9
Membranous Nephropathy*

Membranous nephropathy is a morphologic pattern of diverse etiology. A large number of associated or precipitating factors have been identified in individual cases, but no cause can usually be identified. The glomerular changes consist of varying degrees of glomerular basement membrane reaction to subepithelial deposits, the character and extent of these changes being the basis of morphologic staging. Diagnosis, therefore, relies on the demonstration of either the deposits or the reaction to them and cannot be achieved from the recognition of capillary wall thickening alone. The natural history of idiopathic membranous nephropathy is of progressive membrane change with eventual glomerular destruction and chronic renal failure. In those patients with an identifiable basis, removal of the cause may produce transient or permanent remission. Morphologic identification of the membranous lesion is thus only the first step toward a final clinicopathologic diagnosis.

ETIOLOGY AND PATHOGENESIS

Experimental Membranous Nephropathy

The lesion can be produced in experimental animals by the administration of either exogenous or endogenous antigens. Under certain conditions, repeated injections of foreign soluble antigens (chronic serum sickness) produces subepithelial deposits with no glomerular inflammation (1). This occurs only in animals producing small quantities of antibody and is dependent on the dose of antigen being low, larger doses producing proliferative disease. The circulating complexes in these animals are small, and the antigen can be demonstrated in both the circulating and glomerular complexes. The glomerular lesions regress when antigen administration is ceased. In contrast, the experimental form of membranous nephropathy produced by the administration of endogenous antigen is permanent and is unaffected by either cessation of antigen administration or by various forms of therapy (2). This lesion is produced by the injection of kidney emulsions with adjuvant (active Heymann's nephritis), the antigen re-

*This category of renal disease includes membranous, extramembranous, epimembranous, and perimembranous glomerulonephritis.

152

sponsible for the development of the lesion being derived from the apical portion of the proximal convuluted tubule (3,4). This antigen can be shown in the glomerular deposits (4), but extrarenal deposits cannot be identified (2), and the presence of circulating immune complexes has not been proven. The disease is transferrable to normal animals by serum from those with disease (5) and, similarly, can be induced by a single injection of antibodies against the tubular antigen (passive Heymann's nephritis) (6,7). The mechanism of this passive model could be either complexing of the injected antibody with circulating antigen and subsequent deposition (6) or, alternatively, reaction of the antibody with glomerular components similar or identical to the tubular antigen (7). Such glomerular antigens have, in fact, been identified on visceral epithelial cells, and there is conclusive experimental evidence for in situ formation of complexes (7,7a). Once the complexes have formed, immunologic damage could be perpetuated by the formation and deposition of antibodies to the fixed, foreign protein, as in the heterologous phase of nephrotoxic serum nephritis (6). Heymann's nephritis appears, therefore, to have pathogenetic features in common with both antiglomerular basement membrane disease and the immune complex disorders.

Human Membranous Nephropathy

In a proportion of patients, membranous nephropathy is secondary to infective or neoplastic diseases (8–10). Specific antigens have been identified in the deposits of some patients with these diseases (Table 9-1), and transient or permanent remission may follow successful therapy of the primary disease (8,9). The features in these cases, and in lupus membranous nephropathy, are similar in a number of respects to the chronic serum sickness model. The infective associations are extremely rare, with the exception of hepatitis B in some populations (11), but neoplasms have been found in up to 10% of the adult patients with membranous nephropathy (10). A variety of neoplasms have been implicated, the most common being carcinomas of the lung and large bowel (9). In the majority of patients with membranous nephropathy, no associated condition can be identified, and the antigens implicated in the glomerular immune complexes are unknown. Circulating immune complexes can only rarely be identified in these patients, suggesting analogy with the Heymann model (12). A renal tubular antigen, identical to that found in the experimental disease, has been identified in the deposits of a few patients with membranous (13) and a number of other morphologic lesions (14) but has not been found in the majority of cases of human membranous nephropathy (15,15a). The antigen(s) in the deposits are, therefore, still unknown, but extrapolation from the Heymann lesion suggests that glomerular constituents may be implicated. Membranous nephropathy has also followed exposure to volatile hydrocarbons (16), prolonged heroin addiction (16a) and a number of drugs (Table 9-1), and has usually remitted permanently after withdrawal of the drug concerned. The pathogenesis of these drug-induced lesions is unknown, although experimental models of both gold (17) and mercury membranous (18) lesions have been developed, and circulating immune complexes have been described in one patient with gold nephropathy (19). Many of the drugs showing this association are capable of causing tubular

Table 9-1. Conditions Associated with Membranous Nephropathy [a]

Systemic infections	Hepatitis B[b]
	Syphilis [b]
	Filariasis (Loa Loa)
	Schistosomiasis
	Malaria
	Leprosy
Drugs and toxins	Heavy metals (gold, mercury)
	Penicillamine
	Trimethadione
	Volatile hydrocarbons
	Heroin
Neoplasms	Epithelial tumor [b]
	Lymphoma, leukemia
Systemic connective tissue disorders	Systemic lupus erythematosus [b]
	Mixed connective tissue disease
Miscellaneous	Guillian-Barré syndrome
	Sickle cell disease
	Kidney transplants
	Diabetes mellitus (?)
	Rheumatoid arthritis (?)
	Renal vein thrombosis (?)

[a] See text and ref. 10, 33, and 34 for details.
[b] Specific antigens have been identified in the deposits.

damage, suggesting that release of proximal tubular antigen might initiate the process, but the antigen has not yet been demonstrated in either the serum or the deposits of those patients. Continued study of these secondary forms of membranous nephropathy may provide important information about the pathogenesis and potential reversal of the idiopathic disease.

CLINICAL MANIFESTATIONS AND COURSE

Membranous nephropathy is most common in the fifth to seventh decades but occurs at all ages, with a male predominance of two to three to one (10,20–22). Initial presentation is invariably with signs of altered glomerular permeability, 70–80% of patients having the nephrotic syndrome at onset and the remainder being referred for the investigation of proteinuria (10,22–25). In renal biopsy series, membranous nephropathy is found in 20–30% of nephrotic adults (10,25,26) and 1 to 9% of nephrotic children (10,26–29). The wide range of figures quoted for childhood nephrotics probably reflects differences in referral and selection for biopsy rather than a real variation, and the true incidence is likely to be in the region of 1% (27). Proteinuria may be highly selective, especially in early lesions, but variation is such that this investigation is of little diagnostic value (29). Microscopic hematuria is detectable in most patients, but macroscopic hematuria and other nephritic features are rare (19,21,22). In the absence of systemic manifestations, other investigations do not usually contribute to the diagnosis. Some patients, however, appear to fall into an intermediate position between idiopathic and lupus membranous nephropathy (30), and the presence of hypocomplementemia may be an indication of the presence of lupus, since serum complement values are normal in the idiopathic disease (10). Hypertension may be present at the onset of the disease and develops at some time during the course in up to half the patients (10,22,28). Occasionally, the disease may be first expressed during pregnancy, when it may mimic preeclampsia (26,31). There is considerable variation in the degree of proteinuria in membranous nephropathy. Individual patients may apparently remit for short or long periods, and episodes of nephrotic syndrome may occur for no apparent cause. Even in those patients with only proteinuria at onset, the nephrotic syndrome commonly develops at some time during the evolution of the disease, although proteinuria generally tends to diminish with progression of the glomerular lesions (24). In the vast majority of patients, the nephrotic syndrome caused by membranous nephropathy is unresponsive to corticosteroid therapy (10,20,22,23).

PATHOLOGIC CHARACTERISTICS

The morphologic lesions of membranous nephropathy are an amalgam of subepithelial deposits and membranous reaction (32–34). Either or both of these components must be demonstrated, and the practice of describing all forms of capillary-wall thickening as membranous lesions is disruptive to accurate terminology and should be avoided. On the basis of the glomerular basement membrane reaction, up to six stages have been described, although only four of these stages are commonly used (24,33). At almost any stage, the disease may remit to leave a distorted membrane, which can, with time, show remarkable powers of recovery. Although each of the stages can be recognized by careful light microscopy examination of silver-stained sections, electron microscopy provides the most detailed delineation of the membrane changes. In general, there is a reasonable correlation between the morphologic stage and the duration of the disease (24,32).

Electron Microscopy

The morphologic stages of membranous nephropathy describe events along the path of the incorporation of subepithelial deposits into an altered and greatly thickened membrane. The changes result from the production of new membrane on the epithelial aspect, almost certainly by the epithelial cells, which are a major source of membrane renewal (35). Initially (stage I), the deposits are seen as discrete nodules irregularly distributed along the subepithelial aspect and often completely sparing some loops. These nodules may be dome-shaped, irregularly flattened, or identical to the humps of postinfectious glomerulonephritis, and they often appear to be shaped by the interstices between epithelial foot processes. The foot processes are usually diffusely obliterated, but may occasionally be intact over uninvolved loops. Electron-dense material accumulates in epithelial cytoplasm adjacent to the membrane whenever foot processes are obliterated and may be mistaken by the unwary for deposits in such conditions as epithelial cell disease (Fig. 9-1). The underlying membrane is initially normal, but small protrusions soon appear between the deposits, and continued growth of these protrusions forms spikelike extensions. The majority of initial biopsy specimens show a pattern of relatively regular deposits separated by distinct spikes (stage II) (Fig. 9-2). Epithelial foot processes are almost always diffusely obliterated at this stage, and the cell bodies appear hyperactive with well-developed endoplasmic reticulum, microcystic change, and frequent microvillous projections (Fig. 9-3). Gradually, and often to a varying degree in different areas of the glomerulus, the spikes enlarge and fuse over the external surface of the deposits. The thickened membrane then appears to have three components: an original inner layer of approximately normal width, a central zone of deposits separated by membrane strands, and an outer layer of variably thick membrane separating the deposits from epithelial cells (stage III). Frequently, at this stage, the deposits show varying degrees of apparent resolution with irregular rarefaction, producing a mottled or "moth-eaten" appearance (Fig. 9-4). Individual deposits may contain or be replaced by microvesicular (36) or striated membranous (37) bodies, probably developing from the degeneration of included cytoplasmic components (Figs. 9-5−9-7). After variable periods of time, these changes progress to form a distorted and massively thickened membrane within which deposits may be difficult to distinguish (stage IV) (Fig. 9-8).

Throughout this evolution, there is often considerable variation between glomeruli, and even between individual loops in both the distribution of deposits and the apparent morphologic stage. There is frequently, also, evidence of continuing activity, with apparently fresh subepithelial deposits coexisting even with very advanced membrane lesions. The presence of mesangial or subendothelial deposits is evidence against a diagnosis of idiopathic membranous nephropathy and suggests lupus glomerulonephritis, especially if tubulovesicular bodies are present in endothelial cells (30). In advanced disease, however, irregular capillary wall collapse and segmental insudation may produce an appearance of deposits in almost any location, and diagnosis may, at this stage, be difficult. Rarely, the deposits may assume a parallel fibrotubular or fingerprint pattern, suggesting cryoglobulinemia or lupus, respectively (Figs. 9-9, 9-10). In those cases showing regression, areas of rarefaction are predominant and the deposits progressively disappear. The membrane in these biopsy specimens looks like a ragged chain with lucent areas irregularly distributed between intact outer and inner zones (stage V) (24) (Fig. 9-11). Serial biopsy specimens in such patients reveal gradual reconstruction of the membrane with obscuring of the original pattern, although some irregularity almost always remains (24,28) (Fig. 9-12).

Light Microscopy

Except in the very early stages, the glomeruli are enlarged and show diffuse capillary-wall thickening. In stage I lesions, this thickening is minimal and a

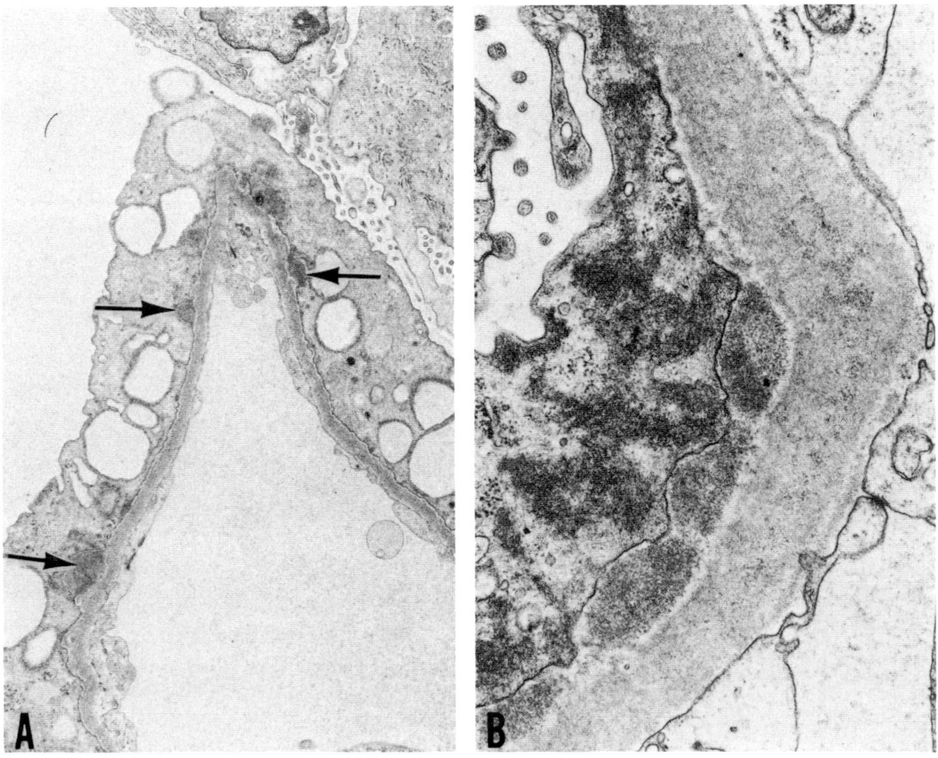

Figure 9-1. Idiopathic membranous nephropathy, stage I. (*a*) Small, sparse subepithelial deposits are present in the capillary loop (arrows). The foot processes are obliterated and the epithelial cell cytoplasm shows microcysts. (*b*) Small dome-shaped subepithelial deposits are separated from the basement membrane by a clear zone. Note the accumulation of electron dense material in the epithelial cell cytoplasm adjacent to the basement membrane ([*a*] ×5,000; [*b*] ×22,600).

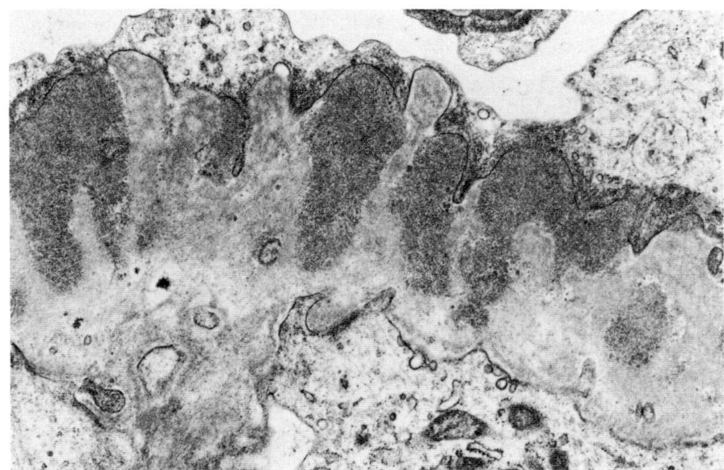

Figure 9-2. Idiopathic membranous nephropathy, stage II. The projections of basement membrane between deposits are responsible for the spikes seen in silver stains (×12,900).

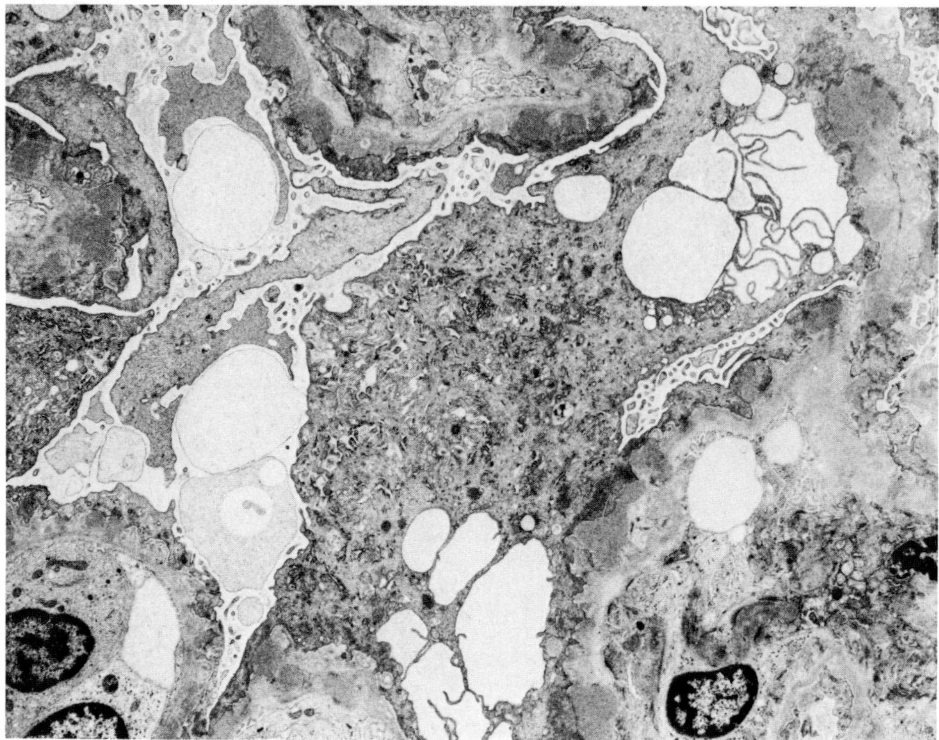

Figure 9-3. Idiopathic membranous nephropathy, stage II. The basement membrane is markedly irregular. There are numerous subepithelial deposits. The foot processes are obliterated and the epithelial cell cytoplasm appears hyperactive, with increase in endoplasmic reticulum, microcystic change, and microvillous projections (×8,700).

diagnosis of "minimal change" may be made if only light microscopy is available (38). Spikes are absent at this stage but careful examination of thin, silver-stained sections frequently reveals some irregularity of the outer membrane contour (Fig. 9-13). With progression into stage II, capillary-wall thickening becomes obvious, and the deposits can often be identified with chromotrope and Masson trichrome stains. The spikes seen at this stage consist of perpendicular extensions of the membrane with rounded or club-shaped ends (Fig. 9-14). In lesions intermediate between stages I and II, the distribution of spikes may be irregular, so that careful examination of several glomeruli may be necessary for their recognition. The incorporation of deposits in stage III occurs by fusion of adjacent spikes to form a double-layered membrane, the two layers separated by transverse bands, which are the residua of the original spikes (Fig. 9-15).

Progressive membrane thickening causes encroachment upon capillary lumina and glomerular obsolescence. This obsolescence may occur as regular glomerular shrinkage but is more often irregular with areas of segmental sclerosis, consolidation, and organizing epithelial proliferation (Fig. 9-16). Segmental sclerosis and hyalinosis may, in fact, occur at any stage during the course and has been associated with a particular tendency to progression into chronic

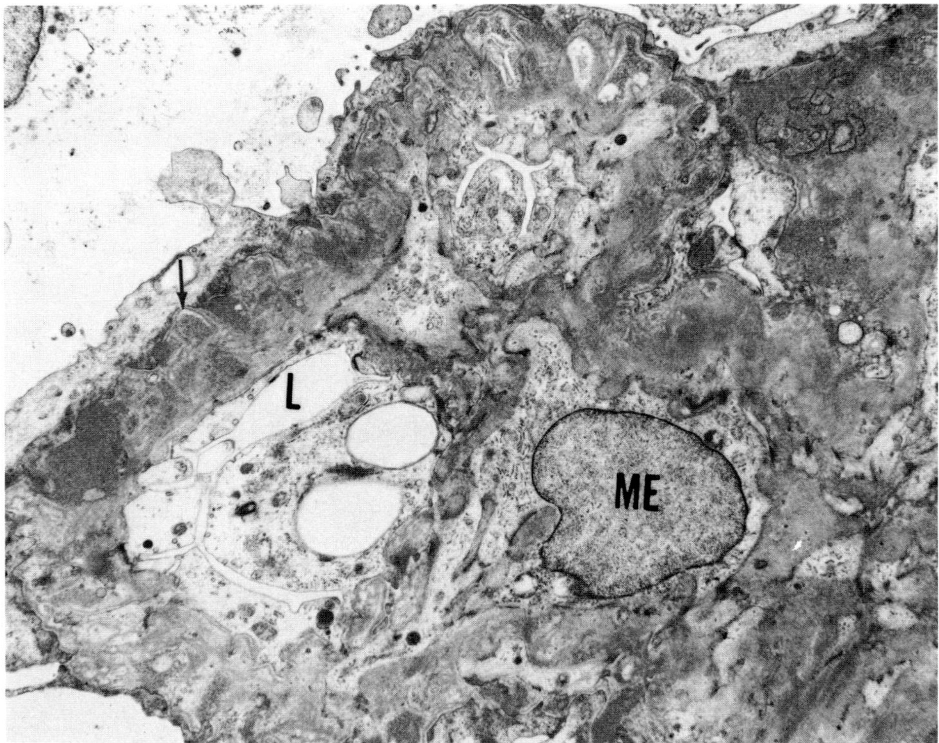

Figure 9-4. Idiopathic membranous nephropathy, stage III. The deposits are surrounded by new basement membrane (arrow) and show varying degrees of resolution. L, capillary lumen; ME, mesangium (×9,000).

renal failure (38a). The final stages of membranous nephropathy may thus be difficult to distinguish from other forms of chronic glomerulonephritis unless the characteristic features can be demonstrated by silver stains or other techniques. Irregular capillary collapse in advanced disease may give an erroneous impression of intracapillary proliferation. Mesangial proliferation can, in fact, be demonstrated by quantitative analysis in many cases of membranous nephropathy (39) and may, in some biopsy specimens, be sufficiently prominent to initially suggest a diagnosis of mesangial proliferative glomerulonephritis. Proliferative and exudative glomerulonephritis has been reported to develop into apparently typical membranous nephropathy in a few patients (40). Conversely, crescentic glomerulonephritis is occasionally superimposed upon an established membranous lesion to produce rapidly progressive deterioration in renal function (41–43). In some (41,42), but not all (43), of these patients, the crescentic disease has been associated with circulating antiglomerular basement membrane antibodies (Fig. 9-17). Progressive disease of any kind causes tubulointerstitial scarring, which accumulates in parallel with the glomerular changes. Interstitial foam cells are commonly seen, as in all forms of chronic proteinuria, but there are no specific extraglomerular lesions.

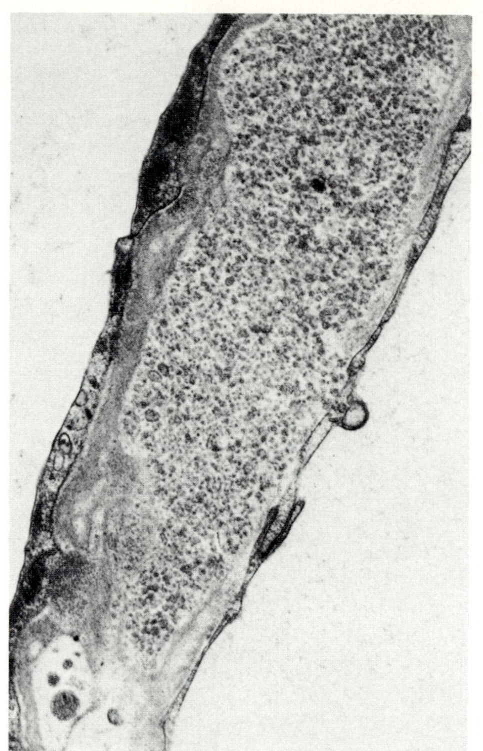

Figure 9-5. Idiopathic membranous nephropathy, with coarse granular deposits within the basement membrane (×14,000).

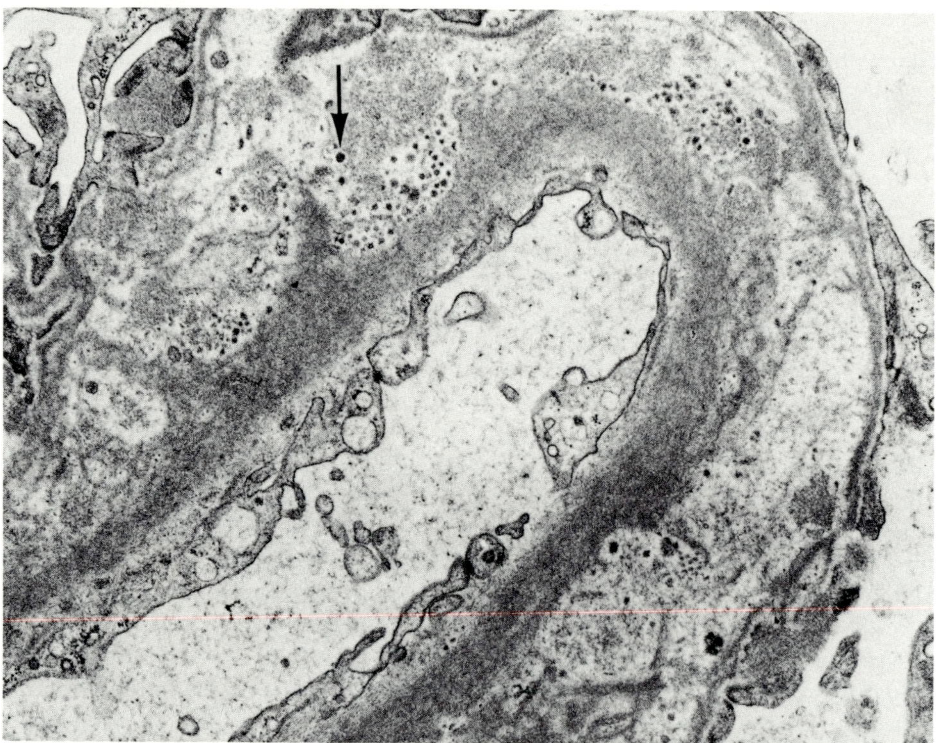

Figure 9-6. Advanced idiopathic membranous nephropathy. The basement membrane is thickened and reticulated. The deposits are disappearing, and numerous spherical structures are seen within them (arrow) (×15,600).

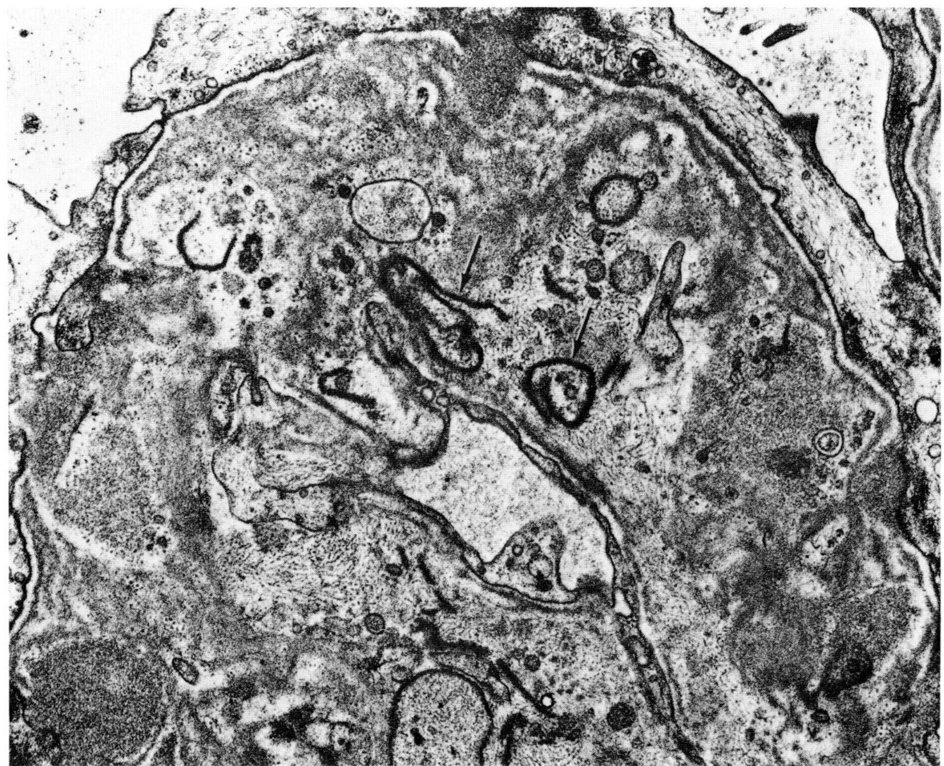

Figure 9-7. Advanced idiopathic membranous nephropathy. The basement membrane is markedly thickened and contains irregular deposits and numerous striated membranous structures (arrows) (×18,000).

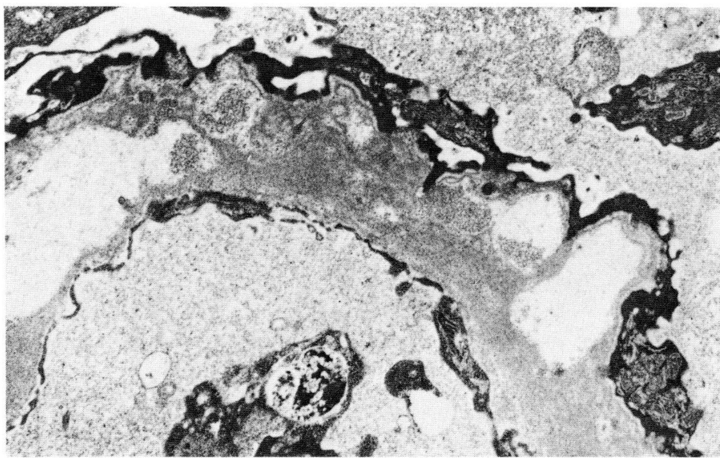

Figure 9-8. Idiopathic membranous nephropathy, stage IV. The basement membrane is thickened and the deposits partially reabsorbed, leaving irregular lucent areas (×8,800).

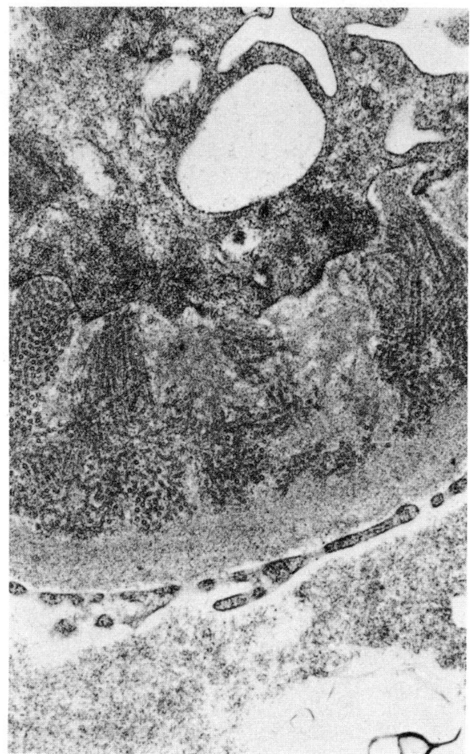

Figure 9-9. Membranous nephropathy. The deposits have a parallel fibrotubular appearance. Cryoglobulins were identified immediately after the biopsy (×48,000).

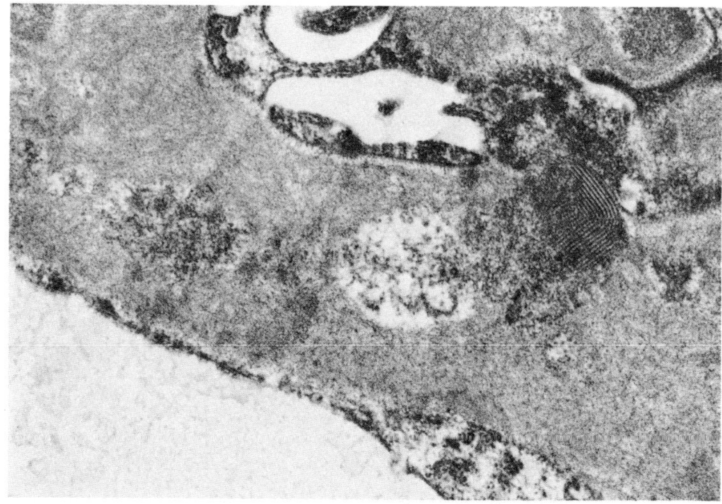

Figure 9-10. Idiopathic membranous nephropathy. The deposits show a fingerprint pattern. No evidence of SLE was demonstrated at time of the biopsy or later (×23,500).

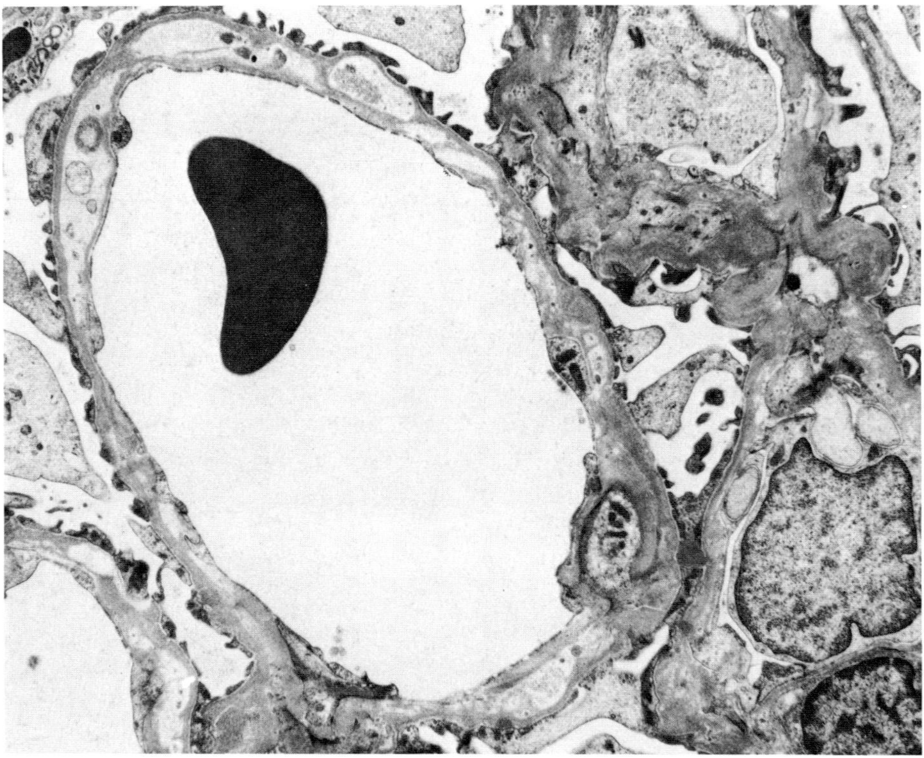

Figure 9-11. Idiopathic membranous nephropathy during regression. The foot processes have been restored. The outer aspect is regular. There are lucent areas irregularly distributed between the outer and inner zones of the basement membrane (×7,000).

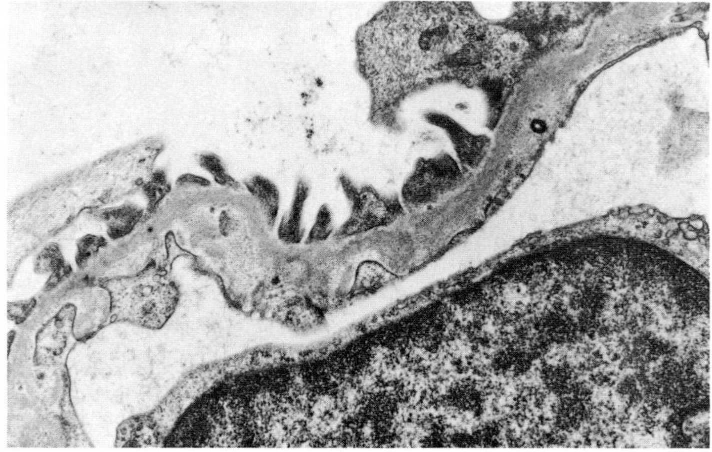

Figure 9-12. Idiopathic membranous nephropathy during remission. The subendothelial aspect is irregular. The basement membrane is normal in thickness and the foot processes are intact (×13,000).

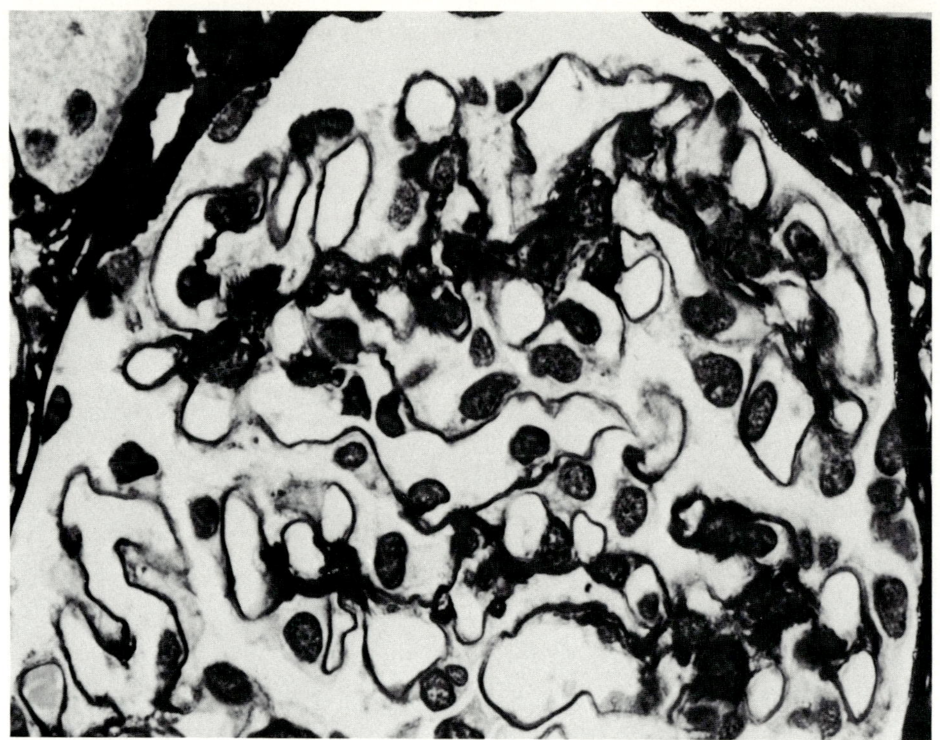

Figure 9-13. Idiopathic membranous nephropathy, stage I. There is no increase in cellularity and the basement membrane is normal in thickness (PASM stain, ×820).

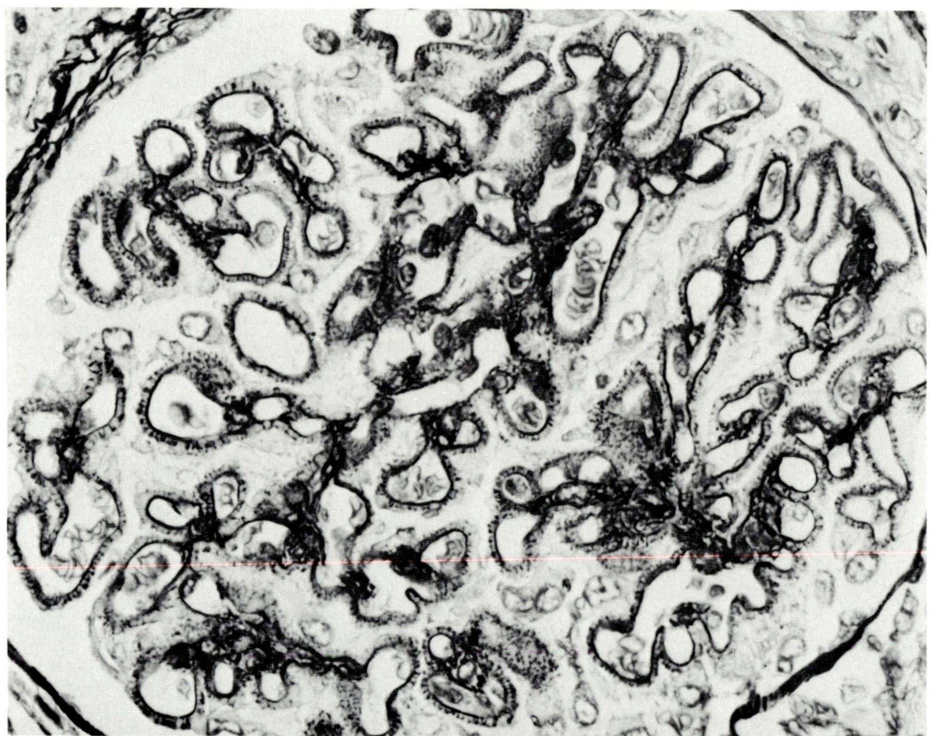

Figure 9-14. Idiopathic membranous nephropathy, stage II. Silver preparation showing "spikes" projecting outward from the basement membrane (PASM stain, ×600).

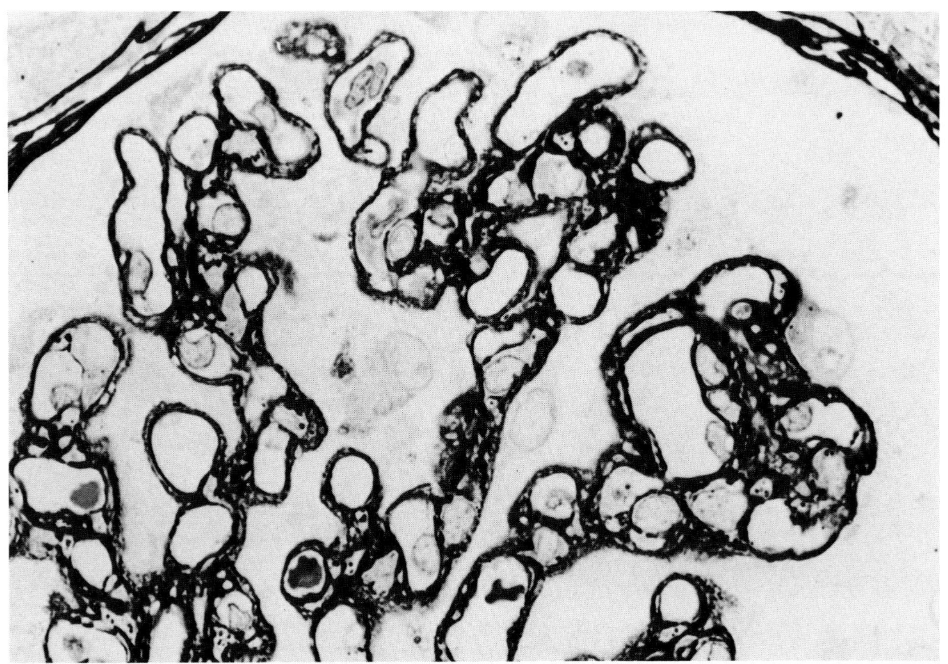

Figure 9-15. Idiopathic membranous nephropathy, stage III. The capillary walls are thickened and formed by two fine parallel bands (PASM stain, ×900).

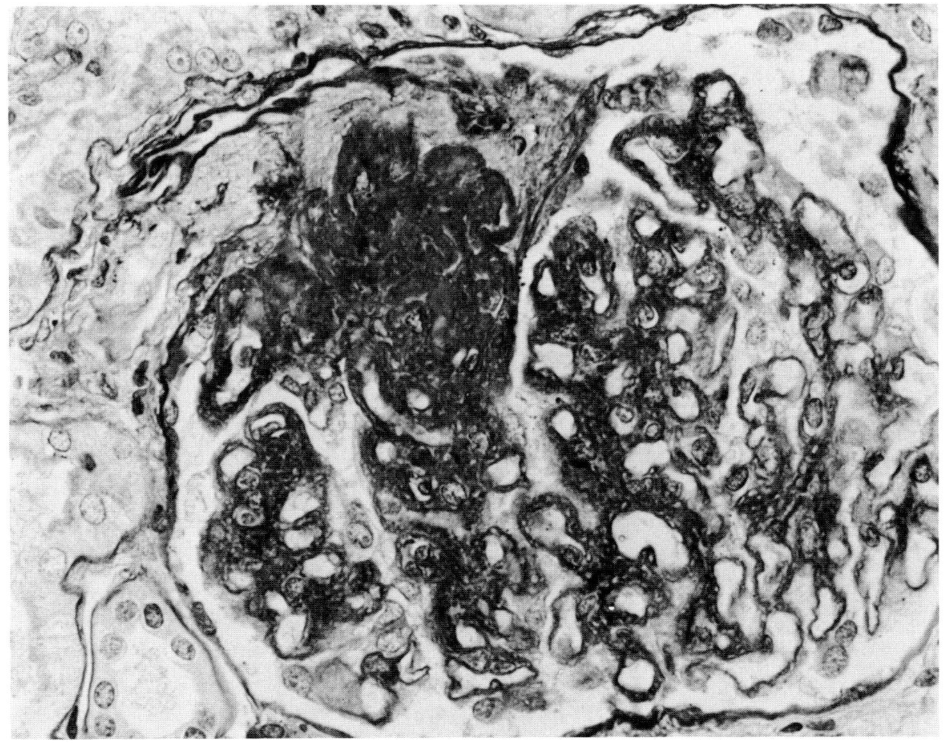

Figure 9-16. Advanced membranous nephropathy with segmental sclerosis (PAS stain, ×625).

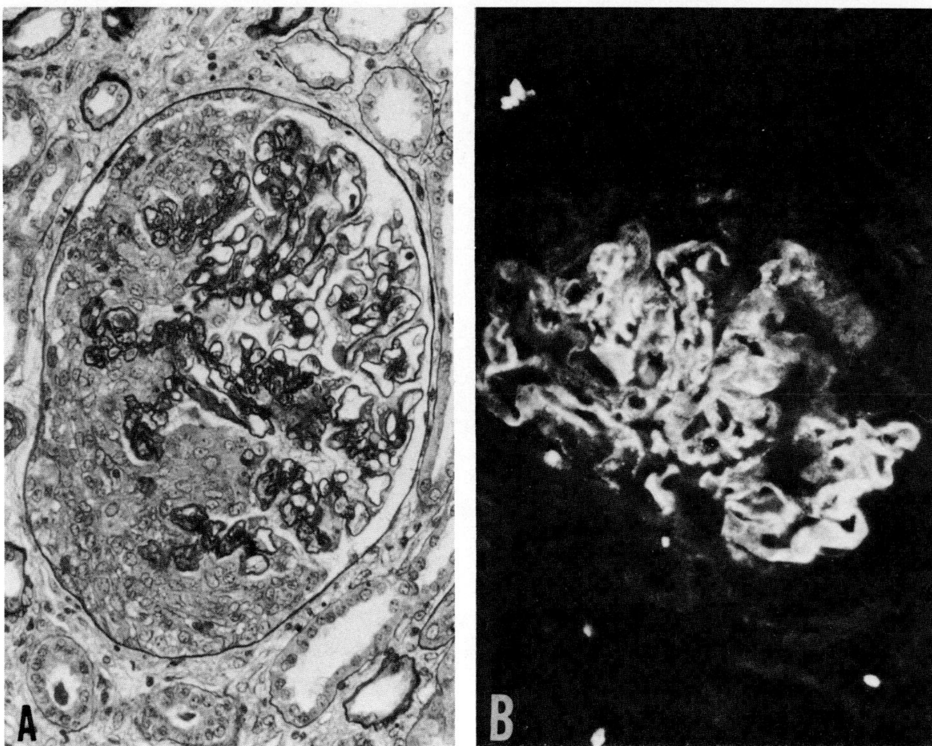

Figure 9-17. (*a*) Membranous nephropathy with superimposed crescentic glomerulone-phritis. (*b*) Immunofluorescent preparation from the same biopsy specimen. The tuft is partially obliterated by crescent. Note the granular staining along the capillary walls (*a*, PAS stain, ×450; *b*, antihuman IgG, ×525).

Immunofluorescence Microscopy

The subepithelial deposits are demonstrated in a highly characteristic pattern of diffuse and granular reactions for IgG along capillary walls (10,44,45) (Fig. 9-18). Reactions for IgA and IgM are usually not prominent and, if intense, raise the possibility of lupus membranous nephropathy (30). Complement components are usually, but not invariably, present in a similar distribution to IgG, C3 being the most frequent, but C1 and C4 occurring in a significant proportion (45). In the majority of biopsy specimens, granularity is coarse and easily recognized with the low power objective, but coalescence of fine granules may occasionally mimic a linear pattern (44) (Fig. 9-19). In the few patients who have developed superimposed antiglomerular basement membrane disease, the direct immunofluorescence pattern has apparently not been clearly linear, and the diagnosis has required the demonstration of circulating antibodies by indirect immunofluorescence or other studies (41,42) (Fig. 9-20). Resolving membranous nephropathy shows progressive reduction in staining intensity and loss of the diffuse reaction pattern. Probably because of nonspecific insudation into membrane defects, irregular reactions for IgM and C3 may replace those for IgG. The typical reactions may also disappear as the disease becomes endstage and may be obscured by nonspecific segmental staining.

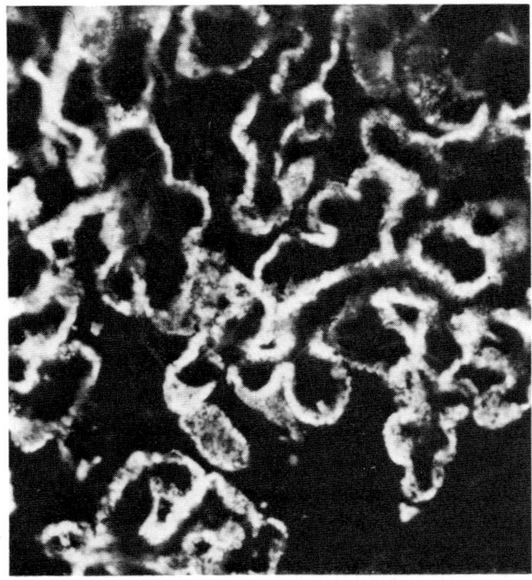

Figure 9-18. Heavy granular IgG deposits in the glomerular basement membrane in membranous nephropathy (antihuman IgG, ×400).

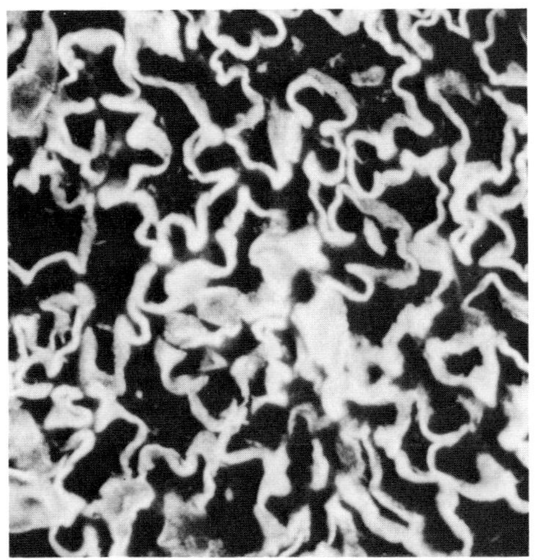

Figure 9-19. Membranous nephropathy with linearlike staining in the capillary walls. No circulating anti-GBM antibodies were demonstrated (antihuman IgG, ×400).

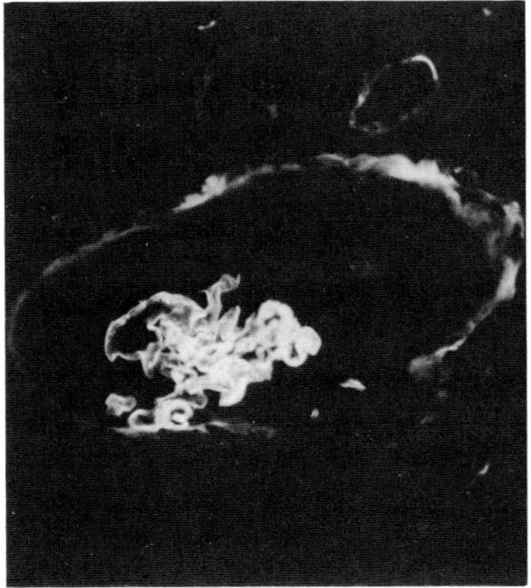

Figure 9-20. Anti-GBM glomerulonephritis complicating membranous nephropathy. There is linear staining along the capillary walls. The tuft is compressed by an epithelial crescent. Circulating anti-GBM was confirmed by radioimmunoassay (antihuman IgG, ×300).

167

DIFFERENTIAL DIAGNOSIS

In the typical and fully developed lesion of membranous nephropathy, there is little difficulty in primary diagnosis. More important is the exclusion of associated and potentially reversible diseases. This is especially important for stage I lesions, where resolution of the deposits could be expected to leave minimal residual damage (45a). Unfortunately, with the exceptions of lupus and gold nephropathy, there are no reliable morphologic methods of distinguishing primary and secondary membranous nephropathy. In lupus nephropathy, unusual immunofluorescent reactions, intracapillary deposits, or tubulovesicular bodies in endothelial cells may suggest the diagnosis while characteristic tubular inclusions indicate previous gold therapy (see below).

Difficulties in diagnosis arise most often when only light-microscopic material is available and usually are caused by misinterpretation of capillary-wall thickening or by poorly stained silver preparations. Spikes can only be seen in thin (2–3 μ) sections and may be obscured by either too heavy or too light impregnation with the silver solution. The methenamine silver technique is capricious in even the most experienced hands, and in laboratories not constantly involved with renal biopsy preparation it may be advisable, if membranous nephropathy is suspected, to stain a number of sections of the biopsy specimen for varying times in the silver solution in parallel with slides of a known membranous lesion. Irregularities on the external aspect of the membrane may mimic spikes, and the diagnosis is best restricted to those biopsy specimens showing widespread spike formation or distinct subepithelial deposits. Even if spikes are visible, the diagnosis is not necessarily established unless other features are typical, since subepithelial deposits in any disease may provoke the same membrane reaction. Widespread spike transformation of the membrane occurs in some cases of glomerular amyloidosis (46), and occasional examples of mixed amyloid and membranous disease have been reported (47). There are occasional biopsy specimens that appear to represent transitions between membranous and other lesions, most commonly mesangiocapillary glomerulonephritis, even when all techniques are available for assessment. Providing that systemic lupus can be excluded, these isolated cases can only be reported descriptively and followed to establish their pattern of progression.

CLINICAL COURSE AND PROGNOSIS

Idiopathic Membranous Nephropathy in Adults

The usual course is of chronic proteinuria with episodes of the nephrotic syndrome, not clearly related to any identifiable precipitating factor, and slow deterioration in renal function. Death or chronic renal failure has been reported to occur in 30%, 60%, and 70% of patients with membranous nephropathy with disease duration of 5, 10, and 15 years, respectively (48), but more recent data based on actuarial records show a survival of 76% at 10 years (48a). The rapidity of deterioration is, however, variable and usually cannot be predicted with certainty at the time of diagnosis, although the disease in females tends to follow a more favorable course (24) and the nephrotic syndrome at onset is often an indication of progressive disease (10,23). In some patients, chronic renal failure appears within three years whereas in others, deterioration may take place over much longer periods (22). The degree of proteinuria is extremely variable and may disappear for some time only to return unabated. The frequency of clinical remission is, therefore, difficult to assess, but permanent remissions are reported in 20–25% of patients (10,20–23,48a). There is controversy over the effects of corticosteroid and immunosuppressive therapy in bringing about these remissions. Most (10,21,23), but not all (49), uncontrolled studies have found no benefit from therapy. The published short-term studies are contradictory, claiming either no benefit from immunosuppressives (50) or a clear improvement in the prognosis of a small group of patients given corticosteroids (51). This variability in both the natural history and therapeutic response of patients with membranous nephropathy suggests that a number of specific disease entities may be hidden within the general diagnosis, and further study may identify groups of patients with more consistent clinical features. Chronic dialysis presents no particular difficulties for patients with the disease and recurrence (52) or de novo development (53) of membranous nephropathy after transplantation is rare.

Idiopathic Membranous Nephropathy in Children

The prognosis of the disease is very much better in children than in adults, especially if presentation is with proteinuria alone. Permanent remission occurs in 30 to 50% of children and only 10% develop chronic renal failure; the remaining cases pursue an indolent and apparently nonprogressive course (10,54). Progressive disease appears to be more likely in older children and in those who have hypertension at presentation (28).

Secondary Membranous Nephropathy

In general, secondary membranous nephropathy resolves after removal of the disease or agent causing the disease. Thus, disease activity may wax and wane in parallel with the control of associated neoplasms (9) or regress after cessation of the inciting drug. Where control of the associated condition is not possible, in such conditions, as sarcoidosis and hepatitis B antigenemia, the renal lesion persists. The list of conditions in Table 9-1 includes only those in which correlation appears to be unequivocal and deliberately omits a number of reported associations which, so far, lack confirmation. The majority of these apparently definite associations are rare, and only four will be considered in more detail.

Gold Nephropathy

Proteinuria occurs in 1.4 to 5% of patients treated with gold and is usually transient, but may become heavy and persistent (55). Occasionally, a form of epithelial cell disease occurs, but the glomerular lesion is usually identical to membranous nephropathy (56). The pathogenesis of this membranous lesion is unknown, but immune complexes have occasionally been demonstrated (19), and the lesion can be reproduced in experimental animals (17). Characteristic gold inclusions with curvilinear arrays can be demonstrated ultrastructurally in the proximal tubules, and occasionally elsewhere (57), but no gold is present in the glomerular deposits (58) (Fig. 9-21). In the majority of patients, proteinuria disappears permanently after gold therapy is ceased, but the morphologic lesion may persist (59), and a few patients appear to develop persistent disease.

Penicillamine Nephropathy

Proteinuria has been reported in 7 to 11% of those patients treated for a variety of diseases with penicillamine (60−62). While often mild and transient, proteinuria may be sufficient to cause the nephrotic syndrome and in these cases is caused by membranous nephropathy. The pathogenesis of the membranous lesion is unknown, but suggestive evidence of circulating immune complexes has been reported in a few patients (62). Occasionally, the membranous lesion has coexisted with glomerular amyloidosis (47). There is a tendency toward progressive resolution after the drug is discontinued, but proteinuria can persist for some time, and it is possible that progressive disease may develop in some of these patients (62).

Syphilis

Proteinuria occurring in congenital or secondary syphilis may be associated with either membranous nephropathy or proliferative glomerulonephritis (63,64). In each lesion, treponemal antigens have been demonstrated in the deposits. The

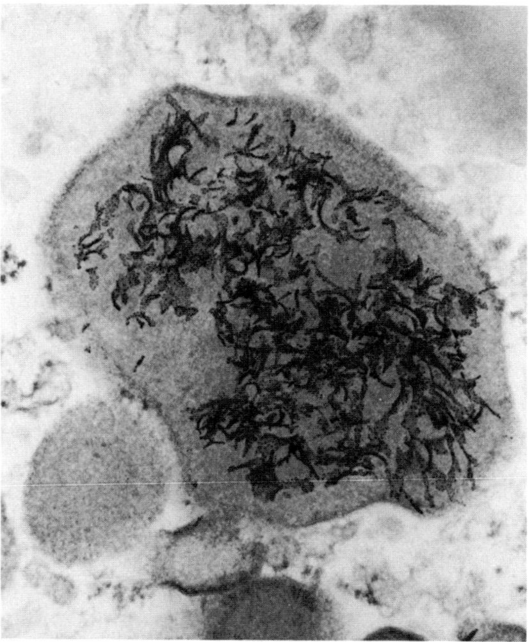

Figure 9-21. Gold particles within a lysosome of a tubular epithelial cell in gold-associated membranous nephropathy (×47,500).

membranous lesions are always arrested at stage I and disappear either spontaneously or with antisyphilitic therapy (Fig. 9-22).

Renal Vein Thrombosis

There has been controversy for many years over the relationship between renal vein thrombosis and membranous nephropathy (65). A variety of other renal diseases, notably mesangiocapillary glomerulonephritis (66), show a relationship with this condition, and recent studies have established that thrombosis is a complication of the glomerular lesion rather than the reverse (65–68). The incidence of thrombosis in membranous nephropathy has been variously estimated as from 7 to 38% (66,68), and the diagnosis may be indicated clinically by such phenomena as loin pain, pulmonary emboli, pyuria, microscopic hematuria, and unusual variations in either renal function or the degree of proteinuria (67,68). Thrombosis may be unilateral or bilateral. Congestion, interstitial edema, and margination of polymorphs in glomerular capillaries are said to be typical morphologic findings but may often be absent (66,68) (Fig. 9-23). Isolated intravascular thrombi may, however, be detected occasionally, and the presence of diffuse interstitial fibrosis may be a clue to indicate the necessity for venography (67). The prognosis for untreated patients is grave; renal function deteriorates rapidly, and death from pulmonary emboli some-

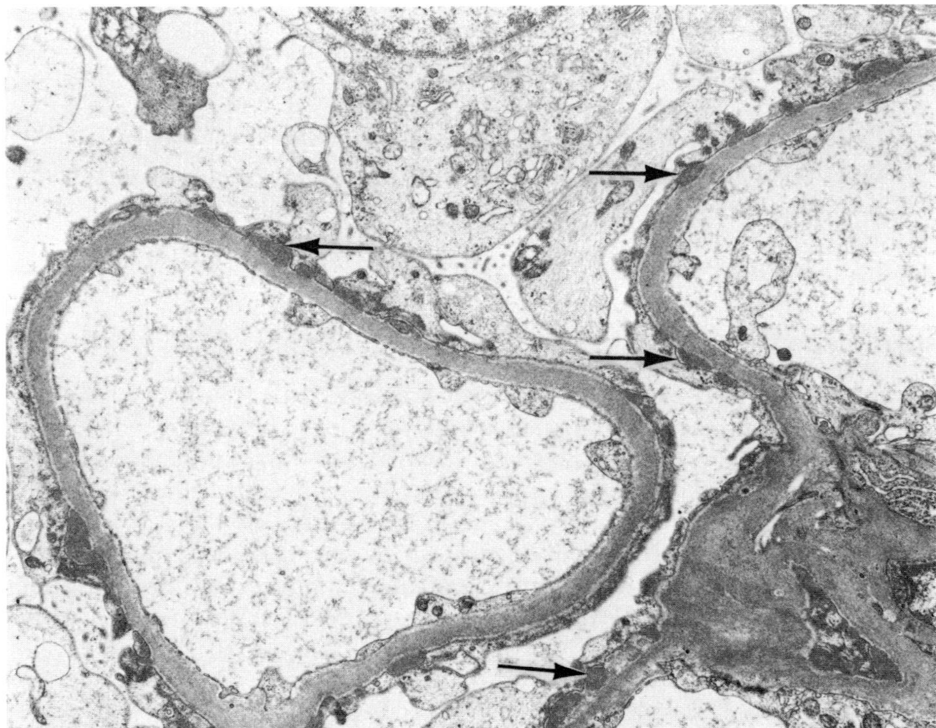

Figure 9-22. Biopsy specimen from a patient with secondary syphilis. A few small subepithelial deposits are present along the loops (arrows) (×7,800).

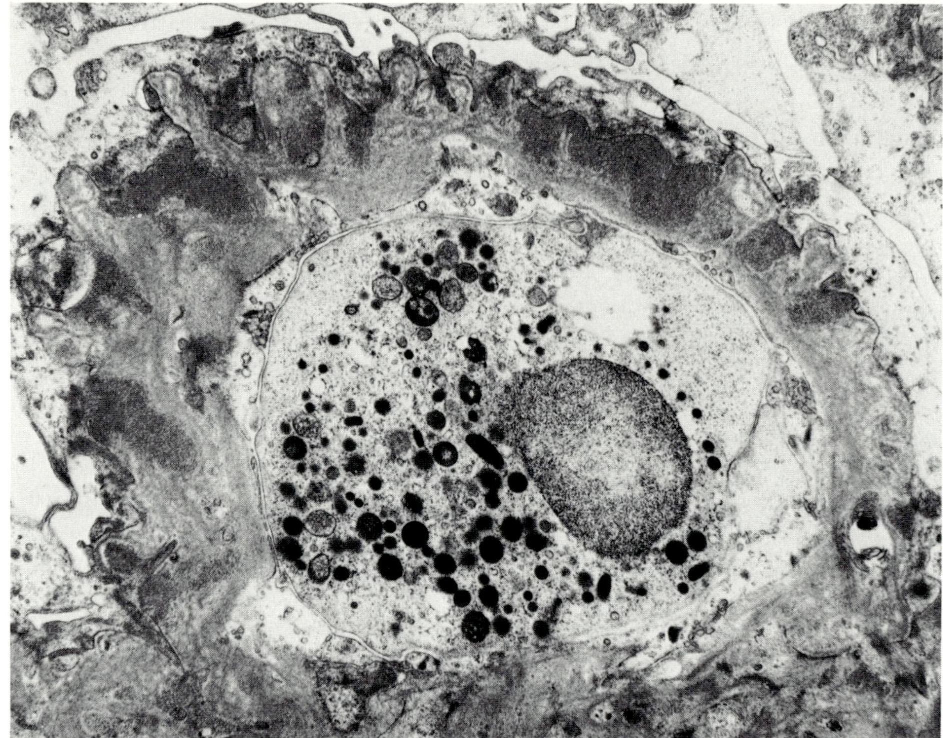

Figure 9-23. Biopsy specimen of a patient with membranous nephropathy and renal vein thrombosis. A neutrophil is present in the capillary lumen ($\times 10{,}200$).

times occurs (68,69). Treatment by either thrombectomy or anticoagulants may arrest the functional deterioration but has no effect on the underlying glomerular lesion (67−69).

SUMMARY

Membranous nephropathy is a glomerular disease with specific morphologic characteristics but varied pathogenesis and behavior. The pathogenesis of the disease in most patients is unknown, but comparison with experimental models suggests that the subepithelial deposits may develop from either circulating immune complexes or those that form in situ. Although there is as yet no definite proof, it is likely that all or most of the secondary examples of membranous nephropathy develop from circulating immune complexes, and that identification and removal of the antigens responsible will lead to cure. In the idiopathic disease, no clear guide to therapy is available, and there is controversy over the value of the various modes of treatment that have been used. This controversy is, in part, due to the heterogeneous patterns of clinical behavior of the lesion. In a significant number of patients with the idiopathic disease, especially children, the disease remits spontaneously, while the remainder may progress rapidly into renal failure or stay apparently static for many years. Progression is sometimes caused by the superimposition of crescentic disease, but is more often produced by advancing membrane damage with glomerulosclerosis, which may be irregular and suggest other forms of glomerulonephritis. Diagnosis is achieved by the identification of either the deposits, which are best shown by electron or immunofluorescence microscopy, or the spiky pattern of membrane reaction, which is easily seen in silver-stained sections. There are no reliable morphologic methods for differentiating between the primary and secondary forms of membranous nephropathy, and the identification of a membranous lesion is only the first stage of establishing a final clinicopathologic diagnosis.

REFERENCES

1. Germuth FG, Rodriguez E: *Immunopathology of the renal glomerulus: immune complex deposit and anti-basement membrane disease.* Boston, Little, Brown and Co, 1973, p. 26.

2. Kupor LR, Lowance DC, McPhaul JJ Jr: Single and multiple drug therapy in autologous immune complex nephritis in rats. *J Lab Clin Med* 87:27, 1976.

3. Heymann W, Hackel DB, Harwood S, et al: Production of nephrotic syndrome in rats by Freund's adjuvant and rat kidney suspensions. *Proc Soc Exp Biol Med* 100:660, 1959.

4. Glassock RJ, Edginton TS, Watson JI, et al: Autologous immune complex nephritis induced with renal tubular antigen. II. The pathogenetic mechanism. *J Exp Med* 127:573, 1968.

5. Sugisaki T, Klassen J, Andres GA, et al: Passive transfer of Heymann nephritis with serum. *Kidney Int* 3:66, 1973.

6. Van Es LA, Blok APR, Schoenfelt L, et al: Chronic nephritis induced by antibodies reacting with glomerular-bound immune complexes. *Kidney Int* 11:106, 1977.

7. Van Damme BJC, Fleuren GJ, Bakker WW, et al: Experimental glomerulonephritis in the rat induced by antibodies directed against tubular antigens. V. Fixed glomerular antigens in the pathogenesis of heterologous immune complex glomerulonephritis. *Lab Invest* 38:502, 1978.

7a. Couser WG, Steinmuller DR, Stilmant MM, et al: Experimental glomerulonephritis in the isolated perfused rat kidney. *J Clin Invest* 62:1275, 1978.

8. O'Regan S, Smith M, Drummond KN: Antigens in human immune complex nephritis. *Clin Nephrol* 6:417, 1976.

9. Eagen JW, Lewis EJ: Glomerulopathies of neoplasia. *Kidney Int* 11:297, 1977.

10. Row PG, Cameron JS, Turner DR, et al: Membranous nephropathy. Long-term follow-up and association with neoplasia. *Quart J Med* 44:207, 1975.

11. Brzosko WJ, Krawczynski K, Nazarewicz T, et al: Glomerulonephritis associated with hepatitis-B surface antigen immune complexes in children. *Lancet* 2:477, 1974.

12. Woodroffe AJ, Foldes M, McKenzie, PE, et al: Serum immune complexes and disease. *Aust NZ J Med* 9:129, 1979.

13. Naruse TL, Kitamura K, Miyakawa Y, et al: Deposition of renal tubular epithelial antigen along the capillary walls of patients with membranous glomerulonephritis. *J Immunol* 110:1163, 1973.

14. Shwayder M, Ozawa T, Boedecker E, et al: Nephrotic syndrome associated with Fanconi syndrome: immunopathogenetic studies of tubulointerstitial nephritis with autologous immune complex glomerulonephritis. *Ann Intern Med* 84:433, 1976.

15. Wilson CB, Dixon FJ: The renal response to immunological injury, in Brenner BM and Rector FC (eds): *The Kidney.* Philadelphia, WB Saunders Co, 1976, vol II, p 892.

15a. Whitworth JA, Leibowitz MC, Kennedy JS, et al: Absence of glomerular renal tubular epithelial antigen in membranous glomerulonephritis. *Clin Nephrol* 5:159, 1976.

16. Ehrenreich T, Yunis SL, Churg J: Membranous nephropathy following exposure to hydrocarbons. *Environ Res* 14:35, 1977.

16a. Llach F, Descouedres C, Massry SG: Heroin associated nephropathy: clinical and morphological studies in 19 patients. *Clin Nephrol* 11:7, 1979.

17. Nagi AM, Alexander F, Barabas AZ: Gold nephropathy in rats: light and electron microscopic studies. *Exp Molec Pathol* 15:354, 1971.

18. Bariety J, Druet P, Laliberte F, et al: Glomerulonephritis with γ-globulin and BC-globulin deposits induced in rats by mercuric chloride. *Am J Pathol* 65:293, 1971.

19. Palosuo T, Provost TT, Milgrom F: Gold nephropathy: serologic data suggesting an immune complex disease. *Clin Exp Immunol* 25:311, 1978.

20. Gluck MC, Gallo G, Lowenstein J, et al: Membranous glomerulonephritis. Evolution of clinical and pathologic features. *Ann Intern Med* 78:1, 1973.

21. Erwin DT, Donadio JV, Holley KE: The clinical course of idiopathic membranous nephropathy. *Mayo Clin Proc* 48:697, 1973.

22. Franklin WA, Jennings, RB, Earle DP: Membranous glomerulonephritis: long-term serial observations on clinical course and morphology. *Kidney Int* 4:36, 1973.

23. Pierides AM, Malasit P, Morley AR, et al: Idiopathic membranous nephropathy. *Quart J Med* 46:163, 1977.

24. Gartner HV, Watanabe T, Ott V, et al: Correlations between morphologic and clinical features in idiopathic perimembranous glomerulonephritis: a study on 403 renal biopsies of 367 patients. *Current Topics Pathol* 65:1, 1977.

25. Hayslett JP, Kashgarian M, Bensch KG, et al: Clinicopathological correlations in the nephrotic syndrome due to primary renal disease. *Medicine (Balt)* 52:93, 1973.

26. Forland M, Spargo BH: Clinicopathological correlations in idiopathic nephrotic syndrome with membranous nephropathy. *Nephron* 6:498, 1969.

27. Nephrotic syndrome in children: prediction of histopathology from clinical and laboratory characteristics at time of diagnosis. A report of the International Study of Kidney Disease in Children. *Kidney Int* 13:159, 1978.

28. Olbing H, Greifer I, Bennett BP, et al: Idiopathic membranous nephropathy in children. *Kidney Int* 3:381, 1973.

29. Habib R, Kleinknecht C: The primary nephrotic syndrome of childhood. Classification and clinicopathologic study of 406 cases. *Pathol Annu* 6:417, 1971.

30. Libit SA, Burke B, Michael AT, et al: Extramembranous glomerulonephritis in childhood: relationship to systemic lupus erythematosus. *J Pediat* 88:394, 1976.

31. Strauch BS, Hayslett JP: Kidney disease and pregnancy. *Br Med J* 4:578, 1974.

32. Jones DB: Nephrotic glomerulonephritis. *Am J Pathol* 33:313, 1957.

33. Ehrenreich T, Churg J: Pathology of membranous nephropathy. *Pathol Annu* 3:145, 1968.

34. Rosen S: Membranous glomerulonephritis: current status. *Human Pathol* 2:209, 1971.

35. Walker F: The origin, turnover and removal of glomerular basement membrane. *J Pathol* 110:233, 1973.

36. Burkholder PM, Hyman LP, Barber TA: Extracellular clusters of spherical microparticles in glomeruli in human renal glomerular diseases. *Lab Invest* 28:415, 1973.

37. Bariety J, Callard P: Striated membranous structures in renal glomerular tufts: an electron microscopic study of 340 human renal biopsies. *Lab Invest* 32:636, 1975.

38. Jao W, Pollak VE, Norris SN, et al: Lipoid nephrosis: an approach to the clinicopathologic analysis and dismemberment of idiopathic nephrotic syndrome with minimal glomerular changes. *Medicine (Balt)* 52:445, 1973.

38a. Ehrenreich T, Churg J: Focal glomerulosclerosis in membranous nephropathy. *Am J Pathol* 87:37a, 1977.

39. Gartner HV, Fischbach H, Wehner N, et al: Comparison of clinical and morphological features of peri- (epi-extra) membranous glomerulonephritis. *Nephron* 13:288, 1974.

40. Richet G, Fillastre JP, Morel-Maroger L, et al: Change from diffuse proliferative to membranous glomerulonephritis: serial biopsies in four cases. *Kidney Int* 5:57, 1974.

41. Klassen J, Elwood C, Grossberg AL, et al: Evolution of membranous nephropathy into anti-glomerular-basement-membrane glomerulonephritis. *N Engl J Med* 290:1340, 1974.

42. Moorthy AV, Zimmerman, SW, Burkholder PM, et al: Association of crescentic glomerulonephritis with membranous nephropathy: a report of three cases. *Clin Nephrol* 6:319, 1976.

43. Hill GS, Robertson J, Grossman R, et al: An unusual variant of membranous nephropathy with abundant crescent formation and recurrence in the transplanted kidney. *Clin Nephrol* 10:114, 1978.

44. Morel-Maroger L, Leathem A, Richet G: Glomerular abnormalities in nonsystemic diseases: relationship between findings by light microscopy and immunofluorescence in 433 renal biopsy specimens. *Am J Med* 53:170, 1972.

45. Verroust PJ, Wilson CB, Cooper NR, et al: Glomerular complement components in human glomerulonephritis. *J Clin Invest* 53:77, 1974.

45a. Törnröth T, Tallqvist G, Pasternack A, et al: Nonprogressive, histologically mild membranous nephropathy appearing in all evolutionary phases as histologically "early" membranous glomerulonephritis. *Kidney Int* 14:511, 1978.

46. Ansell ID, Joekes AM: Spicular arrangement of amyloid in renal biopsy. *J Clin Pathol* 25:1056, 1972.

47. Bohle A, Fischbach H, Gartner H-V, et al: Simultaneous occurrence of perimembranous glomerulonephritis and glomerular amyloidosis. *Virchows Arch (A) Path Anat Histol* 378:315, 1978.

48. Cameron JS: The natural history of glomerulonephritis, in Black DAK (ed), *Renal Disease*, ed 3. Oxford, Blackwell, 1972, p 307.

48a. Noel LH, Zanetti M, Droz D, et al: Long term prognosis of idiopathic membranous glomerulonephritis: study of 116 untreated patients. *Am J Med* 66:82, 1979.

49. Ehrenreich T, Porusch JG, Churg J, et al: Treatment of idiopathic membranous nephropathy. *N Engl J Med* 295:741, 1976.

50. Donadio JV, Holley KE, Anderson CF, et al: Controlled trial of cyclophosphamide in idiopathic membranous nephropathy. *Kidney Int* 6:431, 1974.

51. Coggins CL, Churg J, Spargo BH, et al: US cooperative study of the adult idiopathic nephrotic syndrome. Unpublished observations, 1975.

52. Rubin RJ, Pinn VW, Barnes BA, et al: Recurrent idiopathic membranous glomerulonephritis. *Transplantation* 24:4, 1977.

53. Steinmuller DR, Stilmant MM, Idelson BA: De novo development of membranous nephropathy in cadaver renal allografts. *Clin Nephrol* 9:210, 1978.

54. Habib R, Kleinknecht C, Gubler MC: Extramembranous glomerulonephritis in children: report of 50 cases. *J Pediat* 82:754, 1973.

55. Silverberg DS, Kidd EG, Shnitka TK, et al: Gold nephropathy: a clinical and pathologic study. *Arthritis Rheum* 13:812, 1970.

56. Watanabe I, Whittier FC, Moore J, et al: Gold nephropathy: ultrastructural, fluorescence and microanalytic studies of two patients. *Arch Pathol Lab Med* 100:632, 1976.

57. Stuve J, Galle P: Role of mitochondria in the handling of gold by the kidney. A study of electron microscopy and electron probe microanalysis. *J Cell Biol* 44:667, 1970.

58. Viol GW, Minnielly JA, Bistricki T: Gold nephropathy: tissue analysis by x-ray fluorescent spectrometry. *Arch Pathol Lab Med* 101:635, 1977.

59. Törnröth T, Skrifvars B: The Development and resolution of glomerular basement membrane changes associated with subepithelial immune deposits. *Am J Pathol* 79:219, 1975.

60. Weiss AS, Markenson JA, Weiss MS, et al: Toxicity of D-penicillamine in rheumatoid arthritis: a report of 63 patients including two with aplastic anemia and one with the nephrotic syndrome. *Am J Med* 64:114, 1978.

61. Dische FE, Swinson DR, Hamilton EBD, et al: Immunopathology of penicillamine-induced glomerular disease. *J Rheumatol* 3:145, 1976.

62. Bacon RA, Tribe CR, MacKenzie JC, et al: Penicillamine nephropathy in rheumatoid arthritis: a clinical, pathological and immunological study. *Quart J Med* 45:661, 1976.

63. Gamble CN, Reardan JB: Immunopathogenesis of syphilitic glomerulonephritis: elution of antitreponemal antibody from glomerular immune-complex deposits. *N Engl J Med* 292:449, 1975.

64. Tourville DR, Byrd LH, Kim DU, et al: Treponemal antigen in immunopathogenesis of syphilitic glomerulonephritis. *Am J Pathol* 82:479, 1976.

65. Kaplan BS, Chesney RW, Drummond KN: The nephrotic syndrome and renal vein thrombosis. *Am J Dis Child* 132:367, 1978.

66. Llach F, Koffler A, Finck E, et al: On the incidence of renal vein thrombosis in the nephrotic syndrome. *Arch Intern Med* 137:333, 1977.

67. Cade R, Spooner G, Juncos L, et al: Chronic renal vein thrombosis. *Am J Med* 63:387, 1977.

68. Trew RA, Biava CG, Jacobs RP, et al: Renal vein thrombosis in membranous glomerulonephropathy: incidence and association. *Medicine (Balt)* 57:69, 1978.

69. Duffy JL, Letteri J, Cinque T, et al: Renal vein thrombosis and the nephrotic syndrome: report of two cases with successful treatment of one. *Am J Med* 54:663, 1973.

10
Crescentic Glomerulonephritis

There are few more ominous morphologic patterns in a renal biopsy specimen than numerous circumferential crescents. The crescent is an expression of fulminant glomerular damage and always leaves severe residual scarring. This damage may be caused by a variety of mechanisms, and the recognition of crescentic disease is only the first step toward morphologic classification. Involvement of even a minority of glomeruli by crescents is an indication of potentially serious and progressive disease, but the diagnosis of crescentic glomerulonephritis should be reserved for those biopsy specimens showing extensive involvement. The precise criteria for diagnosis vary in the published accounts of the disease, but an arbitrary figure of 80% has been suggested by the World Health Organization (see Chap. 1). There are a significant number of biopsy specimens in which crescents so dominate the picture that no clue to their etiology can be demonstrated. Such biopsy specimens may reasonably be designated as idiopathic crescentic glomerulonephritis. For the remaining majority, in which other diagnostic features are recognizable, a better approach is to specify both the basic glomerular disease and its crescentic complication.

PATHOGENESIS

Almost any form of glomerular disease may be complicated by the formation of crescents. The ubiquity of this pattern of reaction indicates the probability of a common pathogenetic mechanism. There is general agreement that the most likely mechanism for crescent formation is the escape of fibrin into Bowman's space (1). Fibrin is universally seen by either immunofluorescence or other techniques in human and experimental forms of crescentic glomerulonephritis. In experimental animals, anticoagulation both before (1) and after (2) the induction of glomerulonephritis prevents fibrin accumulation, abolishes crescent formation and ameliorates the severity of the glomerular disease. These observations have led to the widespread use of anticoagulants in human crescentic disease, but the results, though promising, have not been as impressive as in the experimental models (3,4).

There is sufficient alteration of membrane permeability in many forms of glomerulonephritis for fibrinogen to reach Bowman's space, but crescents are relatively uncommon. A direct effect of fibrin has not yet been demonstrated on epithelial cells, and other factors are likely to be implicated in crescent formation. Massive efflux of plasma into Bowman's space could occur via breaks in the glomerular basement membrane, and the cellular injury associated with such damage could activate the coagulation system to produce fibrin and its products. Basement membrane breaks (gaps) are frequently seen in PASM-stained sections of crescentic glomeruli and are regularly demonstrated by electron microscopy (5,6). These local areas of damage are probably produced by the lytic actions of complement and leukocytic enzymes, complement components having been demonstrated adjacent to the breaks in some cases (7). Morphologic evidence strongly favors an epithelial origin of the crescent cells (8), and although tissue culture studies have suggested that these cells may be derived from macrophages (9), labeling studies do not support a macrophage origin (10).

There is abundant evidence from both human and experimental diseases that crescents form within days, perhaps even hours, of glomerular damage. As a general rule, it may be stated that crescentic involvement of a glomerulus will cause permanent scarring, the extent of the scar being directly proportional to the area involved by the crescent. Thus, circumferential crescents cause global sclerosis while localized areas of epithelial proliferation produce segmental effacement of a similar proportion of the glomerulus. Serial biopsy specimens from patients whose disease has been arrested by therapy show remarkable resolution of the active inflammatory changes but the proportion of globally and segmentally scarred glomeruli is almost always closely comparable to the original extent of crescentic disease. Claims for complete disappearance of crescents are unconvincing and are not supported by the photomicrographs published to demonstrate this resolution (11,12,12a).

CLINICAL MANIFESTATIONS AND COURSE

Idiopathic crescentic glomerulonephritis affects all age groups but is most common in older people, and most series show a mild male predominance (4,13–15). Its first appearance is either insidious, with symptoms referable to progressive azotemia, or as a fulminant nephritic syndrome (4,16,17). In some patients, nonspecific upper respiratory or other infections may precede the acute illness, but there are usually no identifiable precipitating factors. The acute presentation may closely resemble that of acute postinfectious glomerulonephritis, although there is more often sustained oliguria and azotemia, or may be with the nephrotic syndrome. The urinary sediment is typical of severe glomerulonephritis, with abundant red cells and protein, but other investigations are of little diagnostic value and serum complement concentrations are almost always normal. Oliguria, or even anuria, often persists for some time so that dialysis is necessary to maintain life. Most patients in earlier series died of renal failure within a few weeks from onset (15,18). There is a clinicopathologic continuum between crescentic glomerulonephritis and the arteritic syndromes, and some patients complain of muscle pains, arthritis, and other systemic features. In such patients, the presence of eosinophilia is a useful (19), but not reliable (18), clue to the diagnosis of arteritis.

PATHOLOGIC CHARACTERISTICS

The crescent is an entirely nonspecific morphologic lesion. Epithelial proliferation is always a complication of underlying glomerular disease and never a primary event. Thus, the first responsibility of the pathologist when faced with a biopsy specimen showing crescents is to establish the primary diagnosis (Table 10-1). Even in those biopsy specimens with no identifiable primary lesion, the next crucial responsibility is to establish the extent of crescentic disease, since prognosis is closely correlated with the percentage of glomeruli involved by crescents (14,17). For this purpose, any degree of crescentic proliferation may be included since, serial sections frequently reveal circumferential crescents around glomeruli which initially appear only segmentally involved. The authors prefer to restrict the term *crescentic glomerulonephritis* to those biopsy specimens with more than 80% glomerular involvement and no apparent cause, designating other cases with a primary diagnosis and a statement of the proportion of glomeruli showing crescents.

Crescents

Crescents range from small groups of cells occupying fractions of Bowman's space to cohesive masses completely surrounding the glomerulus (Figs. 10-1,10-2). Their evolution may be divided into cellular, fibrocellular, and fibrous phases, these appearances frequently coexisting in the same biopsy specimen (8,16). In the cellular phase, polymorphs and fibrin are frequently intermingled with the proliferating cells, which range from spindle to ovoid in form and often contain mitotic figures (13). (Figs. 10-3−10-5). Most cells have voluminous, clear cytoplasm, but some are small and dark, and there may be groups of macrophagelike cells around fragmented basement membrane (8,20) (Fig. 10-6). Occasionally, multinucleate giant cells may be prominent in the crescents, but these carry no etiologic significance (20). A true granulomatous crescentic pattern, however, has occasionally been associated with polyarteritis (21,22) (Fig. 10-7). Ultrastructurally, the cells in the active phase appear to arise from the parietal epithelium and appear clear or dark according to their cytoplasmic content of ribosomes and rough endoplasmic reticulum (8,23) (Figs. 10-8, 10-9).

Within one or two weeks, evidence of organization ushers in the fibrocellular phase. Initially, light microscopic examination discloses strands of PAS- and PASM-positive matrix between the proliferating cells. (Fig. 10-10). This material is identifiable ultrastructurally as basement membrane and is soon admixed with collagen fibers (24) (Fig. 10-11). Accumulating intercellular matrix dissects the masses into groups of smaller cells, which frequently differentiate into glandularlike structures lined by cuboidal epithelium. Finally, segmental crescents are either incorporated into Bowman's capsule as fibrous collars or represented merely by collagenous PAS-negative, glomerular scars (Fig. 10-11). Circumferential crescents transform to globally sclerotic glomeruli in which frequent residual nuclei are the only evidence of the original disease. In the course of crescent development, breaks in Bowman's capsule often develop, and such breaks may provide a clue in sclerotic disease to the previous presence of crescentic proliferation.

Table 10–1. Differential Diagnosis of Crescentic Glomerulonephritis[a]

Diagnosis	Light Microscopy[b]	Immunofluorescence Microscopy[b]	Electron Microscopic Deposits
Postinfectious glomerulonephritis	D, exudative	+	+ (humps)
Bacterial endocarditis glomerulonephritis	F or D ± exudative	+	+ (± humps)
Mesangiocapillary glomerulonephritis	D (mesangiocapillary)	+	+
Dense deposit disease	F or D (intramembranous deposit)	+	+ (intramembranous deposit)
Membranous nephropathy	D (spikes)	+	+
IgA nephropathy and Henoch-Schönlein purpura	F or D	+	+
Lupus glomerulonephritis	F or D (wire loops, hematoxyphil bodies)	+	+
Antiglomerular basement membrane glomerulonephritis	F	+ (linear)	0
Hemolytic uremic syndrome	F	+ (fibrin)	+ (fibrin)
Malignant hypertension	F	+ or 0 (± fibrin)	+ or 0 (± fibrin)
Polyarteritis	F	0	0
Idiopathic	F	0	0

[a] From ref. 26; see other chapters for details.

[b] F = focal; D = diffuse; + = present; 0 = absent.

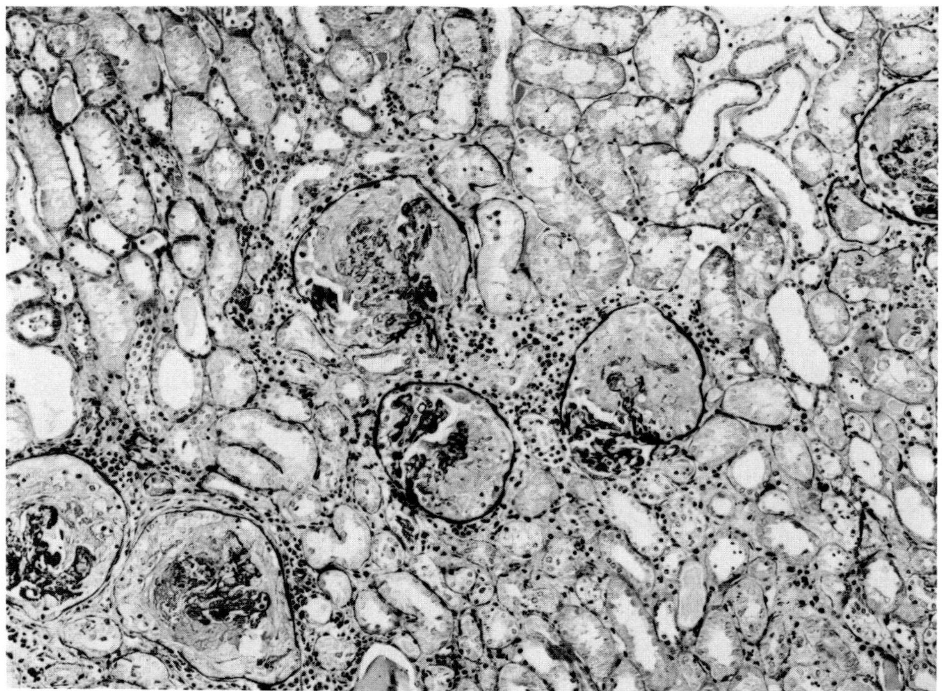

Figure 10-1. Idiopathic crescentic glomerulonephritis. All glomeruli are involved by circumferential crescent (PASM stain, ×120).

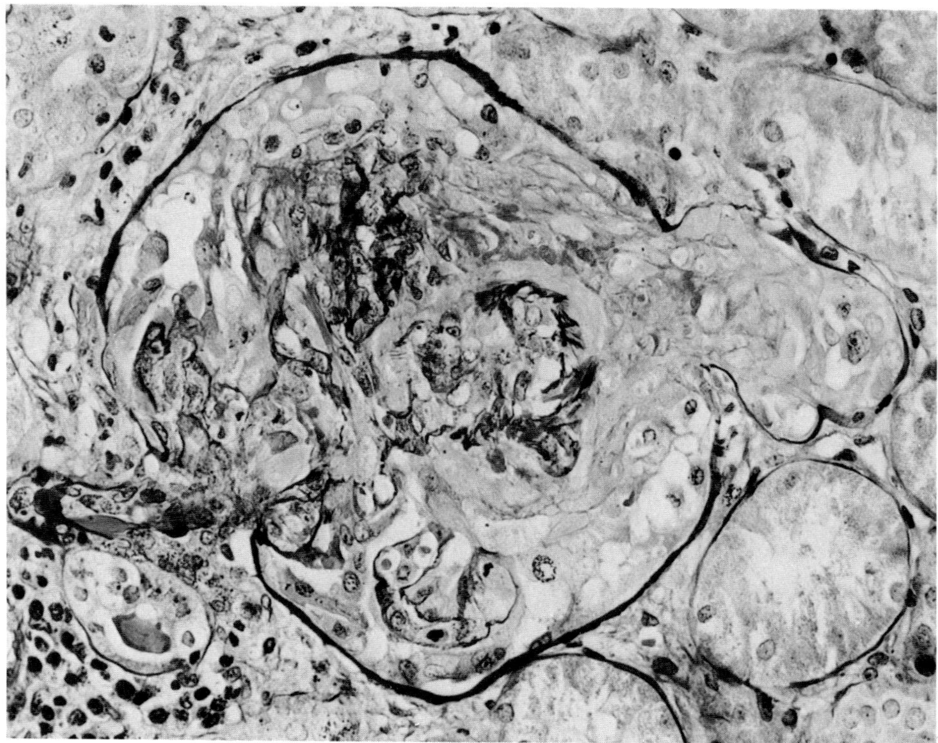

Figure 10-2. Glomerulus with epithelial crescents obliterating the urinary space and extending into the proximal tubule. Note the marked compression of the tuft with interruption of capillary wall (PASM stain, ×350).

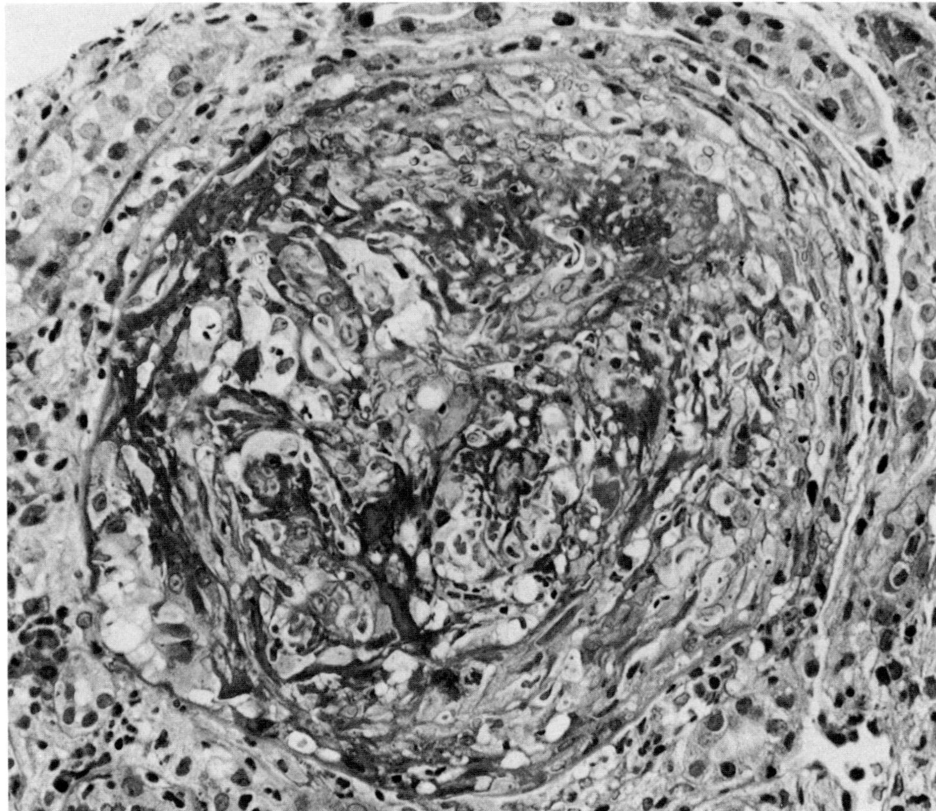

Figure 10-3. Cellular phase of idiopathic crescentic glomerulonephritis. There are polymorphonuclear leukocytes and fibrin intermingled among the proliferating capsular cells. Highly collapsed capillary loops contain polymorphs as well (H&E stain, ×400).

Glomerular Tufts

In those forms of crescentic disease complicating established glomerulonephritis, the diagnostic patterns of the basic disease can usually be identified by light, electron, or immunofluorescence microscopy. In the idiopathic disease, the glomeruli are often completely collapsed, apparently strangled by the surrounding cellular collar (Fig. 10-2). Usually, however, segmental changes can be identified in idiopathic crescentic glomerulonephritis, although these may be visible in only a few of many serial sections. Typically, the segmental lesions show expansion of one or several capillary loops by intracapillary swelling with massive fibrin and polymorph exudation and disruption of the basement membrane. Ultrastructural examination of such areas reveals intraluminal and subendothelial accumulation of fibrin with membrane irregularity or dissolution and, frequently, separation of the adjacent epithelial cells (5,17) (Figs. 10-8, 10-12). Immunofluorescence studies are often negative in the idiopathic disease but may show diffuse granular reactions for immunoglobulins and complement or nonspecific segmental patterns of staining (14,17,25,25a,25b).

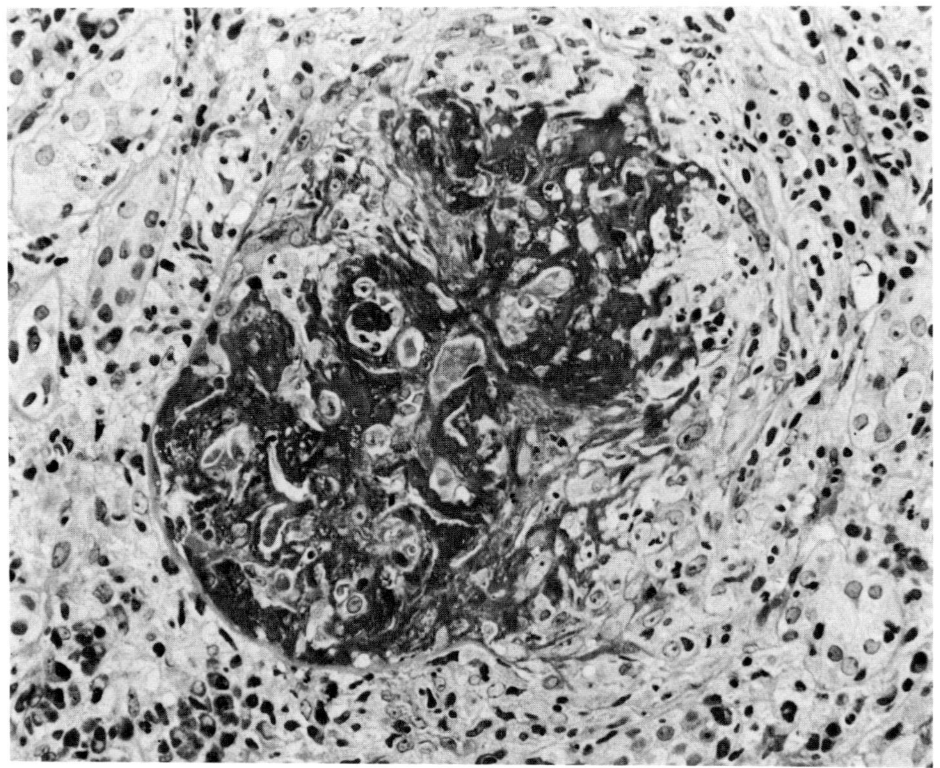

Figure 10-4. The same case as in Figure 10-3. The glomerular tuft is necrotic and the Bowman's capsule disrupted (right). Note severe interstitial inflammation (H&E stain, ×400).

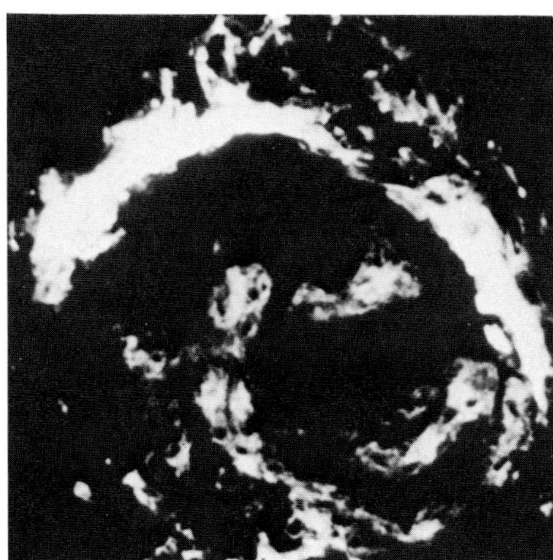

Figure 10-5. The same case as figure 10-3. This immunofluorescent preparation shows massive fibrin deposition within an epithelial crescent and capillary tuft (×300).

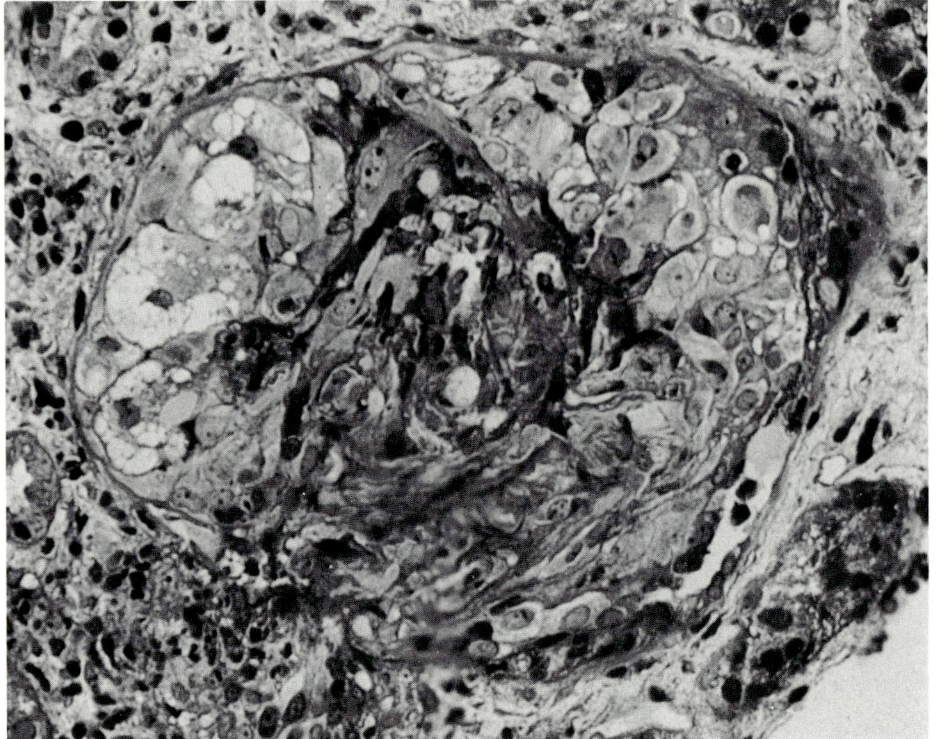

Figure 10-6. Idiopathic crescentic glomerulonephritis with marked collapse of tuft and prominent large proliferating cells with clear cytoplasm (H&E stain, ×400).

Extraglomerular Changes

Crescentic glomerulonephritis is often accompanied by extensive interstitial inflammation which, like glomerular changes, organizes to leave scarring (Fig. 10-4). Especially if eosinophils are frequent in this infiltrate or interstitial granulomata can be seen, a careful search for necrotizing arteritis is indicated (19).

DIFFERENTIAL DIAGNOSIS

In the majority of biopsy specimens showing crescentic glomerulonephritis, an underlying glomerular lesion can be demonstrated (26) (Table 10-1). Usually, intracapillary proliferation is clearly visible in spite of crescentic disease, but in some cases the tuft changes may be obscured (27). The most difficult diagnostic problem is the exclusion of microscopic polyarteritis (18). As already mentioned, crescentic glomerulonephritis and polyarteritis share many features, and clear differentiation may be impossible. A number of patients with crescentic disease have symptoms highly suggestive of arteritis, but no vascular lesions appear in biopsy specimens, while arteritic changes have been found in other patients in whom such symptoms are absent (25b). The arteritic lesions may be extraordinarily sparse, even with exhaustive postmortem study, and a reasonable com-

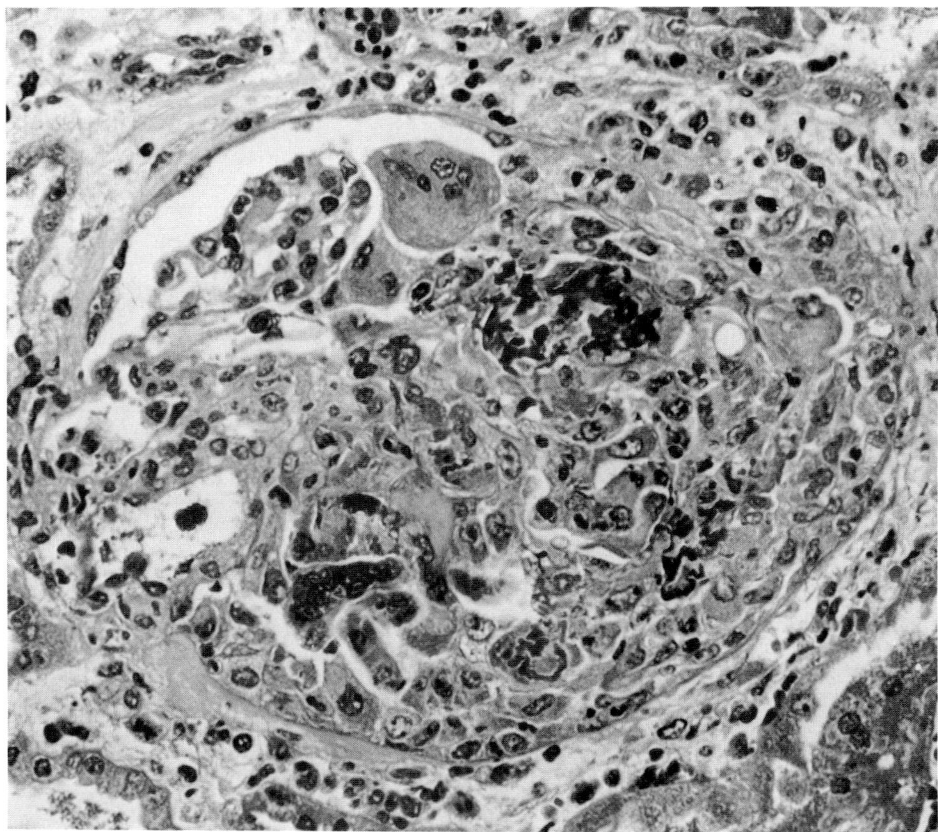

Figure 10-7. Idiopathic crescentic glomerulonephritis with multinucleated giant cells (H&E stain, ×450).

promise is probably to regard all cases of idiopathic crescentic glomerulonephritis as potential examples of polyarteritis. In a significant proportion of patients, careful examination of serial biopsy sections will demonstrate vasculitic lesions.

PROGNOSIS AND THERAPY

The prognosis of crescentic glomerulonephritis depends on the cause of the glomerular disease, the extent of crescentic involvement, and the renal function at presentation. Those patients with oligoanuria at onset and/or 100% crescents rarely recover, whereas those with lesser degrees of glomerular obliteration may show substantial recovery (14,17,28). Various combinations of anticoagulants, corticosteroids, and immunosuppressive agents have been reported to cause significant improvement in various forms of crescentic disease (3,28,29), especially those associated with definite vasculitis (30), and promising results have been reported with plasmapheresis (31). Even when the acute disease is controlled, however, extensive residual scarring usually leads to severe hypertension, which may, in turn, cause renewed deterioration in renal function.

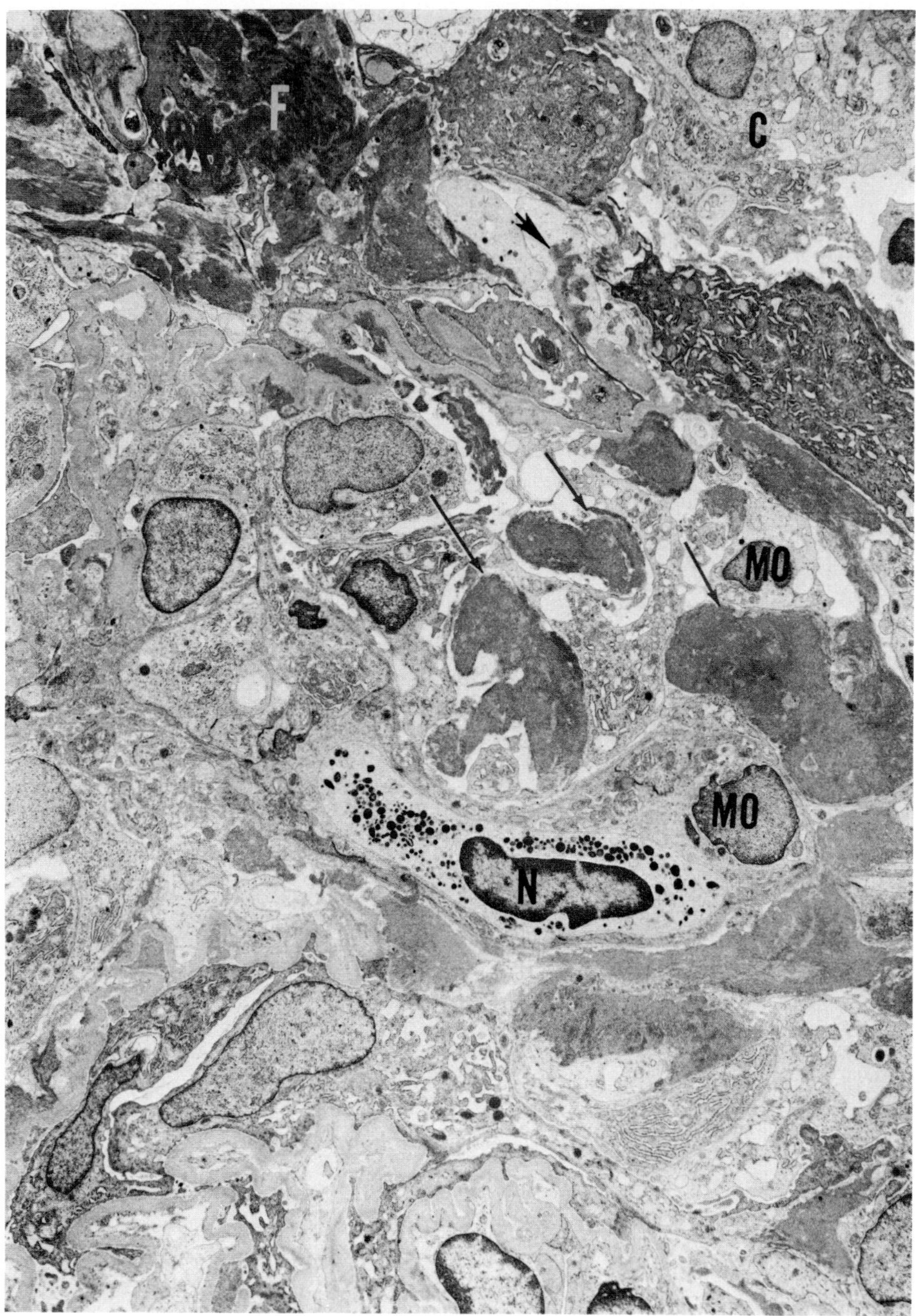

Figure 10-8. Active idiopathic crescentic glomerulonephritis. The capillary loop is filled with fibrin in different stages of polymerization (arrows), monocytes (MO), and neutrophilic leukocytes (N). Fibrin (F) is also found in the urinary space. A portion of a crescent is present on the right upper corner (C). The endoplasmic reticulum of crescent cells is variably developed. The glomerular basement membrane is focally disrupted (arrow head) (×3,450).

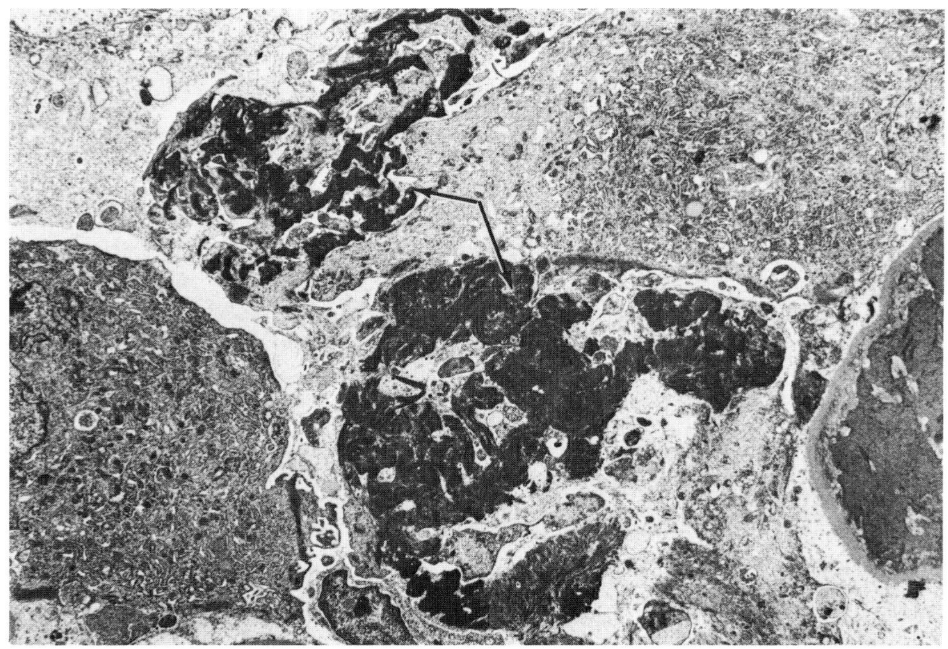

Figure 10-9. Strands of fibrin (arrows) are present between the proliferated epithelial cells. The latter have well-developed endoplasmic reticulum (×8,100).

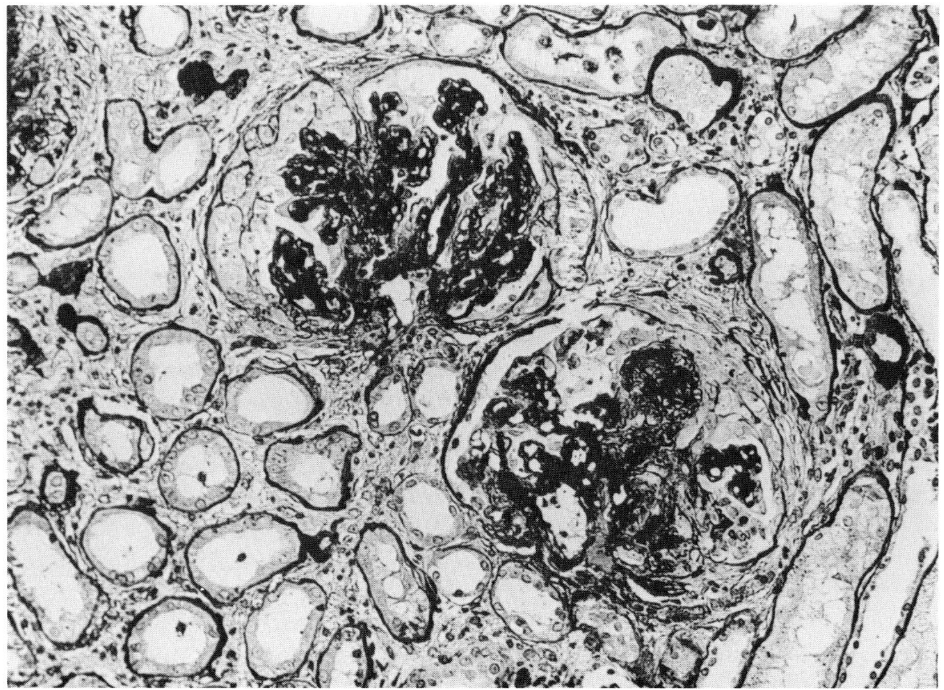

Figure 10-10. Organizing crescentic glomerulonephritis (PASM stain, ×225).

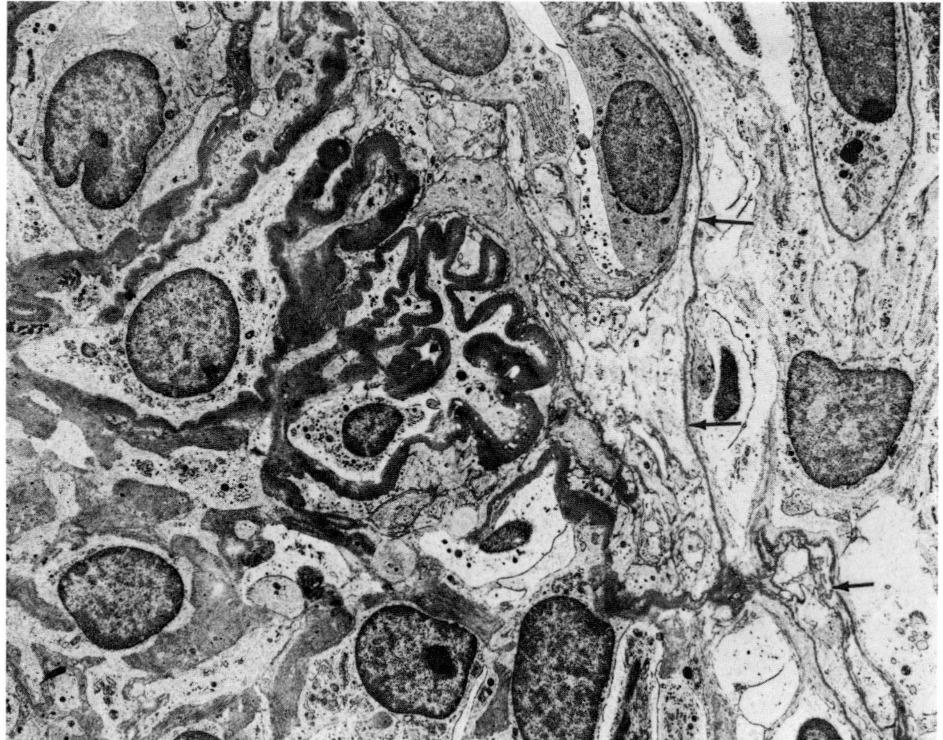

Figure 10-11. Electron micrograph illustrating organized crescent. Scanty thin strands of basement membrane-like material are recognized between capsular epithelial cells (arrows). The glomerular tuft is markedly collapsed (×2,600).

Idiopathic crescentic glomerulonephritis very occasionally affects transplanted kidneys, either as recurrent (7) or de novo (32) disease, but transplantation in those patients proceeding to chronic renal failure is usually successful.

SUMMARY

Crescentic glomerulonephritis is a heterogeneous collection of clinicopathologic entities that are unified by the presence of epithelial proliferation in Bowman's space. The formation of crescents is probably related to the presence of extracapillary fibrin, which escapes via breaks in the glomerular basement membrane. The natural history of the crescent is of progressive fibrosis with compression and, finally, obliteration of glomeruli. An assessment of the percentage of involved glomeruli is, therefore, important, in order to provide the physician with an approximate indication of the likely degree of future scarring. Although crescents appear morphologically similar in whichever disease they complicate, the prognosis for continued crescent formation varies according to the underlying glomerular lesion. Accurate and specific recognition of this underlying disease is, therefore, essential to allow effective therapeutic intervention. Only in those cases with no diagnostic features in the glomerular tuft is a diagnosis of crescentic glomerulonephritis appropriate.

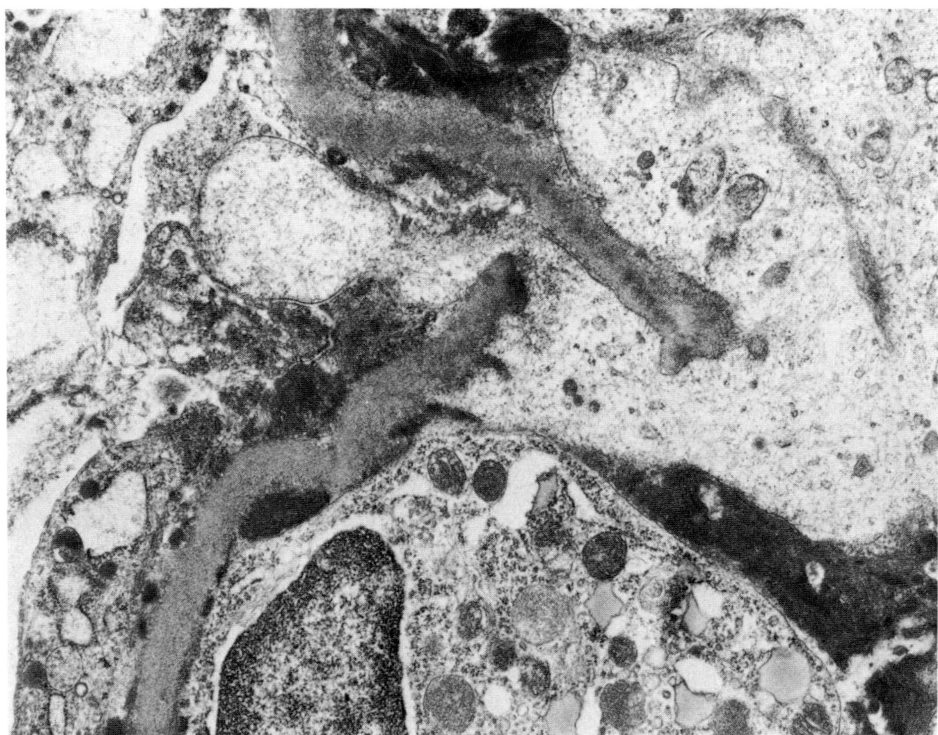

Figure 10-12. Thrombosed capillary with break of the basement membrane ($\times$14,400).

REFERENCES

1. Vassalli P, McCluskey RT: The pathogenetic role of the coagulation process in glomerular diseases of immunologic origin. *Adv Nephrol* 1:47, 1971.

2. Naish P, Penn GB, Evans DJ, et al: The effect of defibrination on nephrotoxic serum nephritis in rabbits. *Clin Sci* 42:643, 1972.

3. Kincaid-Smith P, Saker BM, Fairley KF: Anticoagulants in "irreversible" acute renal failure. *Lancet* 2:1360, 1968.

4. Morrin PAF, Hinglais N, Nabarra B, et al: Rapidly progressive glomerulonephritis: a clinical and pathological study. *Am J Med* 65:446, 1978.

5. Stejskal J, Pirani CL, Okada M, et al: Discontinuities (gaps) of the glomerular capillary wall and basement membrane in renal diseases. *Lab Invest* 28:149, 1978.

6. Min KW, Györkey F, Györkey P, et al: The morphogenesis of glomerular crescents in rapidly progressive glomerulonephritis. *Kidney Int* 5:47, 1974.

7. Davis CA, McEnery PT, Maby S, et al: Observations on the evolution of idiopathic rapidly progressive glomerulonephritis. *Clin Nephrol* 9:91, 1978.

8. Morita T, Suzuki Y, Churg J: Structure and development of the glomerular crescent. *Am J Pathol* 72:349, 1973.

9. Thomson NM, Holdsworth SR, Glasgow EF, et al: The macrophage in the development of experimental crescentic glomerulonephritis: studies using tissue culture and electron microscopy. *Am J Pathol* 94:223, 1979.

10. Cattell V, Jamieson SW: The origin of glomerular crescents in experimental nephrotoxic serum nephritis in the rat. *Lab Invest* 39:584, 1978.

11. McCluskey RT, Baldwin DS: Natural history of acute glomerulonephritis. *Am J Med* 35:213, 1963.

12. Heptinstall RH: *Pathology of the Kidney* ed 2. Boston, Little, Brown and Co, 1974, Vol 1, p 378.

12a. Faarup P, Norgaard T, Elling F, et al: Structural changes in kidneys of patients with oliguric extracapillary glomerulonephritis during immunosuppressive therapy. *Acta Pathol Microbiol Scand (A)*, 86:409, 1978.

13. Rosen S: Crescentic glomerulonephritis: occurrence, mechanisms and prognosis. *Pathol Annu* 10:37, 1975.

14. Whitworth JA, Morel-Maroger L, Mignon F, et al: The significance of extracapillary proliferation: clinicopathological review of 60 patients. *Nephron* 16:1, 1976.

15. Bailestock D, Tange JD: Acute necrotizing glomerulonephritis: the clinical features and pathology in nine cases. *Aust Ann Med* 8:281, 1959.

16. Bacani RA, Velasquez F, Kanter A, et al: Rapidly progressive (nonstreptococcal) glomerulonephritis. *Ann Intern Med* 69:463, 1968.

17. Sonsino E, Nabarra B, Kazatchkine M, et al: Extracapillary proliferative glomerulonephritis, so called malignant glomerulonephritis. *Adv Nephrol* 2:121, 1972.

18. Harrison CV, Loughridge LW, Milne MD: Acute oliguric renal failure in acute glomerulonephritis and polyarteritis nodosa. *Quart J Med* 33:39, 1964.

19. Chumbley LC, Harrison EG, Deremee RA: Allergic granulomatosis and angiitis (Churg-Strauss syndrome): report and analysis of 30 cases. *Mayo Clin Proc* 52:477, 1977.

20. Olsen S: Extracapillary glomerulonephritis: a semiquantitative light microscopical study of 59 patients. *Acta Pathol Microbiol Scand (A)* (suppl 249) 82:7, 1974.

21. McManus JFA, Hornsby AT: Granulomatous glomerulonephritis associated with polyarthritis: report of a case. *Arch Pathol* 40:84, 1952.

22. Buchanan N, Berkowitz F, Gold C, et al: Granulomatous glomerulonephritis and fulminant polyarteritis nodosa in a child. *S Afr Med J* 50:1057, 1976.

23. Bohmann S-O, Olsen S, Petersen VP: Glomerular ultrastructure in extracapillary glomerulonephritis. *Acta Pathol Microbiol Scand (A)* (suppl 249) 82:29, 1974.

24. Gabbert H, Thoenes W: Formation of basement membrane in extracapillary proliferation in rapidly progressive glomerulonephritis. *Virchows Arch B Cell Pathol* 25:265, 1977.

25. Olsen S, Petersen VP, Hansen ES: Immunofluorescence studies of extracapillary glomerulonephritis. *Acta Pathol Microbiol Scand (A)* (suppl 249) 82:20, 1974.

25a. McLeish KR, Yum MN, Luft FC: Rapidly progressive glomerulonephritis in adults: clinical and histologic correlations. *Clin Nephrol* 10:43, 1978.

25b. Stilmant MM, Bolton WK, Sturgill BC, et al: Crescentic glomerulonephritis without immune deposits: clinicopathologic features. *Kidney Int* 15:184, 1979.

26. Spargo BH, Ordóñez NG, Ringus JL: The differential diagnosis of crescentic glomerulonephritis: the pathology of specific lesions with prognostic implications. *Human Pathol* 8:187, 1977.

27. Elfenbein IB, Baluarte HJ, Cubillas-Rojas M, et al: Quantitative morphometry of glomerulonephritis with crescents: diagnostic and predictive value. *Lab Invest* 32:56, 1975.

28. Arieff AI, Pingerra WF: Rapidly progressive glomerulonephritis treated with anticoagulants. *Arch Intern Med* 129:77, 1972.

29. Brown CB, Wilson D, Turner DR, et al: Combined immunosuppression and anticoagulation in rapidly progressive glomerulonephritis. *Lancet* 2:1166, 1974.

30. Friedman A, Kincaid-Smith P: Arteritis with impaired renal function, in Kincaid-Smith P, Mathew TH, Becker EL (eds): *Glomerulonephritis: Morphology, Natural History and Treatment.* New York, John Wiley & Sons, 1972, Vol II, p 1047.

31. Lockwood CM, Rees AJ, Pinching AJ, et al: Plasma-exchange and immunosuppression in the treatment of fulminating immune-complex glomerulonephritis. *Lancet* 1:63, 1977.

32. Merrill JP: The genesis of glomerulonephritis in renal transplants. *Adv Nephrol* 4:65, 1974.

11
Antiglomerular Basement Membrane Disease

Goodpasture, in 1919, reported the coexistence of "glomerular nephropathy" and pulmonary hemorrhage in a young man whom he considered to have fulminant influenza (1). In 1958, Stanton and Tange described several patients with the combination of pulmonary hemorrhage and crescentic glomerulonephritis and coined the eponym "Goodpasture's syndrome" on the grounds of "brevity and precedence" (2). By 1965, this eponym was established in the medical literature, and the immune nature of the syndrome was demonstrated by the finding of linear immunofluorescence along both glomerular and alveolar basement membranes (3,4). Within two years, the presence and nephrotoxicity of antiglomerular basement membrane (anti-GBM) antibodies were confirmed (5) and, subsequently, antibodies eluted from glomeruli were shown to attach to alveolar as well as glomerular basement membranes (6). The existence, clinical features, and pathogenesis of the syndrome thus appeared to be clearly defined.

The specificity of the syndrome, however, was soon challenged. The clinical combination of glomerulonephritis and pulmonary hemorrhage was shown to be caused by a variety of disorders (7), and cases of anti-GBM glomerulonephritis without pulmonary disease were recognized with increasing frequency (5,8–10). The true frequency of pulmonary hemorrhage in the disease remains uncertain since considerable blood loss may accumulate in the lungs without hemoptysis (3), and clinical renal involvement may apparently be delayed for some years after the onset of pulmonary symptoms (3,9). Clinically, the disease appears to be a spectrum, with most patients having combined pulmonary and renal disease, while some show renal disease alone and a minority have only pulmonary hemorrhage. Further clinical and experimental studies are likely to elucidate the mechanisms by which particular disease patterns are determined. For the moment, however, the disease complex is best described as anti-GBM glomerulonephritis and specified as of the Goodpasture type if pulmonary hemorrhage can be identified.

PATHOGENESIS

The glomerular basement membrane (GBM) is a complicated chemical mixture of proteins, carbohydrates, and lipids (11) within which at least seven distinct antigens have been identified (12). Many of these antigens are not restricted to the glomerulus, since both experimental and human anti-GBM antibodies can be shown to adhere, in vitro, to a variety of basement membranes throughout the body (13). Within the various antigenic constituents there are two major components, termed collagen and noncollagen proteins, of which the noncollagen component appears to contain the nephritogenic fraction in both animals and man (13). Precise chemical characterization of this fraction has not yet been achieved.

Experimental Anti-GBM Glomerulonephritis

Studies of the pathogenesis of anti-GBM disease (13,14) have used two principal experimental models, one produced by passive administration of antibodies raised in another animal or species (Masugi or nephrotoxic serum nephritis), the other induced by active immunization with GBM antigens (Steblay or autoimmune glomerulonephritis). Although each of these models is associated with a linear immunofluorescence pattern, the mechanisms of glomerular damage are distinct. In nephrotoxic serum nephritis, glomerular injury occurs in two separate phases: an immediate, but usually transient, reaction to the infused antibody (heterologous phase) and a delayed, more severe, reaction caused by host antibodies fixing to the foreign antibody along the GBM (autologous phase). Circulating antibodies to the foreign protein can be demonstrated in the autologous phase, but there is no evidence of specific anti-GBM activity. Glomerular injury in autoimmune glomerulonephritis is monophasic and is caused by the cross-reactivity of host GBM with the antibodies produced against the injected GBM antigens. Circulating anti-GBM antibodies can, therefore, be demonstrated in this model, and the disease is transferrable to other animals by either cross-circulation or the infusion of globulin fractions. In each system, glomerular injury is focal and segmental with crescent formation. Pulmonary hemorrhage is inconstant in nephrotoxic serum nephritis but is an integral feature of many models of autoimmune glomerulonephritis. Indeed, a syndrome analogous to human Goodpasture's disease can be produced in some animals by infusion of either glomerular or alveolar basement membrane antigens.

Human Anti-GBM Glomerulonephritis

Anti-GBM disease in man appears analogous to the Steblay model of autoimmune glomerulonephritis. There is little doubt that both pulmonary and renal lesions are caused by fixation of circulating antibody, although the factors mediating inflammation are uncertain. The most controversial aspect of anti-GBM disease is the mechanism of antibody formation. Theoretically, this could occur by either release into the circulation of native GBM antigens or the formation of cross-reactive antibodies following exposure to agents with similar antigenic constituents. Human urine contains small quantities of GBM antigens, and infusion into experimental animals of these antigens, which increase in concentration after glomerular injury, induces anti-GBM glomerulonephritis (15). Induction of anti-GBM antibodies from urinary antigens would be supported by the superimposition of anti-GBM disease upon other forms of glomerular disease, but this is, in fact, a very rare occurrence, having been reported only with membranous nephropathy (16,17), cortical necrosis (18), and the nail-patella syndrome (19). Alternatively, release of antigens from pulmonary alveoli has been suggested by the frequent prodromal respiratory infections in patients with anti-GBM disease, and a report of significant exposure to potentially tissue-toxic hydrocarbon fumes in one series (20). Hydrocarbon exposure has not been a feature in most series, however, and there is no firm evidence for antigen release in respiratory infection. Tissue infection might also provide a source of cross-reacting antigenic material, since antigenic similarities have been demonstrated between the GBM and streptococcal cell walls (9). Streptococcal infections do not, in fact, frequently precede anti-GBM disease (9), and the few reports of viral material in the secretions (9) and tissues (21,22) of patients with the disease have not been supported by evidence of common antigenicity between the GBM and viral proteins.

Thus, the factors promoting the formation of anti-GBM antibody remain unknown. Taking into account the prolonged circulation of these antibodies (9), the phenomena so far examined may, in fact, represent mechanisms of disease precipitation rather than antibody formation (23). The antigenic similarities between basement membranes throughout the body suggest that a very wide variety of injuries might theoretically release antigens capable of inducing the formation of nephritogenic antibodies. The relative rarity of anti-GBM disease, in the face of such a source of antigenic material, raises the possibility of varying capacity among the population for the formation of anti-GBM antibodies. There is insufficient information in the literature to assess the incidence of anti-GBM disease among different population groups. Some support for this hypothesis is, however, provided by the occasional reports of familial anti-GBM disease (9,24), the occurrence of the disease in a set of identical twins (25) and an apparent association with the HLA group DRW2 (25a). Further studies of affected individuals and population groups may clarify the factors involved in antibody formation.

CLINICAL MANIFESTATIONS AND COURSE

Anti-GBM disease is rare, forming less than 5% of most biopsy series (26,27), and predominantly affects young men. Compiled data from three recent series, in which the diagnosis was achieved by the demonstration of circulating antibodies (9,10,28), shows a mean age at onset of 28.5 years and a male preponderance of 80%. There is, however, a wide range and the disease has been documented from the first to the seventh decades. The major presenting feature in all but one series (28) has been rapidly progressive renal failure, with or without hemoptysis. Lesser numbers of patients were referred for the investigation of proteinuria, the nephrotic syndrome, and a variety of other phenomena (9,10). In the one dissenting series (28), most patients had hematuria or the nephrotic syndrome, but this experience appears to be unique. A significant number of patients with the more usual florid presentation have, however, had proteinuria and/or microscopic hematuria documented some months before referral. It is, therefore, reasonable to expect an occasional biopsy specimen taken for the routine investigation of an abnormal urinary sediment to show the features of anti-GBM disease.

Hemoptysis may be the sole or predominant factor precipitating appearance of the disease but, on the other hand, may be absent. Approximately half of the patients with anti-GBM disease in two recent series presented with the classical Goodpasture syndrome (9,10). The precise incidence of lung hemorrhage in the disease remains to be determined, and subclinical pulmonary phenomena may be present in the majority of patients. In those patients with overt pulmonary disease, usually manifest as hemoptysis, nephritis may antedate or postdate the pulmonary appearance. Thus, in one series of 32 patients with Goodpasture's disease, 12 patients presented with the combined syndrome, 12 with hemoptysis, and 8 with nephritis (9). Isolated renal or pulmonary disease preceded the development of the full syndrome by up to 13 months in some of these patients. Pulmonary hemorrhage may be so massive and repeated as to cause death or may be relatively inconspicuous. The only indication of pulmonary disease initially may be the presence of unexplained iron deficiency anemia or an abnormal chest roentgenogram (10). In such patients, pulmonary hemorrhage may be confirmed by examination of the sputum for hemosiderophages or by the recently described carbon monoxide studies (29).

The clinical course of patients with anti-GBM disease is variable, the obvious determining factors being the presence and severity of pulmonary hemorrhage and the duration of antibody circulation. Presuming that pulmonary hemorrhage is not fatal, as it was in many of the early reports, renal disease may remain active for many months. In the most carefully studied series (9), the mean duration of antibody circulation was 8 months in patients with Goodpasture's syndrome and 7 months in patients with apparently isolated renal disease, but the range was from 4 to 25 months. Clearly, these patients were studied only from the clinical onset of disease, and anti-GBM antibodies may well have been present for much longer periods. This hypothesis is supported by the demonstration of exacerbations and remissions of disease activity independent of alterations in circulating antibody concentrations (23). The exacerbations in such patients appeared to correlate with a variety of nonspecific infections and other events. Thus, the factors determining the clinical course in patients with anti-GBM disease remain uncertain. Generally, disease activity gradually wanes over a period of months and can be titered by serial estimations of circulating antibody concentration by either specific assay or indirect immunofluorescence. This predictable course may, however, be punctuated by episodes of pulmonary hemorrhage or renal deterioration not clearly related to changes in antibody concentration.

PATHOLOGIC CHARACTERISTICS

Light Microscopy

Glomerular involvement is characteristically irregular. Depending on the extent of the disease, glomerular changes may range from minor segmental disease to complete crescentic obliteration. The characteristic lesion is a focal and segmental necrotizing glomerulonephritis. (Figs. 11-1–11-3). A portion of the tuft is effaced by disruption of glomerular capillaries with abundant fibrin in Bowman's space and intense local proliferation of epithelial cells. Polymorphs may be abundant but intracapillary proliferation is usually minimal. In biopsy specimens

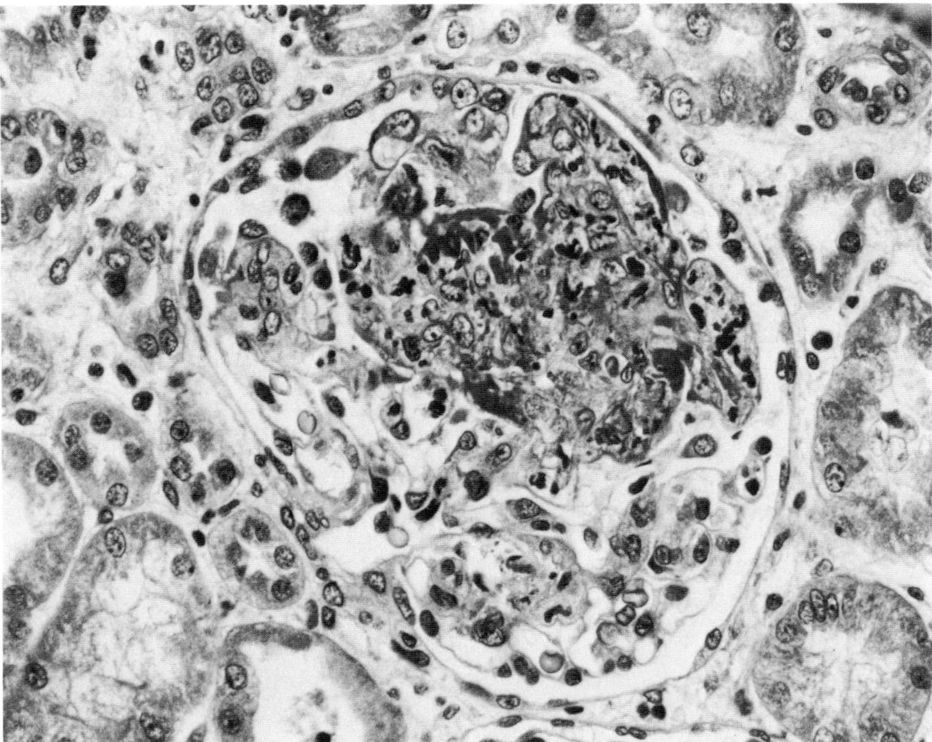

Figure 11-1 Glomerulus in a renal biopsy specimen of a patient with Goodpasture's syndrome, showing a localized area of cell proliferation with polymorphonuclear leukocytes and necrosis (H&E stain, ×535).

showing more advanced disease, an irregular pattern can usually be identified. This irregularity shows itself in both the distribution and apparent duration of the lesions. Even in universal crescentic disease, careful examination of multiple sections usually discloses glomeruli in which the segmental character of the inflammation is apparent. Similarly, especially in those patients with a history of repeated hemoptyses, the lesions may show varying degrees of organization. This organization may be expressed as segmental or global areas of sclerosis or as varying degrees of fibrous replacement of crescents (Fig. 11-4). Multinucleate giant cells may occasionally be visible in the crescents (30) (Fig. 11-2). In addition to the glomerular lesions, interstitial edema with an intense mononuclear inflammatory infiltrate may be seen. Anti-GBM disease has rarely been associated with necrotizing arteritis (8), but the blood vessels in the majority of patients show no significant abnormality. None of these morphologic features is in any way specific, and the diagnosis of anti-GBM glomerulonephritis cannot be achieved by light microscopy alone.

Electron Microscopy

There are no diagnostic ultrastructural appearances in anti-GBM disease. Suggestive changes include the presence of a subendothelial lucent zone (31) and diffuse increase in density of the GBM (6,32), but each of these findings is

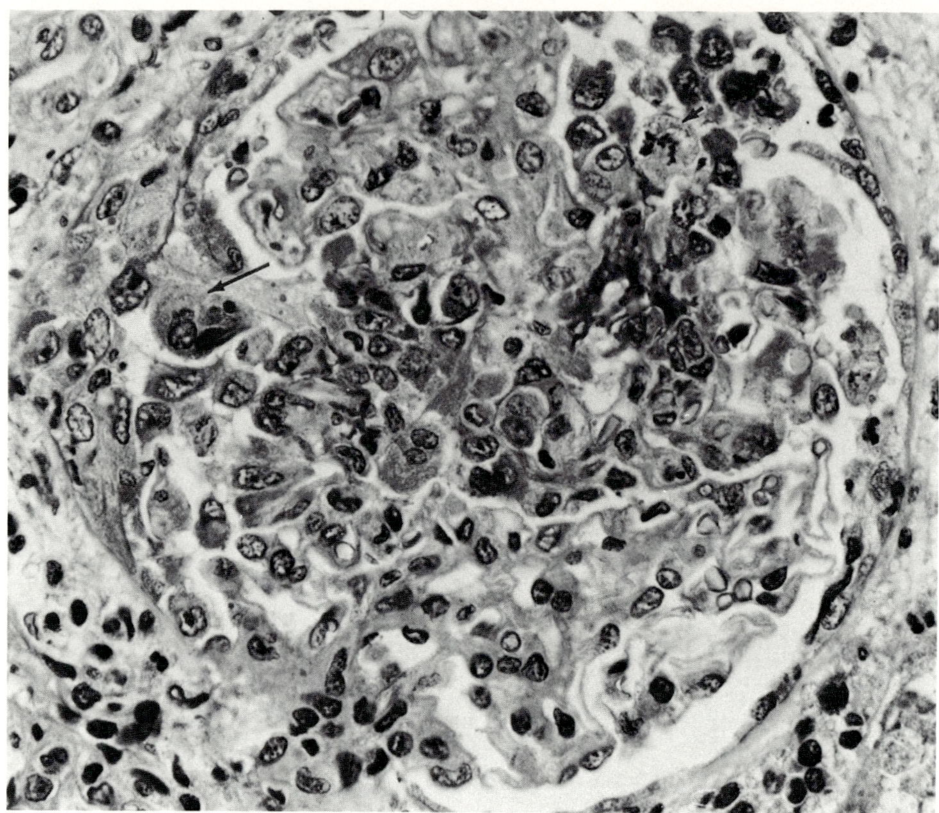

Figure 11-2. Glomerular epithelial proliferation with crescent formation (left) in Goodpasture's syndrome. Note the presence of multi-nucleated giant cells (arrows) and mitotic figure (arrow head) (H&E stain, ×600).

essentially nonspecific (Fig. 11-5). Membrane breaks are frequently seen in anti-GBM glomerulonephritis (31,32) as in other crescentic disease (33) (Fig. 11-6). Intranuclear inclusions suggestive of viruses have occasionally been described (21,22). Generally, however, the ultrastructural appearances in biopsy specimens from patients with anti-GBM disease are nonspecific, showing only the sequelae of inflammatory damage. Specifically, distinct deposits are almost always absent. Recently, two reports have described subepithelial deposits in patients with anti-GBM disease, possibly analogous to those occasionally seen in the autologous phase of nephrotoxic serum nephritis (34,35). Immunofluorescence microscopy in these cases revealed a combined linear and granular pattern, and the mixed pattern is probably the result of two separate pathogenetic mechanisms operating in the same patient.

Immunofluorescence Microscopy

Anti-GBM disease was first characterized by its smooth, continuous pattern of reaction for IgG. In the active stages of the disease, this reaction occurs equally in all glomeruli, although it may be distorted in those glomeruli compressed by

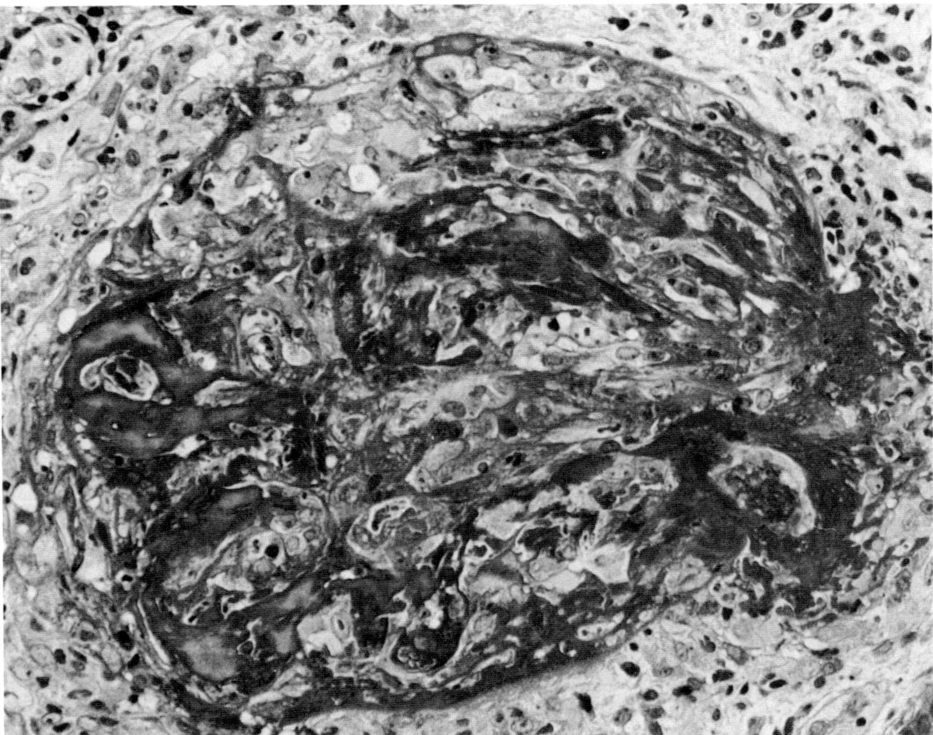

Figure 11-3. Necrotizing crescentic glomerulonephritis in the renal biopsy specimen of a patient with anti-GBM glomerulonephritis (H&E stain, ×450).

crescents. This distortion may include areas of apparent discontinuity of the membrane analogous to the membrane gaps demonstrated by light and electron microscopy. Later in the disease, the linear reactions become less intense and may be discontinuous. The predominant immunoglobulin is almost always IgG, and reactions for other immunoglobulins are rarely conspicuous (35a) (Figs. 11-7, 11-8). Complement is found in approximately three-quarters of biopsy specimens from patients with anti-GBM disease (9) and is usually distributed in an irregular interrupted or granular rather than linear pattern. There are no clinicopathologic differences between patients with and without complement reactions by immunofluorescence (36). Fibrin reactions are always found among crescents but are usually not significant in glomerular tufts. Linear IgG reactions frequently occur along tubular basement membranes and are positively correlated with the intensity of interstitial inflammation (37). The immunofluorescent reactions for IgG are quite characteristic and false-negative reactions have been reported only once (38). In this report, immunofluorescent studies were negative on the initial renal biopsy of a patient with typical Goodpasture's disease, but typical linear reactions were demonstrated on tissue from the bilateral nephrectomy specimens examined six months later. The mechanisms for the negative reactions in this patient, in whom circulating antibodies were demonstrated by hemagglutination, are unknown. Apparently false-positive reactions are seen in a number of conditions, which are discussed below.

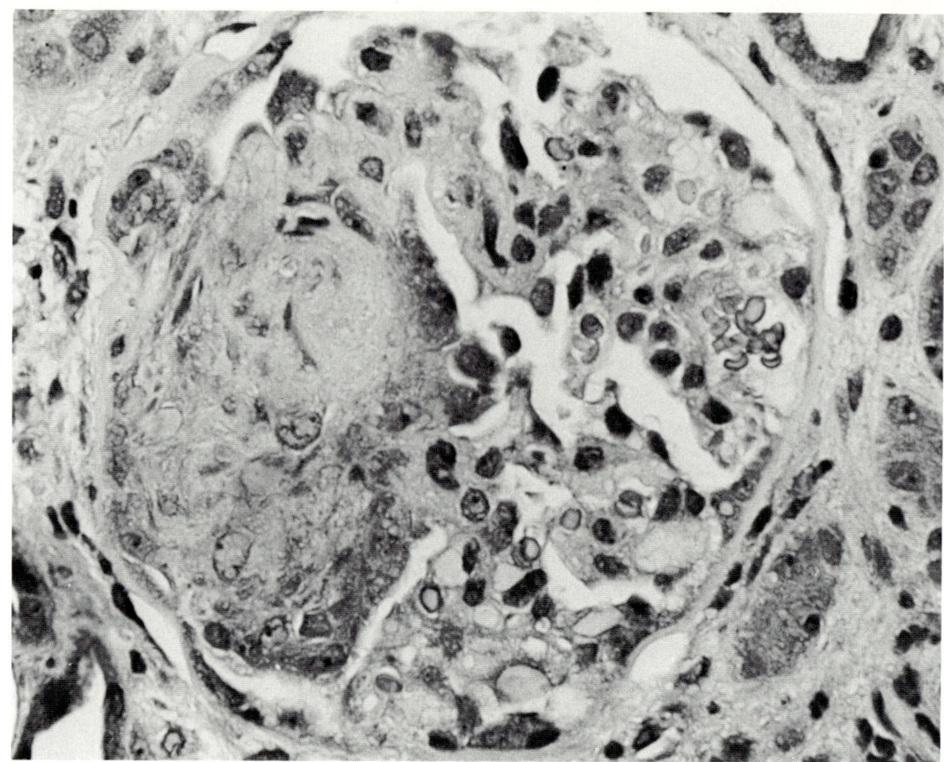

Figure 11-4. Segmented area of sclerosis adherent to Bowman's capsule, presumably a healed necrotic lesion in a patient with Goodpasture's syndrome (H&E stain, ×600).

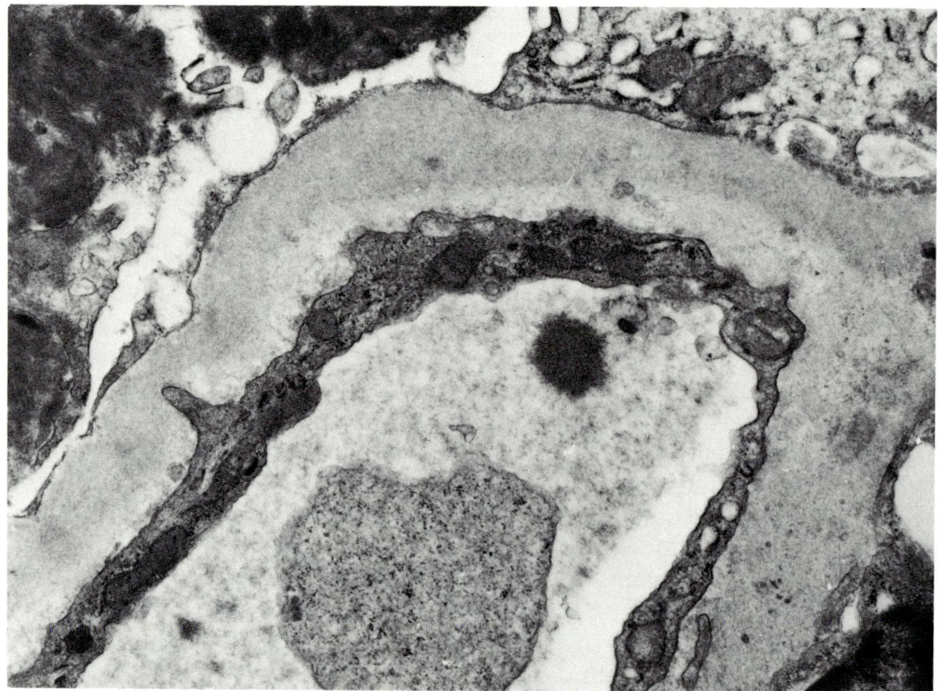

Figure 11-5. Electron micrograph from a patient with Goodpasture's syndrome, showing an electron-lucent zone on the endothelial side of the basement membrane. A large amount of fibrin is present in the urinary space (left upper corner) (×14,875).

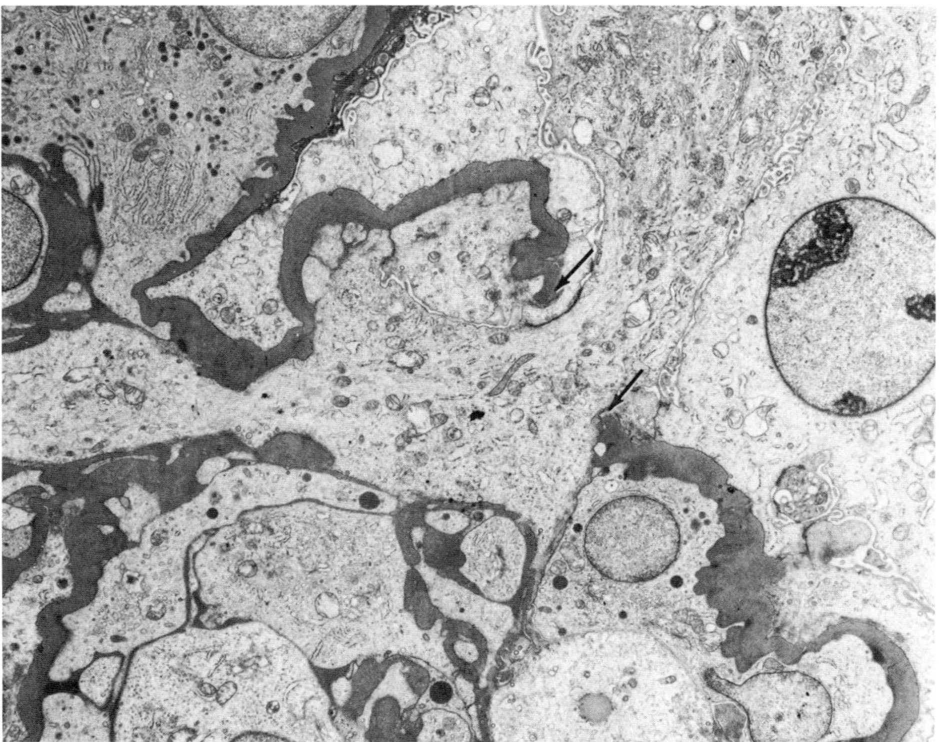

Figure 11-6. Disruption of the glomerular basement membrane (arrows) in a case of Goodpasture's syndrome (×6,500).

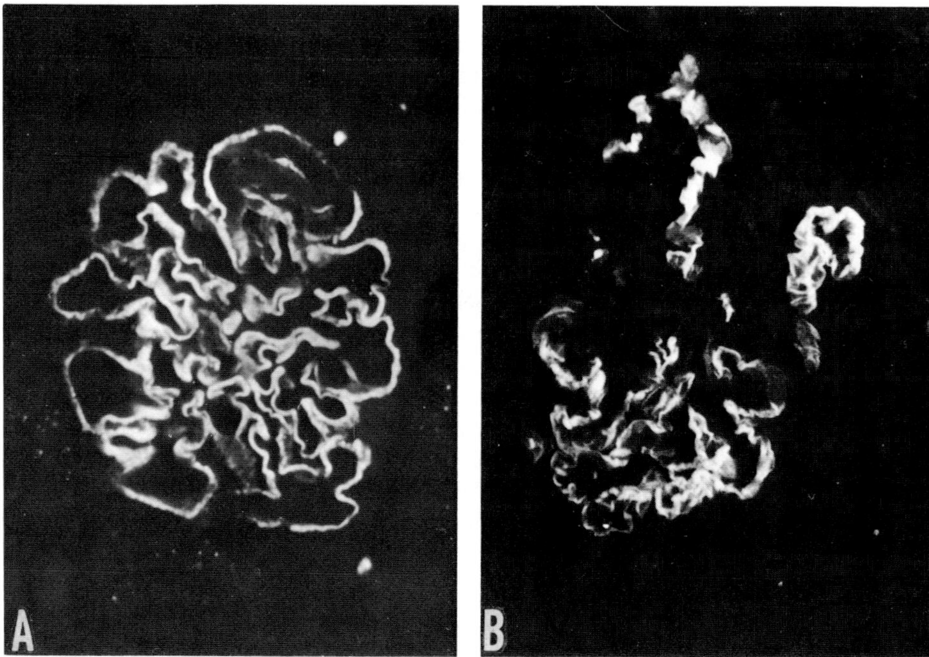

Figure 11-7. (*a*) Uniform linear IgG deposits along the glomerular capillary walls, in a case of anti-GBM glomerulonephritis. (*b*) A more advanced stage; the glomerular tuft is collapsed and the basement membrane is wrinkled and irregular (antihuman IgG, ×220).

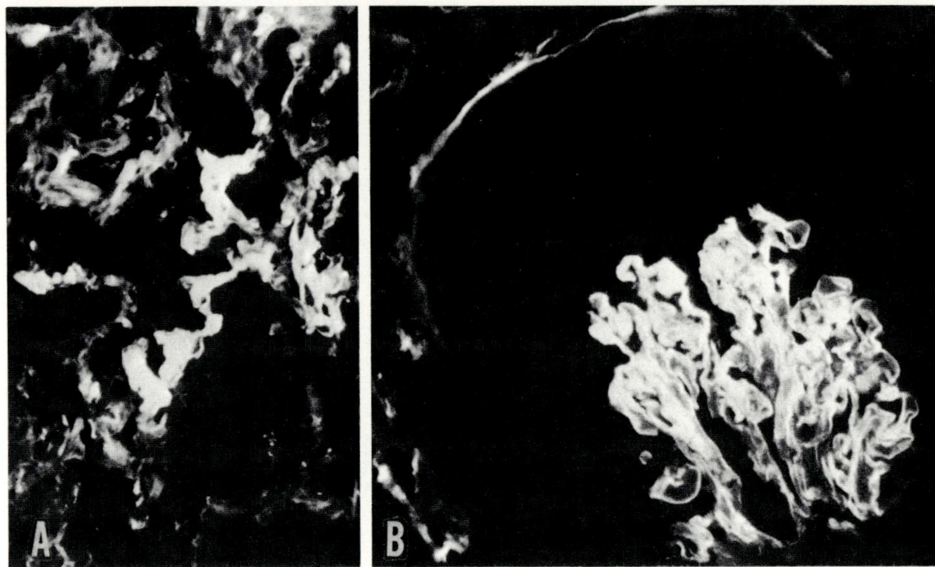

Figure 11-8. (*a*) Linear fluorescence along the alveolar walls in a patient with Goodpasture's syndrome. (*b*) Renal biopsy specimen from the same patient showing linear staining of the glomerular basement membrane and Bowman's capsule. The tuft is compressed by an epithelial crescent (antihuman IgG, ×335).

DIFFERENTIAL DIAGNOSIS

The tissue diagnosis of anti-GBM disease requires the demonstration of linear immunofluorescence reactions for IgG. Unfortunately, this immunofluorescent pattern is not specific for the disease. Linear patterns have been described in diabetic glomerulosclerosis, lupus glomerulonephritis, kidneys perfused before transplantation, and in autopsy kidneys (27). Circulating antibodies cannot be demonstrated in patients with these "false-positive" reactions, and the staining probably reflects an increase, for varying reasons, in the IgG normally bound in the GBM (12). The demonstration of linear IgG is, therefore, highly suggestive of anti-GBM disease but is only the first step towards specific diagnosis. This requires the demonstration of circulating anti-GBM antibodies by either direct radioimmunoassay or indirect immunofluorescence. The assay is only available in a few centers (27,28), but indirect immunofluorescence is a relatively simple, if somewhat insensitive, technique, which can be performed in most laboratories (39).

Recently, in several studies, the relationship between anti-GBM disease and idiopathic pulmonary hemosiderosis (IPH) have been examined. The clinical similarities between these syndromes have suggested some pathogenetic link, especially since minor renal lesions have occasionally been seen in patients with IPH (40). Circulating anti-GBM antibodies with linear reactions along both alveolar and glomerular basement membranes have been shown in a few patients who had been clinically diagnosed as having IPH (27,41). In each of these patients, pulmonary hemorrhage was the presenting feature, and there was little clinical or morphologic evidence of renal disease even though linear GBM reactions were present. Similar findings were seen in one patient in another study purporting to investigate the differences in pulmonary morphology between the two syndromes (42), and other intermediate forms have been described (43). Such phenomena indicate the difficulty of definition of the two disorders. On the one hand, combined pulmonary-renal disorders occur with glomerulonephritic lesions of varying type and no evidence of GBM antibodies (7,44,45). On the other hand, anti-GBM antibodies may be associated with apparently isolated clinical syndromes affecting either the lungs or kidneys as well as with the classical combined clinical syndrome. Clearly, the mechanisms determining pulmonary and renal damage require clarification, and more detailed investigation is needed of those patients with apparently isolated anti-GBM glomerulonephritis.

PROGNOSIS AND THERAPY

All the early reports of Goodpasture's syndrome emphasized its explosive progression into renal failure, often with life-threatening pulmonary hemorrhage. In subsequent studies, it has become clear that anti-GBM disease is variable in both its manifestations and its progression and has a clinical spectrum ranging from isolated hemoptysis with minimal renal disease to rapidly progressive renal destruction, with or without pulmonary disease. There is, at this stage, insufficient information to assess either the therapy or long-term outlook of those patients whose major manifestation is hemoptysis, although some have certainly died from overwhelming hemorrhage (43).

In those patients with severe renal disease, with or without pulmonary hemorrhage, there is general agreement that recovery is unlikely without therapeutic intervention (9,10,23). There is, however, controversy over the most appropriate and effective forms of therapy. The administration of corticosteroids and immunosuppressive agents is standard practice in anti-GBM disease and has been associated not only with recovery (46) but also with progression (9,10,23). Bilateral nephrectomy was, for a time, recommended to control pulmonary hemorrhage, and was effective in some (47), but not all (9), patients. Recently, plasma exchange therapy (plasmapheresis) had become popular, since it offers the opportunity to remove toxic antibodies from the circulation. The first reports on the benefit of plasmapheresis have been encouraging, but not all patients respond and more experience will be necessary before its value is established (48,49,49a).

TRANSPLANTATION

Recurrence of anti-GBM glomerulonephritis in the transplanted kidney was recognized early in the study of the disease (5). Linear antibody deposition was demonstrated 75 minutes after restoration of the blood flow to the graft and segmental glomerular lesions developed later, but renal function remained intact. In later reports, however, crescentic glomerulonephritis occurred requiring transplant nephrectomy (9,50). This experience naturally led to caution in proposing patients with the disease for transplantation, and a negative assay for circulating antibodies was usually regarded a prerequisite. The indirect immunofluorescence assay may be a satisfactory screening technique for this purpose, but recurrent disease has been reported in the presence of a negative assay

(51) and more sensitive tests may be required. Several patients have, however, undergone transplantation while antibodies were present in the circulation and have remained free of disease, even though linear immunofluorescence could be demonstrated in the glomeruli of the graft (9,52,53). Recurrent disease is thus not a necessary consequence of persistent anti-GBM antibody, either in the circulation or in the graft. Whether the development of recurrent glomerulonephritis is dependent on antibody concentration or on other factors remains uncertain, but a delay of some months after the last detectable positive assay seems a reasonable method of minimizing the risk (54). Apparently de novo glomerulonephritis of anti-GBM type has occasionally been reported in the transplanted kidney (55).

SUMMARY

The mechanisms of anti-GBM disease have been illustrated in detail by both experimental and human investigation. The morphologic lesions are produced by the deposition of circulating antibodies, which share reactivity with glomerular and alveolar basement membranes. Thus the characteristic clinical syndrome in anti-GBM disease is combined glomerulonephritis and pulmonary hemorrhage. However, the factors determining the capacity of these antibodies to cause inflammation are presently uncertain. The morphologic lesions are characteristically irregular: focal and segmental glomerulonephritis and unevenly distributed pulmonary hemorrhage. In either organ, the damage may be great enough to cause death or permanent disability, but there is a curious and poorly explained unpredictability about organ involvement. Renal disease may be predominant in some patients and pulmonary disease in others, and a number show combinations of the two that may change from day to day. Anti-GBM disease can be suspected by the demonstration of linear reactions for IgG along the GBM, but certain diagnosis requires the demonstration of specific antibodies either in the circulation or by elution. Progression to renal failure is common, but may be prevented by techniques such as plasmapheresis. Recurrence of the disease has occurred in transplanted kidneys. The mechanisms promoting antibody formation are poorly understood, and further studies are needed to clarify many features of the disease.

REFERENCES

1. Goodpasture EW: The significance of certain pulmonary lesions in relation to the etiology of influenza. *Am J Med Sci* 158:863, 1919.
2. Stanton MC, Tange JD: Goodpasture's syndrome (pulmonary hemorrhage associated with glomerulonephritis). *Aust Ann Med* 7:132, 1958.
3. Scheer RL, Grossman MA: Immune aspects of the glomerulonephritis associated with pulmonary hemorrhage. *Ann Intern Med* 60:1009, 1964.
4. Sturgill BC, Westervelt FB: Immunofluorescence studies in a case of Goodpasture's syndrome. *JAMA* 194:172, 1965.
5. Lerner RA, Glassock RJ, Dixon FJ: The role of anti-glomerular basement membrane antibody in the pathogenesis of human glomerulonephritis. *J Exp Med* 126:989, 1967.
6. Poskitt TR: Immunologic and electron microscopic studies in Goodpasture's syndrome. *Am J Med* 49:251, 1970.
7. Thomas HM III, Irwin RS: Classification of diffuse intrapulmonary hemorrhage. *Chest* 68:483, 1975.

8. Lewis EJ, Cavallo T, Harrington JT, et al: An immunopathologic study of rapidly progressive glomerulonephritis in the adult. *Human Pathol* 2:185, 1971.

9. Wilson CB, Dixon FJ: Anti-glomerular basement membrane antibody-induced glomerulonephritis. *Kidney Int* 3:74, 1973.

10. Sissons JGP, Evans DJ, Peters DK, et al: Glomerulonephritis associated with antibody to glomerular basement membrane. *Br Med J* 4:11, 1974.

11. Misra RP: The glomerular basement membrane, in Black DAK (ed): *Renal Disease*, ed 3. Oxford, Blackwell Scientific Publications, 1972, p 187.

12. Marquardt H, Wilson CB, Dixon FJ: Isolation and Immunological characterization of human glomerular basement membrane antigens. *Kidney Int* 3:57, 1973.

13. Wilson CB, Dixon FJ: The renal response to immunological injury, in Brenner BM, Rector FC (eds), *The Kidney*. Philadelphia, WB Saunders Co, 1976, Vol II, p 838.

14. Unanue ER, Dixon FJ: Experimental glomerulonephritis: immunologic events and pathogenetic mechanisms. *Adv Immunol* 6:1, 1967.

15. Lerner RA, Dixon FJ: The induction of acute glomerulonephritis in rabbits with soluble antigens isolated from normal homologous and autologous urine. *J Immunol* 100:1277, 1968.

16. Klassen J, Elwood C, Grossberg AL, et al: Evolution of membranous nephropathy into antiglomerular-basement-membrane glomerulonephritis. *N Engl J Med* 290:1340, 1974.

17. Moorthy AV, Zimmerman SW, Burkholder PM, et al: Association of crescentic glomerulonephritis with membranous nephropathy: a report of three cases. *Clin Nephrol* 6:320, 1976.

18. Hume DM, Sterling WA, Weymouth RJ, et al: Glomerulonephritis in human renal transplants. *Transplant Proc* 2:361, 1970.

19. Curtis JJ, Bhathena D, Leach RP, et al: Goodpasture's syndrome in a patient with the nail-patella syndrome. *Am J Med* 61:401, 1976.

20. Beirne GJ, Brennan JT: Glomerulonephritis associated with hydrocarbon solvents. *Arch Environ Health* 25:365, 1972.

21. Duncan DA, Drummond KN, Michael AF, et al: Pulmonary hemorrhage and glomerulonephritis: report of six cases and study of the renal lesion by the fluorescent antibody technique and electron microscopy. *Ann Intern Med* 62:920, 1965.

22. Tsai CC, Kissane JM, Germuth FG Jr: Paramyxovirus-like structures in Goodpasture's syndrome. *Lancet* 2:601, 1974.

23. Rees AJ, Lockwood CM, Peters DK: Enhanced allergic tissue injury in Goodpasture's syndrome by intercurrent bacterial infection. *Br Med J* 2:723, 1977.

24. Gossain VV, Gerstein AR, Janes AW: Goodpasture's syndrome: a familial occurrence. *Am Rev Respir Dis* 105:621, 1972.

25. D'Apice AJF, Kincaid-Smith P, Becker GJ, et al: Goodpasture's syndrome in identical twins. *Ann Intern Med* 88:61, 1978.

25a. Rees AJ, Peters DK, Compston DAS, et al: Strong association between HLA-DRW2 and antibody-mediated Goodpasture's syndrome. *Lancet* 1:966, 1978.

26. Morel-Maroger L, Leathem A, Richet G: Glomerular abnormalities in nonsystemic diseases: relationship between findings by light microscopy and immunofluorescence in 433 renal biopsy specimens. *Am J Med* 53:170, 1972.

27. Wilson CB, Dixon RJ: Diagnosis of immunopathologic renal disease. *Kidney Int* 5:389, 1974.

28. McPhaul JJ, Mullins JD: Glomerulonephritis mediated by antibody to glomerular basement membrane: immunological, clinical and histopathological characteristics. *J Clin Invest* 57:351, 1976.

29. Ewan PJ, Jones HA, Rhodes CG, et al: Detection of intrapulmonary hemorrhage with carbon monoxide uptake: application in Goodpasture's syndrome. *N Engl J Med* 295:1391, 1976.

30. Kalowski S, McKay DG, Howes EL Jr, et al: Multinucleated giant cells in antiglomerular basement membrane antibody-induced glomerulonephritis. *Nephron* 16:415, 1976.

31. Bohman SO, Olsen S, Petersen VP: Glomerular ultrastructure in extracapillary glomerulonephritis. *Acta Path Microbiol Scand (A)* (suppl 249) 82:29, 1974.

32. Germuth FJ Jr, Choi IJ, Taylor JJ, et al: Antibasement membrane disease: I. The glomerular lesions of Goodpasture's disease and experimental disease in sheep. *Johns Hopkins Med J* 131:367, 1972.

33. Stejskal J, Pirani CL, Okada M, et al: Discontinuities (gaps) of the glomerular capillary wall and basement membrane in renal diseases. *Lab Invest* 28:149, 1973.

34. Agoda LCV, Striker GE, George CRP, et al: The appearance of nonlinear deposits of immunoglobulins in Goodpasture's syndrome. *Am J Med* 61:407, 1976.

35. Pasternack A, Törnröth T, Linder E: Evidence of both anti-GBM and immune complex mediated pathogenesis in the initial phase of Goodpasture's syndrome. *Clin Nephrol* 9:77, 1978.

35a. Border WA, Baehler RW, Bhathena D, et al: IgA antibasement membrane nephritis with pulmonary hemorrhage. *Ann Intern Med* 91:21, 1979.

36. Verroust PJ, Wilson CB, Cooper NR, et al: Glomerular complement components in human glomerulonephritis. *J Clin Invest* 53:77, 1974.

37. Andres G, Brentjens J, Kohli R, et al: Histology of human tubulointerstitial nephritis associated with antibodies to renal basement membranes. *Kidney Int* 13:480, 1978.

38. Eisenger AJ, Lewis WHP, Henari FZ, et al: Immunofluorescence in a case of Goodpasture's syndrome. *Nephron* 11:1, 1973.

39. McPhaul JJ, Dixon FJ: The presence of anti-glomerular basement membrane antibodies in peripheral blood. *J Immunol* 103:1168, 1969.

40. Soergel KH, Sommers SC: Idiopathic pulmonary hemosiderosis and related syndromes. *Am J Med* 32:499, 1962.

41. Mathew TH, Hobbs JB, Kalowski S, et al: Goodpasture's syndrome: normal renal diagnostic findings. *Ann Intern Med* 82:215, 1975.

42. Donald KJ, Edwards RL, McEvoy JDS: Alveolar capillary basement membrane lesions in Goodpasture's syndrome and idiopathic pulmonary hemosiderosis. *Am J Med* 59:642, 1975.

43. Zimmerman SW, Varanasi UR, Hoff B: Goodpasture's syndrome with normal renal function. *Am J Med* 66:163, 1979.

44. Lewis EJ, Schur PH, Busch GJ, et al: Immunopathologic features of a patient with glomerulonephritis and pulmonary hemorrhage. *Am J Med* 54:507, 1973.

45. Yum MN, Lampton LM, Bloom PM, et al: Asymptomatic IgA nephropathy associated with pulmonary hemosiderosis. *Am J Med* 64:1056, 1978.

46. Cohen LH, Wilson CB, Freeman RH: Goodpasture's syndrome: recovery after severe renal insufficiency. *Arch Intern Med* 136:835, 1976.

47. Siegel RR: The basis of pulmonary disease resolution after nephrectomy in Goodpasture's syndrome. *Am J Med Sci* 259:201, 1970.

48. Plasmapheresis in glomerulonephritis, editorial. *Br Med J* 1:434, 1979.

49. Pinching AJ, Peters DK: Plasma exchange in nephritis. *J Roy Soc Med* 72:395, 1979.

49a. McKenzie PE, Taylor AE, Woodroffe AJ, et al: Plasmapheresis in glomerulonephritis. *Clin Nephrol* 12: 97, 1979.

50. Dixon FJ, McPhaul JJ Jr, Lerner RA: Recurrence of glomerulonephritis in the transplanted kidney. *Arch Intern Med* 123:559, 1969.

51. Beleil OM, Coburn JW, Shinaberger JH, et al: Recurrent glomerulonephritis due to antiglomerular basement membrane-antibodies in two successive allografts. *Clin Nephrol* 1:377, 1973.

52. Cove-Smith JR, McLeon AA, Blamey RW, et al: Transplantation, immunosuppression and plasmapheresis in Goodpasture's syndrome. *Clin Nephrol* 9:126, 1978.

53. McPhaul JJ Jr, Lordon RE, Thompson AL Jr, et al: Nephritogenic immunopathologic mechanisms and human renal transplants: the problem of recurrent glomerulonephritis. *Kidney Int* 10:135, 1976.

54. Cameron JS, Turner DR: Recurrent glomerulonephritis in allografted kidneys. *Clin Nephrol* 7:47, 1977.

55. Gluckman JC, Beaufils H, Berger J, et al: Rapidly progressive glomerulonephritis with linear fluorescence in a kidney transplant. *Clin Nephrol* 1:40, 1973.

12
Vasculitis

The nomenclature and classification of the vasculitides is an etymologic quagmire: few who enter the area emerge unscathed. This chapter does not venture to preempt those who have categorized the various forms of vasculitis (1,2). Instead, an attempt is made to outline some of the major clinical and pathologic features of those patients with vasculitic renal disease. Furthermore, this review is restricted to those forms of vasculitis that are characterized by necrosis of the vessel wall. In this context, the pathologist may encounter renal vasculitis or its complications in several clinical settings (Table 12-1). The morphologic lesions in a number of these situations are identical and the appropriate designations require consideration of the clinical features.

PATHOGENESIS

The morphologic lesion of necrotizing vasculitis is nonspecific. An exactly similar pattern can occur adjacent to acutely inflamed areas or in circulations exposed to a sudden and severe increase in perfusion pressure. There is little doubt, therefore, that many pathogenetic factors are likely to be involved in the various vasculitides or that these conditions may be linked only by a common morphology. The most attractive experimental model, however, is the necrotizing vasculitis occurring in the immune elimination phase of acute serum sickness (3,4). Complement and immune complexes can initially be detected within the vascular lesions, but they rapidly disappear, so that proof of an immune origin may not be possible in lesions of more than a few days duration. Damage is probably caused both by deposition of preformed complexes and by complexing of circulating antibody with antigen that has previously diffused into the vascular

Table 12-1. Necrotizing Arteritis Involving the Kidney

Systemic vasculitis (polyarteritis):
   classical, microscopic
Accompanying crescentic glomerulonephritis
Occurring in systemic, predominantly nonvasculitic disease
Accompanying predominantly cutaneous vasculitis
"Specific" vasculitic diseases:
   allergic granulomatosis, temporal arteritis, Wegener's granulomatosis

---

wall. Diffusion of sufficient antibody to cause such a localized Arthus's reaction can only occur during the phase of high serum concentration of antigen produced in the acute model, and vasculitis is not a feature of chronic serum sickness.

Systemic vasculitis may also be produced experimentally by direct infective vascular damage by several organisms (4). The association of vasculitic syndromes with a variety of immunologic phenomena has, however, fostered the general belief that at least some forms are immune complex in type (5). Support for this belief has come from the presence of hepatitis B antigenemia in up to 40% of patients with "polyarteritis," and the demonstration of the antigen in both the tissue and circulating immune complexes of some of these patients (4,6,7). Circulating immune complexes and/or cryoglobulins have also been identified in a number of patients with vasculitis syndromes unassociated with hepatitis B (7). Necrotizing vasculitis has been reported in association with amphetamine abuse (8) and with a variety of other drugs, including sulphonamides, penicillin, thiouracil and diphenylhydantoin (9). At this time, only the association with hepatitis B appears to fulfill the criteria for acceptance as an immune complex disease, and other mechanisms, such as defects in cell-mediated immune function in Wegener's granulomatosis (10), may prove to be responsible for some vasculitic syndromes.

SYSTEMIC VASCULITIS (POLYARTERITIS)

Polyarteritis was originally described as an acute systemic syndrome characterized by palpable vascular aneurysms (nodosa), but the concept of the disease has broadened to such an extent that the term has little specificity. Currently, some pathologists describe as polyarteritis any form of necrotizing vasculitis, but the term is used here to define a disease causing necrotizing inflammation of muscular arteries and arterioles without identifiable associated conditions. Within this general group, two variants can be recognized: a disorder affecting predominantly medium-sized arteries, sometimes with nodose swellings (classical polyarteritis), and a syndrome differing only by involvement of smaller arteries, arterioles, and glomeruli (microscopic polyarteritis) (11). Each of these variants increases in incidence with age and is more common in men than in women (12). Typically, the patient has an acute illness characterized by fever, arthralgia, muscle pains, and specific vasculitic phenomena such as peripheral neuropathy. Renal involvement occurs in approximately 80% of patients and differs in its features according to the pattern of arteritis (12). Classical polyarteritis causes renal infarcts, which may be manifest as loin pain, with or without hematuria, in the acute stage, and may cause hypertension later. Microscopic polyarteritis typically appears with rapidly progressive renal failure, but may be more subtle and not be detected until symptoms of developing azotemia call attention to other systemic phenomena. The natural history of either variety is of progression to death over months or years (12,13). Therapy with corticosteroids and immunosuppressive agents can, however, arrest this course and, if continued long enough, can cause apparent cure (3,14).

PATHOLOGIC CHARACTERISTICS

Vasculitis

Necrotizing arteritis of any type is characterized by segmental or circumferential destruction of the vessel wall by massive insudation of fibrin with admixed polymorphs and, in some cases, eosinophils. There is often a collar of surrounding mononuclear or polymorphonuclear inflammation ("periarteritis"), and the lumen may be occluded by thrombus. In classical polyarteritis the involved vessels are typically of arcuate or larger type whereas interlobular arteries and arterioles are principally affected in the microscopic form (Figs. 12-1–12-7). A typical feature of polyarteritis is a remitting and exacerbating clinical course, and this fluctuation is morphologically reflected by the presence in tissues of both acute and healed vasculitic lesions. Healed lesions may be recognized by areas of mural fibrosis that often coexist with intimal thickening and are most easily recognized by segmental disappearance of the elastic lamina in sections stained with techniques demonstrating elastica (Fig. 12-5). Immunofluorescence techniques have demonstrated globulins and complement in the lesions of those cases associated with hepatitis B (6) but, in our experience, no specific reactions are usually demonstrable.

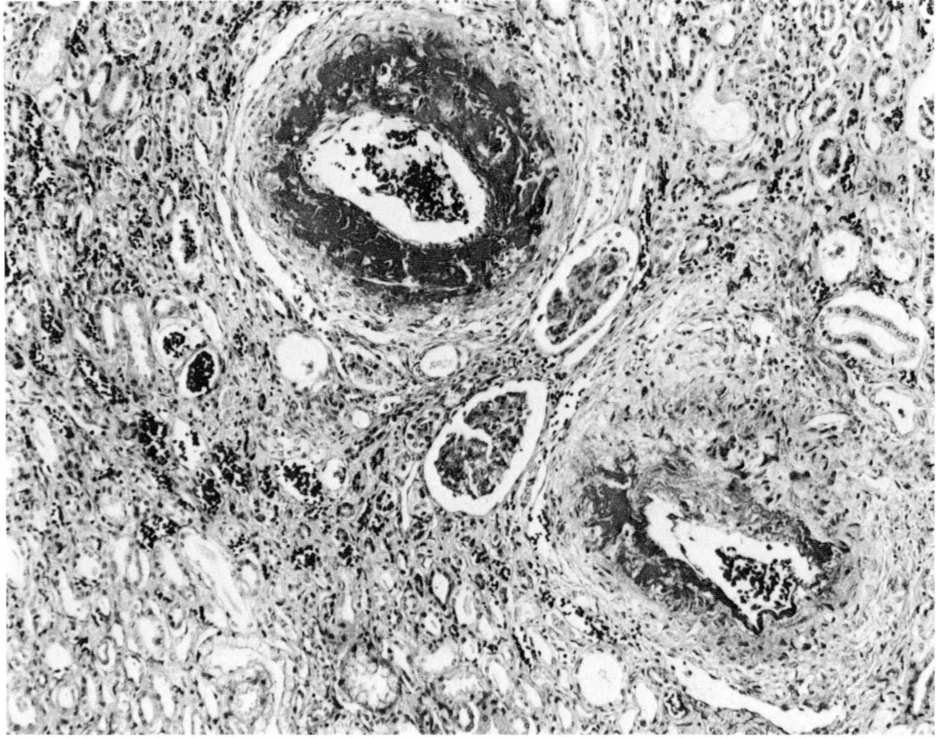

Figure 12-1. Fibrinoid necrosis involving medium-size arteries in classical polyarteritis nodosa. Note the ischemic changes present in the renal parenchyma (H&E stain, ×100).

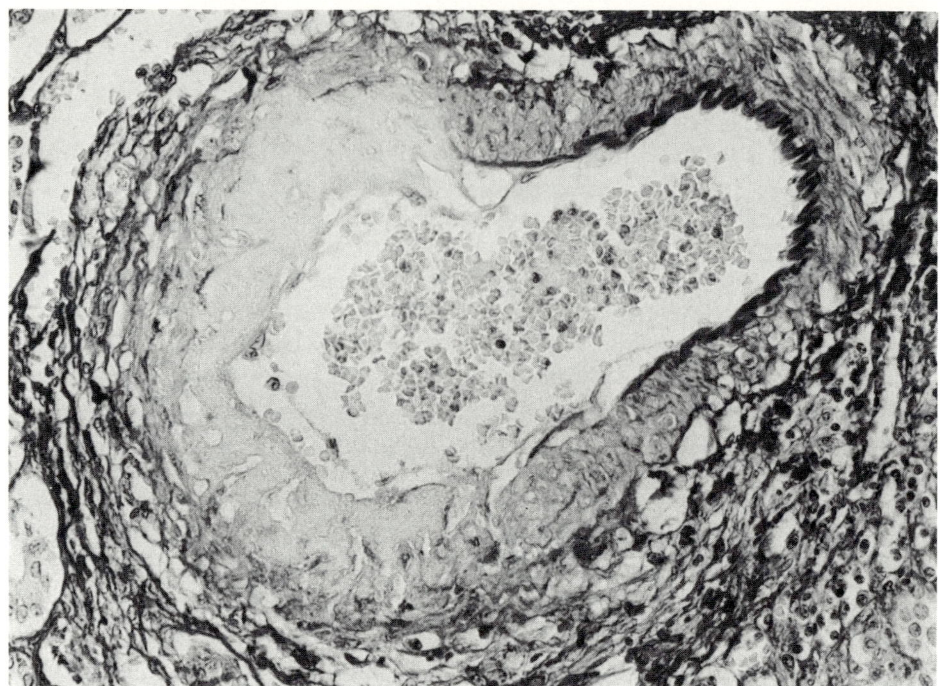

Figure 12-2. Arcuate artery showing focal necrosis of the wall with partial destruction of internal elastic lamina (Van Gieson stain, ×250).

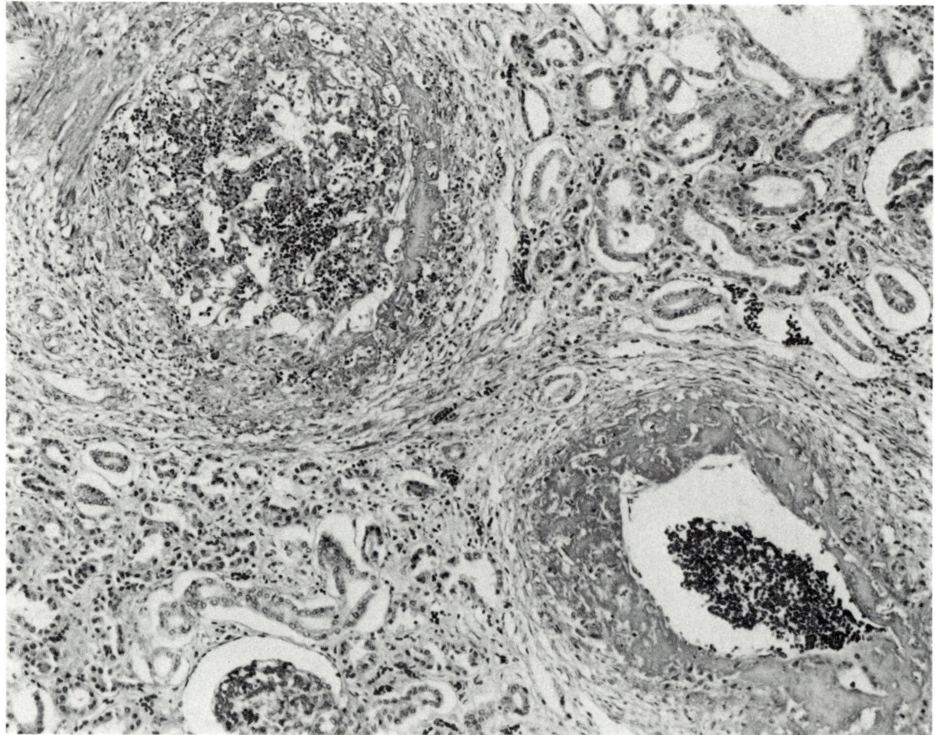

Figure 12-3. The same case as Figure 10-1, showing circumferential necrosis of the vascular walls and partially recanalized thrombus (left upper corner) (H&E stain, ×120).

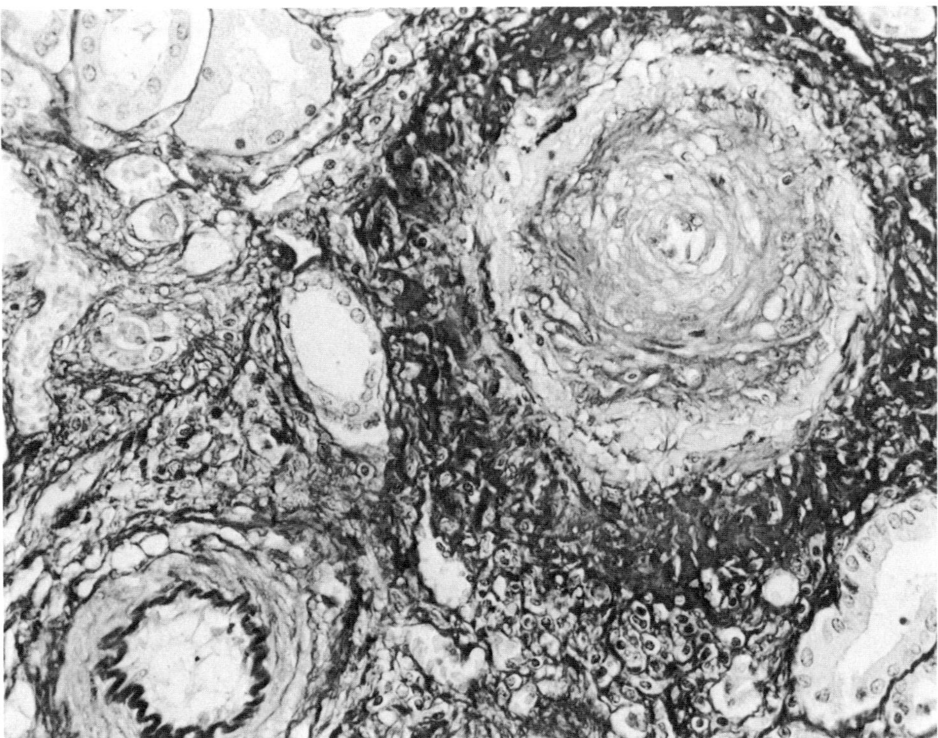

Figure 12-4. Healing phase of arteritis in arcuate artery from a case of classical polyarteritis nodosa. Necrosis of the wall is still present, but the intima is markedly thickened by fibroblastic proliferation. The artery in the left lower corner is normal (H&E stain, ×300).

Glomerulonephritis

The glomeruli in classical polyarteritis show only ischemic shrinkage (Fig. 12-1). In the microscopic form, however, there is a focal and segmental glomerulonephritis that is often necrotizing in type and may be associated with crescents (11,15). Usually, there is minimal endocapillary proliferation, and the initial phase of the lesion appears to be capillary thrombosis with subsequent dissolution of the capillary wall, exudation into Bowman's space, and crescent formation (Figs. 12-8, 12-9). In common with the differing ages of the vasculitic lesions, varying degrees of glomerular scarring and organization may coexist with fresh damage, sometimes even in the same glomerulus. In the glomerulonephritis complicating microscopic polyarteritis, no deposits can be identified by electron or immunofluorescence microscopy. Thus, the discovery of a segmental glomerulonephritis without deposits is strong presumptive evidence for vasculitis and is an indication to search for confirmatory features by either biopsies of other tissues or angiography (8). Biopsy specimens from patients with hepatitis B-associated polyarteritis have been reported to show other patterns of glomerular disease, including mesangial proliferative and mesangiocapillary glomerulonephritis (6).

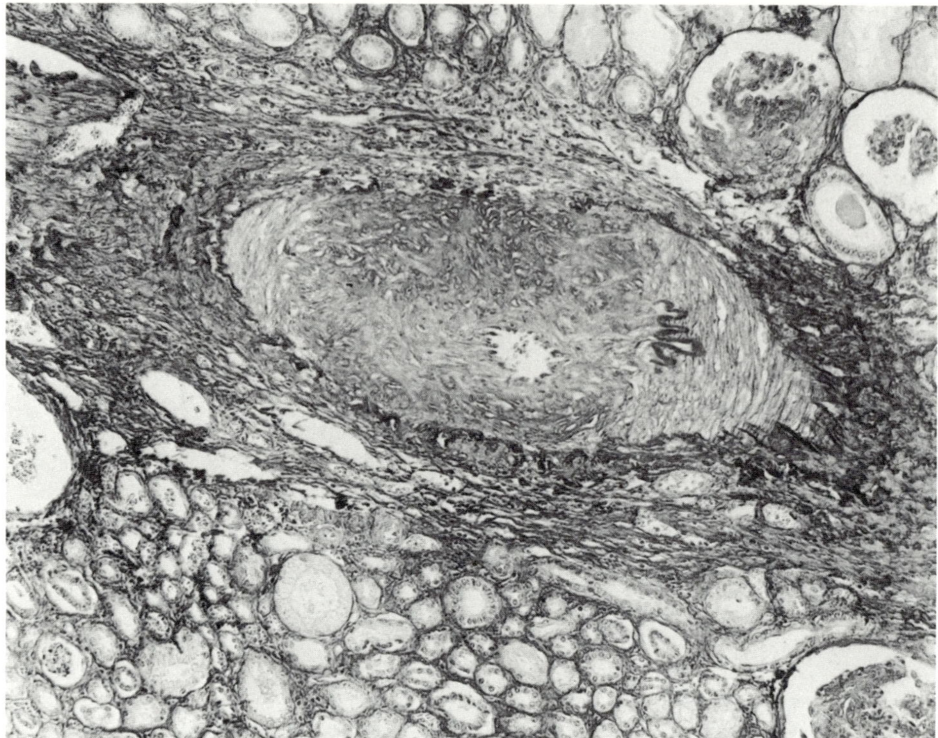

Figure 12-5. Arcuate artery in chronic healed stage from a patient with the classical form of polyarteritis nodosa. There is fibrosis replacement and marked obliteration of the lumen. Only fragments of internal elastic lamina remain (Van Gieson stain, ×130).

VASCULITIS ACCOMPANYING CRESCENTIC GLOMERULONEPHRITIS

As already discussed, the possibility of vasculitis exists whenever segmental, crescentic glomerulonephritis is encountered. If no immunofluorescent or electron microscopic deposits are demonstrable, a thorough examination of serial sections cut through the entire biopsy specimen is indicated. Vasculitic lesions are frequently found in these instances, but they may be present in only one of many sections. Even if no lesions can be demonstrated, the diagnosis cannot be excluded since evidence of vasculitis may be present in only a few of the blocks taken from all organs at autopsy (15). Typical necrotizing vasculitis has been reported only rarely in association with crescentic glomerulonephritis caused by antiglomerular basement membrane disease (16) and acute postinfectious glomerulonephritis (17).

VASCULITIS ACCOMPANYING OTHER SPECIFIC DISEASE ENTITIES

Necrotizing arteritis may be an occasional complication in a wide variety of diseases including systemic lupus, rheumatoid arthritis, dermatomyositis and infective endocarditis (2,4). The morphologic characteristics of the vascular le-

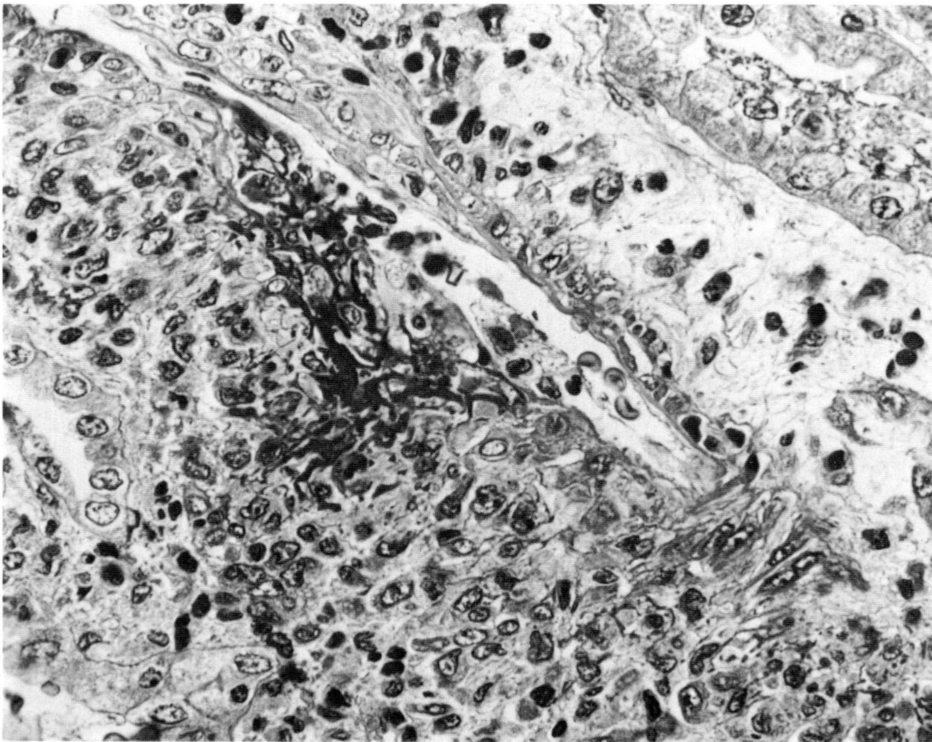

Figure 12-6. Small artery showing necrosis and inflammatory infiltrate in microscopic polyarteritis nodosa (H&E stain, ×325).

sions in these diseases do not differ from those already described, and diagnosis depends on the recognition of the associated clinical or pathologic features.

PREDOMINANTLY CUTANEOUS VASCULITIS

Although any of the conditions so far discussed may occasionally involve the skin, cutaneous vasculitis is usually one of a series of diseases with distinct clinical features (18,19). Some of these are specifically cutaneous syndromes, but others are more or less commonly associated with visceral involvement. In those syndromes associated with necrotizing vasculitis, there is usually predominant involvement of arterioles and venules with extensive breakdown of polymorph nuclei to produce karyorrhectic fragments (leukocytoclastic vasculitis) (20,21). The skin lesions occurring in this form may be of either urticarial or palpable purpuric type, and there is often associated hypocomplementemia with characteristics of classical pathway activation. This clinical and morphologic syndrome may occur in cryoglobulinemia, systemic lupus, and the Henoch-Schönlein syndrome, which are discussed elsewhere, but often has no identifiable associated disease. Renal involvement is reported in a number of papers discussing cutaneous vasculitis (18–20) but without satisfactory documentation. In the urticarial form of hypocomplementemic cutaneous vasculitis, however, several cases of

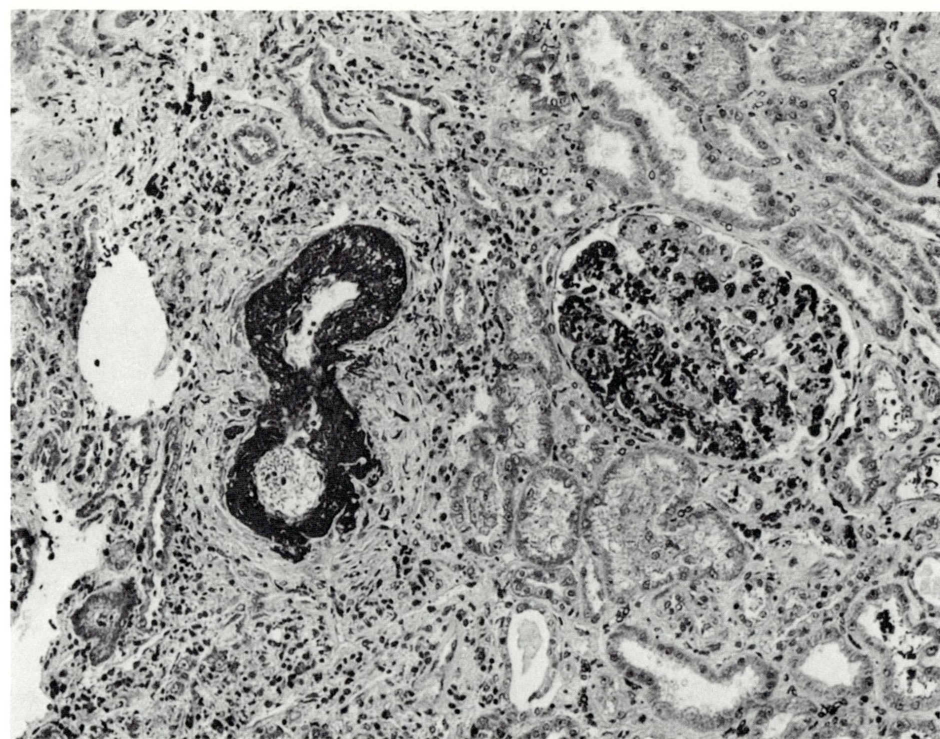

Figure 12-7. Biopsy specimen from a patient with microscopic polyarteritis nodosa, showing a necrotic interlobular artery surrounded by inflammatory infiltrate. The glomerulus is congested and nearly infarcted (H&E stain, ×243).

proliferative glomerulonephritis have been described (22,23). These cases showed diffuse mesangial and endothelial proliferation with granular immunofluorescent reactions for IgG, IgM, IgA, C1, and C3, and ultrastructural deposits in various locations.

"SPECIFIC" VASCULITIC DISEASES

Until more is known about the pathogenesis of the various vasculitic lesions, disease entities cannot be reliably characterized. Instead, syndromes are defined by the more or less constant constellations of clinical and pathologic features. Among the many such syndromes, the uncertain entity of polyarteritis has already been discussed. In this section, several other conditions associated with renal damage are briefly reviewed.

Eosinophilic Granulomatosis

In 1951, Churg and Strauss described a series of patients with systemic vasculitis occurring on a background of asthma, fever, and eosinophilia (24). Soon after,

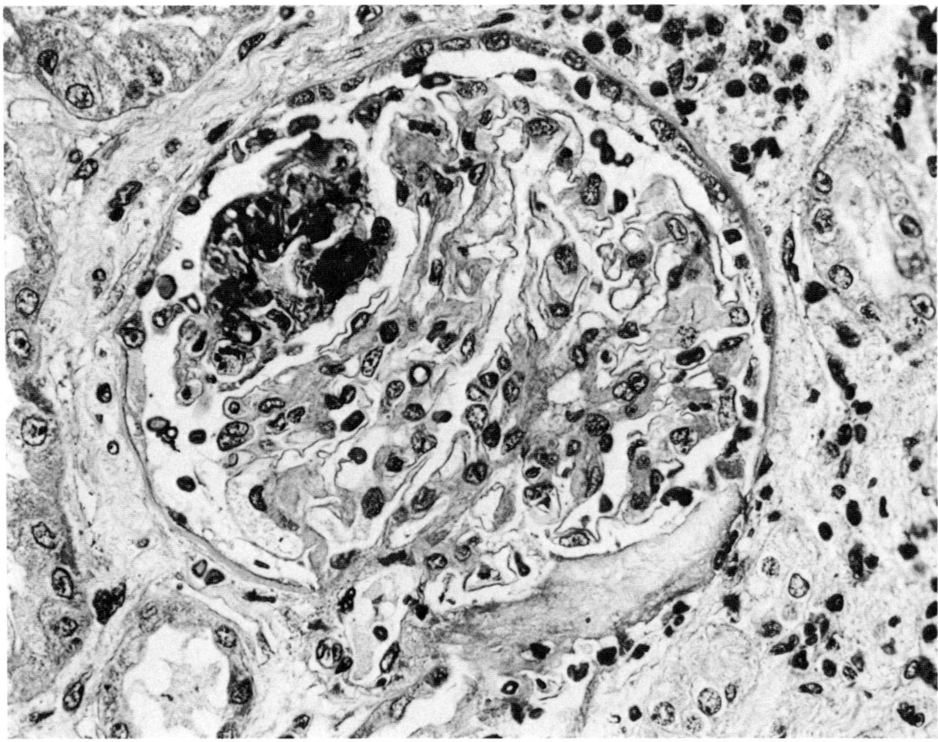

Figure 12-8. Glomerulus from a case of microscopic type polyarteritis nodosa, showing a well-circumscribed small area of capillary collapse and thrombosis at the periphery of the tuft (H&E stain, ×600).

Rose and Spencer defined similar characteristics by dividing a series of patients into those with and without lung involvement (25). Aside from the characteristic clinical features, this relatively rare syndrome is defined by tissue eosinophilia, the granulomatous nature of some vasculitic lesions, and the occurrence of necrotizing interstitial inflammation. Hematuria and proteinuria are relatively common, but renal failure rarely occurs in this condition (26). Renal involvement may be glomerular, vascular, or interstitial. The glomerulonephritis and vasculitis usually closely resemble those of microscopic polyarteritis, but may be granulomatous in type. Interstitial disease may be characterized either by diffuse eosinophilic infiltration or by necrotic, granulomatous nodules.

Temporal (Giant-Cell) Arteritis

Giant-cell arteritis characteristically affects the temporal arteries of the elderly and is often associated with a vague systemic illness termed polymyalgia rheumatica (27). Extracranial involvement is probably more common than previously recognized, but renal involvement by vasculitis and necrotizing glomerulonephritis is rare (28). Rarely, disseminated giant-cell arteritis occurs in the absence of temporal artery involvement and may affect both glomeruli and renal blood vessels (29). An association of necrotizing vasculitis, usually of con-

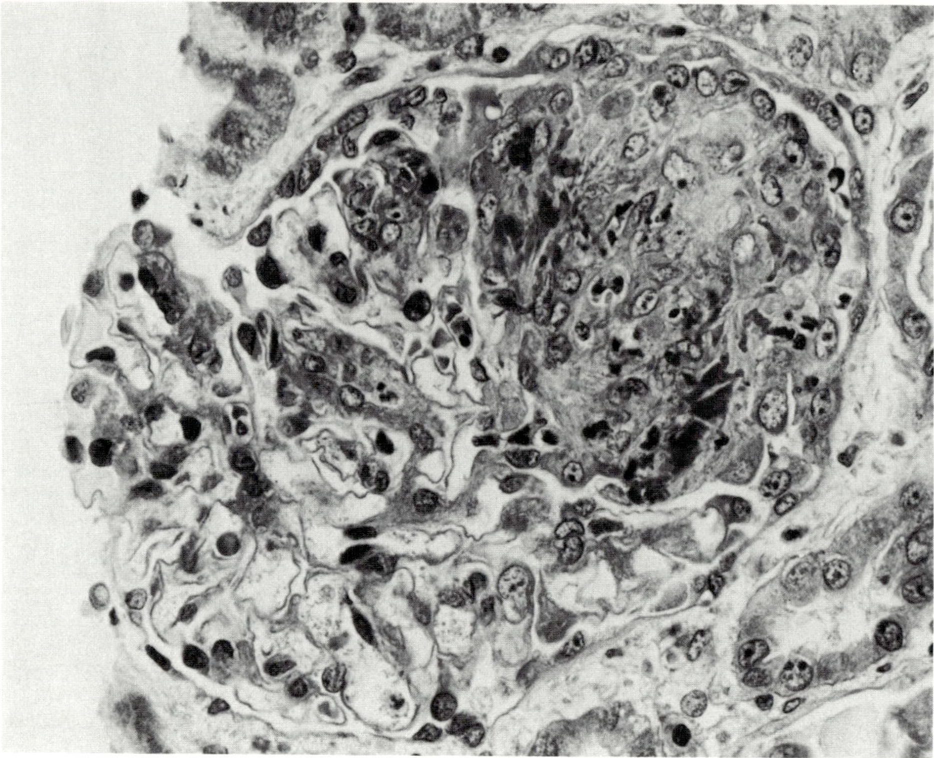

Figure 12-9. Necrotizing segmental glomerulonephritis in a case of microscopic polyarteritis nodosa (H&E, ×600).

ventional type, with a necrotizing and granulomatous pattern of glomerulonephritis, has also been rarely reported (30,31).

Wegener's Granulomatosis

Wegener's granulomatosis is a syndrome of necrotizing granulomata in the upper respiratory tract and lung with systemic necrotizing vasculitis (32). A separate group of patients has been identified with identical pulmonary lesions but no evidence of systemic involvement (localized Wegener's granulomatosis) (33). In addition, there is a range of pulmonary lesions that may mimic the clinical and pathologic features of Wegener's lung disease, but appear to represent separate entities (33). Differentiation between some of these separate lesions and true Wegener's may, however, be difficult, and accurate classification is impeded by the fact that systemic involvement may be delayed for many years (34). Wegener's granulomatosis may occur at any age, but it is most common in the fourth and fifth decades and affects males more often than females (35). Presentation is usually with upper respiratory symptoms followed by pulmonary disease and systemic phenomena related to the vasculitis. In most patients, renal involvement is simultaneous with the other clinical features and is manifest either by an active urinary sediment or progressive renal failure. The glomerular lesions are identical to those of microscopic polyarteritis, consisting of focal and segmental necrotizing glomerulonephritis, often with crescents (36) (Figs. 12-10, 12-11). Granular reactions of IgG and subepithelial deposits have occasionally been described (35,36), but in our experience no deposits can be identified, and others have reported similar negative findings (37). Necrotizing vasculitis of arterioles and small arteries can often be detected in the renal biopsy specimen if serial sections are examined, and there may be pronounced interstitial inflammation with small necrotizing granulomata (Fig. 12-11). The mean survival period for patients with untreated Wegener's granulomatosis is five months, most patients dying in renal failure, but complete remission can be induced by corticosteroid and immunosuppressive therapy (3,35).

SUMMARY

The vasculitides are a heterogenous group of conditions unified by a common morphology. Their classification is empirical and is based on the distribution and size of the vessels involved, together with associated clinical syndromes. There is evidence that some of these conditions may be produced by immune complexes, but the pathogenesis is generally obscure. Vasculitis of large vessels tends to be

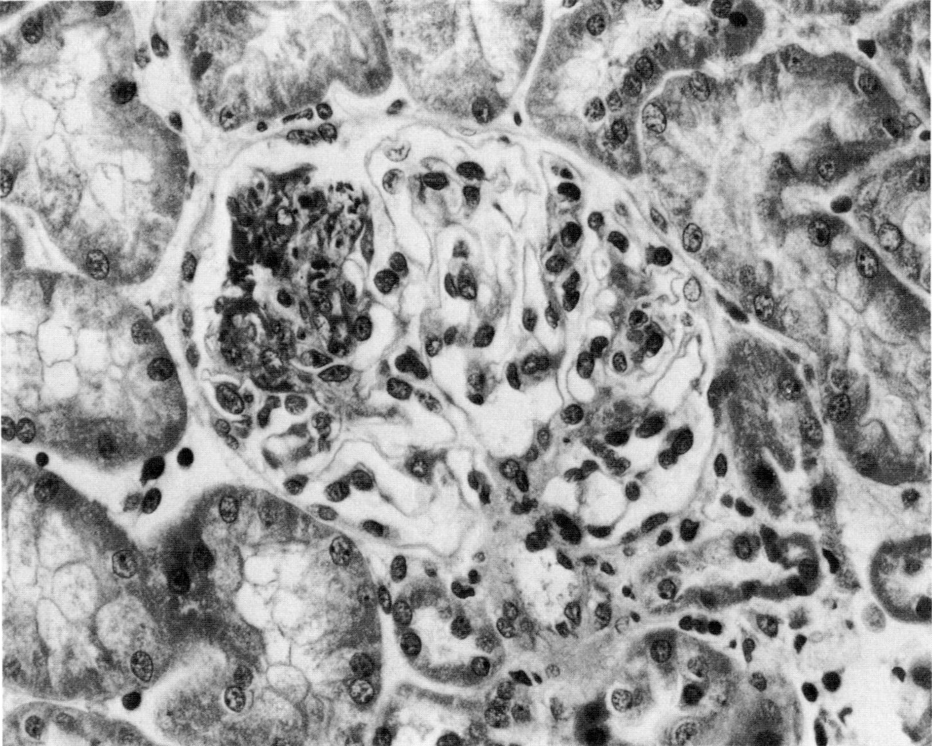

Figure 12-10. Renal biopsy specimen from a patient with Wegener's granulomatosis, showing necrotizing changes confined to periphery of the tuft (H&E stain, ×450).

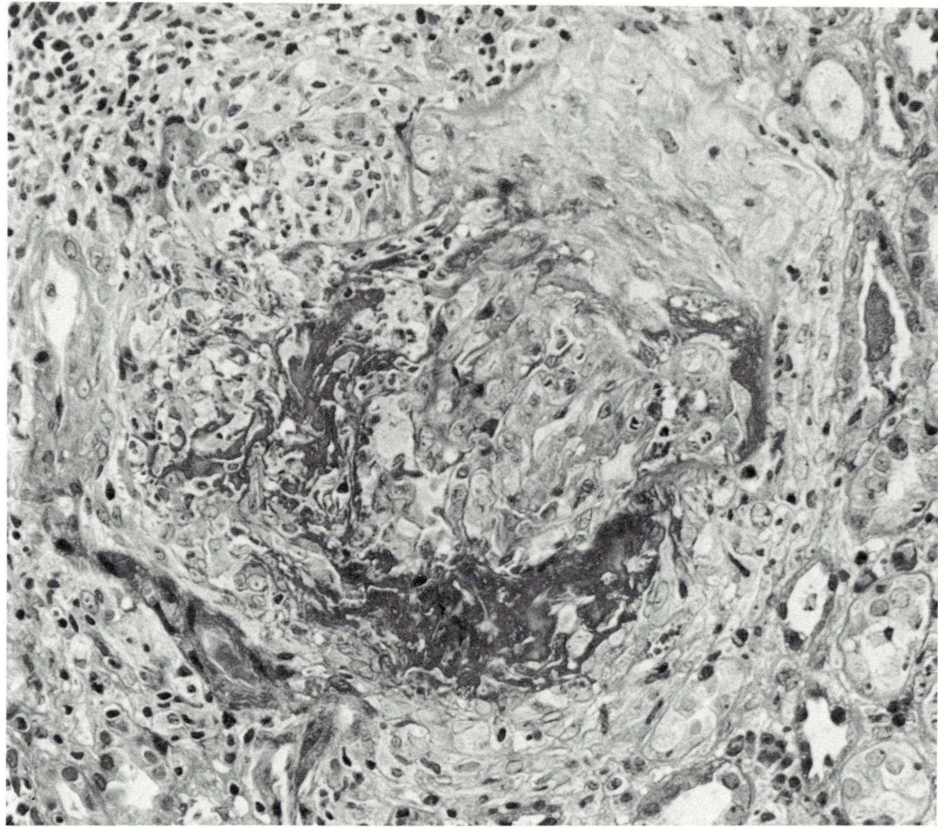

Figure 12-11. Wegener's granulomatosis. The glomerular tuft can not be distinguished due to marked crescentic proliferation, necrosis, and acute inflammation, which extends into the surrounding tissue (H&E stain, ×600).

associated with vascular occlusion and infarcts, whereas involvement of smaller vessels tends to extend to the glomerulus. In common with the vascular lesions, the glomerulonephritis is irregular in distribution and often in development, so that scarred areas may coexist with fresh, segmental damage. The presence of vasculitis requires consideration whenever a focal and segmental glomerulonephritis is seen, especially if there are no immunofluorescence or electron microscopic deposits. In such cases, examination of the clinical setting and of serial sections of the biopsy may confirm or support the diagnosis but, frequently, definitive diagnosis is not possible.

REFERENCES

1. Zeek PM: Periarteritis nodosa: a critical review. *Am J Clin Pathol* 22:777, 1952.
2. Alarcon-Segovia D: The necrotizing vasculitides: a new pathogenetic classification. *Med Clin NA* 61:241, 1977.
3. Fauci AS, Hayes BG, Katz P: The spectrum of vasculitis: clinical, pathologic, immunologic and therapeutic considerations. *Ann Intern Med* 89:660, 1978.

4. Christian CL, Sergent JS: Vasculitis syndrome: clinical and experimental models. *Am J Med* 61:385, 1976.

5. Conn DL, McDuffie FC, Holley KE: Immunologic mechanisms in systemic vasculitis. *Mayo Clin Proc* 51:511, 1976.

6. Michalak T: Immune complexes of hepatitis B surface antigen in the pathogenesis of polyarteritis nodosa: a study of seven necropsy cases. *Am J Pathol* 90:619, 1978.

7. Fye KH, Becker MJ, Theofilopoulos AN, et al: Immune complexes in hepatitis B antigen-associated periarteritis nodosa: detection in antibody-dependent cell-mediated cytotoxicity and the Raji cell asssay. *Am J Med* 62:783, 1977.

8. Halpern M, Citron BP: Necrotizing angiitis associated with drug abuse. *Am J Roentgenol Radium Ther Nucl Med* 111:663, 1971.

9. Heptinstall RH: *Pathology of the kidney,* ed 2. Boston, Little, Brown, and Co, 1974, Vol II, p 626.

10. Shillitoe EJ, Lehner T, Lessof MH, et al: Immunologic features of Wegener's granulomatosis. *Lancet* 1:281, 1974.

11. Davson J, Ball J, Platt R: The kidney in periarteritis nodosa. *Quart J Med* 17:175, 1948.

12. Rose GA: The natural history of polyarteritis. *Br Med J* 2:1148, 1957.

13. Frohnert PP, Sheps SG: Long-term followup study of periarteritis nodosa. *Am J Med* 43:8, 1967.

14. Friedman A, Kincaid-Smith P: Arteritis with impaired renal function, in Kincaid-Smith P, Mathew TH, Becker EL (eds): *Glomerulonephritis: morphology, natural history and treatment.* New York, Wiley & Sons, 1973, Part II, p 1047.

15. Harrison CV, Loughridge LW, Milne MD: Acute oliguric renal failure in acute glomerulonephritis and polyarteritis nodosa. *Quart J Med* 33:39, 1964.

16. Lewis EJ, Cavallo T, Harrington JT, et al: An immunopathologic study of rapidly progressive glomerulonephritis in the adult. *Human Pathol* 2:185, 1971.

17. Ingelfinger JR, McCluskey RT, Schneeberger EE, et al: Necrotizing arteritis in acute poststreptococcal glomerulonephritis. *J Pediat* 91:228, 1977.

18. Winkelmann RK, Ditto WB: Cutaneous and visceral syndromes of necrotizing or "allergic" angiitis: a study of 38 cases. *Medicine (Balt)* 43:59, 1964.

19. Cream JJ: Clinical and immunological aspects of cutaneous vasculitis. *Quart J Med* 45:255, 1976.

20. Sams WM Jr, Thorne EG, Small P, et al: Leukocytoclastic arteritis. *Arch Dermatol* 112:219, 1976.

21. Soter NA, Mihm MC, Gigli I, et al: Two distinct cellular patterns in cutaneous necrotizing angiitis. *J Invest Dermatol* 66:344, 1976.

22. McDuffie FC, Sams WM Jr, Maldonado JE, et al: Hypocomplementemia with cutaneous vasculitis and arthritis: possible immune complex syndrome. *Mayo Clin Proc* 48:340, 1973.

23. Feig PU, Soter NA, Yager HM, et al: Vasculitis with urticaria, hypocomplementemia and multiple system involvement. *JAMA* 236:2065, 1976.

24. Churg J, Strauss L: Allergic granulomatosis, allergic angiitis and periarteritis nodosa. *Am J Pathol* 27:277, 1951.

25. Rose GA, Spencer H: Polyarteritis nodosa. *Quart J Med* 20:43, 1957.

26. Chumbley LC, Harrison EG, Deremee RA: Allergic granulomatosis and angiitis (Churg-Strauss syndrome): report and analysis of 30 cases. *Mayo Clin Proc* 52:477, 1977.

27. Hamilton CR, Shelley WM, Tumulty PA: Giant cell arteritis: including temporal arteritis and polymyalgia rheumatica. *Medicine (Balt)* 50:1, 1971.

28. O'Neill WM Jr, Hammar SP, Bloomer HA: Giant cell arteritis with visceral angiitis. *Arch Intern Med* 136:1155, 1976.

29. Lie JT: Disseminated visceral giant cell arteritis: histopathologic description and differentiation from other granulomatous vasculitides. *Am J Clin Pathol* 69:229, 1978.

30. McManus JFA, Hornsby AT: Granulomatous glomerulonephritis associated with polyarthritis: report of a case. *Arch Pathol* 40:84, 1952.

31. Buchanan N, Berkowitz F, Gold C, et al: Granulomatous glomerulonephritis and fulminant polyarteritis nodosa in a child. *S Afr Med J* 50:1057, 1976.

32. Godman GC, Churg J: Wegener's granulomatosis: pathology and review of the literature. *Arch Pathol* 58:533, 1954.

33. Liebow AA: Pulmonary angiitis and granulomatosis, the J Burns Amberson lecture. *Am Rev Resp Dis* 108:1, 1973.

34. Saldana MJ, Patchefsky AS, Isreal HI, et al: Pulmonary angiitis and granulomatosis: the relationship between histological features, organ involvement and response to treatment. *Human Pathol* 8:391, 1977.

35. Fauci AS, Wolff SM: Wegener's granulomatosis: studies in eighteen patients and a review of the literature. *Medicine (Balt)* 52:535, 1973.

36. Horn RG, Fauci AS, Rosenthal AS, et al: Renal biopsy pathology in Wegener's granulomatosis. *Am J Pathol* 74:423, 1974.

37. Howell SB, Epstein WV: Circulating immune complexes in Wegener's granulomatosis. *Am J Med* 60:259, 1976.

13
Systemic Lupus Erythematosus

Like syphilis in the skin, lupus in the kidney is the great mimic. Almost any pattern of glomerular change may occur, and these patterns may alter during the course of the disease. Since systemic lupus is the prototype of human immune complex disease (1), this variation provides a unique opportunity to study the mechanism of immune glomerular damage. Much of the literature describing lupus nephropathy emanates from major medical centers, and the experience in such centers may not be representative of lupus in the community (2). In most studies, however, renal involvement has been reported in 50–80% of patients with lupus, depending on the criteria used for diagnosis (3–5). In these patients, renal damage may be the principal site of disease or only a minor facet. Some workers believe that the detection and management of lupus nephropathy is possible by clinical criteria alone (6). Most, however, consider that documentation of the degree of renal involvement by renal biopsy is the most sensitive and reliable guide to prognosis and therapy. This view is reinforced by the biopsy demonstration of significant renal disease in patients exhibiting no clinical criteria of kidney involvement (7). Thus, renal biopsy is an integral component of the initial investigation of patients with lupus in many medical centers.

PATHOGENESIS

A variety of immune aberrations occur in systemic lupus (8). Specific antibodies to nuclear components and to other normal body structures can be identified in the serum and immune complexes are demonstrable in both the circulation and tissues (9,10). Evidence of complex deposition is present in many extrarenal tissues, indicating that many of the systemic complications of lupus are mediated by this mechanism (11–14). The clinical and serologic phenomena in human lupus are remarkably similar to those occurring in several animal models, especially the $NZ(B \times W)F_1$ hybrid strain of mice (10,15). These mice spontaneously develop antibodies to nuclear components and suffer from a progressive glomerulonephritis that is almost identical in pattern to that of systemic lupus. As in human lupus, the progressive disease is almost entirely restricted to female mice. Intensive investigation of this and other experimental models has demonstrated immune complexes in glomeruli and other tissues containing, in addition to nuclear antigen and antibodies, components of C-type virus (16). Genetic factors are clearly implicated in the frequency and type of disease in these animals as well as in the expression of a variety of changes in lymphocytic function. Whether the continued presence of the virus is the cause or merely a secondary effect of these changes is uncertain, but the abnormalities in lymphocyte function appear to be crucial in the development of disease. The principal cellular defect is inhibition of the actions of suppressor T cells, allowing unbridled activity of B cells with consequent increased production of a variety of antibodies and lymphocytic infiltration of tissue (15).

In human lupus, similar genetic and lymphocytic factors appear to be implicated. There is a clear familial distribution of the disease and a variety of serologic abnormalities have been found in apparently unaffected relatives (8). Antilymphocytc antibodies occur frequently, and there is suggestive, but not yet conclusive, evidence of a suppressor T-cell defect analogous to that found in the mouse (8,15). This is reflected in the production of antibodies to various nuclear components and to other tissues. Further, there is immunofluorescence evidence for the presence of C-type viral antigen and antibody in both renal and extrarenal deposits of human lupus (14,17–19).

The nuclear antigens identified in the serum and deposits of patients with lupus are of several types (9). Antibodies to native DNA, single- and double-stranded DNA, nucleoprotein, and extractable nuclear antigen have been demonstrated in serum, and there is evidence for the participation of several immune complex systems involving these nuclear components. Recently, refined techniques allowing specific identification of the circulating factors have indicated that immune complexes containing double-stranded DNA are of special importance in the production of renal disease (20,21). This peculiarity would explain the rarity of nephritis and other tissue complications in the drug-induced lupus syndromes, which are usually characterized by antibodies to single-stranded DNA. The production of disparate immune complex systems is likely to lead to a variety of glomerular disease patterns, as in chronic experimental serum sickness (22). The predominant site of deposition in lupus glomerulonephritis is usually the mesangial-subendothelial region, probably indicating large and poorly soluble complexes, but intramembranous and subepithelial deposits may be seen and are sometimes predominant. The exclusive presence of subepithelial deposits in membranous lupus nephropathy may reflect a different pattern of antibody response, causing the formation of small, nonprecipitating complexes that are more prone to capillary wall localization (23). Alternatively, large complexes formed with antibodies of high avidity, and having the capacity to fix abundant complement, are well correlated with intracapillary localization (24–26). These primary mechanisms may be augmented by one or a number of secondary systems such as in situ formation of immune complexes by complexing of circulating antibodies with DNA bound to the glomerular basement membrane (24a), and the production of antiglobulins (9). As in chronic serum sickness, continued deposition may produce exhaustion of the glomerular capacity to dispose of complexes, with consequent spillage of deposits into tubulointerstitial regions (27).

The pathogenesis of lupus and its complications remains uncertain. Present evidence suggests that defects in cellular immune function allow the formation of antibodies against nuclear and other antigens with the subsequent formation of immune complexes. Viruses, probably of C-type, are likely to be implicated in the disease, but whether the immune aberrations are produced by these agents or predispose to infection is uncertain. There is no doubt that the renal complications of the disease are caused by immune complex deposition, the nature of these complexes determining the character of the lesions. Cyclic production and deposition of complexes are reflected in changes in the activity of renal disease and in the degree of hypocomplementemia which results from the immune reactions.

CLINICAL MANIFESTATIONS

Systemic lupus is a disease of young women. In North America, the annual incidence of new cases is 7.6 per 100,000 population, and there is a fivefold to tenfold excess of the disease in women, with most patients showing symptoms in the second to fourth decades (28–30). There is a higher incidence among blacks than among whites, but the disease is rare in Asians. Initially, appearance may be with a wide variety of localized or systemic signs, but most common are skin rash, photosensitivity, and nondeforming arthritis. Manifestation or exacerbation of the disease may be precipitated by severe photosensitivity following sun exposure, presumably because of the release of damaged cutaneous nucleoproteins. A series of 14 criteria for the diagnosis has been recommended by the American Rheumatism Association (29). As already discussed, there is a familial tendency to the development of lupus and allied diseases, but no specific association with any HLA type has as yet been demonstrated.

Renal involvement occurs in the majority of lupus patients attending medical centers and may be the initial presenting feature in 6% (30). Most often proteinuria and microscopic hematuria are found during routine assessment, but appearance may be with the nephritic or nephrotic syndromes or, rarely, acute renal failure. (4,29,31,32). Renal disease may be absent when the patient is first seen and develop later, usually within the first two years, but is rarely delayed for more than five years after onset (30). Significant glomerulonephritis is usually associated with hypocomplementemia, affecting both C3 and early acting components, and with circulating antibodies to nuclear components (9). Severe renal damage may, however, occur in patients with neither clinical nor laboratory evidence of renal disease (7). The classic method of laboratory diagnosis in the past was the LE cell, produced by the in vitro action of antinuclear antibodies against polymorphs, but this test has recently been largely replaced by direct tests for antinuclear antibodies (29). The immunofluorescent demonstration of immunoglobulins and complement along the dermoepidermal junction of clinically normal skin has been recommended as an indication of significant renal disease (33). The relationship between this test and glomerular involvement is not, however, absolute, and positive reactions have been demonstrated in patients with atypical forms of glomerulonephritis and no systemic features of lupus (34). Lupus-like syndromes occur after treatment with a variety of drugs, most commonly hydralazine, procainamide, methyldopa, and isoniazid, but renal disease in these syndromes is rare and usually not clinically significant (35).

PATHOLOGIC CHARACTERISTICS

The morphologic manifestations of lupus in the kidney are protean, and various classifications have been proposed using light (3,31,36), electron (37), and immunofluorescence (38) microscopic criteria. None of these classifications is entirely satisfactory by itself. However, since each technique provides significant prognostic information, a modification of the most widely used approach (see Table 13-1) is satisfactory for routine use (31). The frequencies of each of these morphologic patterns will clearly differ between individual series depending on the criteria for biopsy, and the experience of several centers is included in Table 13-1. With the usual exception of membranous nephropathy, these patterns form a continuum and can be described together.

Light Microscopy

Glomerular Lesions

Cellular proliferation in lupus glomerulonephritis is typically mesangial and often irregular. Mild glomerular involvement is characterized by diffuse mesangial expansion, with or without hypercellularity, and there is often superimposed segmental proliferation (Fig. 13-1). If strict criteria are applied, few biopsy specimens from patients with lupus show a truly focal pattern; usually, the pattern is of diffuse mesangial proliferation with areas of accentuation and segmental inflammation. Such segmental areas may show only intracapillary swelling and proliferation, but there is frequently polymorph infiltration with karyorrhexis and obvious deposit (Figs. 13-2−13-4). This deposit is most often subendothelial and takes the form of thickened, refractile capillary walls (wire loops), but small subepithelial spikes may demonstrate the extension of deposit through the membrane (Fig. 13-5). The point at which focal or irregular involvement becomes diffuse is not specified in most publications, but significant damage to more than half the glomeruli is probably a reasonable compromise (36). Even when all glomeruli are involved, the pattern is often irregular, with minimally altered segments alternating with areas of severe damage manifest by necrosis, wire loops and occlusion of capillary lumina by hyaline "thrombi." Especially in

Table 13-1. Light Microscopic Patterns in Biopsy Specimens from Patients with Systemic Lupus

	Frequency Range%[a]	Mean %
Glomerular lesions		
Minimal or no abnormality	4−37	16
Mesangial proliferative glomerulonephritis	2−30	16
Focal segmental proliferative glomerulonephritis	5−36	20
Diffuse proliferative glomerulonephritis	12−58	38
Membranous nephropathy	6−26	10
Extraglomerular lesions		
Interstitial nephritis	—	—
Necrotizing arteritis and variants	—	—

[a]Data compiled from refs. 3,4,31,36,38,40,41,42,43.

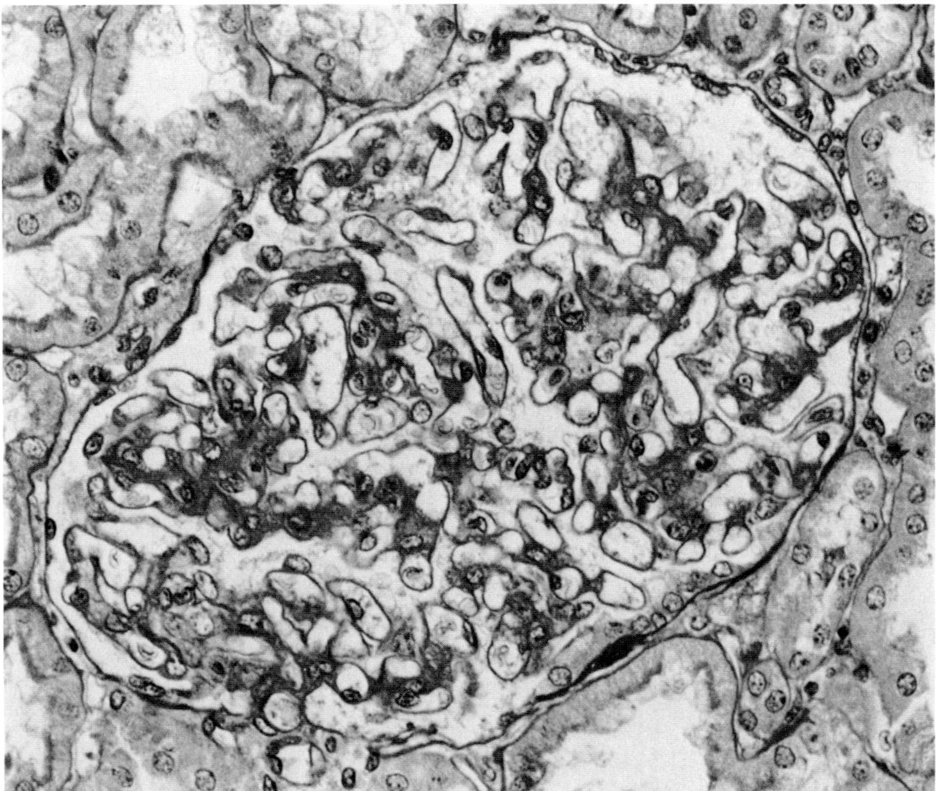

Figure 13-1. Renal biopsy specimen from a patient with mild lupus nephritis showing mild mesangial expansion (H&E stain, ×500).

necrotic areas, the fragmented nuclei may have the lilac tinge of hematoxyphil bodies. These bodies range in size from tiny fragments to irregularly rounded masses approximating the diameter of normal nuclei and are regarded as the only pathognomic feature of lupus tissue damage (44) (Figs. 13-4, 13-6).

Careful study of multiple sections will disclose hematoxyphil bodies in the majority of biopsy specimens with severe glomerulonephritis, but they are only very rarely an obvious feature of the glomerular lesions. The most advanced forms of lupus glomerulonephritis, especially when it first appears in association with an acute nephritic or nephrotic syndrome, show enhanced lobulation with diffuse endocapillary proliferation, wire loops, hyaline "thrombi," and focal or diffuse crescents (Figs. 13-7 – 13-9). Areas of mesangial interposition are common, and a pattern indistinguishable from mesangiocapillary glomerulonephritis is occasionally seen (Fig. 13-10). Because the disease is frequently episodic, active proliferation and inflammation may coexist with the sclerotic residua of previous damage such as segmental scars and adhesions to Bowman's capsule (Fig. 13-11). The pattern of lupus membranous nephropathy is in no way different from that of the idiopathic disease, but as will be discussed, varying degrees of membranous transformation of proliferative lesions may produce a similar morphologic appearance (Fig. 13-12).

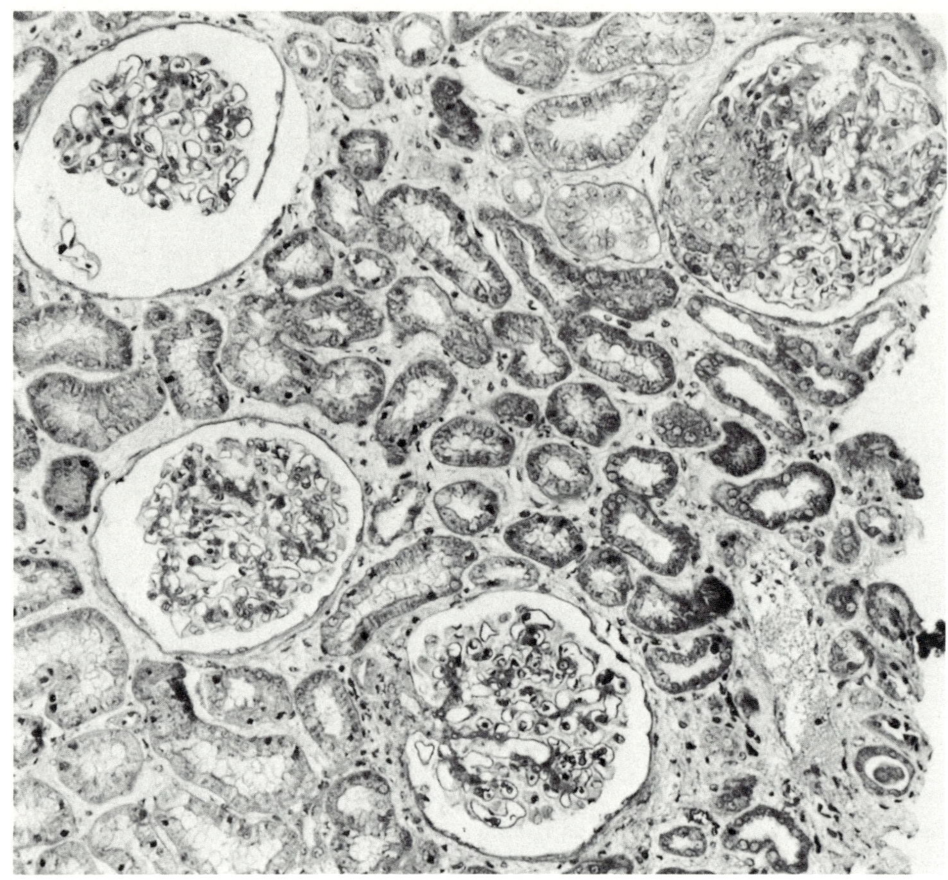

Figure 13-2. Focal lupus glomerulonephritis. The glomerulus in the upper right corner shows segmental hypercellularity while the remainder are normal (H&E stain, ×210).

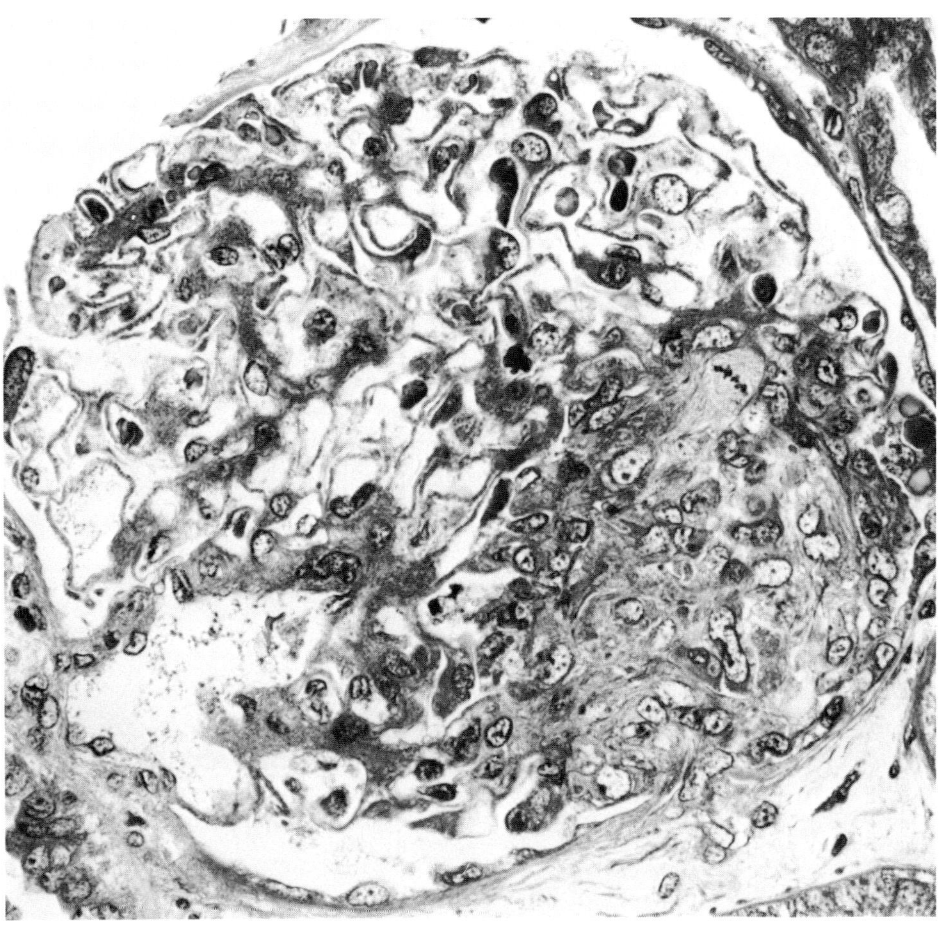

Figure 13-3. Higher magnification of the involved glomerulus shown in Figure 13-2. One glomerular lobule is adherent to Bowman's capsule. Note the presence of a mitotic figure (H&E stain, ×675).

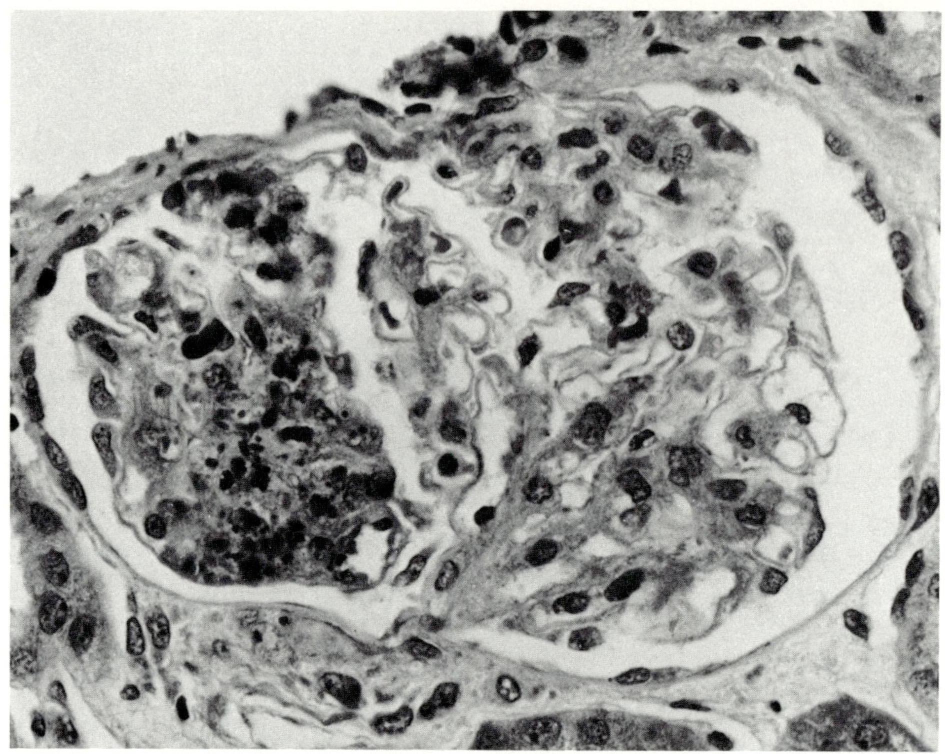

Figure 13-4. Biopsy from a patient with active focal lupus glomerulonephritis, showing a well-circumscribed area of necrosis containing numerous small hematoxyphil bodies (H&E stain, ×680).

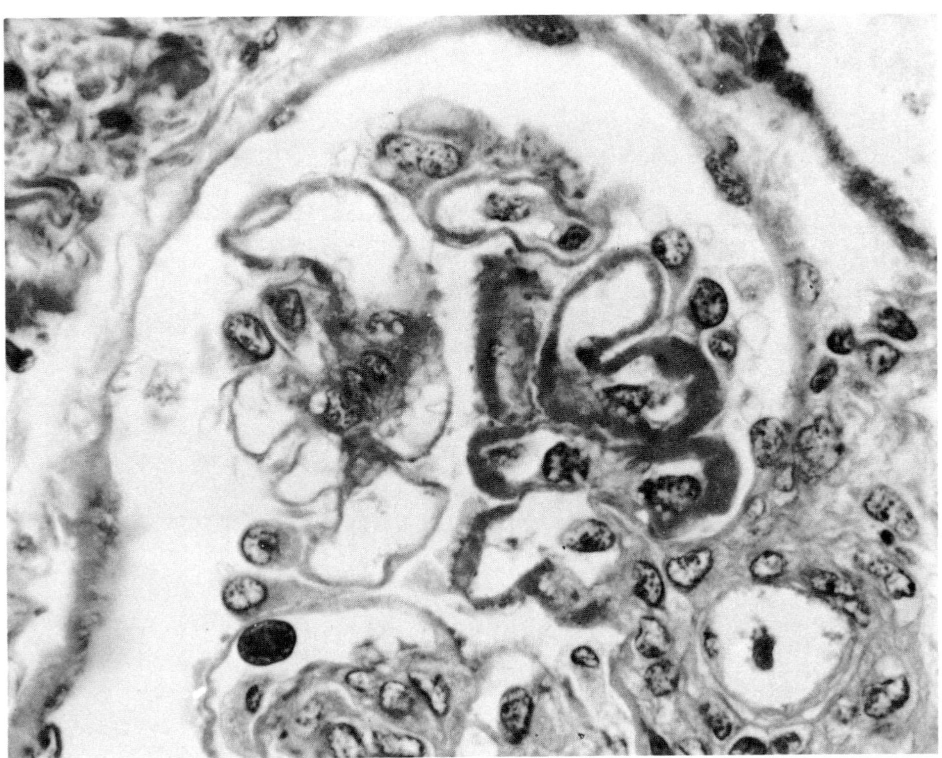

Figure 13-5. Glomerulus showing several "wire-loop" lesions (H&E stain, ×660).

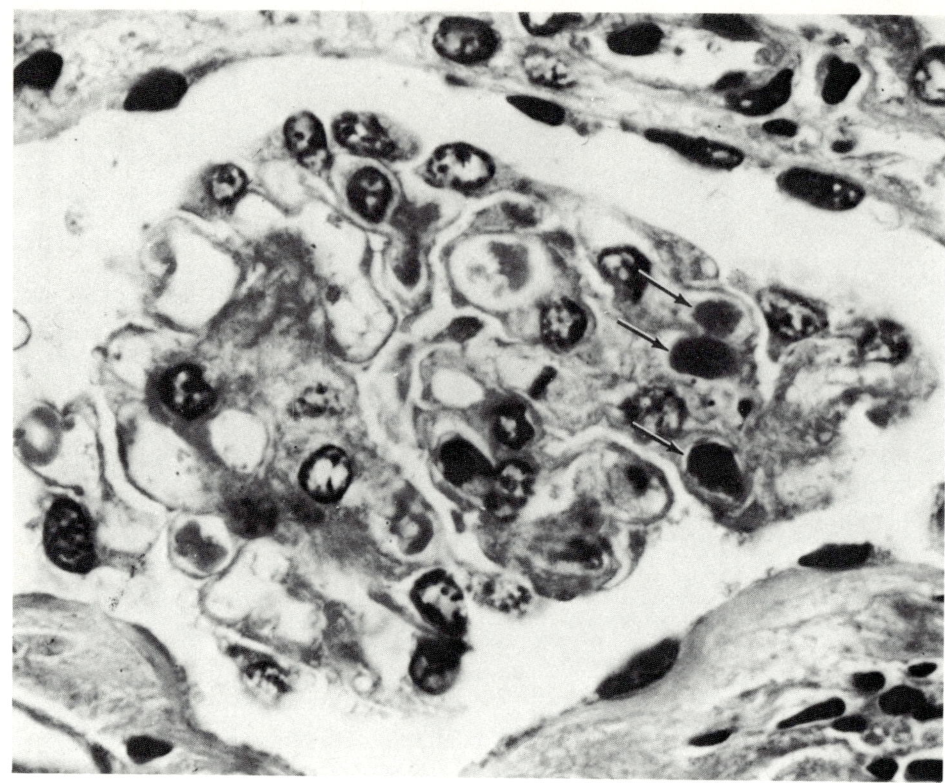

Figure 13-6. Glomerulus demonstrating three isolated hematoxyphil bodies (arrows) (H&E stain, ×700).

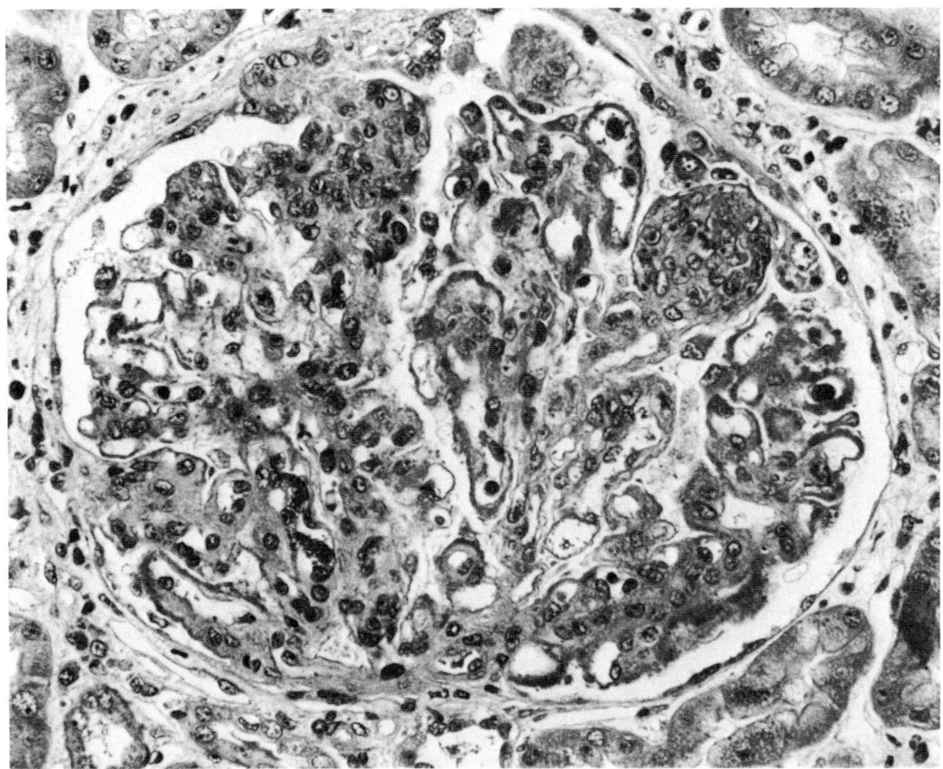

Figure 13-7. Diffuse proliferative glomerulonephritis. There is mesangial and endothelial cell proliferation involving several glomerular lobules (H&E stain, ×400).

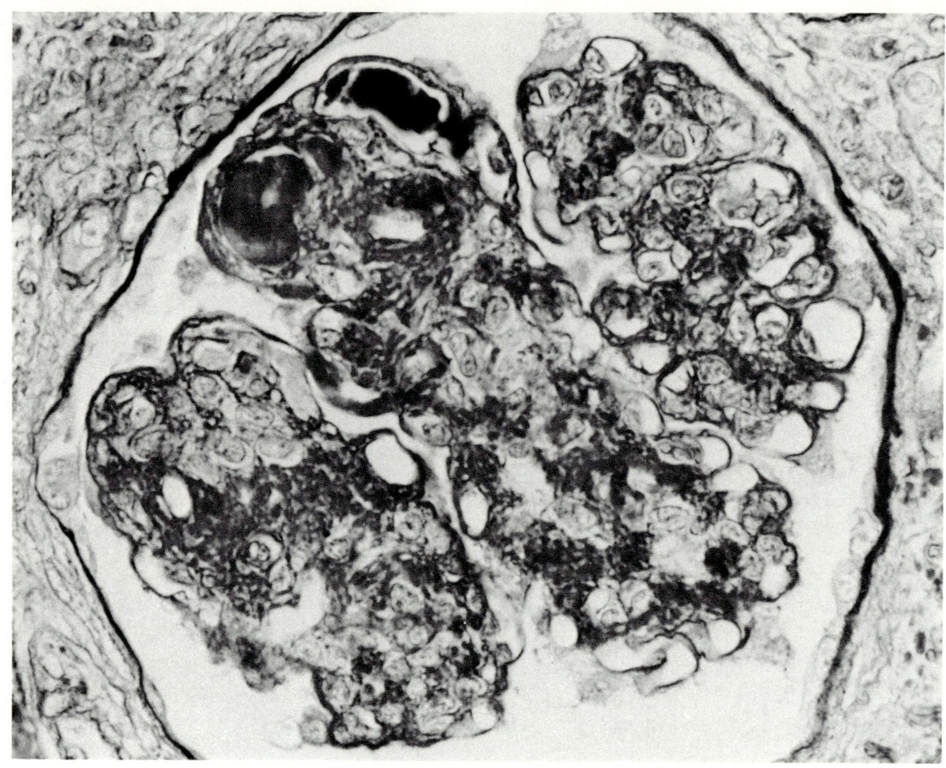

Figure 13-8. Glomerulus showing large mesangial deposits and hyaline thrombi (upper loops) (PAS stain, ×650).

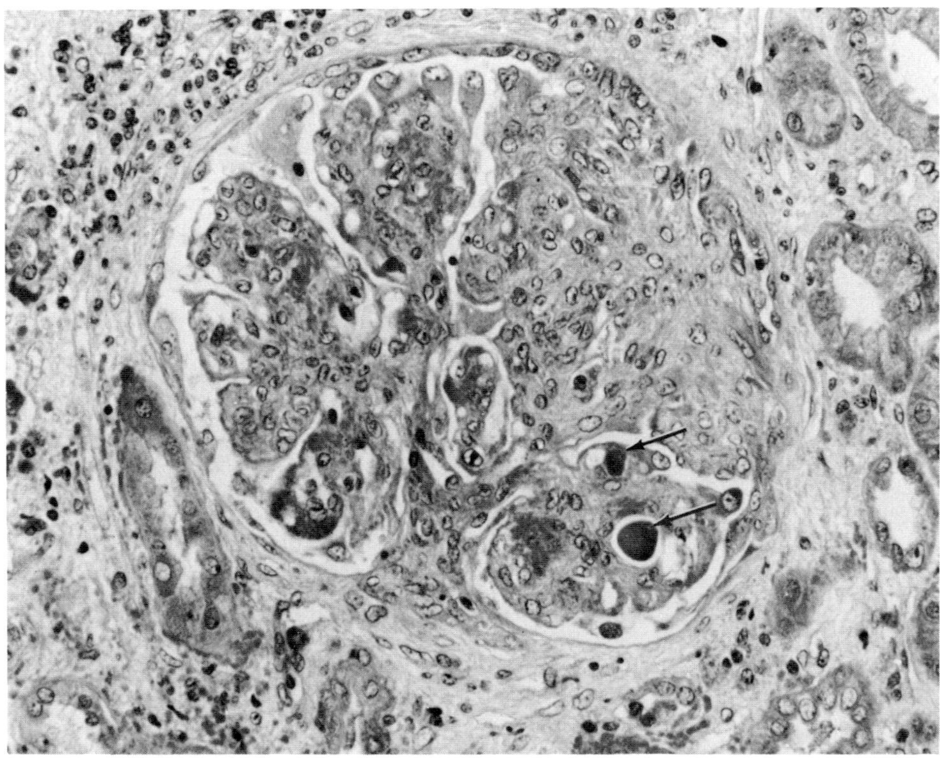

Figure 13-9. Biopsy specimen from a patient with active lupus nephritis showing capillary proliferation with an epithelial crescent and two hyaline thrombi (arrows). The interstitium is prominent and is infiltrated by mononuclear inflammatory cells (H&E stain, ×450).

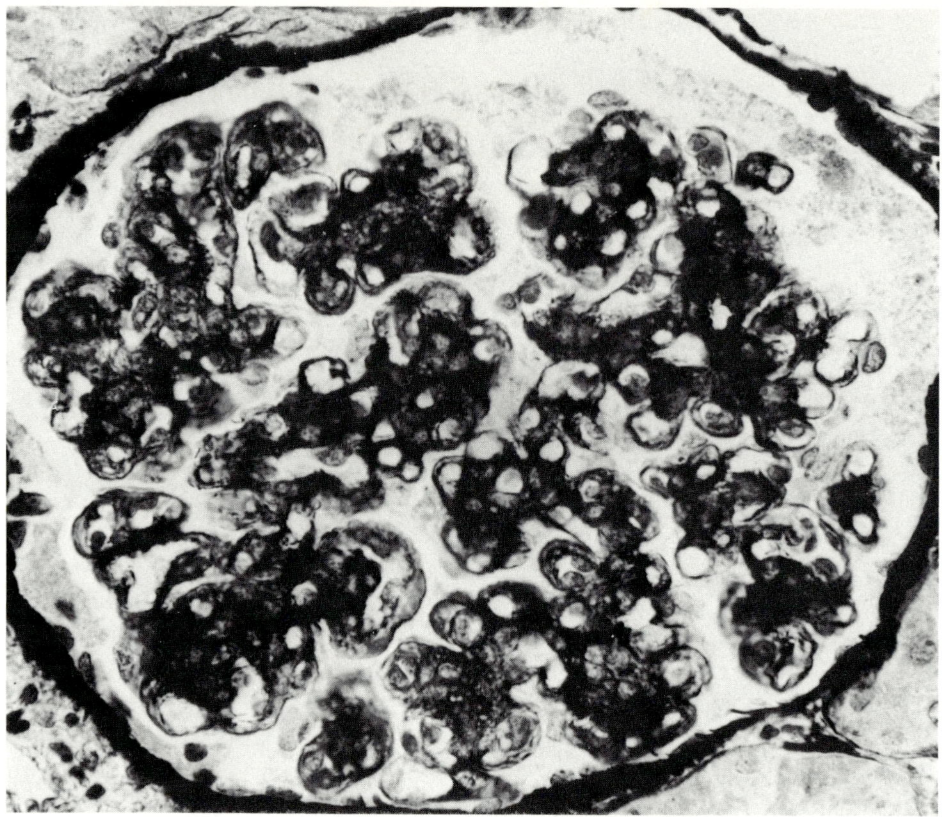

Figure 13-10. Diffuse lupus glomerulonephritis with prominent mesangial interposition producing a double contour appearance to the capillary loops indistinguishable from mesangiocapillary glomerulonephritis (PASM stain, ×540).

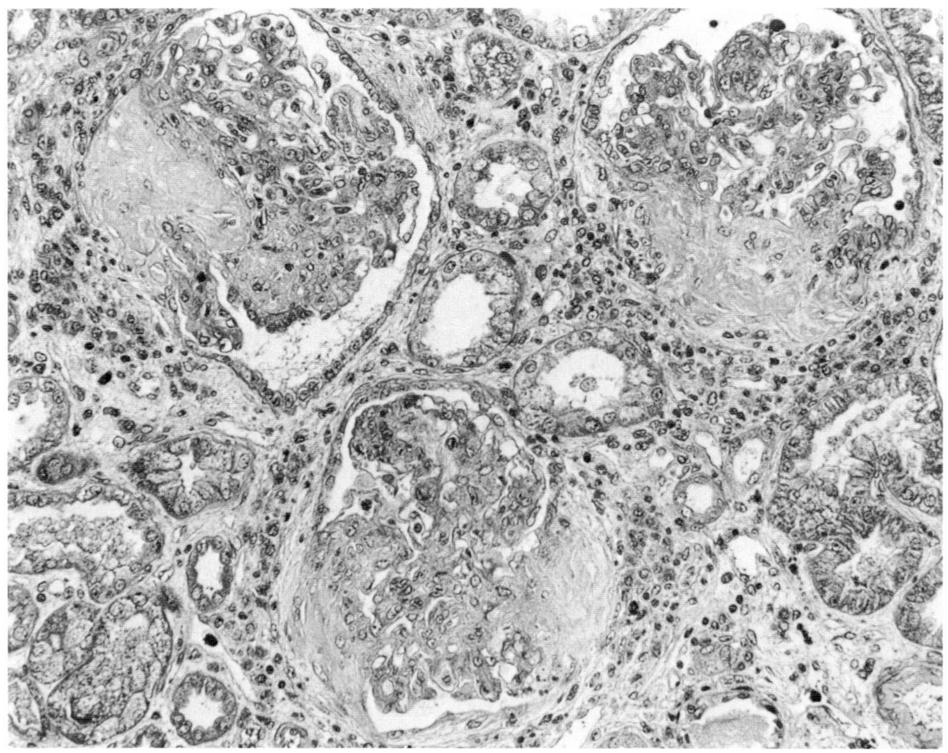

Figure 13-11. Biopsy specimen from a patient with active lupus glomerulonephritis. The glomeruli show segmental sclerosis with adhesions to Bowman's capsule and cell proliferation. The interstitium appears infiltrated by mononuclear inflammatory cells (H&E stain, ×240).

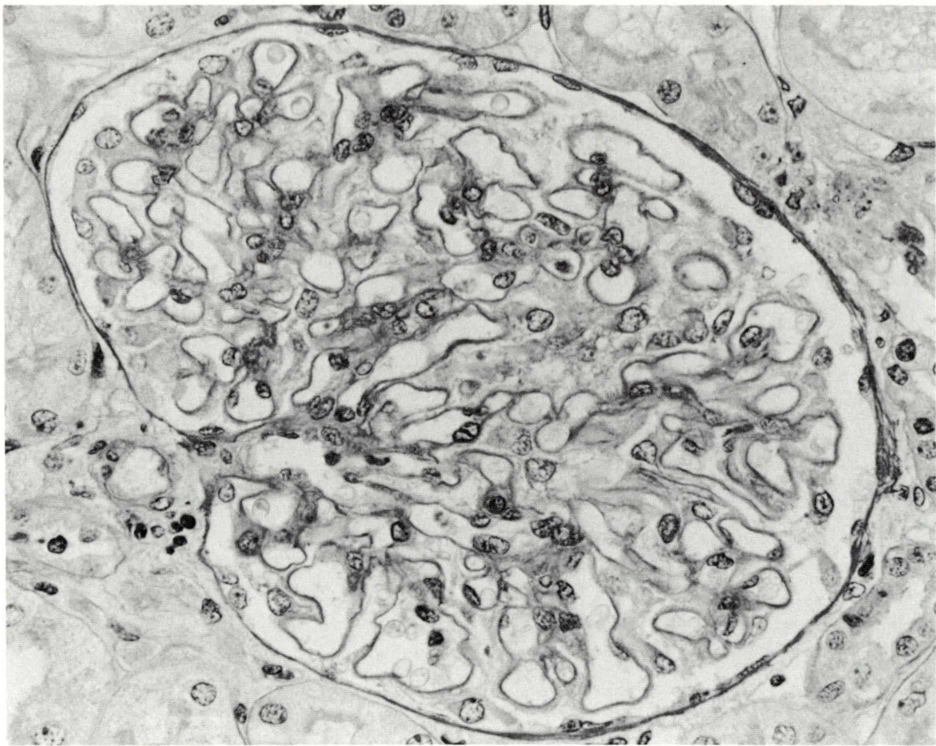

Figure 13-12. Mild diffuse capillary wall thickening in a patient with lupus membranous nephropathy (PAS stain, ×625).

Interstitial Inflammation

Interstitial inflammation is almost invariable in significant lupus glomerulonephritis and is related to extraglomerular deposition of immune complexes (27) (Figs. 13-9, 13-11). Occasionally, interstitial nephritis may be the major morphologic feature, with progressive inflammatory and fibrotic damage coexisting with minor glomerular lesions (45).

Arteritis

Arteritis is occasionally part of the renal and extrarenal tissue complications of systemic lupus (46). In many cases, the vascular lesions are indistinguishable from other forms of necrotizing arteritis, but some patients show mainly fibrin insudation into the wall with luminal thrombosis and minimal mural inflammation. This pattern closely resembles the arteriolar lesions of the hemolytic-uremic syndrome and is usually associated with a fulminant presentation in acute renal failure (31,32).

Electron Microscopy

There is a close correlation between the site and extent of the deposits in lupus glomerulonephritis and the severity of inflammation (37,47,48). Generally, exclusively mesangial deposits correspond to minor or mesangial proliferative light microscopic patterns while increasing extension into subendothelial regions is associated with progressively more severe segmental or global inflammation. Mesangial deposits are often found in biopsy specimens showing no significant light microscopic change (5,49) (Fig. 13-13). The presence of more than occasional subendothelial deposits in biopsy specimens showing only mesangial disease by light microscopy is an indication to express caution about the prognosis, for such patients may have an enhanced potential to develop more serious glomerulonephritis. In established proliferative lupus glomerulonephritis, deposits are characteristically seen in all locations, though the mesangial and endothelial regions are principally involved (Figs. 13-13−13-16). Large subendothelial deposits frequently coexist with both intramembranous and subepithelial densities, presumably reflecting the several patterns of immune complexes in the disease. With persistent inflammation, and especially after therapy, the subepithelial deposits may become the predominant feature (Fig. 13-17). The subendothelial deposits in severe glomerulonephritis are often massive, sufficient even to occlude capillary lumina, and tangential cutting of these large masses probably produces the apparent "thrombi" seen by light microscopy (Fig. 13-18). Areas of true fibrin deposition may be seen but are rarely extensive. Hematoxyphil bodies are found principally in mesangia and consist of degenerate nuclear chromatin and cytoplasmic organelles within membrane sacs (44)

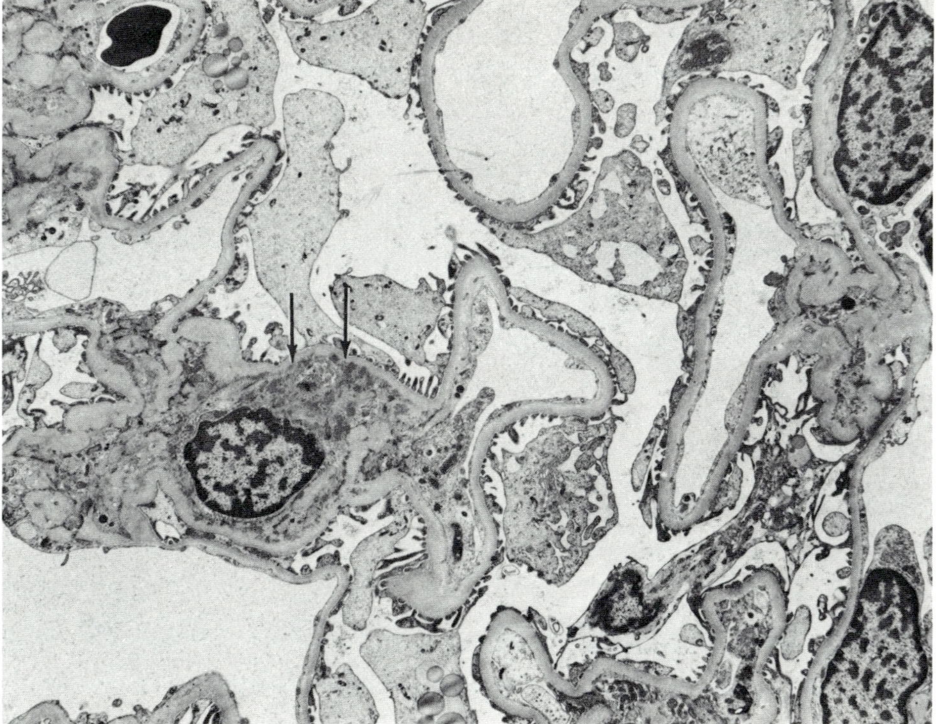

Figure 13-13. Electron micrograph of a biopsy specimen from a patient with lupus nephritis showing mesangial deposits (arrows). No significant glomerular changes were seen by light microscopy (×4,000).

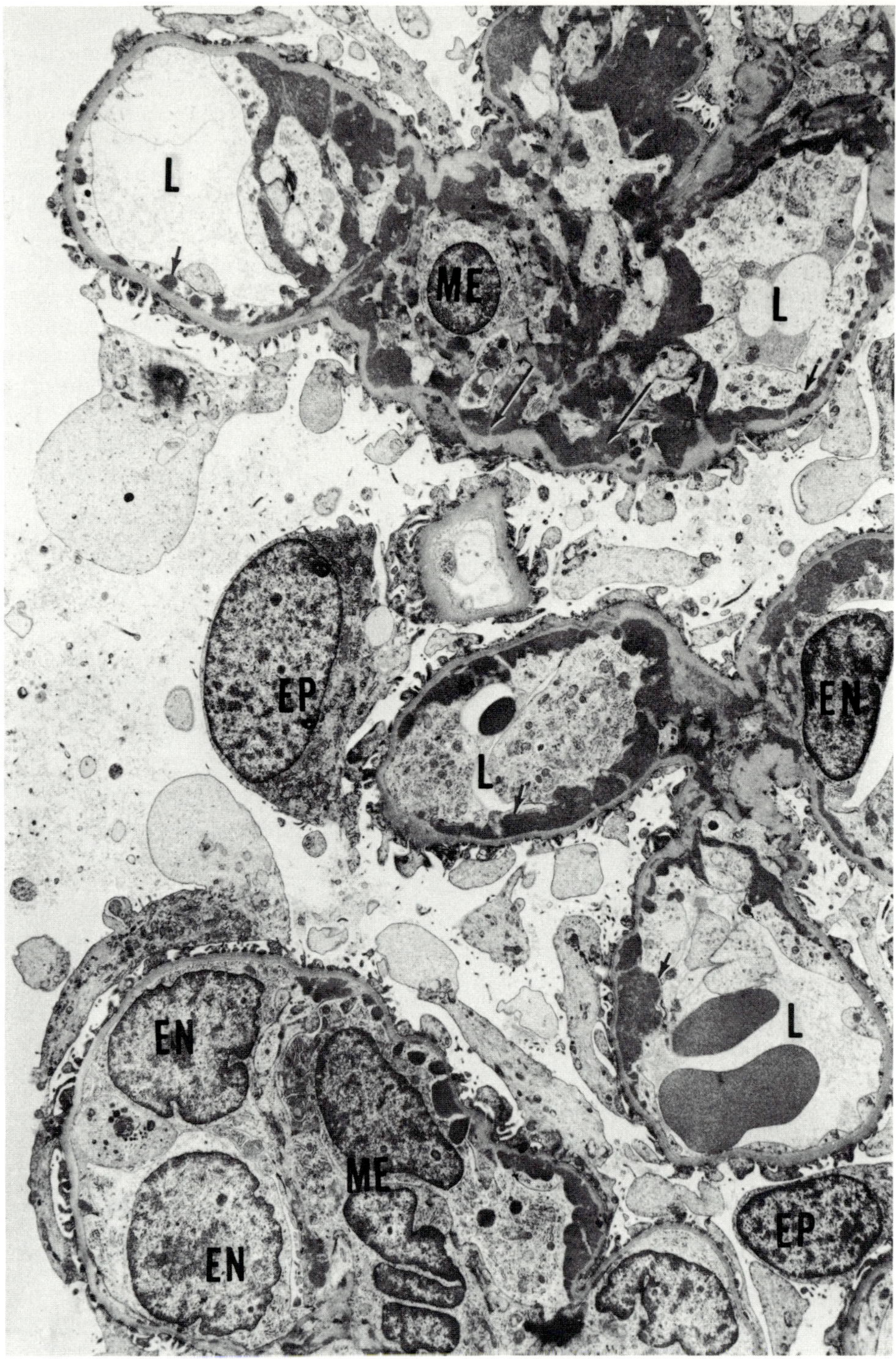

Figure 13-14. Portion of a glomerulus from a patient with active lupus glomerulonephritis showing large amounts of mesangial (arrows) and subendothelial (arrow heads) deposits. L, capillary lumen; EP, epithelial cell; EN, endothelial cell; ME, mesangium (×3,800).

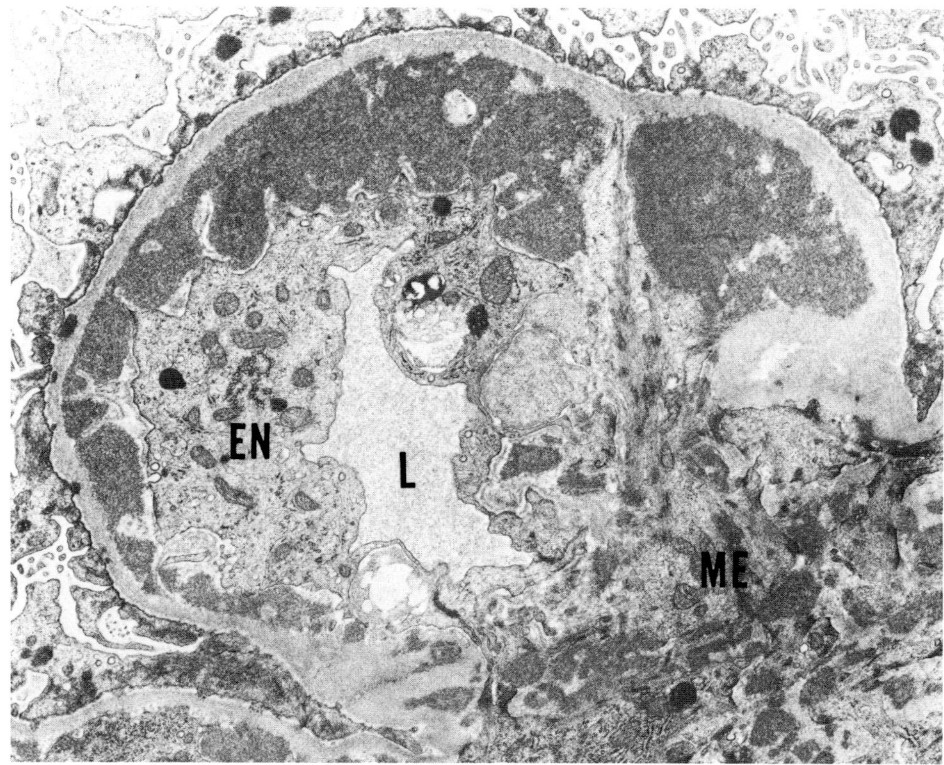

Figure 13-15. Capillary loop showing massive accumulation of deposits in the mesangium and subendothelial regions. The deposits in this latter location represent the "wire-loop" lesion seen by light microscopy. L, capillary lumen; EN, endothelial cell; ME, mesangium (×7,000).

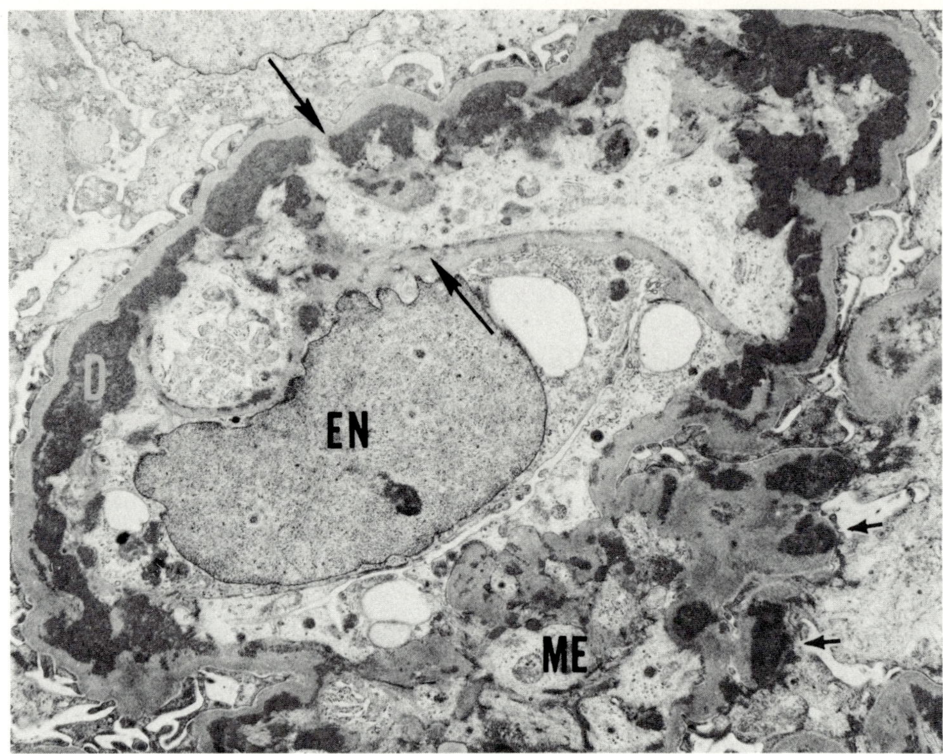

Figure 13-16. Portion of a glomerulus showing mesangial interposition at the periphery of the loop (arrows) with prominent subendothelial deposits (D). In addition there are moderate amounts of subepithelial (arrow heads) and mesangial (middle lower) deposits. EN, endothelial cell; ME, mesangium (×6,100).

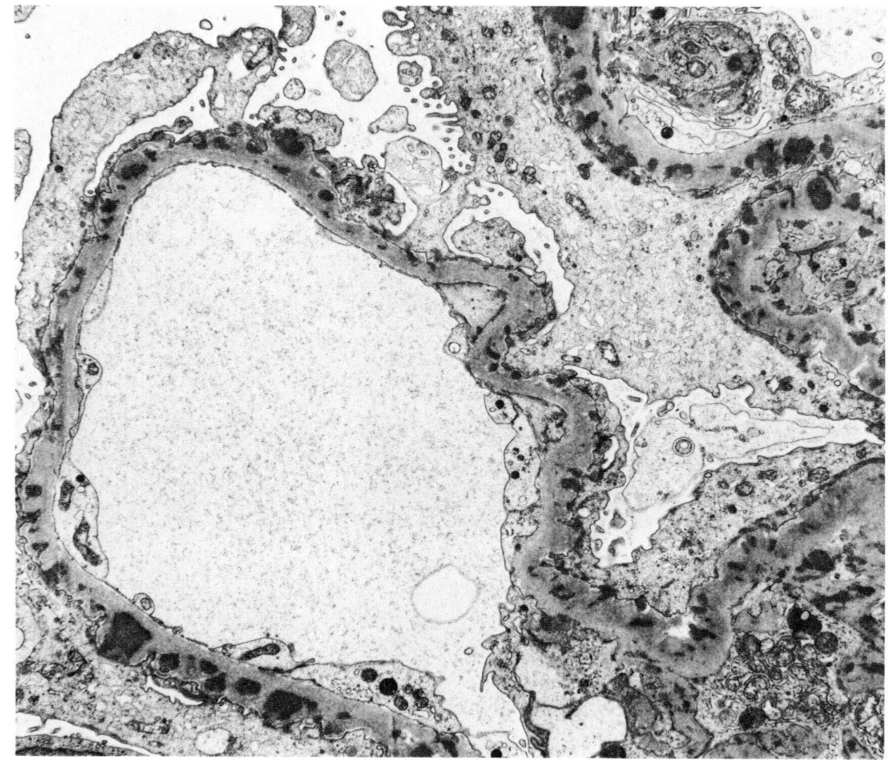

Figure 13-17. Membranous lupus nephropathy with subepithelial and intramembranous deposits. The foot processes are obliterated (×4,600).

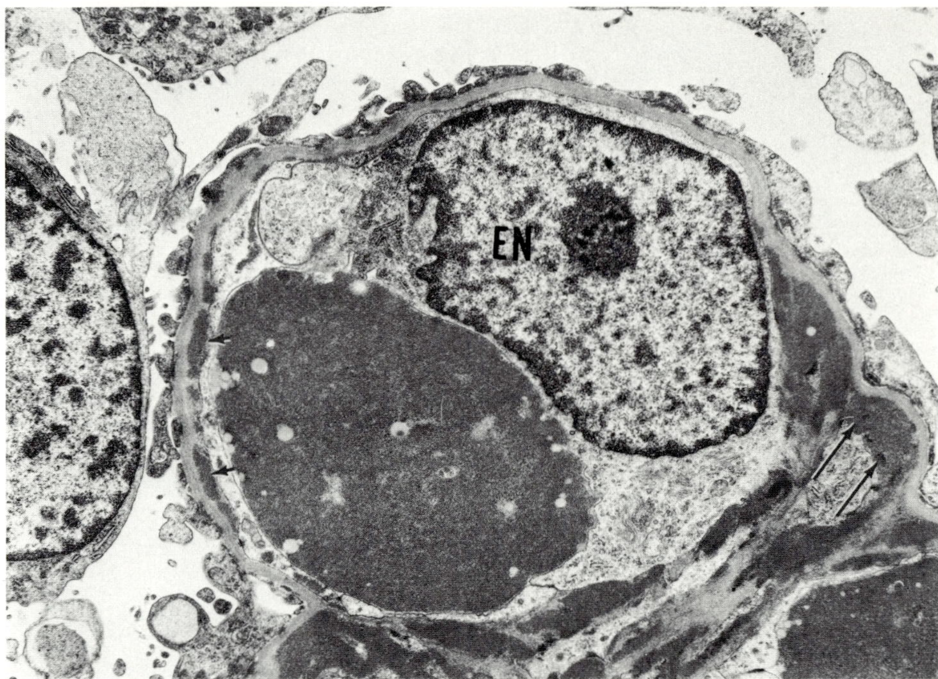

Figure 13-18. Electron micrograph of hyaline thrombi (middle and lower right corner.) In addition there are mesangial (arrows) and subendothelial (arrow heads) deposits. EN, endothelial cell (×7,500).

(Fig. 13-19). Careful examination of the tissue around glomeruli usually demonstrates deposits along tubular basement membranes and in the walls of interstitial capillaries (Fig. 13-20).

Organized Deposits
In a minority of biopsy specimens, some or all of the deposits exhibit an organized structure with either a fingerprint or microtubular configuration (50) (Fig. 13-21). These patterns may be seen in either glomerular or extraglomerular locations and are sometimes present in only a minority of the deposits (Fig. 13-22). Similar patterns occur in extrarenal deposits (11,12), and the organized structure probably reflects particular forms of crystallization within the immune complexes, although there is some evidence to suggest included phospholipids in these configurations (51). The organized pattern is highly characteristic of lupus glomerulonephritis, but has been produced in several experimental models of immune complex glomerulonephritis and is probably not a specific diagnostic appearance (52,53).

Tubulovesicular Bodies (Myxovirus-like, Microtubular, Glomiform Bodies)
Interwoven tubules and vesicles can be identified in glomerular and interstitial capillary endothelial cells in most biopsy specimens from patients with lupus (54) (Figs. 13-20, 13-23). Rarely, they are also present in mesangial and visceral epithelial cells (Fig. 13-24). These structures are also present in extrarenal loca-

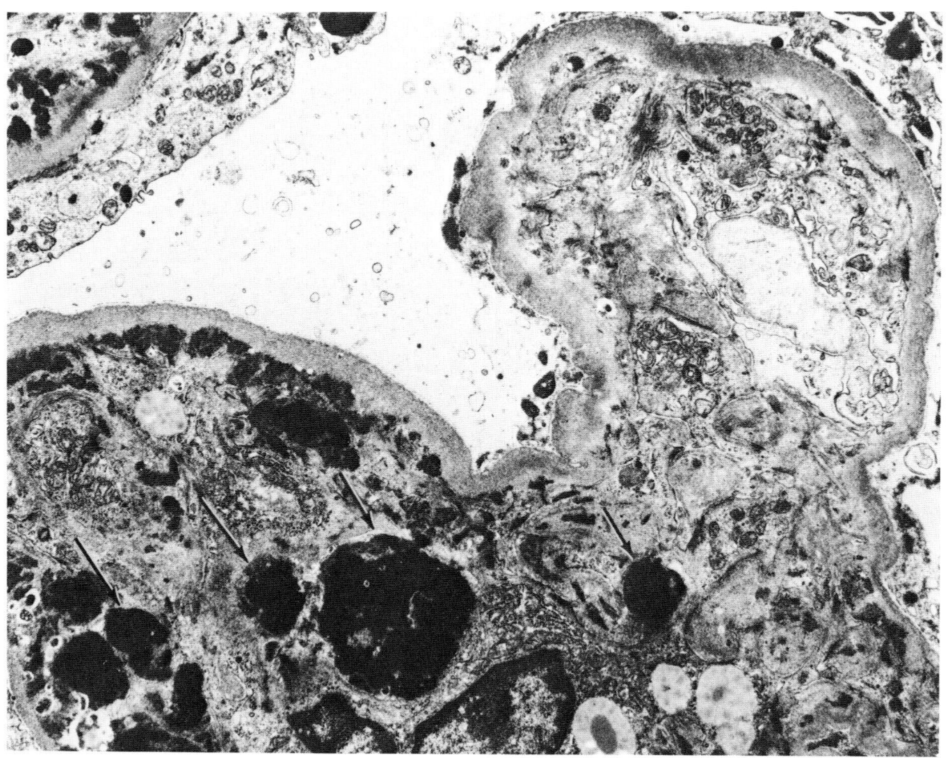

Figure 13-19. Electron micrograph of a portion of a glomerulus showing hematoxyphil bodies in the mesangium (arrows) (×6,200).

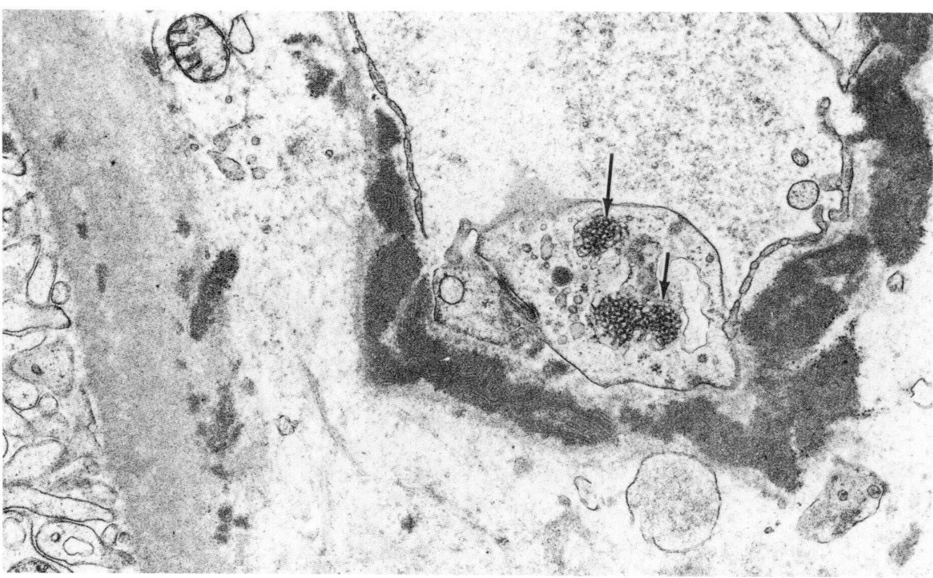

Figure 13-20. Electron micrograph showing deposits around the tubular basement membrane and peritubular capillary. The endothelial capillary cell contains clusters of tubulovesicular bodies (arrows) (×17,700).

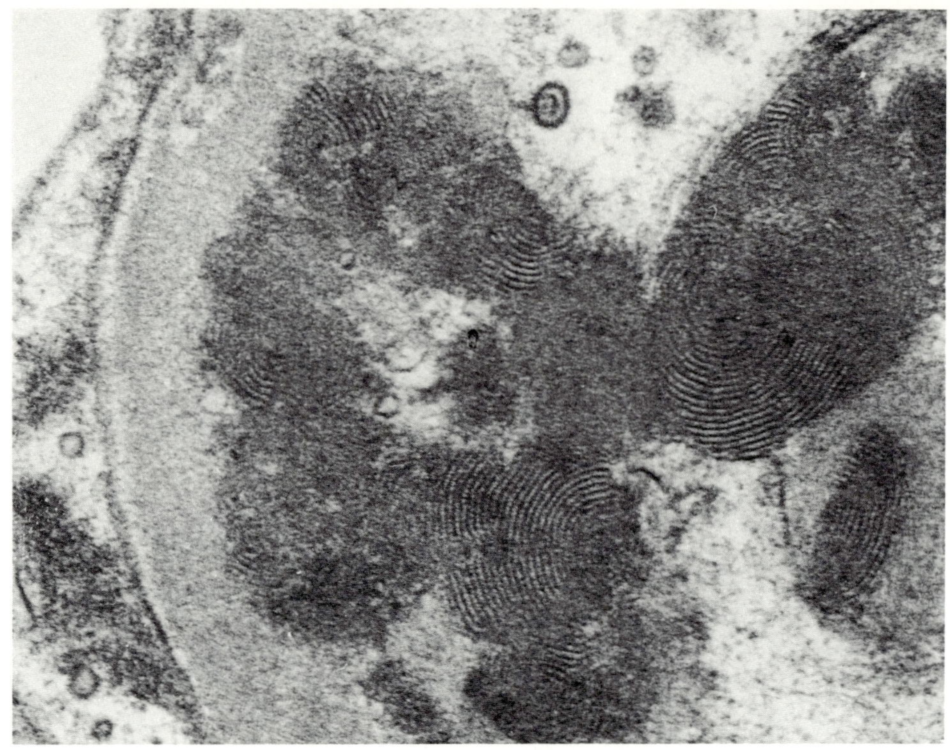

Figure 13-21. Electron-dense deposits with fingerprint configuration (×48,000).

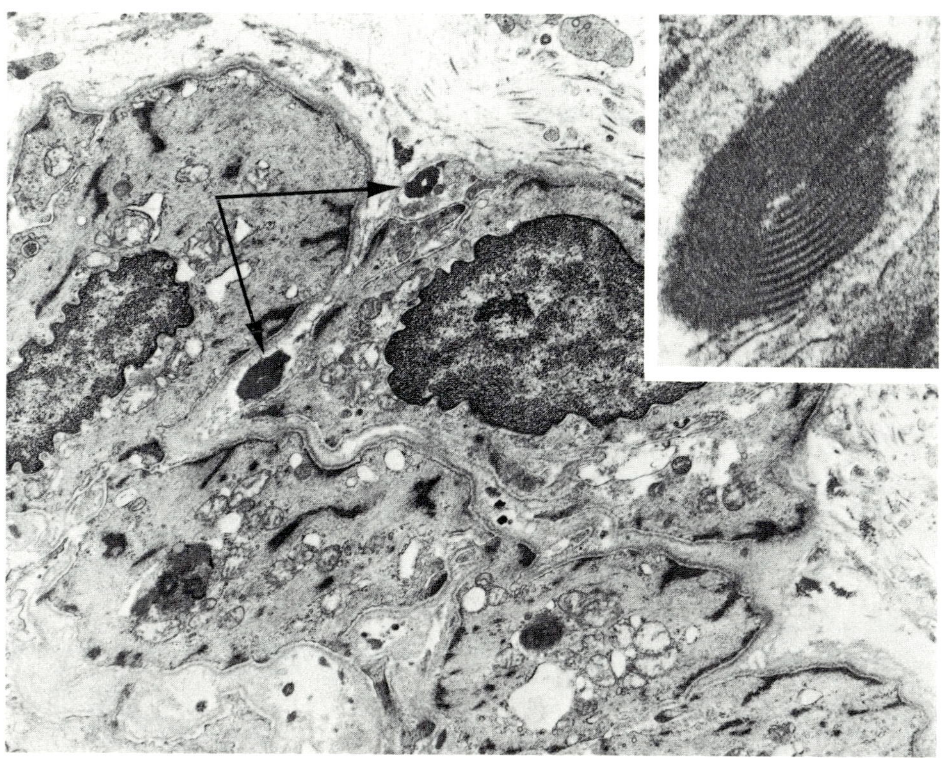

Figure 13-22. Electron micrograph of a blood vessel from a patient with diffuse active lupus glomerulonephritis showing deposits with a fingerprint appearance (arrows) (×8,600; insert, ×47,000).

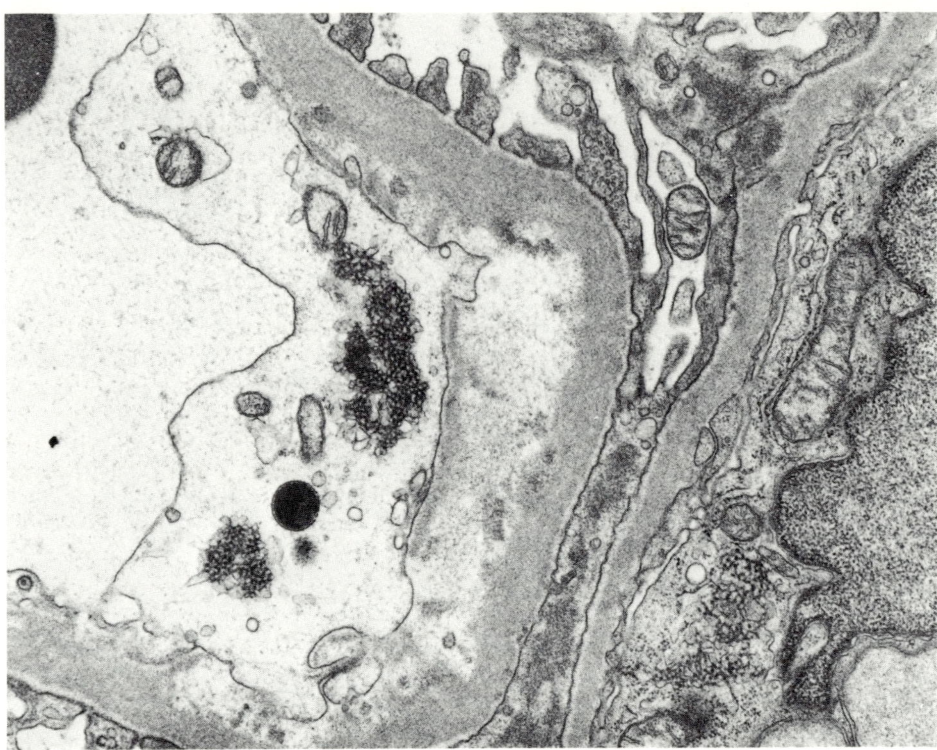

Figure 13-23. Capillary loop showing tubulovesicular bodies in the endothelial cell. The subendothelial electron-lucent area probably represents reabsorbed deposits (×19,625).

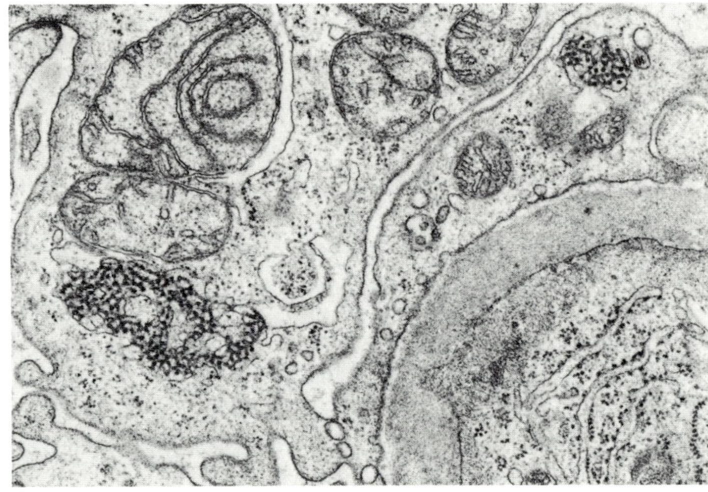

Figure 13-24. Clusters of tubulovesicular bodies in a visceral epithelial cell (×4,800).

tions in lupus patients and show no relationship to the severity of the disease (55). Careful examination of renal biopsy specimens with a wide variety of diseases will reveal similar structures in up to a quarter of patients, and their presence in small numbers has no diagnostic specificity (56). Large numbers of tubulovesicular bodies are, however, quite suggestive of lupus, and serial serologic studies are indicated if they are abundant (54, 57). Although the bodies superficially resemble profiles of a paramyxovirus, there is no evidence to confirm a viral origin, and studies indicating a glycoprotein structure suggest that they arise from contorted tubules of endoplasmic reticulum (58,59).

Immunofluorescence Microscopy

The patterns and intensity of the immunofluorescent reactions correlate closely with the light microscopic changes (38). Purely mesangial reactions generally are associated with minimal or mesangial proliferative lesions, while extension of staining onto capillary walls correlates with the development of segmental disease (Figs. 13-25–13-27). Diffuse reactions throughout all mesangia and along all capillary walls are typically associated with severe, diffuse glomerulonephritis (Fig. 13-28). These diffuse reactions usually show segmental accentuation with broad strips of capillary wall deposit corresponding to wire loops and intralumi-

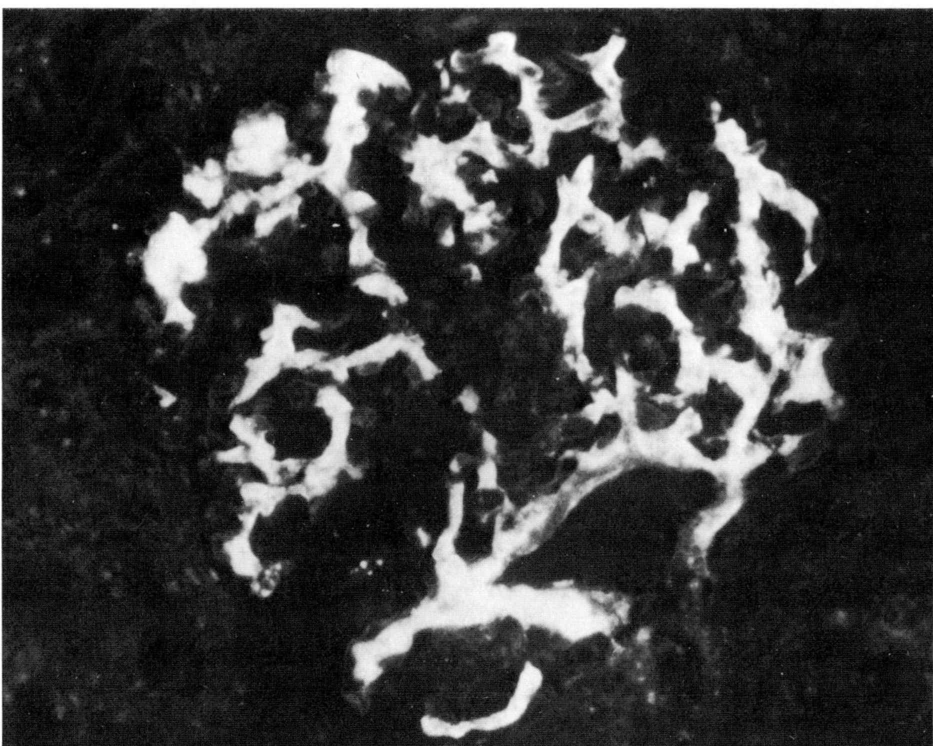

Figure 13-25. Mesangial proliferative lupus glomerulonephritis showing mesangial fluorescent deposits (antihuman IgG, ×500).

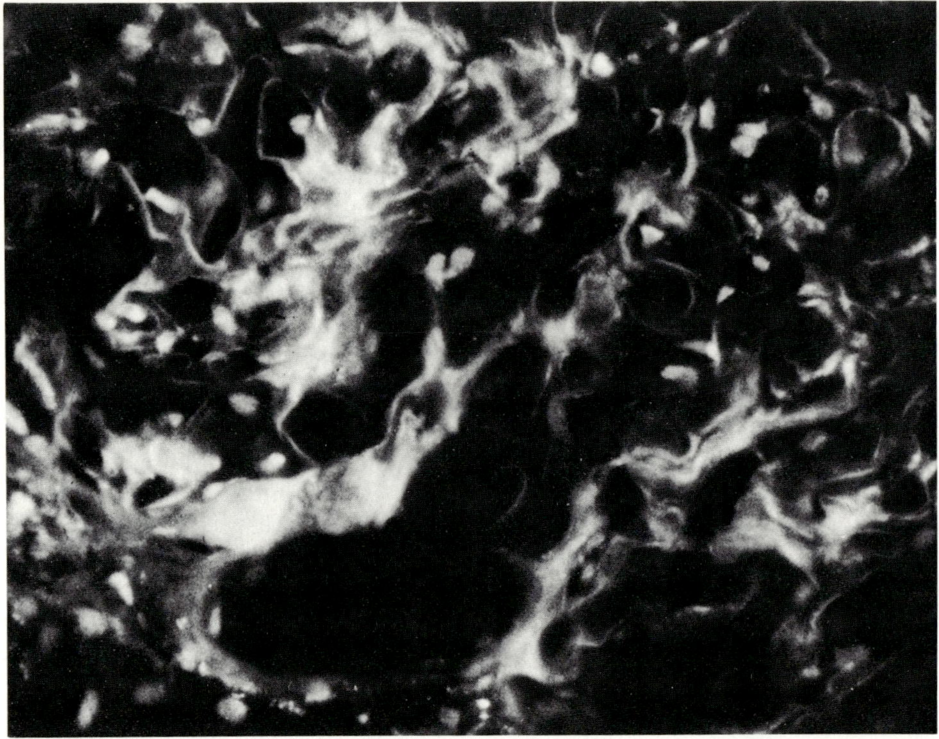

Figure 13-26. Glomerulus showing moderate mesangial and peripheral linearlike fluorescence. Strong antinuclear staining is also present (antihuman IgG, ×600).

nal plugs representing hyaline "thrombi." (Fig. 13-29). The purely capillary wall pattern of lupus membranous nephropathy is similar to that of the idiopathic disease, although reactions for IgA and early acting complement components are more common in lupus (Fig. 13-30). In all types of lupus nephropathy, the reactions are almost invariably granular, but a linear pattern of IgG has rarely been reported (60). The predominant immunoglobulin is usually IgG, though both IgA and IgM are often abundant and either may occasionally be the principal reaction. Both C3 and early acting complement components are generally present, with the C1 reactions often being especially intense, possibly because of interaction with DNA molecules (9). In severe disease, fibrin may be present either in the glomeruli or in superimposed crescents. The characteristic feature of severe lupus glomerulonephritis is a "full-house" pattern of immunofluorescence, reactions occurring with all reagents. While negative results occur in some patients, the majority have some deposits (38). Studies of lupus patients with no overt renal involvement have confirmed the frequency of positive reactions, usually mesangial in distribution (5,7,49). In addition to the glomerular deposits, granular reactions for IgG and C3 are common along tubular basement membranes and in the interstitium (27,61). The identification of extraglomerular reactions, especially for IgG, is an indication to consider lupus in the differential diagnosis. As has already been discussed, C-type viral antigen and antibody have been identified in the deposits of lupus patients (14,17–19).

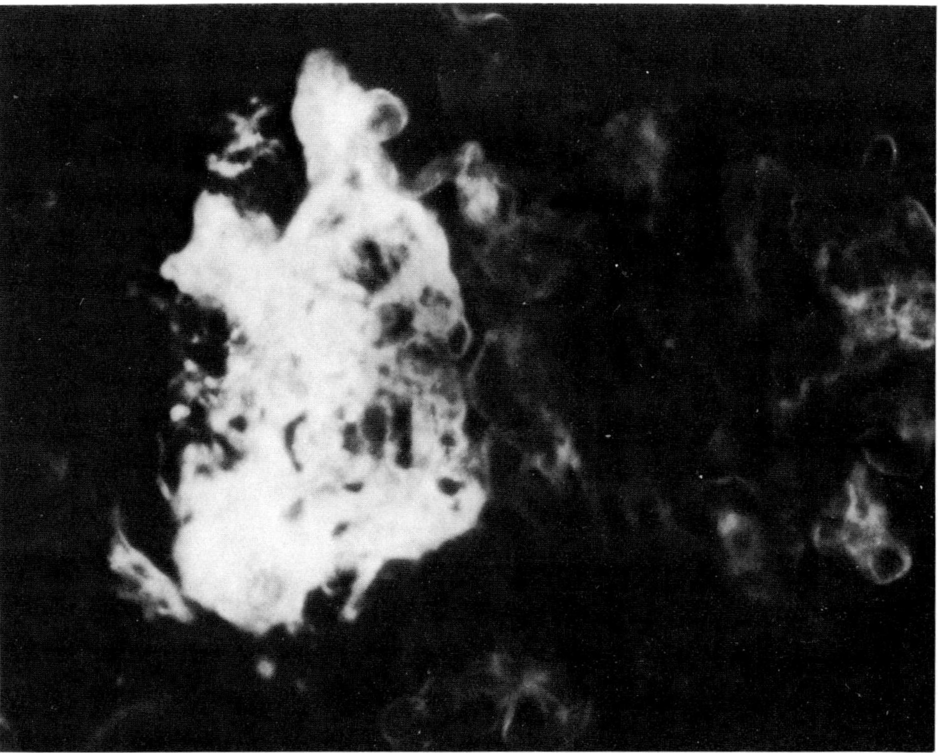

Figure 13-27. Segmental deposits of fibrinogen from a patient with focal necrotizing lupus glomerulonephritis ($\times 500$).

CLINICOPATHOLOGIC CORRELATIONS AND EVALUATION

Although significant renal disease may occur without overt clinical or laboratory signs, there is usually a close correlation between the severity of glomerulonephritis and its clinical expression. Thus, mesangial proliferative glomerulonephritis tends to be associated with proteinuria while hematuria is more common with increasing degrees of segmental activity, especially if there is superimposed necrosis. Similarly, the degree of proteinuria generally corresponds to the severity of inflammation, except in the membranous form (62). Generally, the presence of the nephrotic syndrome or of overt nephritic features in a patient with lupus indicates a strong probability of serious renal disease. Morphologic severity is clearly related to the degree of hypocomplementemia but corresponds less well with other serologic abnormalities (39,63).

The morphologic changes are merely the expressions of the type and extent of immune complex deposition at the time of biopsy and may therefore alter during the course of the disease. Progression of minor lesions to more significant patterns of damage occurs in a significant proportion of patients and, conversely, severe inflammatory changes may resolve with effective therapy (31,36,39,42,43). Almost any pattern of progression may occur, but among the most important is an occasional tendency for the deposits in proliferative lesions to assume a subepithelial position so that the picture closely resembles mem-

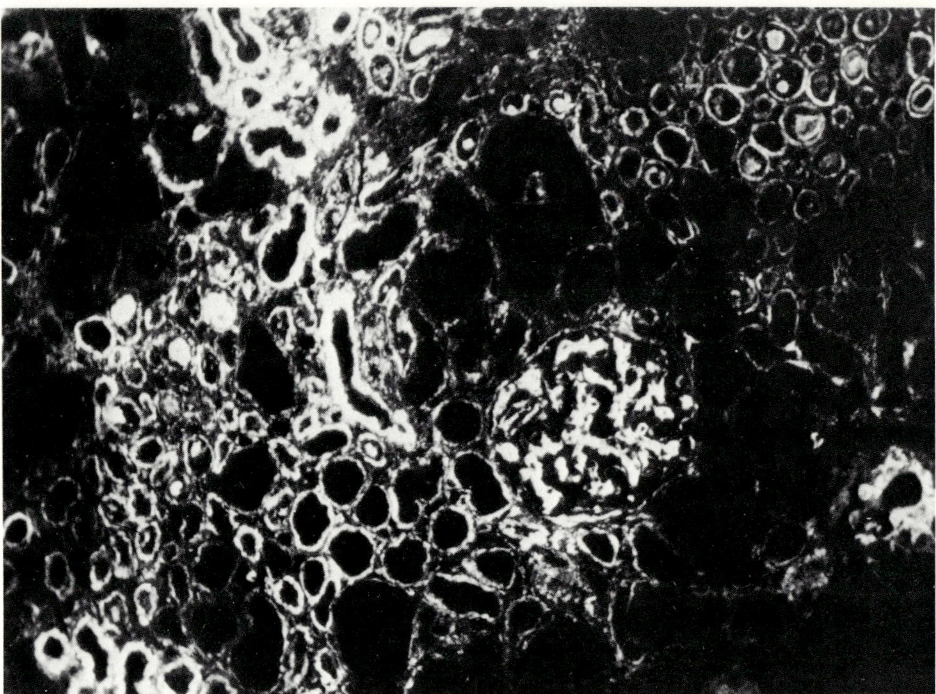

Figure 13-28. Severe lupus nephritis showing large amounts of mesangial and peripheral deposits in glomeruli as well as along tubular basement membranes, blood vessels, and interstitium (antihuman IgG, ×140).

branous nephropathy (64). This transformation is especially likely to occur after therapy, with transformation of the DNA antibodies from precipitating to non-precipitating type (64a) and the frequency of membranous nephropathy in some studies may have been artificially inflated by the inclusion of patients with treated proliferative disease. Recognition of this pseudomembranous pattern is important, because the patients retain the potential for explosive exacerbation of proliferative disease if treatment is suspended (63). For this reason, the diagnosis of lupus membranous nephropathy in a treated patient should only be made after thorough examination to include the presence of intracapillary deposit. Generally, effective therapy does not cause the membranous pattern but rather causes resolution of most deposits with diminution of immunofluorescent reactions and the production of ultrastructural lucencies in the basement membrane. Cellular proliferation and exudation are controllable by therapy, but sclerosis is permanent and may accumulate to produce chronic renal failure (31,39).

PROGNOSIS

Renal disease is, with involvement of the central nervous system, the major prognostic determinant in patients with lupus (2,30). Renal failure was the cause

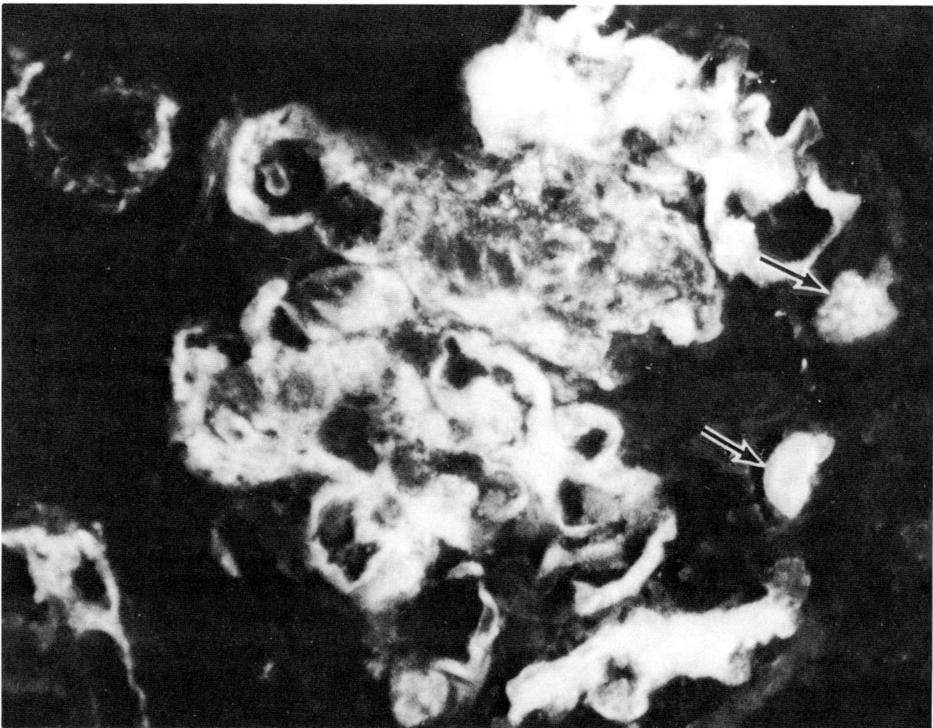

Figure 13-29. Coarse endomembranous deposits in several loops corresponding to the wire-loop lesion as seen by light microscopy. In addition, one capillary loop appears occluded by deposits, corresponding to the hyaline thrombi seen light microscopically in this biopsy specimen (arrows) (antihuman IgG, ×550).

of death in up to 38% of patients, but the incidence of renal death has drastically declined with the introduction of effective therapy and the control of infective complications. Analysis of survival data from series published before 1970 is, therefore, hazardous, and the reported variations in prognosis for the various renal lesions may reflect the inclusion of patients treated in an earlier therapeutic era. Currently, the five-year survival rates for the several forms of lupus glomerulonephritis are: mesangial proliferative, 100%; focal proliferative, 60–87%; diffuse proliferative, 38–83%; and membranous, 80–100% (4,31,39–41). Since the five-year survival of all patients with lupus is 77–95%, only the diffuse and (in some series) focal proliferative patterns are now major threats to life (2,30). This profound alteration from previous experience has been brought about by the judicious use of corticosteroid and immunosuppressive therapy (65), with plasmapheresis being used in some centers for particular cases (66). While these forms of therapy undoubtedly control the acute inflammatory features of lupus nephropathy, sclerotic lesions are unaffected and slow progression to renal failure can still occur if extensive scarring has developed (31,39). Transplantation in such patients has been successful and recurrent lupus glomerulonephritis has not been recorded (67).

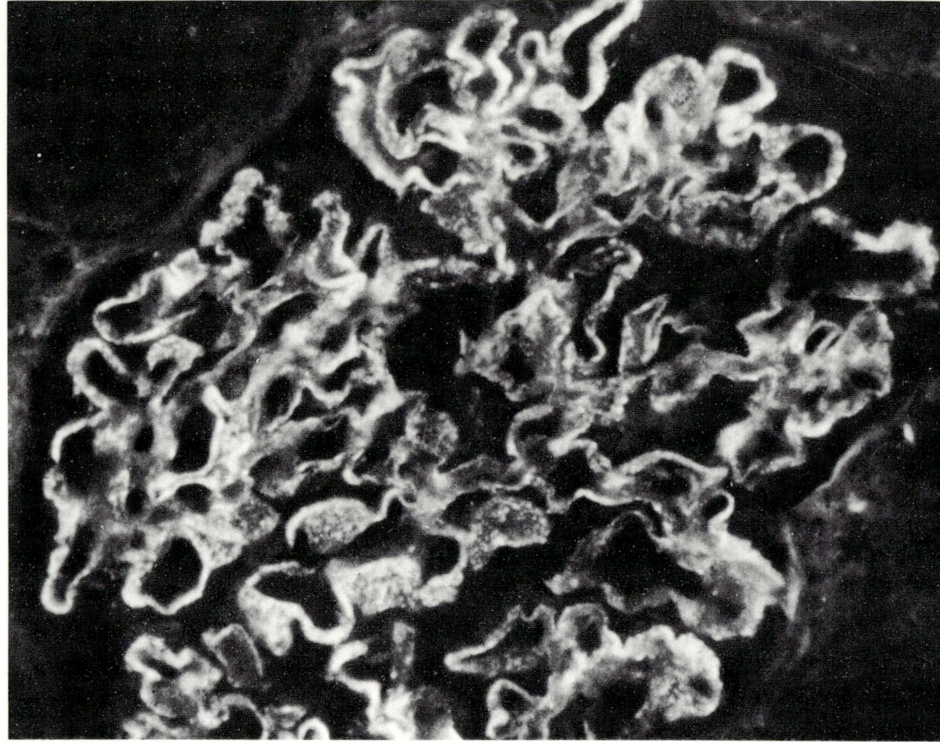

Figure 13-30. Granular fluorescent deposits along capillary loops in a case of lupus membranous nephropathy (antihuman IgG, ×540).

SUMMARY

Lupus glomerulonephritis is produced by the deposition of immune complexes containing nuclear and viral material. The participation of several immune complex systems produces two general patterns of renal disease, proliferative glomerulonephritis occurring with mesangial and subendothelial deposition and membranous nephropathy resulting from subepithelial localization. The severity of the proliferative forms of glomerulonephritis is closely correlated with the extent of deposit demonstrated by either electron or immunofluorescence microscopy, and the clinical expressions of these changes generally conform to their morphologic degree. Because there is variation in the presence and type of the immune complexes in patients with lupus, the glomerular lesions are not fixed and may change drastically within short periods of time. Probably, most lupus patients have some degree of glomerular damage, but severe glomerulonephritis is present in only about one-third, and modern therapy can halt the previously inexorable progress of this disease. Because many medical centers include renal biopsy as an integral part of the initial investigation of lupus patients, the pathologist has the opportunity to examine the patterns of immune complex deposition and their morphologic effects.

REFERENCES

1. Koffler D, Agnello V, Thoburn R, et al: Systemic lupus erythematosus: prototype of immune complex nephritis in man. *J Exp Med* 134:169s, 1971.

2. Dubois EL, Wierzchowiecki M, Cox MB, et al: Duration and death in systemic lupus erythematosus: an analysis of 249 cases. *JAMA* 227:1399, 1974.

3. Pollak VE, Pirani CL: Renal histologic findings in systemic lupus erythematosus. *Mayo Clin Proc* 44:630, 1969.

4. Fish AJ, Blau EB, Westberg NG, et al: Systemic lupus erythematosus during the first two decades of life. *Am J Med* 62:99, 1977.

5. Cavallo T, Cameron WR, Lapenas D: Immunopathology of early and clinically silent lupus. *Am J Pathol* 87:1, 1977.

6. Fries JF, Porta J, Liang MH: Marginal benefit of renal biopsy in systemic lupus erythematosus. *Arch Intern Med* 138:1386, 1978.

7. Mahajan SK, Ordóñez NG, Feitelson PJ, et al: Lupus nephropathy without clinical renal involvement. *Medicine (Balt)* 56:493, 1977.

8. Bach J-F, Bach MA, Tron F: New conceptions of autoimmunity and of systemic lupus erythematosus. *Adv Nephrol* 6:5, 1976.

9. Agnello V: The immunopathogenesis of lupus nephritis. *Adv Nephrol* 6:119, 1976.

10. Cochrane CG, Koffler D: Immune complex disease in experimental animals and man. *Adv Immunol* 16:185, 1973.

11. Grishman E, Churg J: Ultrastructural of dermal lesions in systemic lupus erythematosus. *Lab Invest* 22:189, 1970.

12. Grishman E, Churg J: Connective tissue in systemic lupus erythematosus: demonstration of disseminated vascular and extravascular "wire-loop" deposits. *Arch Pathol* 91:156, 1971.

13. McIntosh RM, Koss MM: The choroid plexus: immunologic injury and disease. *Ann Intern Med* 81:111, 1974.

14. Ordóñez NG, Panem S, Aronson A, et al: Viral immune complexes in systemic lupus erythematosus. C-type viral complex deposition at extra-renal sites. *Virchows Arch (B) Cell Pathol* 25:355, 1977.

15. Talal N, Pillarisetty R, Papoian R, et al: Experimental lupus: a disorder of immunologic regulation. *Adv Nephrol* 6:37, 1976.

16. Imamura M, Mellors RC, Strand M, et al: Murine type C viral envelope glycoprotein gp69/71 and lupus-like glomerulonephritis of New Zealand mice: an immunoperoxidase study. *Am J Pathol* 86:375, 1977.

17. Panem S, Ordóñez NG, Kirsten WH, et al: C-Type virus expression in systemic lupus erythematosus. *N Engl J Med* 295:470, 1976.

18. Panem S, Ordóñez NG, Katz AI, et al: Viral immune complexes in systemic lupus erythematosus: Specificity of C-type viral complexes. *Lab Invest* 39:413, 1978.

19. Panem S, Ordóñez NG, Dalton H, et al: Viral immune complex in systemic lupus erythematosus, C-type viral complex deposition in skin. *J Dermatol Invest* 71:260, 1978.

20. Friou GJ: Double-stranded DNA: an antigen of unique significance, editorial. *J Lab Clin Med* 91:545, 1978.

21. Steinmann CR, Grishman E, Spiera H, et al: Binding of double-stranded DNA by serum from patients with systemic lupus erythematosus: correlation with renal histology. *Am J Med* 62:319, 1977.

22. Germuth FG, Rodriguez E: *Immunopathology of the Renal Glomerulus. Immune Complex Deposit and Anti-Basement Membrane Disease,* Boston, Little, Brown and Co, 1973, p 113.

23. Friend PS, Kim Y, Michael AF, et al: Pathogenesis of membranous nephropathy in systemic lupus erythematosus: possible role of nonprecipitating DNA antibody. *Br Med J* 1:25, 1977.

24. Winfield JB, Faiferman I, Koffler D: Avidity of anti-DNA antibodies in serum and IgG glomerular eluates from patients with systemic lupus erythematosus. Association of high avidity antinative DNA antibody with glomerulonephritis. *J Clin Invest* 59:90, 1977.

24a. Izui S, Lambert P, Miescher P: In vitro demonstration of particular affinity of glomerular basement membrane and collagen for DNA. *J Exp Med* 144:428, 1976.

25. Asano Y, Nakamoto Y: Avidity of antinative DNA antibody and glomerular immune complex localization in lupus nephritis. *Clin Nephrol* 10:134, 1978.

26. Sontheimer RD, Gilliam JN: DNA antibody class, subclass and complement fixation in systemic lupus erythematosus with and without nephritis. *Clin Immunol Immunopathol* 10:459, 1978.

27. Brentjens JR, Sepulveda M, Baliah T, et al: Interstitial immune complex nephritis in patients with systemic lupus erythematosus. *Kidney Int* 7:342, 1975.

28. Fessel WJ: Systemic lupus erythematosus in the community. Incidence, prevalence, outcome and first symptoms; the high prevalence in black women. *Arch Intern Med* 134:1027, 1974.

29. Schur PH: Lupus erythematosus. *Adv Nephrol* 6:63, 1976.

30. Estes D, Christian CL: The natural history of systemic lupus erythematosus by prospective analysis. *Medicine (Balt)* 50:58, 1971.

31. Baldwin DS, Bluck MC, Lowenstein J, et al: Lupus nephritis. Clinical course as related to morphologic forms and their transitions. *Am J Med* 62:12, 1977.

32. Ponticelli C, Imbasciati E, Brancaccio D, et al: Acute renal failure in systemic lupus erythematosus. *Br Med J* 3:716, 1974.

33. Gilliam JN, Cheatum DE, Hurd ER, et al: Immunoglobulin in clinically uninvolved skin in systemic lupus erythematosus: association with renal disease. *J Clin Invest* 53:1434, 1974.

34. Lief PD, Barland P, Bank N: Diagnosis of lupus nephritis by skin immunofluorescence, in the absence of extrarenal manifestations of systemic lupus erythematosus. *Am J Med* 63:441, 1977.

35. Whittle TS, Ainsworth SK: Procainamide-induced systemic lupus erythematosus: renal involvement with deposition of immune complexes. *Arch Pathol Lab Med* 100:469, 1976.

36. Sinniah R, Feng PH: Lupus nephritis: correlation between light, electron microscopic and immunofluorescent findings and renal function. *Clin Nephrol* 6:340, 1976.

37. Comerford FR, Cohen AS: The nephropathy of systemic lupus erythematosus. An assessment by clinical, light and electron microscopy criteria. *Medicine (Balt)* 46:425, 1967.

38. Hill GS, Hinglais N, Tron F, et al: Systemic lupus erythematosus. Morphologic correlations with immunologic and clinical data at the time of the biopsy. *Am J Med* 64:61, 1978.

39. Morel-Maroger L, Mery J-Ph, Droz D, et al: The course of lupus nephritis: contribution of serial renal biopsies. *Adv Nephrol* 6:79, 1976.

40. Cheatum DE, Hurd ER, Strunk SW, et al: Renal histology and clinical course of systemic lupus erythematosus. A prospective study. *Arthritis Rheum* 16:670, 1973.

41. Lee P, Urowitz MB, Bookman AA, et al: Systemic lupus erythematosus. A review of 110 cases with reference to nephritis, the nervous system, infections, aseptic necrosis and prognosis. *Quart J Med* 46:1, 1977.

42. Mahajan SK, Ordóñez NG, Spargo BH, et al: Changing histopathology patterns in lupus nephropathy. *Clin Nephrol* 10:1, 1978.

43. Ginzler EM, Nicastri AD, Chen CK, et al: Progression of mesangial and focal to diffuse lupus nephritis. *N Engl J Med* 291:693, 1974.

44. Cohen AH, Zamboni L: Ultrastructural appearance and morphogenesis of renal hematoxylin bodies. *Am J Pathol* 89:105, 1977.

45. Case records of the Massachusetts General Hospital. *N Engl J Med* 294:100, 1976.

46. Case records of the Massachusetts General Hospital. *N Engl J Med* 298:1143, 1978.

47. Dujovne I, Pollak VE, Pirani CL, et al: The distribution and character of glomerular deposits in systemic lupus erythematosus. *Kidney Int* 2:33, 1972.

48. Grishman E, Porush JG, Lee SL, et al: Renal biopsies in lupus nephritis. Correlation of electron microscopic findings with clinical course. *Nephron* 10:25, 1973.

49. Weis LS, Pachman LM, Potter EV, et al: Occult lupus nephropathy: a correlated light, electron and immunofluorescent microscopic study. *Histopathol* 1:401, 1977.

50. Churg J, Grishman E: Ultrastructure of immune deposits in renal glomeruli. *Ann Intern Med* 76:479, 1972.

51. Wood C: Crystalline phospholipid deposits in renal glomeruli in glomerulonephritis. *Am J Pathol* 66:592, 1972.

52. Okumura K: Induction of a disease resembling systemic lupus erythematosus in C57BI GJ mice by prolonged immunization with egg albumin. *Acta Pathol Jap* 23:695, 1973.

53. Hard RC, Moncure CW, Still WJS: Renal lesions with organized deposits and lipid as part of the Host versus Graft syndrome in parent/F1 mouse chimeras. *Lab Invest* 28:468, 1973.

54. Garancis JC, Komorowski RA, Bernhard GC, et al: Significance of cytoplasmic microtubules in lupus nephritis. *Am J Pathol* 64:1, 1971.

55. Imamura M, Block SR, Mellors RC: Electron microscopic study of distinctive structures in peripheral blood lymphocytes obtained from twins with lupus erythematosus. *Am J Pathol* 81:561, 1975.

56. Bariety D, Richer DD, Appay MD, et al: Frequency of intraendothelial "viruslike" particles: an electron microscopy study of 376 human renal biopsies. *J Clin Pathol* 26:21, 1973.

57. Libit SA, Burke B, Michael AF, et al: Extramembranous glomerulonephritis in childhood: relationship to systemic lupus erythematosus. *J Pediat* 88:394, 1976.

58. Schaff Z, Barry DW, Grimley PM: Cytochemistry of tubuloreticular structures in lymphocytes from patients with systemic lupus erythematosus and in cultured human lymphoid cells. Comparison to a paramyxovirus. *Lab Invest* 29:577, 1973.

59. Hruban Z, Wong T-W, Itabashi M, et al: Glomiform and fibrillar cytoplasmic inclusions. *Virchows Arch (B) Cell Pathol* 20:91, 1976.

60. Koffler D, Angello V, Carr RI, et al: Variable patterns of immunoglobulin and complement deposition in the kidney of patients with systemic lupus erythematosus. *Am J Pathol* 56:305, 1969.

61. Lehman DH, Wilson CB, Dixon FJ: Extraglomerular immunoglobulin deposits in human nephritis. *Am J Med* 58:765, 1975.

62. Donadio JV, Burgess JH, Holley KE: Membranous lupus nephropathy: a clinicopathologic study. *Medicine (Balt)* 5:527, 1977.

63. Appel AE, Sabley LB, Golden RA, et al: The effect of normalization of serum complement and anti-DNA antibody on the course of lupus nephritis: a two year prospective study. *Am J Med* 64:274, 1978.

64. Hayslett JP, Kashgarian M, Cook CD, et al: The effect of azathioprine on lupus glomerulonephritis. *Medicine (Balt)* 51:393, 1972.

64a. Friend PS, Michael AF: Hypothesis: immunologic rationale for the therapy of membranous lupus nephropathy. *Clin Immunol Immunopathol* 10:35, 1978.

65. Pollak VE: Treatment of lupus nephritis. *Adv Nephrol* 6:136, 1976.

66. Verrier JJ, Cumming RH, Bucknall RC, et al: Plasmapheresis in the management of acute systemic lupus glomerulonephritis? *Lancet* 1:709, 1976.

67. Cameron JS, Turner DR: Recurrent glomerulonephritis in allografted kidneys. *Clin Nephrol* 7:47, 1977.

14
Progressive Systemic Sclerosis

Progressive systemic sclerosis (PSS) is the systemic expression of cutaneous scleroderma. There is, in fact, a clinical spectrum ranging from static and localized skin thickening to rapidly progressive and systemic disease, the factors controlling the breadth of this spectrum being unknown. Various clinical classifications have been proposed (1,2) and have proved prognostically valuable, but the disease shows no respect for artificial divisions and may move from one category to another. The clinical features of PSS are produced by differing combinations of excessive collagen deposition and vascular disease, the former causing deformity and morbidity and the latter being the mechanism for most of the systemic complications. Among these systemic effects the most feared is a characteristic and peculiarly aggressive form of acute renal failure. Recently, it has become clear that the renal manifestations of PSS may be more indolent than previously thought, and that they may be mediated by mechanisms similar to those producing peripheral Raynaud's changes. The precise mechanisms of these vascular changes, however, and ways by which the changes might be either prevented or reversed have so far eluded investigation.

PATHOGENESIS

The etiology of PSS is unknown. Familial disease is rare and there are no constant HLA markers to suggest a genetic basis (3). The connective tissue changes may, occasionally, follow exposure to silica, cement, or polyvinyl chloride (3,4), but they usually appear spontaneously. Extensive studies of the altered dermis in PSS have revealed no abnormalities other than an excess of newly formed collagen and a capacity for increased collagen production by fibroblasts in tissue culture, with, possibly, a reduction in collagen degradation (5,6). Both local and systemic factors appear to control the dermal fibrosis since normal skin becomes altered when transplanted to abnormal areas (7), and resolution of the dermal changes has followed the control of rapidly progressing renal failure (8). Although a number of serologic abnormalities have been demonstrated in patients with PSS, none of these appears to be clearly correlated with the tissue changes. There is, however, fragmentary evidence for cell-mediated immune mechanisms

254

in the production of cutaneous fibrosis. Mononuclear inflammatory infiltrates are ubiquitous in early lesions, and lymphocytes from PSS patients transform after exposure to collagen with the release of lymphokines, which are chemotactic for fibroblasts and monocytes (3,9).

There is abundant evidence that morphologic and functional vascular alterations that occur in patients who have PSS. The capillary circulation in affected and unaffected skin is both depleted and morphologically abnormal, and abnormal capillaries have been demonstrated in noncutaneous tissues (3,5,10). The archetypal clinical evidence of arterial disease in PSS is Raynaud's phenomenon, which is produced by intense vasospasm, this spasm occurring in normal vessels but being more protracted in vessels with morphologic changes (11). There is good reason to believe that the renal complications of PSS are mediated by changes similar to those in the digital arteries. The renal circulation is impeded by vascular spasm which correlates closely with cold-induced Raynaud's changes, and the renal failure syndrome is considerably more frequent in the colder seasons (11). In all locations, arteries show a similar morphologic pattern of stenosing intimal fibrosis, which is similar, in some respects, to the picture seen with organization of luminal thrombi (12). This similarity has suggested that the tonic and morphologic vascular changes might be sequelae of intravascular coagulation, possibly initiated by diffusion into vessels of newly formed collagen and propagated by the development of intimal changes (5). The vasoconstriction can be temporarily relieved by a variety of drugs, but therapeutic control has not yet been achieved. Clinically, the vascular and connective tissue manifestations of PSS are closely related, but linking pathogenic pathways have not yet been demonstrated. Other mechanisms, such as increased blood viscosity (3), are likely to be implicated, but the precise factors mediating tissue damage are presently unknown.

CLINICAL MANIFESTATIONS

PSS is predominantly a disease of women in the fourth to sixth decades of life, but it may occur in both sexes and at all ages (12−14). Initial signs and symptoms usually are Raynaud's phenomenon, hand swelling, and skin changes (14). Typically, the affected skin is thickened, tethered, and tightly drawn over the underlying tissues, producing stiffening and reduced mobility. These characteristic clinical features may, occasionally, be associated with other "connective tissue diseases," such as rheumatoid arthritis and either cutaneous or systemic lupus erythematosus (15,16). Similarly, a range of serologic abnormalities, common to many of the connective tissue diseases, may occur in PSS. These include hypergammaglobulinemia, elevated sedimentation rate, rheumatoid factor and LE cells (15,17,18). Antinuclear antibodies can be identified in 10 to 60% of patients with PSS and may be of varying type, although the speckled pattern is most common (3,18). Recently, immunodiffusion studies have identified a nonhistone nuclear protein that appears to be highly characteristic of the disease (19). None of these serologic findings correlates well with either the extent or severity of

PSS, but eosinophilia has been associated with an especially aggressive clinical course (20).

The incidence of renal disease differs among individual series, probably because of varying patient selection. Thus, mortality statistics are likely to show a relatively high incidence of renal and other complications, while data from dermatologic clinics may provide an opposite view (8). Generally, all complications are more frequent in patients with diffuse, rather than localized, skin involvement (2), but occasional patients may have severe systemic complications with only minimal skin disease (21). Renal disease has been reported in 5–45% of patients with PSS (13), the wide range reflecting both differing patient groups and varying criteria. The best known, but least common, pattern of renal involvement is a catastrophic and rapidly progressive form of acute renal failure, which is often associated with malignant hypertension and systemic vasoconstriction. Renal damage of this pattern progresses inexorably over one or two months to either death or permanent azotemia (11,13,22). Because renal destruction is produced by vascular intimal fibrosis with ischemia and endothelial damage, hyperreninemia is frequent and a microangiopathic hemolytic anemia may occur (23,24). Hyperreninemia correlates closely with the presence of vascular lesions on biopsy specimens and is often, but not invariably, an ominous harbinger for the development of progressive renal failure (24a,24b). Although malignant hypertension is usual with this aggressive form of renal failure, blood pressure may be normal or only mildly raised (11). Less fulminant renal damage, manifested by varying combinations of proteinuria, hypertension, and azotemia, is rather more frequent than the acute form. Proteinuria may be isolated but is more commonly associated with hypertension and is usually less than 1 gm/day (13). The nephrotic syndrome has only occasionally been reported in association with PSS (11). Hypertension is usually mild, in contrast to the aggressive disease, and may remain static for several years without renal decompensation. Azotemia may develop slowly in association with hypertension or proteinuria or may, on the other hand, appear suddenly as the aggressive pattern of disease supervenes upon these other features. The presence of any of these clinical features of renal disease is an indication of a poor prognosis. The onset of renal disease is usually within six years of onset of PSS (13,22) but may be delayed for up to 23 years (25).

PATHOLOGIC CHARACTERISTICS

The characteristic renal changes in PSS correlate closely with the aggressive pattern of acute renal failure. All the changes are essentially identical regardless of the presence or absence of malignant hypertension (11,16). While the morphologic changes illustrate the degree of vascular stenosis in vivo, it must be remembered that many of the severe vascular changes identified by arteriography cannot be identified in nephrectomy or autopsy specimens, indicating that vasospasm plays a major role that cannot be identified morphologically (11). Further, severe vascular changes have occasionally been documented in patients with persistently normal renal function and blood pressure (24b).

Light Microscopy

The major changes in the acute phase of renal failure are in interlobular arteries (Figs. 14-1–14-4). These show striking intimal thickening by loose, myxoid, fibrous tissue with concentrically arranged nuclei (11,26). Red cells may be seen within the endothelial cushions, and fibrin may be present on or just beneath the endothelium (Fig. 14-3). The muscular wall of the artery is usually attenuated and stretched around the excessive intima, and periarterial fibrosis may be prominent (11) (Fig. 14-1). Distally, the arterioles frequently show massive fibrin insudation, which may continue uninterrupted into glomeruli. The arcuate and interlobar arteries are minimally involved in acute PSS renal damage but, in chronic disease, may show nonspecific, sclerotic intimal thickening that cannot be reliably distinguished from normal age changes (Fig. 14-5). The glomeruli are typically small, in acute damage, with irregular basement membrane wrinkling in an ischemic pattern (Figs. 14-2, 14-4). Segmental lesions may occasionally occur either by extension of the fibrinoid arteriolar changes or by segmental ischemic sclerosis. Juxtaglomerular hyperplasia may be prominent, especially in patients with malignant hypertension and hyperreninemia (11,23). Varying degrees of tubular atrophy with interstitial fibrosis may occur with longstanding disease, but

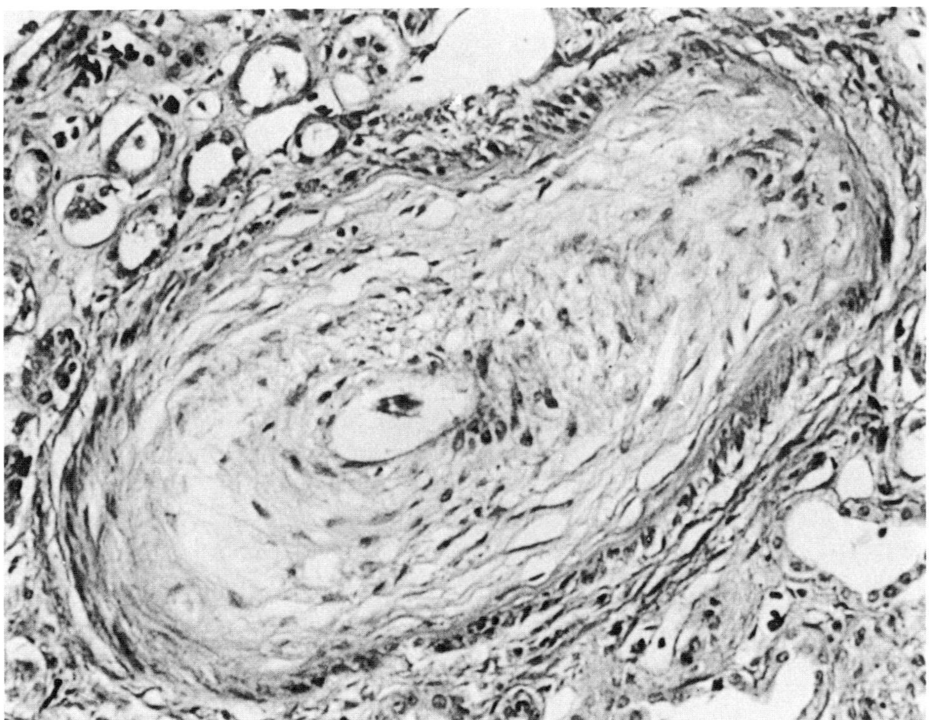

Figure 14-1. Interlobular artery showing intimal loose fibrous thickening and luminal narrowing in PSS. The muscular wall is thin and shows adventitial fibrosis (H&E stain, ×280).

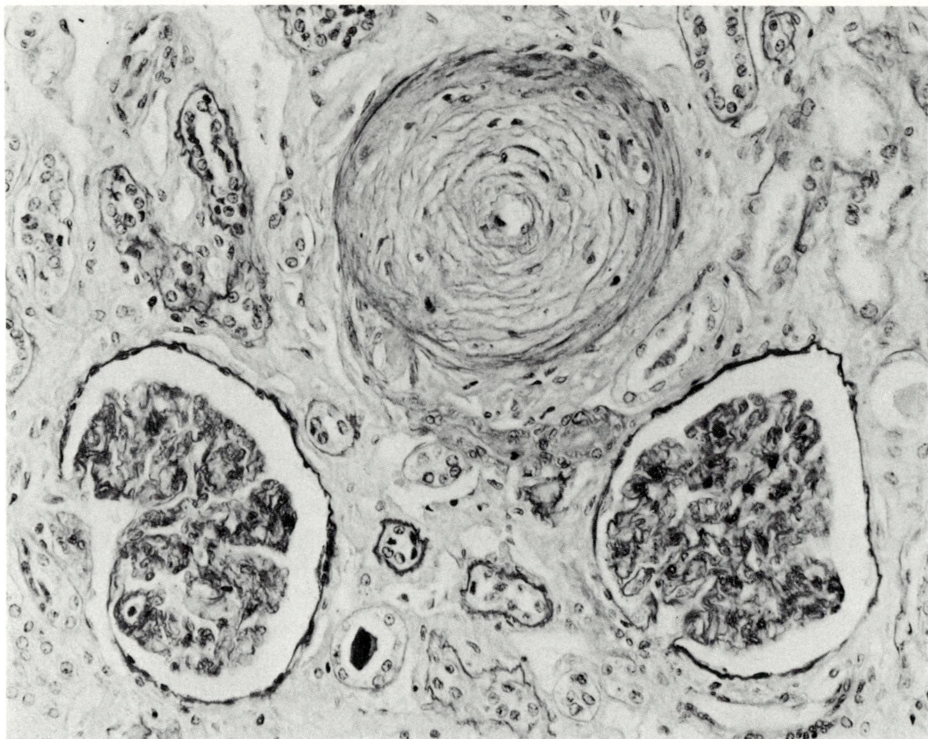

Figure 14-2. Concentric loose myxoid intimal proliferation of interlobular artery. The glomeruli are normocellular and the capillary walls are thickened and folded (PAS stain, ×250).

these are not usually prominent. Instead, rapidly advancing vascular occlusion may produce multiple small cortical infarcts.

Electron Microscopy

Affected blood vessels show intimal widening by amorphous, electron-lucent material, corresponding to myxoid ground substance and containing frequent myointimal cells (26). With time, the intima may become increasingly occupied by concentric layers of basement membrane material, which produce a light microscopic pattern of onion-skin thickening. The glomeruli show ischemic wrinkling, similar to that seen in malignant hypertension, with a broad and irregular zone of subendothelial lucency, which may contain fibrin strands and variably dense deposit (12,26) (Figs. 14-6, 14-7).

Immunofluorescence Microscopy

Within the thickened vascular intima, reactions are usually found for immunoglobulins (especially IgM), complement, (especially C1), and fibrin, all being most intense in acute disease (27−29) (Fig. 14-8). These are almost certainly nonspecific indications of altered endothelial permeability and provide no evi-

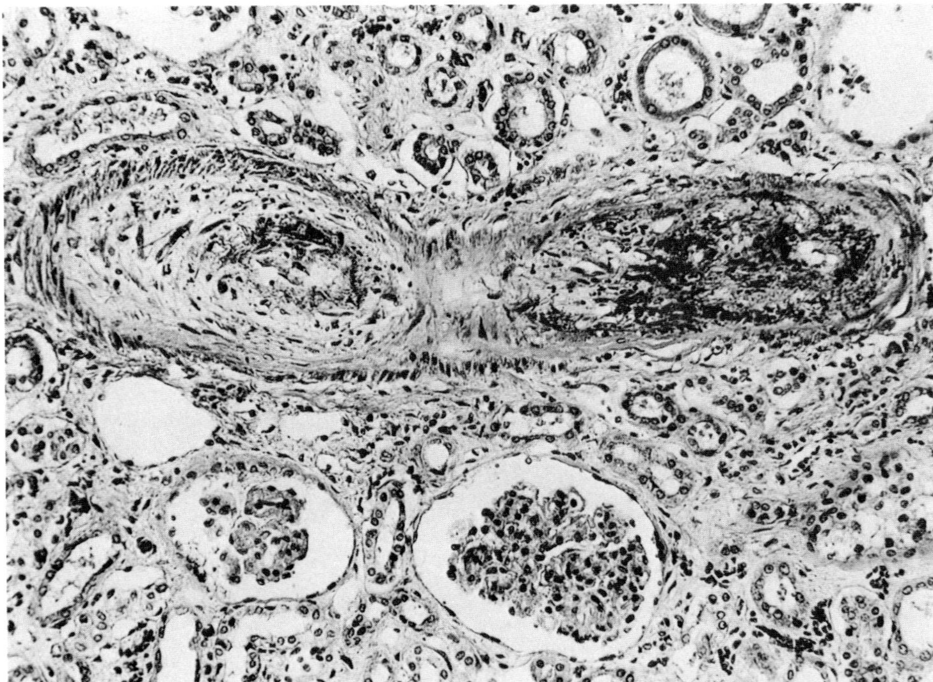

Figure 14-3. Interlobular artery with hemorrhage and fibrin deposition in the hyperplastic intimal tissue (H&E stain, ×190).

dence for an immune pathogenesis. Similar reactions may extend into glomeruli, but glomerular staining is usually less impressive than that seen in the vessels.

DIFFERENTIAL DIAGNOSIS

The morphologic pattern of basophilic intimal thickening affecting renal arteries is almost identical in PSS, malignant hypertension, the hemolytic uremic syndrome, and vascular transplant rejection (30). Reliable differentiation between these lesions is not possible by light, electron, or immunofluorescence microscopy, although some features, such as cortical infarction and periarterial fibrosis, are said to favor PSS (11,12). Similarly, there may be clinical difficulty in distinguishing between PSS and the hemolytic uremic syndrome or malignant hypertension when skin changes are minor (21). The morphologic features described are not, therefore, characteristic for any one diagnostic entity but rather are expressions of similar patterns of vascular damage that may be initiated by a variety of mechanisms.

Mixed Connective Tissue Disease

This recently described clinical entity may show many overlapping clinical features with PSS (31) but is distinguished by more frequent joint and muscle

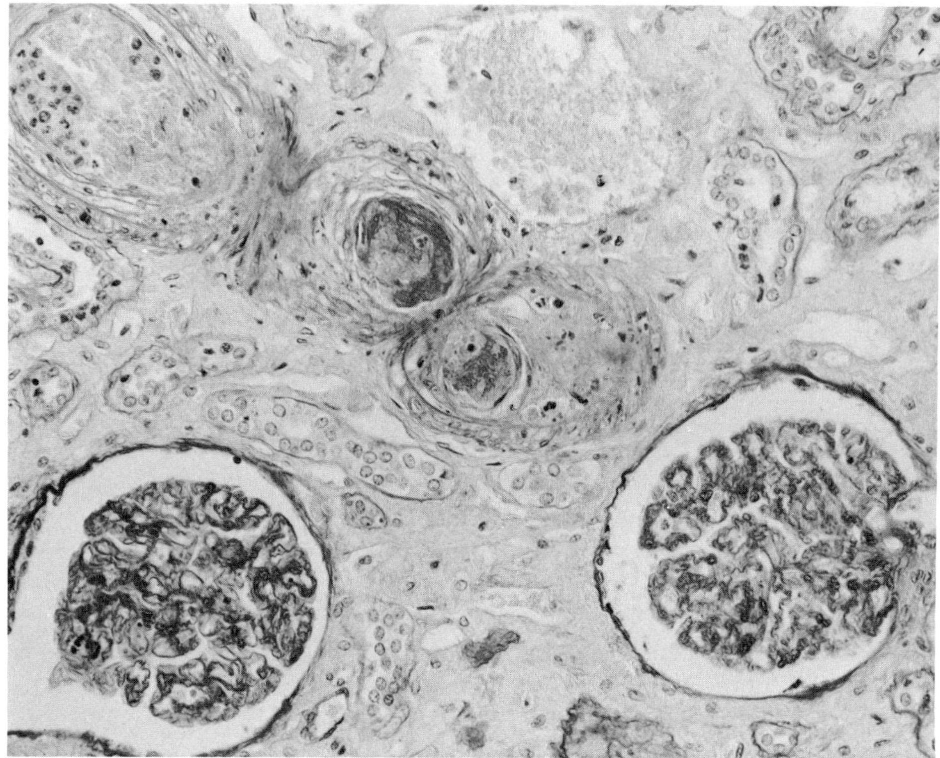

Figure 14-4. Interlobular artery with thrombosis. The glomeruli are normocellular and show marked ischemic changes (PAS stain, ×260).

involvement, a characteristic pattern of skin immunofluorescence (32), and circulating antibodies to nuclear ribonucleoprotein (33). Renal disease occurs in 20% of patients with this disease and may have varying patterns. Proliferative glomerulonephritis, either focal or diffuse, has been described, but the usual glomerular lesion has been membranous nephropathy (34,34a). Vascular changes like those of PSS have not been described.

PROGNOSIS AND THERAPY

The overall survival in patients with PSS varies with the extent of involvement but may be as high as 70% and 55% for 5 or 10 years, respectively, in prospective series (2). Retrospective series, based upon mortality data, give a more gloomy picture with such figures as 48% and 35% for 5- and 10-year survival (35). The major causes of death in all series are complications affecting the kidneys, lungs, and heart (2,15,35). Any sign of renal involvement implies a poor prognosis, 60% of patients with such signs dying in one series compared with 10% not having these signs (11). Most of the patients in this study died within one year of the appearance of renal signs, and the mean survival of those developing acute renal failure was one month.

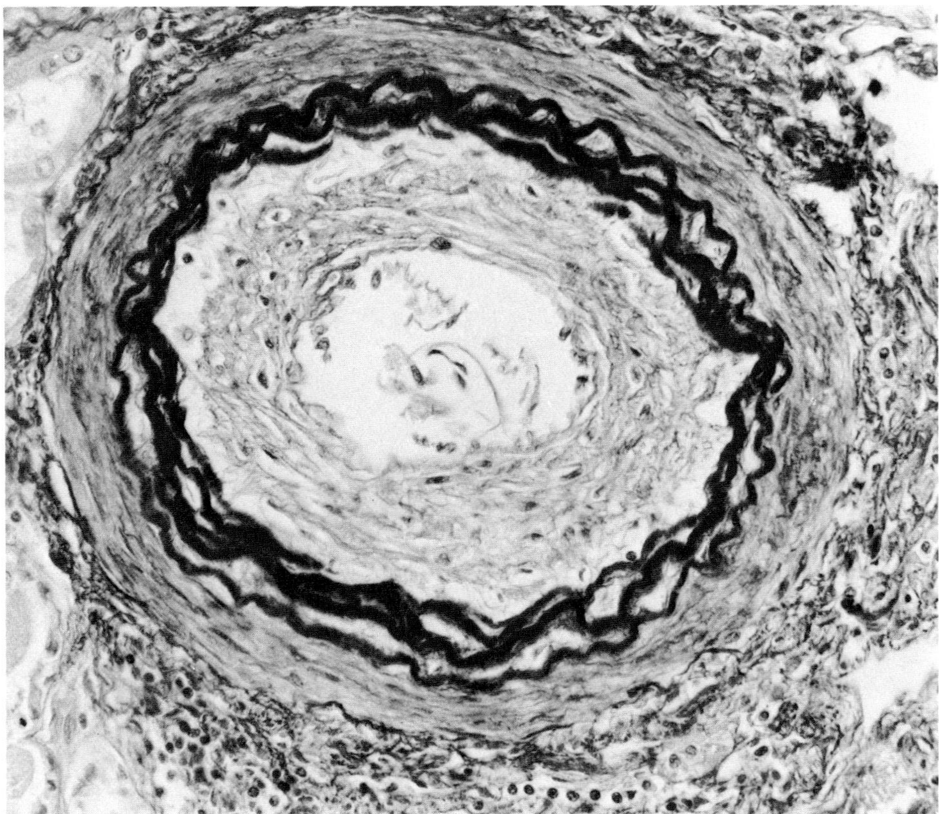

Figure 14-5. Arcuate artery exhibiting marked myointimal proliferation and reduplication of the internal elastic lamina in chronic PSS (elastic Van Gieson stain, ×300).

No therapy has clearly reproducibly affected cutaneous fibrosis in PSS (36) or reversed renal changes (14). Once established, accelerating renal damage may cause death from malignant hypertension with hyperreninemia and systemic vasoconstriction unless the deterioration can be stemmed by either urgent bilateral nephrectomy (22) or aggressive hypotensive therapy (8). Several patients have been successfully maintained on long-term dialysis after control of this acute state (22), but difficulty in vascular access (13) and advancing pulmonary or gastrointestinal complications (37) have been major problems. Transplantation has been successful in a few patients (22,38), but recurrence of vascular lesions has recently been reported (28,39,40) in the grafts. In view of the close resemblance between the morphologic features of vascular rejection and PSS, these reports are difficult to interpret, and more experience is required before the value of transplantation in PSS is established.

SUMMARY

Renal disease in PSS is relatively common and is a major cause of morbidity and mortality. Involvement of the kidney may be initially indolent but usually be-

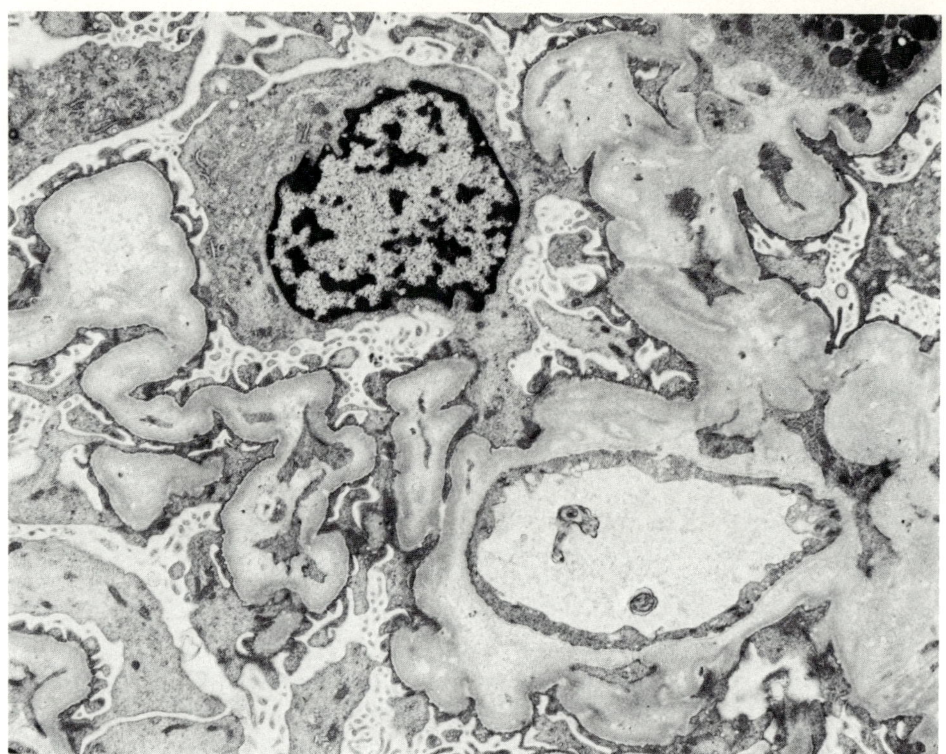

Figure 14-6. Marked ischemic collapse of the glomerular capillary loops in PSS (×4,700).

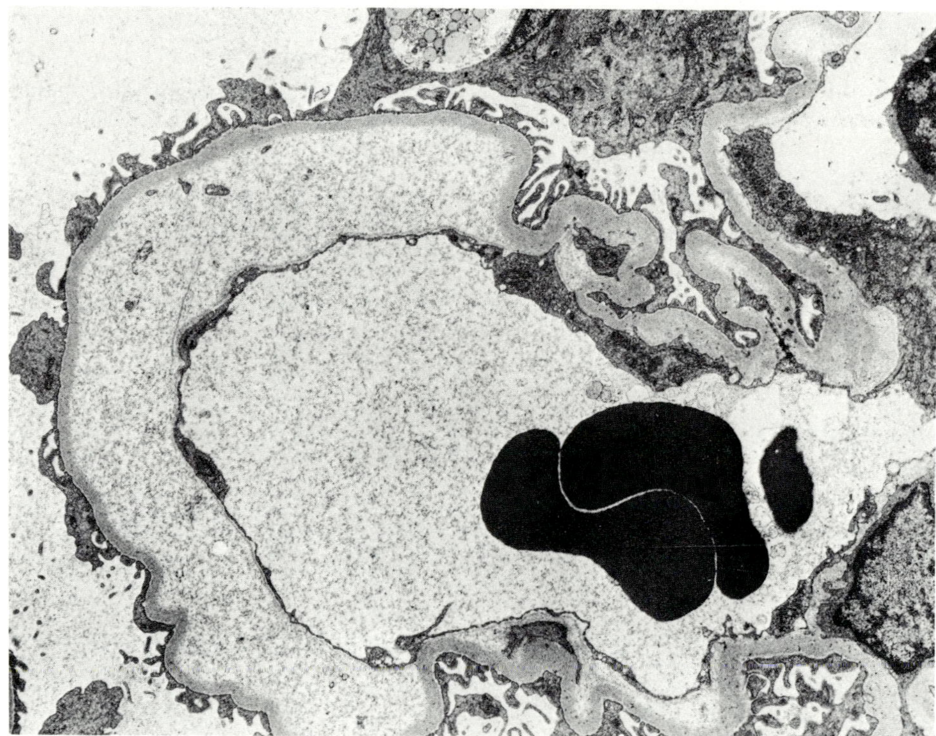

Figure 14-7. Glomerular capillary loop demonstrating translucent subendothelial zone with particulate electron dense material (×6,700).

262

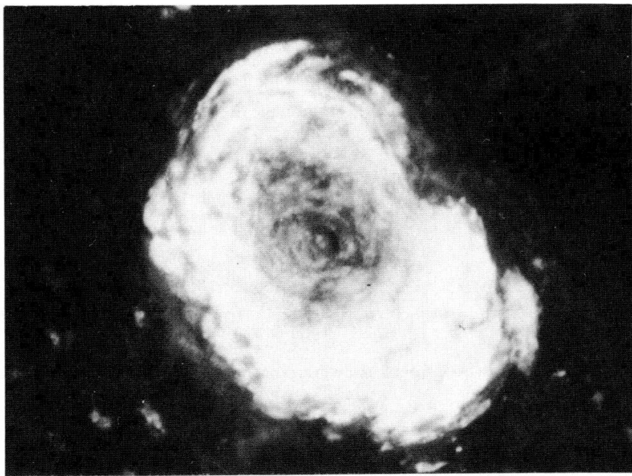

Figure 14-8. Interlobular artery with subintimal fibrinogen deposition (×250).

comes rapidly progressive and cannot be arrested once established. The major sites of damage are the interlobular arteries, which show spastic contraction by angiography and develop stenosing intimal thickening. This thickening has a characteristic, but not specific, myxoid appearance and often contains immuno-fluorescent fibrin, immunoglobulins, and complement. Whether these reactions imply active coagulation as a cause of the thickening or are merely expressions of insudation is unknown, but there is little evidence of a humoral immune pathogenesis. The changes, both morphologic and functional, are similar in digital and renal arteries, suggesting that vasospasm plays a major role in their production. The mechanisms producing this vasospasm are, however, unknown. Glomerular changes are secondary in PSS and are ischemic in character. Treatment of end-stage PSS renal disease by dialysis and transplantation has been successful in some patients, but a number of problems have been encountered. In particular, evidence suggestive of recurrent vascular lesions has been reported, although differentiation of these lesions from vascular rejection is extremely difficult. The similarities of the vascular disease in PSS, vascular rejection, malignant hypertension, and the hemolytic uremic syndrome suggest interlocking pathogenetic pathways for these diseases.

REFERENCES

1. Winkelmann RK: Classification and pathogenesis of scleroderma. *Mayo Clin Proc* 46:83, 1971.

2. Barnett AJ: Scleroderma (progressive systemic sclerosis): progress and course based on a personal series of 118 cases. *Med J Aust* 2:129, 1978.

3. Penny R: Scleroderma: pathogenetic factors and current management. *Aust NZ J Med* 8(suppl 1):143, 1978.

4. Jayson MIV: Vinyl chloride diseases. *Ann Rheum Dis* 36(suppl 2):39, 1977.

5. Jayson MIV: Collagen changes in the pathogenesis of systemic sclerosis. *Ann Rheum Dis* 36(suppl 2):26, 1977.

6. Perez-Tamayo R: Pathology of collagen degradation. *Am J Pathol* 92:509, 1978.

7. Fries JF, Hoopes JE, Shulman LE: Reciprocal skin grafts in systemic sclerosis (scleroderma). *Arthritis Rheum* 14:571, 1971.

8. Wasner C, Cooke R, Fries JF: Successful medical treatment of scleroderma medical crisis. *N Engl J Med* 299:873, 1978.

9. Stuart JN, Postlethwaite AE, Kang AH: Evidence for cell-mediated immunity to collagen in progressive systemic sclerosis. *J Lab Clin Med* 88:601, 1976.

10. Norton WL, Nardo JM: Vascular disease in progressive systemic sclerosis (scleroderma). *Ann Intern Med* 73:317, 1970.

11. Cannon PJ, Hasser M, Case DB, et al: The relationship of hypertension and renal failure in scleroderma (progressive systemic sclerosis) to structural and functional abnormalities of the renal cortical circulation. *Medicine (Balt)* 53:1, 1974.

12. Kincaid-Smith P: Participation of intravascular coagulation in the pathogenesis of glomerular and vascular lesions. *Kidney Int* 7:242, 1975.

13. Oliver JA, Cannon PJ: The kidney in scleroderma. *Nephron* 18:141, 1977.

14. Rodnan GP: The natural history of progressive systemic sclerosis (diffuse scleroderma). *Bull Rheum Dis* 13:301, 1963.

15. Dubois EL, Chandor S, Friou GJ, et al: Progressive systemic sclerosis (PSS) and localized scleroderma (morphea) with positive LE cell test and unusual systemic manifestations compatible with systemic lupus erythematosus (SLE): presentation of 14 cases including one set of identical twins, one with scleroderma and the other with SLE. Review of the literature. *Medicine (Balt)* 50:199, 1973.

16. D'Angelo WA, Fries JF, Masi AT, et al: Pathologic observations in systemic sclerosis (scleroderma). A study of fifty-eight autopsy cases and fifty-eight matched controls. *Am J Med* 46:428, 1969.

17. Clark JA, Winkelmann RK, Ward LE: Serologic alterations in scleroderma and sclerodermatomyositis. *Mayo Clin Proc* 46:104, 1971.

18. Jordon RE, Deheer D, Schroeter A, et al: Antinuclear antibodies: their significance in scleroderma. *Mayo Clin Proc* 46:111, 1971.

19. Tan EN: Immunospecificities of the antinuclear antibodies. *Arthritis Rheum* 20(suppl 187):1977.

20. Don IJ, Khettry U, Canoso JJ: Progressive systemic sclerosis with eosinophilia and a fulminating course. *Am J Med* 65:346, 1978.

21. Case records of the Massachusetts General Hospital. *N Engl J Med* 299:466, 1978.

22. Leroy EC, Fleischmann RM: The management of renal scleroderma: experience with dialysis, nephrectomy and transplantation. *Am J Med* 64:974, 1978.

23. Stone RA, Tisher CC, Hawkins HK, et al: Juxtaglomerular hyperplasia and hyperreninemia in progressive systemic sclerosis complicated by acute renal failure. *Am J Med* 56:119, 1974.

24. Salyer WR, Salyer DC, Heptinstall RH: Scleroderma and microangiopathic hemolytic anemia. *Ann Intern Med* 78:895, 1973.

24a. Gavras H, Gavras I, Cannon PJ, et al: Is elevated plasma renin activity of prognostic importance in progressive systemic sclerosis? *Arch Intern Med* 137:1554, 1977.

24b. Kovalchik MT, Guggenheim SJ, Silverman MH, et al: The kidney in progressive systemic sclerosis: a prospective study. *Ann Intern Med* 89:881, 1978.

25. Levine RJ, Boshell BR: Renal involvement in progressive systemic sclerosis (scleroderma). *Ann Intern Med* 52:517, 1960.

26. Sinclair RA, Antonovych TT, Mostofi FK: Renal proliferative arteriopathies and associated glomerular changes. A light and electron microscopic study. *Human Pathol* 7:565, 1976.

27. Lapenas D, Rodnan GP, Cavallo T: Immunopathology of renal vascular lesion of progressive systemic sclerosis (scleroderma). *Am J Pathol* 91:243, 1978.

28. McCoy RC, Tisher CC, Pepe PF, et al: The kidney in progressive systemic sclerosis. Immunohistochemical and antibody elution studies. *Lab Invest* 35:124, 1976.

29. Gerber MA: Immunohistochemical findings in the renal vascular lesions of progressive systemic sclerosis. *Human Pathol* 6:343, 1975.

30. Bohle A, Helmchen KE, Grund HV: Malignant nephrosclerosis in patients with hemolytic uremic syndrome. *Curr Topics Pathol* 65:81, 1977.

31. Sharp GC, Irvin WS, Tan EM, et al: Mixed connective tissue disease—an apparently distinct rheumatic disease syndrome associated with a specific antibody to an extractable nuclear antigen (ENA). *Am J Med* 52:148, 1972.

32. Levinton PM, Weary PE, Ginliano VJ: The immunofluorescence "band" test in mixed connective tissue disease. *Ann Intern Med* 83:53, 1975.

33. Brook AS: Mixed connective tissue disease. *Aust NZ J Med* 8(suppl 1):130, 1978.

34. Bennett RM, Spargo BH: Immune complex nephropathy in mixed connective tissue disease. *Am J Med* 63:534, 1977.

34a. Jones MB, Osterhole RK, Wilson BB, et al: Fatal pulmonary hypertension and resolving immune-complex glomerulonephritis in mixed connective tissue disease: a case report and review of the literature. *Am J Med* 65:855, 1978.

35. Medsger TA, Masi AT, Rodnan GP, et al: Survival with systemic sclerosis (scleroderma). A life-table analysis of clinical and dermographic factors in 309 patients. *Ann Intern Med* 75:369, 1971.

36. Allison AC: Effects of agents interacting with microtubules on collagen synthesis and breakdown. *Ann Rheum Dis* 36(suppl 2):65, 1977.

37. Shapiro CB, Lerner NE, Ackad AS, et al: Malignant hypertension and uremia in scleroderma: efficacy of nephrectomy and hemodialysis. *Clin Nephrol* 8:321, 1977.

38. Keane WF, Danielson B, Raij L: Successful renal transplantation in progressive systemic sclerosis. *Ann Intern Med* 85:199, 1976.

39. Woodhall PB, McCoy RC, Gunnells JC, et al: Apparent recurrence of progressive systemic sclerosis in a renal allograft. *JAMA* 236:1032, 1976.

40. Merino GE, Sutherland DER, Kjellstrand CM, et al: Renal transplantation for progressive systemic sclerosis with renal failure. A case report and review of previous experience. *Am J Surg* 133:745, 1977.

15
Hemolytic Uremic Syndrome

Hemolysis and uremia may coexist in a number of situations, but an apparently specific hemolytic uremic syndrome (HUS) in children was described by Gasser in 1955 (1). Several subgroups have since been distinguished within this pediatric syndrome, and a similar clinical and morphologic picture has been recognized in adults. The morphology of pediatric and adult HUS is essentially identical, but the prognoses and precipitating factors differ. There is accumulating evidence for a wide variety of pathogenetic mechanisms in HUS, and the term describes a number of similar clinicopathologic phenomena rather than designating a specific disease (2).

PATHOGENESIS

HUS is the clinical expression of coagulation within glomeruli and small renal blood vessels. In addition to causing impairment of renal function, the fibrin strands in these coagula damage passing red cells and platelets to produce a microangiopathic pattern of hemolysis (3). This pattern of Coombs-negative hemolysis with fragmented red cells and thrombocytopenia is characteristic of HUS but also occurs in a number of other conditions. Some of these conditions are known to be mediated by disseminated intravascular coagulation, and a similar process, analogous to the experimental Schwartzman reaction, was postulated by early students of HUS (4). The Schwartzman reaction may be either generalized or localized to one tissue, according to the experimental protocol, and is produced by two sequential injections of endotoxin (5). Each type is characterized by an initial phase of intense vasoconstriction with subsequent intravascular coagulation and tissue damage, the major manifestation of the generalized reaction being renal cortical necrosis. The abolition of vasoconstriction by blockade of adrenergic vascular receptors prevents the development of coagulation and cortical necrosis, but the reaction, once initiated, is self-perpetuating, since fibrin products are both thrombogenic and vasospastic (6). Only one injection of endotoxin is needed to produce the reaction in pregnant animals.

The relevance of this experimental system to HUS is uncertain. Thrombi occur in many organs in the generalized Schwartzman reaction, but hematologic and autopsy data in HUS provide conflicting evidence of systemic coagulation

266

(7,8). Systemic thrombosis appears to be rare in children (9) but relatively common in adults, especially those with HUS following pregnancy or the use of oral contraceptives (10,11). Changes in coagulation factors are well documented in these situations, apparently reflecting a sustained state of low-grade intravascular coagulation, and this systemic syndrome closely resembles the Schwartzman reaction in pregnant animals (12,13). Intravascular coagulation may be precipitated by platelet or red-cell disruption, extravascular tissue damage or endothelial injury (14). Damage to platelets, red cells, and extravascular tissues certainly occurs in HUS and may be a secondary mechanism for continuing activity, but it can rarely be implicated as the primary event. Most interest in the pathogenesis of HUS has centered around the role of endothelium.

Vascular endothelium possesses a variety of mechanisms for the minimization and control of thrombosis, the most important probably being the production of a prostaglandin product, prostacyclin (PGI_2), which is a potent inhibitor of platelet aggregation (15). Endotoxin is directly toxic to endothelium (16) and has been directly implicated in the pathogenesis of some, but not most, cases of HUS associated with bacterial infection (17), but not in the majority of sporatic cases (7). Similarly, various viruses may localize in endothelial cells and HUS commonly follows episodes of proven or suspected viral infection (7). The possibility of immune-mediated endothelial damage has also been suggested by the demonstration of hypocomplementemia and immunofluorescent deposits of immunoglobulin and complement in many patients with HUS (18). Similar immunofluorescence reactions, however, occur in the Schwartzman reaction, probably via nonspecific insudation, and the enzymes involved in coagulation are capable of cleaving complement components (19,20). Recent evidence suggests that patients with HUS may lack a plasma factor, whose replacement aborts the syndrome, and that this factor may activate prostacyclin (21). Any of these mechanisms for endothelial damage might inhibit prostacyclin production and predispose to the development of HUS. The recent report of a patient with a congenital defect in the production of prostacyclin or a similar factor suggests that environmental or genetic influences might contribute to the occurrence of endemic and familial HUS (22).

The etiology and pathogenesis of HUS, therefore, remain unknown. Although coagulation is clearly a significant component of the established lesion, it is presently uncertain whether the coagulation system is activated primarily or as a secondary event. Recent evidence suggests that endothelial damage is likely to be the common initiating mechanism and that impairment of normal homeostatic activities causes thrombosis and intense vasoconstriction. A variety of injurious stimuli may lead to endothelial damage, and the subsequent events may depend on the reparative capacity of the host. The development of severe changes could be potentiated by preexisting hypercoagulable states or genetic defects in prostacyclin production.

CLASSIFICATION AND CLINICAL MANIFESTATIONS

HUS is defined by the coexistence of an acute nephropathy with microangiopathic hemolysis and thrombocytopenia (7,8). Detailed study of many patients with this syndrome has revealed a number of more or less well-defined subgroups (Table 15-1). The most important subdivision is by the age at onset since the prognosis in children, in whom the syndrome is much more common, is considerably better than in adults.

HUS in Children

HUS may occur throughout childhood and has been reported in a 25-day-old infant, but it is most common in the first four years of life (7,8,23). The sexes are affected equally. No country is immune from HUS, but the incidence in Argentina, South Africa, Holland, and the west coast of the USA is considerably higher than elsewhere, and the syndrome appears to be endemic in these regions (7). Sporadic small and large epidemics of HUS have also been reported, some associated with *Salmonella* or *Shigella* dysentery (7,17). Presentation is biphasic with an initial prodrome period followed by the abrupt onset of nephropathy. The prodrome generally persists for 5 to 7 days, but varies from 1 to 15 days, and usually consists of vomiting and diarrhea, although a minority of patients have coryzal symptoms (7,8,23). A variety of specific organisms have been isolated from patients with HUS, but cultures are usually negative (7). The acute nephropathy is introduced by pallor, oliguria, hypertension, proteinuria, and microscopic hematuria. Macroscopic hematuria sometimes occurs and some patients may develop the nephrotic syndrome. The characteristic microangiopathic blood picture appears at this stage, and purpura may accompany the thrombocytopenia. Hypocomplementemia is frequent, with depression of both early and late components, and there is a single report of circulating C3 nephritic factor (18,24). Hepatosplenomegaly is found in about half the patients, and a similar proportion have severe central nervous system manifestations such as coma, convulsions, and hemiplegia. Minor cerebral signs such as irritability,

Table 15.1. Classification of Hemolytic Uremic Syndrome

Primary
  Childhood
    Sporadic
    Endemic
    Epidemic
  Adult
    Sporadic
    Postpartum
    Estrogen and oral contraceptive therapy
  Familial
    Sporadic
    Endemic
  Recurrent

Secondary
  Common component of renal lesions
  Rare associations

somnolence, and disorientation are present in the majority. The nephropathy has been divided into three categories, according to the presence and duration of oliguria, with the majority of patients being equally divided between the first two groups (7,8). Patients with mild nephropathy have no or transient oliguria and few systemic manifestations, while those with severe nephropathy are anuric for varying periods and a rare, third group show a progressive and inexorable decline in renal function.

Adult HUS

Adult HUS is largely restricted to women in the postpartum period or exposed to exogenous estrogen, either alone or as part of an oral contraceptive preparation (10,11,25). Occasional cases occur in either sex with neither of these precipitating factors and show a similar prodrome to the childhood patients (10). The onset of HUS may be delayed for up to two years post partum, but it usually occurs in the first weeks or months and may either be preceded by a typical prodrome or develop abruptly with vaginal bleeding, purpura, oliguria, and hypertension (25). The syndrome has occasionally developed during pregnancy (26) and shows no constant relationship with preceding preeclampsia. The onset of HUS in women taking oral contraceptives may be apparently spontaneous but usually follows an increase in estrogen dosage or the change from a low-dose to a high-dose estrogen preparation (27). We have seen one male patient with fatal HUS occurring after the prescription of estrogen for carcinoma of the prostate.

Familial HUS

HUS is familial in 3% of patients and may show two patterns (7,23). A genetic predisposition is suggested by the occurrence of HUS in several members of one family, in one or several generations, and a dominant pattern of inheritance has been suggested (28,29). More commonly, siblings in endemic areas are affected simultaneously, suggesting environmental influences (30).

Recurrent HUS

One or multiple recurrences of HUS have been reported in a few patients, usually in nonendemic areas and often in a setting of familial disease (31). The recurrent syndrome in these patients is frequently atypical and may be fatal.

Secondary HUS

Clinical and morphologic features almost identical to HUS occur in some patients with malignant hypertension, progressive systemic sclerosis, and transplant rejection, presumably secondary to vascular spasm and endothelial damage. Acute lupus nephritis may occasionally resemble HUS, and there are isolated reports of an association with Addison's disease (33) and of the development of HUS in a patient with membranous nephropathy (34).

PATHOLOGIC CHARACTERISTICS

Light Microscopy

The principal site of damage resulting from HUS is the glomerulus, but blood vessels and tubules may also be extensively damaged (35–38). The changes in adults and children are essentially identical aside from a tendency toward more frequent and severe vascular lesions in adults (37). Initially, small arteries and arterioles show focal damage characterized by insudation of fibrin and red cells, with or without thrombosis (Figs. 15-1, 15-2). Fibrin may suffuse throughout the wall or be restricted to the intima and is occasionally accompanied by frequent polymorphs (Figs. 15-3, 15-4). There may be sufficient damage to cause aneurysmal dilatation, most often in afferent arterioles (Figs. 15-5, 15-6). Extensive vascular occlusion may cause focal or extensive cortical necrosis, but nonspecific tubular degenerative changes are more commonly seen and are associated with interstitial edema and mononuclear inflammation. The pattern of vascular necrosis progresses into a stage of intense and basophilic intimal thickening which greatly restricts the vascular lumina. This mucoid intimal change may be seen very early in the disease but usually develops over several weeks (Figs. 15-4, 15-7, 15-8). Organization of these vascular changes, often in association with severe hypertension, produces an initially hyperplastic and later

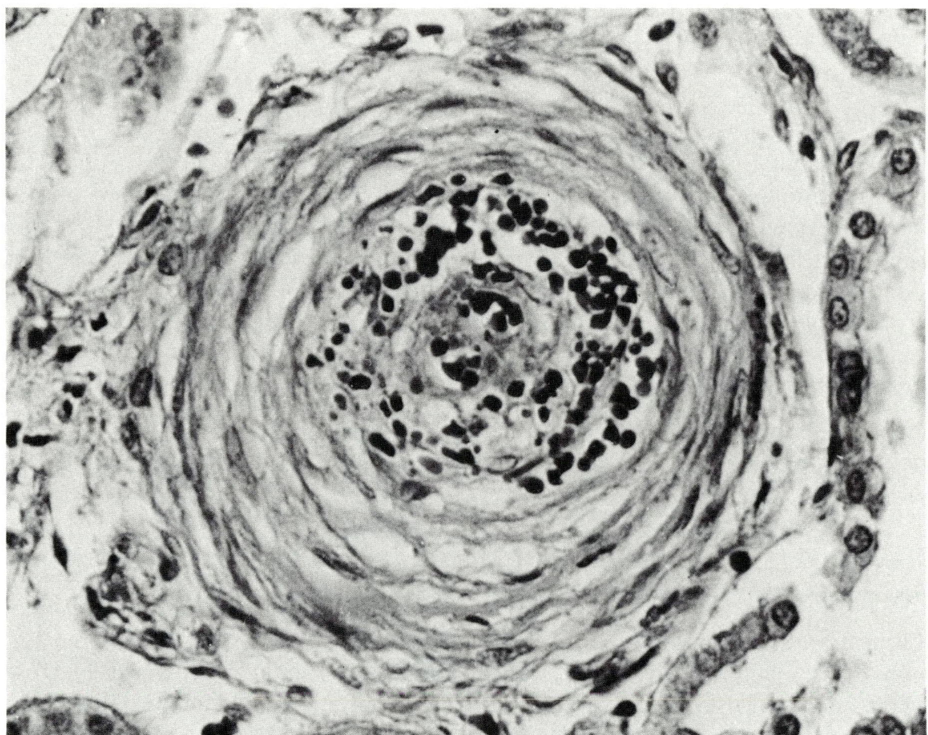

Figure 15-1. Interlobular artery showing stenosing intimal proliferation with hemorrhage into the intima (H&E stain, ×625).

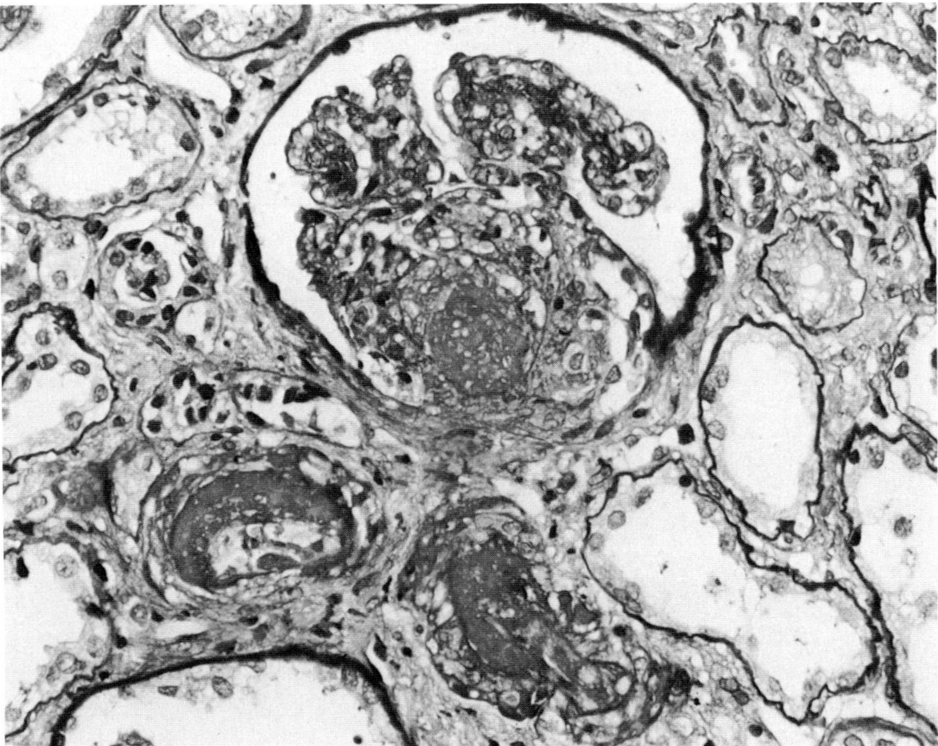

Figure 15-2. Renal biopsy specimen from a patient with hemolytic uremic syndrome showing widespread thickening and splitting of the capillary walls. The afferent arteriole is occluded by a thrombus, which extends into the glomerular tuft (PAS stain, ×375).

collagenous pattern of intimal thickening, which is indistinguishable from that seen in other chronic renal diseases.

A variety of glomerular changes may coexist in the same biopsy specimen or even in the same glomerulus. Some glomeruli appear wrinkled and collapsed while others show segmental or global swelling. Proliferation is usually not conspicuous, but there is irregular mesangial and endothelial swelling, sometimes resembling focal glomerulonephritis, and scattered crescents may be seen (Fig. 15-9). In the early stages, there is no increase in matrix, and the affected areas appear foamy or merge into apparently infarcted zones characterized by aneurysmal capillary dilatation (Fig. 15-10). Thrombi vary considerably in frequency and distribution, being very extensive in some biopsy specimens and almost completely absent from others (Fig. 15-11). The most characteristic abnormality is an irregular thickening of capillary walls produced by the apparent splitting of the basement membrane with an empty or weakly PAS-positive intervening space (Fig. 15-2). This pattern may be segmental or global and often appears to develop without mesangial interposition, although continuity with the mesangium can usually be seen in some areas. Cellular swelling abates as the syndrome subsides, but the capillary wall changes remain and are associated with a progressive increase in matrix. Thus, biopsy specimens taken more than one

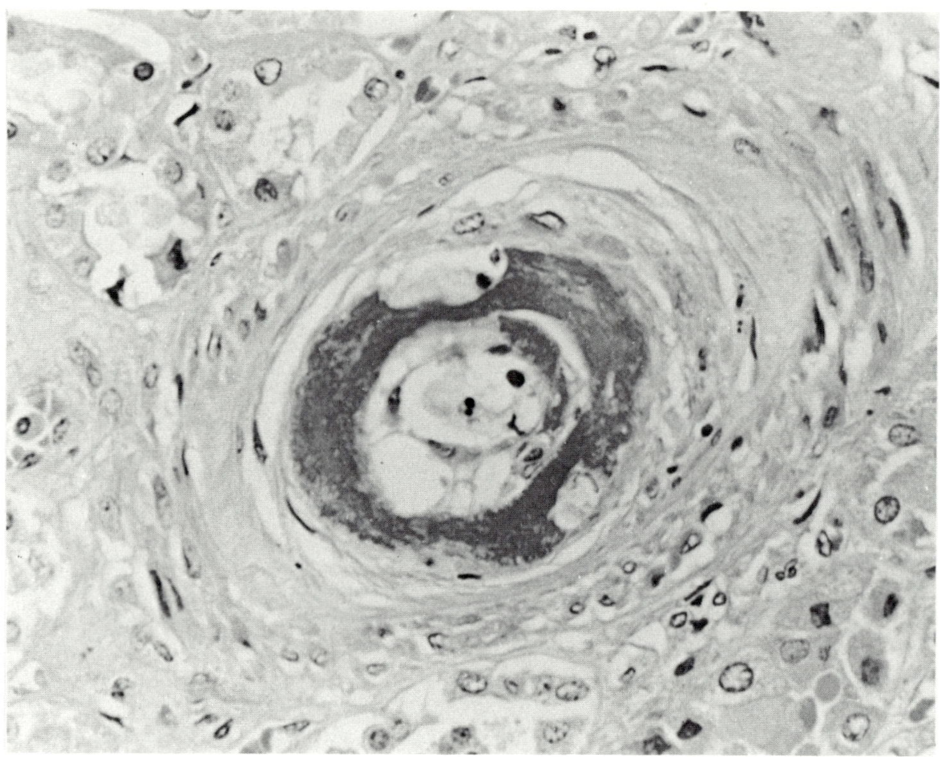

Figure 15-3. Interlobular artery from a patient with hemolytic uremic syndrome showing fibrinlike material in the intima and edema with narrowing of the lumen (H&E stain, ×500).

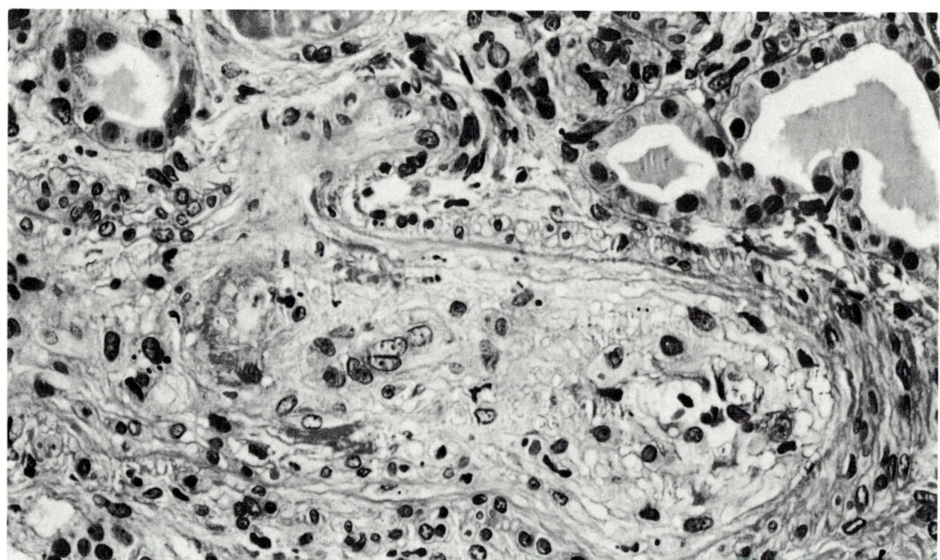

Figure 15-4. Interlobular artery with proliferated intima containing red blood cells and fibrin among vacuolated intimal cells. There are mononuclear inflammatory cells in the interstitium and around the vascular wall. The tubules are dilated and contain proteinaceous casts (H&E stain, ×235).

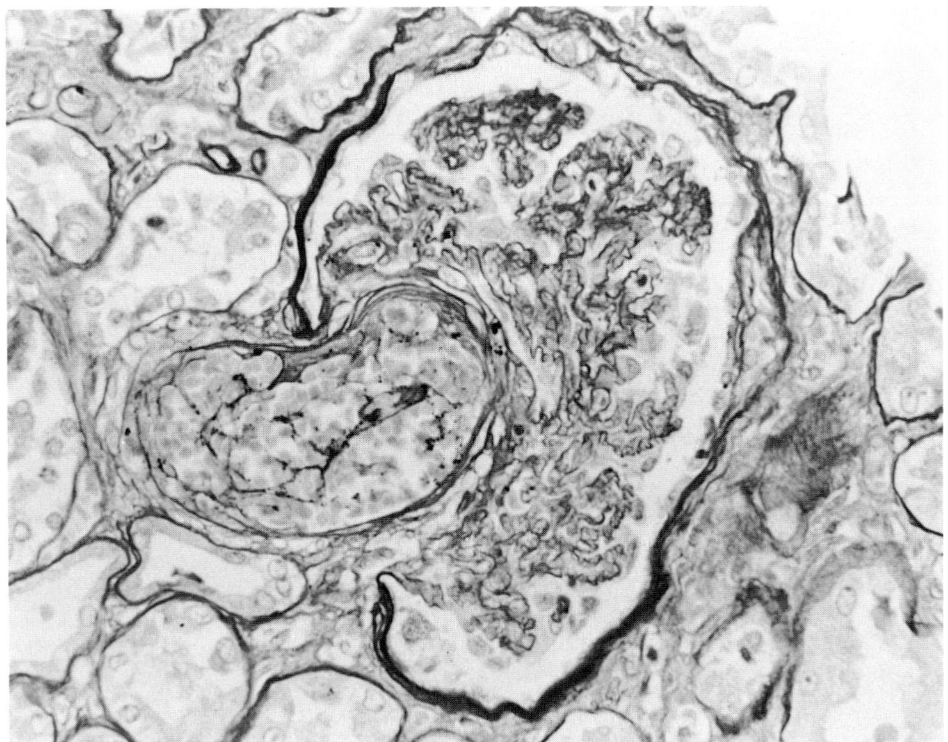

Figure 15-5. Aneurysmal dilatation of the afferent arteriole in hemolytic uremic syndrome (PAS stain, ×450).

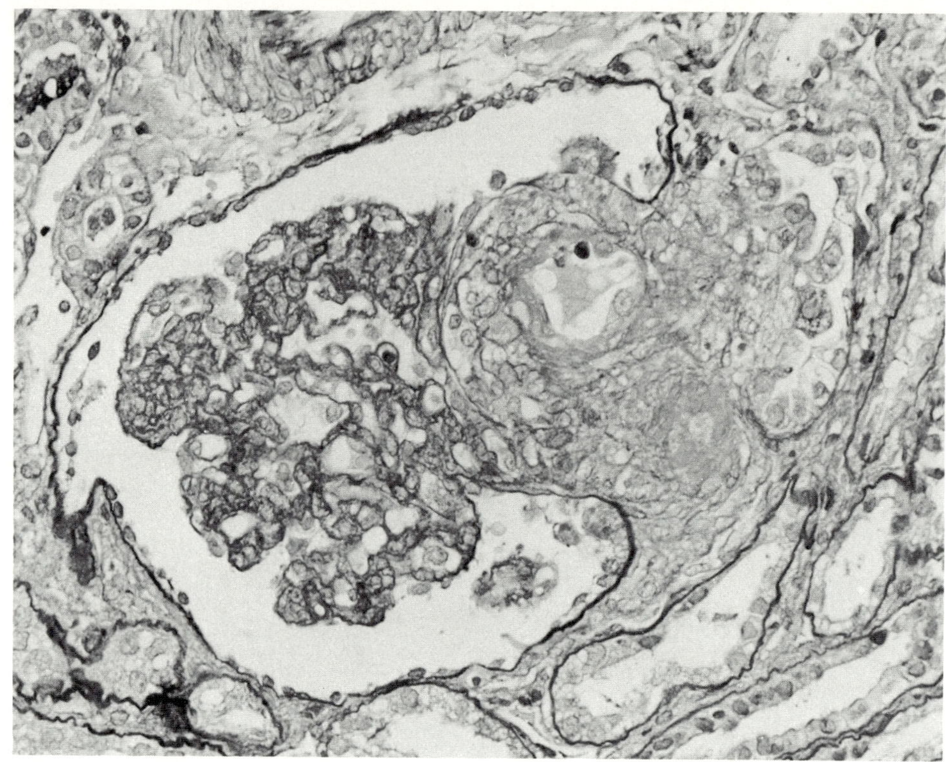

Figure 15-6. Glomerulus with aneurysmal dilatation of the afferent arteriole and marked endothelial proliferation, forming a "glomeruloid body" (PAS stain, ×400).

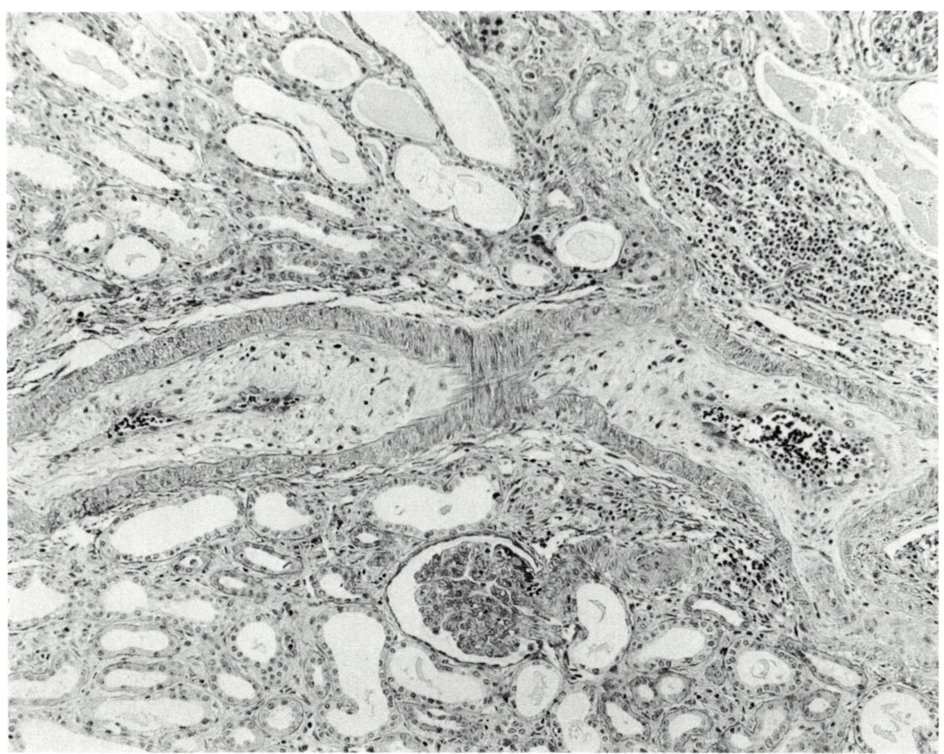

Figure 15-7. Hemolytic uremic syndrome in a woman three weeks postpartum. The interlobular artery is almost obliterated by loose, mucinous subintimal proliferation. In addition, there is tubular atrophy and lymphocytic interstitial infilatration (H&E stain, ×130).

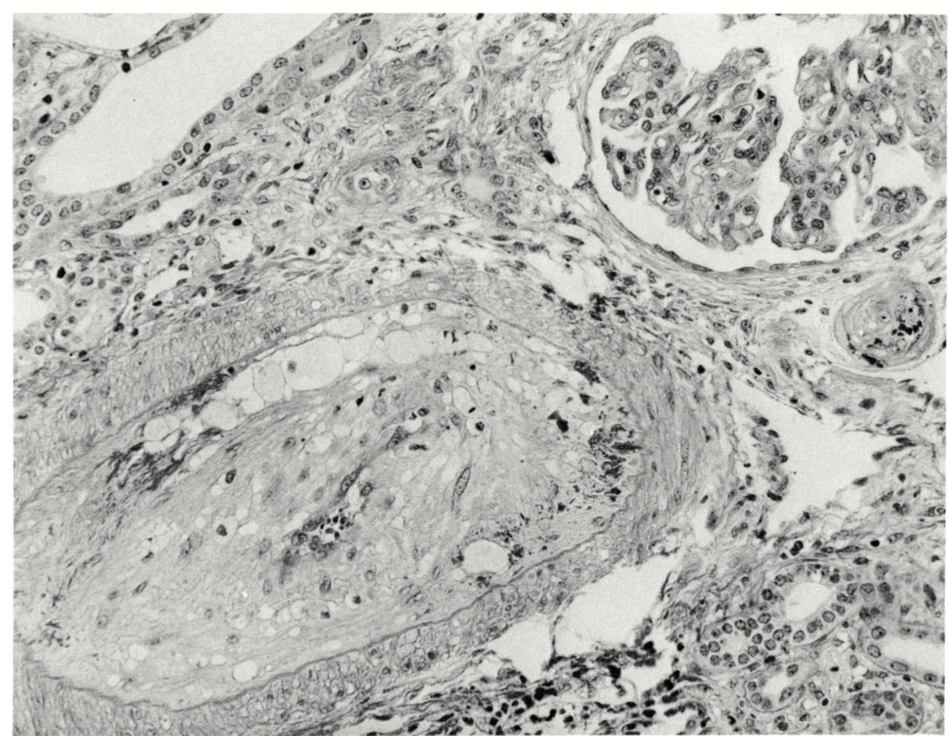

Figure 15-8. Interlobular artery and afferent arteriole with prominent mucinous subintimal proliferation. Some cells have foamy cytoplasm (H&E stain, ×310).

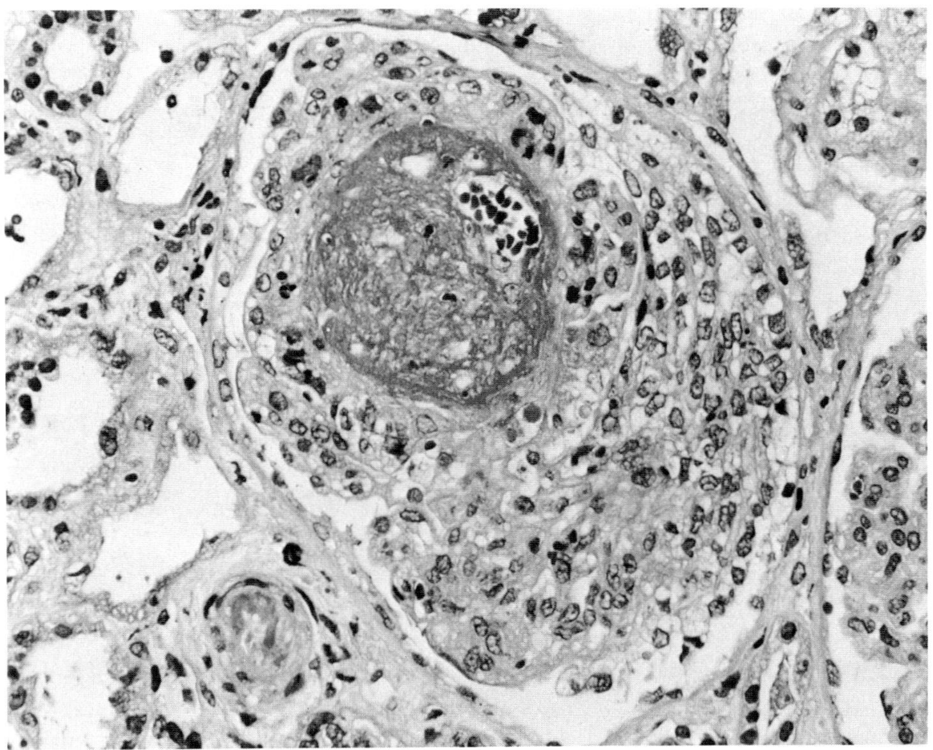

Figure 15-9. Glomerulus with thrombosis and crescentic proliferation of epithelial cells. The afferent arteriole is occluded by thrombus (H&E stain, ×375).

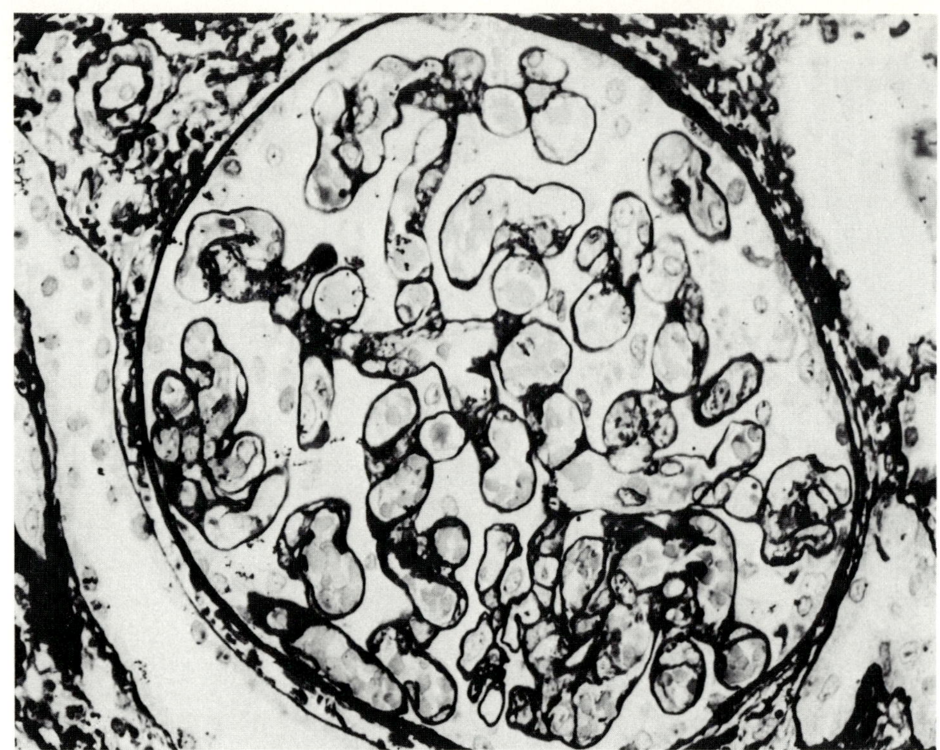

Figure 15-10. Renal biopsy specimen from a patient with hemolytic uremic syndrome showing dilatation with segmental splitting of glomerular capillaries (PASM stain, ×550).

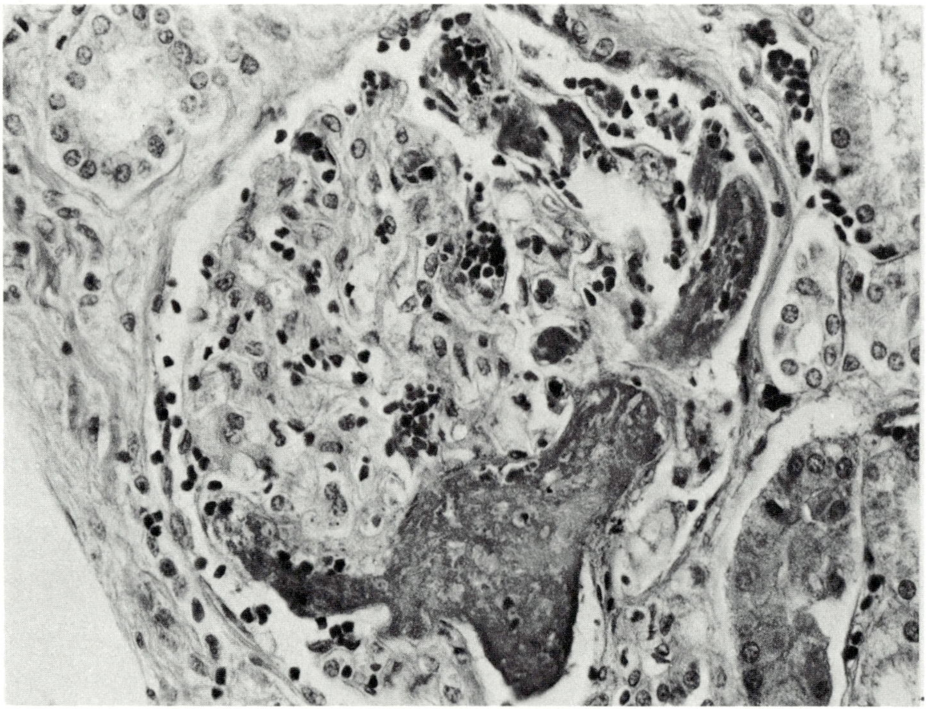

Figure 15-11. Thrombus of the glomerular hilum with peripheral extension to the capillary loops (H&E stain, ×450).

month after onset show widespread "splitting" of capillary walls with irregularly increased mesangial matrix and segmental adhesions or organizing crescents. These evolving changes may be complicated by, and at times even submerged in, extensive membrane wrinkling caused by vascular stenosis. The final glomerular pattern in progressive HUS may not be distinguishable from other forms of progressive disease.

Electron Microscopy

There is cellular hypertrophy and swelling with the accumulation of lucent sub-endothelial and mesangial deposits (35−39) (Fig. 15-12). The subendothelial change varies from slight separation of endothelial cells from the basement membrane to massive accumulation, which causes stenosis of the capillary lumen (Figs. 15-13,15-14). The material causing this separation is generally electron-lucent, but contains areas of fluffy, dense material, irregularly dispersed fibrils, and in severely affected areas, tactoids of fibrin, red cells, and other blood elements (Figs. 15-12, 15-13). The red cells often appear irregular in shape and density. Mesangial areas are expanded by similar lucent material, correlating with the foamy light microscopic appearance, and may be completely disrupted (39). An irregular layer of membranelike material, possibly endothelial in origin, separates the endothelial cells from the lucent deposit and forms the double contour seen by light microscopy. Later the subendothelial deposit is gradually

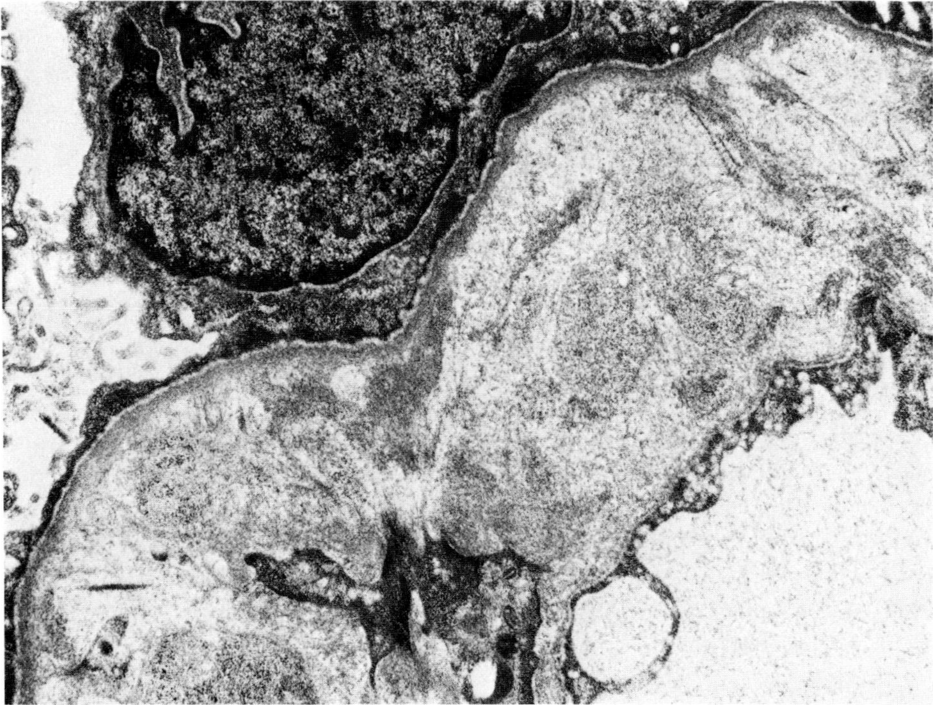

Figure 15-12. Peripheral loop showing lucent subendothelial zone containing finely particulate electron-dense granules (×13,000).

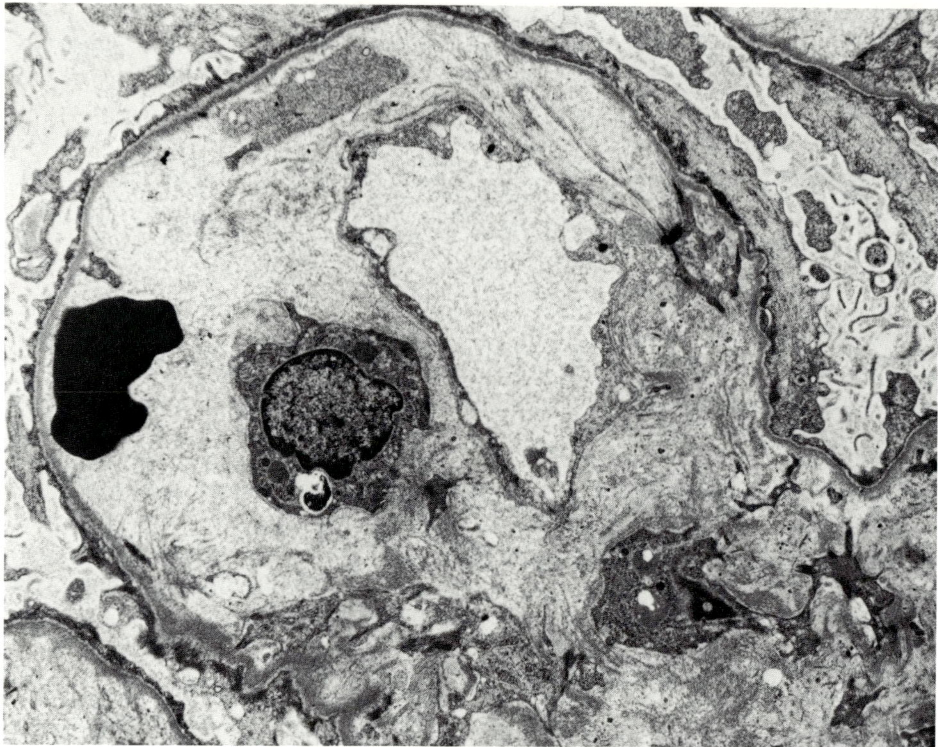

Figure 15-13. The capillary lumen is stenosed by marked widening of the subendothelial space, which contains irregularly dense amorphous material and a red blood cell. The foot processes are obliterated and show moderate villous formation (×8,200).

replaced by new membrane, causing massive and irregular thickening of the basement membrane. The capillary lumina are further compromised by striking endothelial swelling, or ballooning, and mesangial hypertrophy, with frequent cytoplasmic organelles and phagolysosomes (Fig. 15-15). Thrombosed capillaries appear as masses of fibrin with admixed red cells, platelets, and other formed elements (Fig. 15-16). The endothelial lining is interrupted in thrombosed capillaries, and in those showing aneurysmal dilatation, causing denudation with attenuation or even rupture of the basement membrane. Epithelial cells are generally hypertrophic with extensive obliteration of foot processes, especially in regions of collapse, and focal proliferation in relation to membrane rupture (Figs. 15-13, 15-14). The changes in small blood vessels mirror those in the glomeruli. There is endothelial swelling, with focal ulceration and expansion of the intima by lucent material, or disruption of the wall by insuded plasma and red cells.

Immunofluorescence Microscopy

Reactions may be limited to either glomeruli or blood vessels but usually occur in both and are most common for IgM, C3, and fibrin (18,35,40). In the blood vessels, deposits may extend throughout the wall or be limited by the elastic

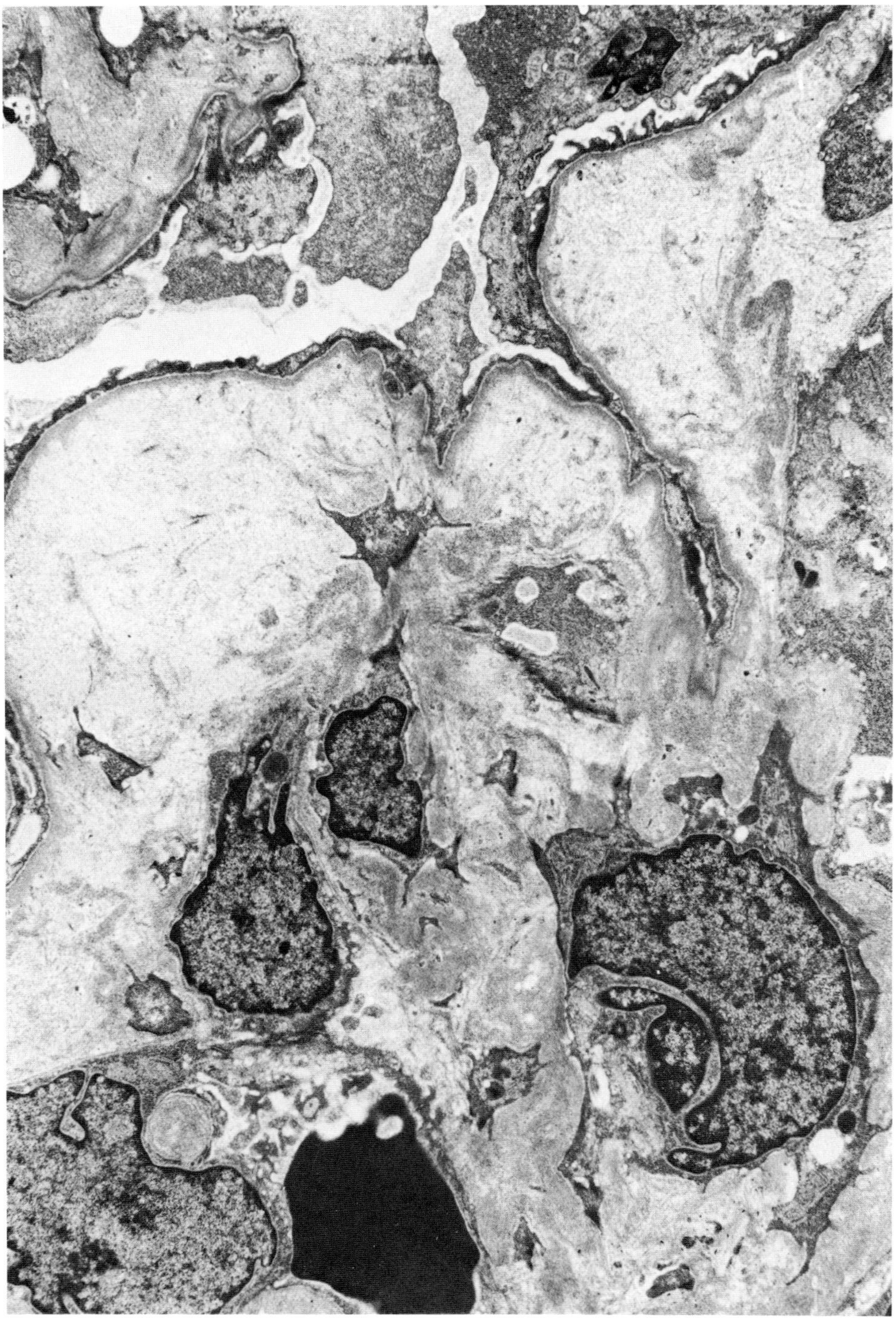

Figure 15-14. Portion of a glomerulus from a patient with hemolytic uremic syndrome showing a prominent subendothelial electron-lucent zone with obliteration of the capillary lumen. The epithelial foot processes are extensively obliterated (×8,000).

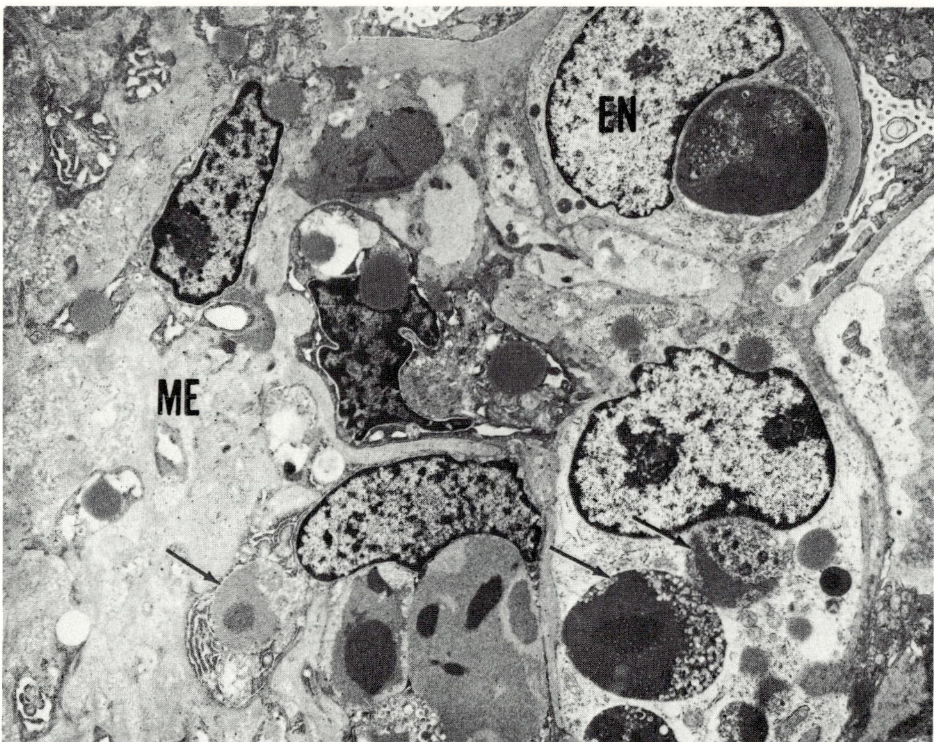

Figure 15-15. Glomerulus from a patient with hemolytic uremic syndrome showing endothelial swelling, mesangial hypertrophy, and numerous phagolysosomes (arrows) (EN, endothelial cell; ME, mesangium; ×7,000).

lamina. Glomerular reactions are typically irregular and are seen both in mesangia and along capillary walls, often with segmental smudging or accentuation in areas of infarction or thrombosis (Figs. 15-17, 15-18). Early acting complement components are often present, and immunoglobulins other than IgM are occasionally detected. Similar reactions have been described in the skin (40).

DIFFERENTIAL DIAGNOSIS

The fully developed lesions of HUS are highly characteristic but not specific. Distinguishing reliably between HUS and progressive systemic sclerosis or malignant hypertension depends on careful consideration of the clinical data and may be extremely difficult, although the presence of widespread subendothelial lucent deposits favors HUS. In children, the diagnosis is usually straightforward, but the differentiation of HUS in adults from malignant hypertension may be impossible, and confusion between these conditions almost certainly postponed recognition of the postpartum syndrome. Extensive arteriolar damage with admixed polymorphs may occasionally suggest necrotizing arteritis, but the glomerular lesions are usually sufficiently characteristic to prevent misdiagnosis.

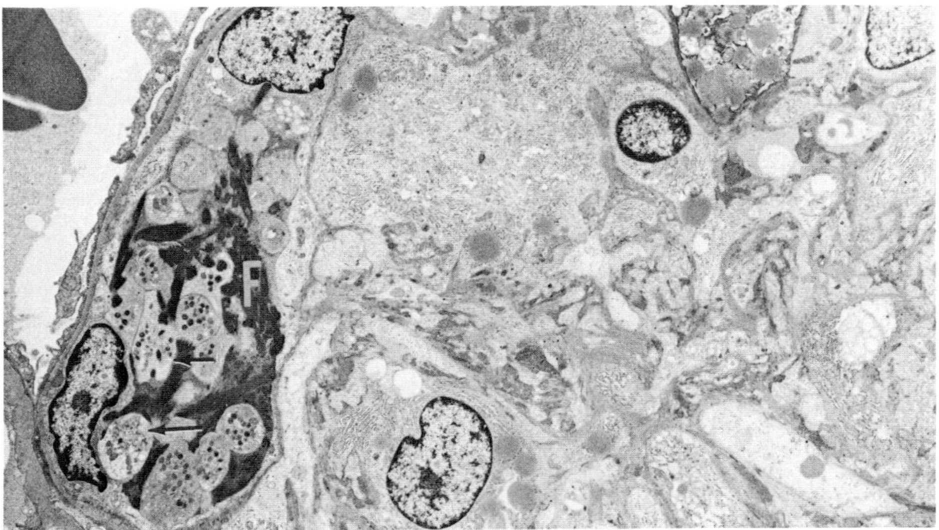

Figure 15-16. Capillary lumen occluded by platelets (arrows) and fibrin (F). The mesangium is hypertrophic and contains numerous lysosomal granules (×4,300).

CLINICAL COURSE AND PROGNOSIS

HUS in Children

The prognosis correlates directly with the severity of the nephropathy, which is, in turn, related to the intensity of extrarenal manifestations (7,8). There is some evidence to suggest that serious sequelae are more common in children with nongastrointestinal prodromes (41). Mildly affected patients show gradual return of normal renal output and function with resolution of microangiopathy over several weeks and permanent recovery. The occurrence of anuria or prolonged oliguria until recently was regarded as a grave prognostic sign, but the majority of such patients now recover completely with dialysis and appropriate supportive therapy. There is no satisfactory evidence to support the use of anticoagulants or thrombolytic agents (7). Hypertension may be severe during the active phase of the syndrome and continues after convalescence in some patients. A small percentage is left with varying degrees of chronic renal failure, which is usually associated with hypertension and may gradually progress. This percentage appears to be higher in endemic areas where a persistently active glomerular lesion has been described that may cause chronic renal failure some years after the acute disease (8,42). The overall mortality varies in different reports but is probably less than 5% (7).

HUS in Adults

The prognosis in adults with HUS is grave, most entering permanent chronic renal failure soon after onset. Complete recovery is rare and any residual renal function may gradually disappear over the course of a year in association with severe hypertension. As in children, the acute mortality has been greatly reduced by prompt dialysis, and most patients now survive with chronic renal failure. The

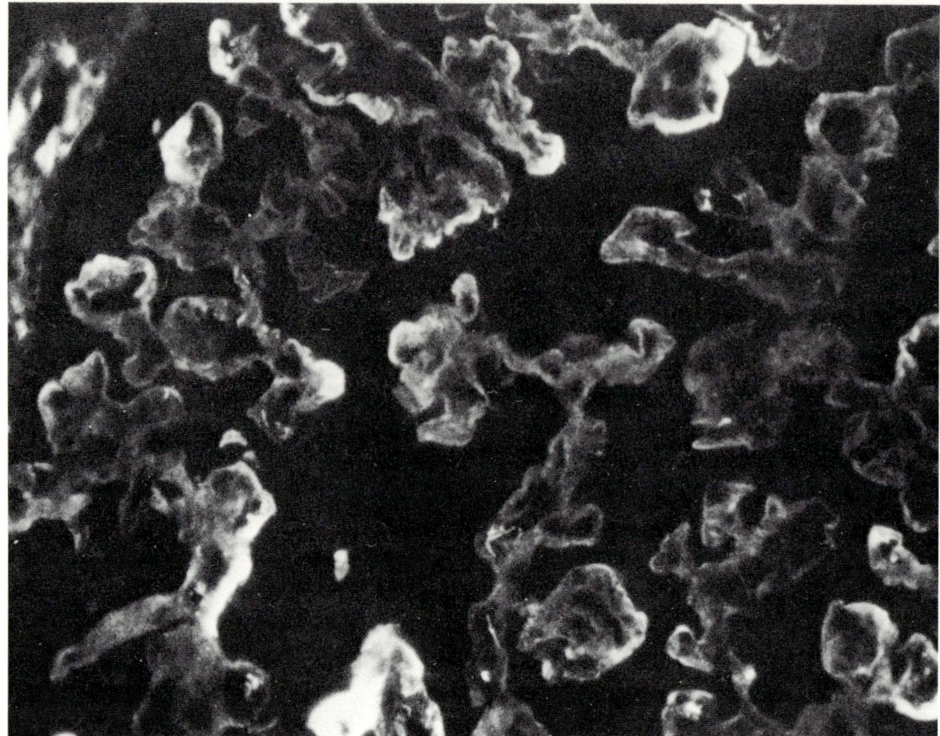

Figure 15-17. Glomerulus from the same biopsy specimen as in figure 15-10, showing irregular fluorescence along capillary loops (Antihuman fibrinogen, ×650).

activity of the syndrome gradually wanes over several weeks and significant systemic complications are uncommon, although pulmonary thrombotic or embolic episodes may occur, and cardiac damage was common in one series (43). While some investigators believe in the value of anticoagulants (44), most consider that neither these nor other agents affect the eventual outcome. Plasma exchange or infusion has recently been reported to cause resolution of the syndrome (21), but this observation has not yet been confirmed.

TRANSPLANTATION

Transplantation has been used successfully for both adults and children with chronic renal failure following HUS. Differentiating between transplant rejection and recurrent HUS may be difficult (45), but there is only one convincing report of recurrent disease (46), although another patient died after a massive and generalized Schwartzman-like reaction within hours of transplantation (10). Apparently de novo HUS has also been reported in a transplanted patient following a viral prodrome (46a).

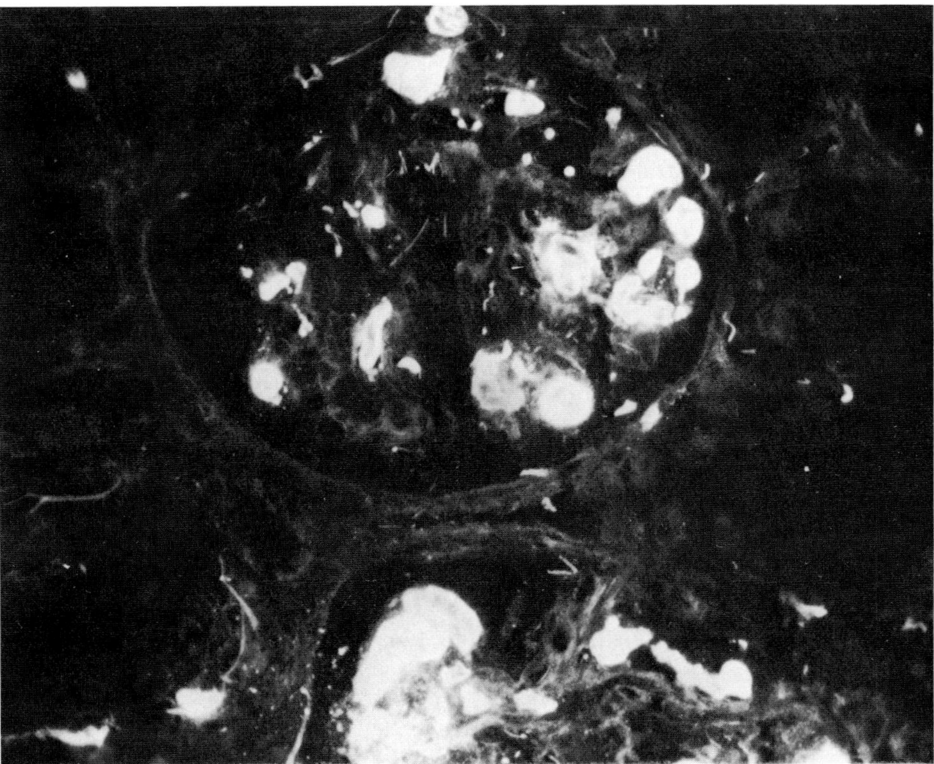

Figure 15-18. Thrombosis of glomerular capillaries in a case of hemolytic uremic syndrome (antihuman fibrinogen, ×250).

THROMBOTIC THROMBOCYTOPENIC PURPURA (TTP)

TTP is a rare syndrome defined by the coexistence of fever, purpura, central nervous system abnormalities, and microangiopathic hemolysis (47). The syndrome is most common in women in their 30s, but it may occur at any age, and is probably a nonspecific clinical phenomenon with many causes (48,49). Renal disease occurs in 88% of patients with TTP and is characterized by episodes of proteinuria, microscopic hematuria, and azotemia (47). Early reports included patients who would now be categorized as having HUS, and recent studies have not confirmed earlier descriptions (50) of vascular and glomerular lesions in TTP identical to those already described for HUS. The usual pattern is of sporadic thrombi in glomerular capillaries, arterioles, and small arteries with vascular endothelial proliferation but minimal glomerular reaction (49). Endothelial proliferation in afferent arterioles may be florid and associated with aneurysmal dilatation to produce nodules with a glomerulus-like structure. These "glomeruloid bodies" are not, however, specific for TTP and may be found in patients with disseminated intravascular coagulation from any cause (51). The prognosis for patients with TTP was previously regarded as almost hopeless, but improved survival has been reported recently with the use of plasma exchange or infusion and other measures (48,52).

DISSEMINATED INTRAVASCULAR COAGULATION

Disseminated intravascular coagulation may be produced by many mechanisms and causes damage to many tissues (14,53). Acute renal failure is a common complication, and its association with a microangiopathic blood picture may suggest the diagnosis of HUS. The morphologic features in the kidney are, however, quite distinct. Autopsy studies of disseminated intravascular coagulation describe glomerular thrombi and glomeruloid bodies but no other lesions (51,53,54) (Fig. 15-19). In our experience, renal biopsy specimens from these patients have shown either nonspecific tubular changes only or irregular mesangial swelling with a characteristic pattern of confluent necrosis of the cells lining tubular segments, usually near the corticomedullary junction. A similar pattern of confluent necrosis has been described in association with eclampsia and "endotoxin shock" (54). No fibrin could be demonstrated in these biopsy specimens, but the mesangial swelling may have been caused by the phagocytosis of coagulation products (13).

CORTICAL NECROSIS

Cortical necrosis is a rare condition that is typically seen in association with complications of pregnancy (see p. 316) but may occur with systemic sepsis, severe trauma, or other diseases (55,56). The necrosis varies in extent and usually spares the juxtamedullary regions, so that residual renal function is present in up to 50% of patients and may allow survival without the necessity for chronic dialysis (55). There is a clear correlation between the proportion of glomeruli destroyed and both the duration of oliguria and survival (55). Although patchy infarction may be seen in patients with HUS, the glomerular lesions typical of this syndrome do not occur in cortical necrosis, and the two conditions appear to be quite distinct (Figs. 15-20, 15-21).

SUMMARY

Coagulation is a feature of many renal diseases and may be associated with a variety of morphologic and functional changes. These changes show the greatest variety in HUS, which is a heterogeneous clinical syndrome with many pathogenetic mechanisms. Glomerular disease is predominant in HUS and is characterized by cellular swelling and basement membrane duplication, but extensive vascular insudation or swelling may occur. The syndrome differs in children and adults. In children it usually follows an apparent or proven viral prodrome and is self-limiting if the acute renal failure can be controlled by dialysis. By contrast, adult HUS typically occurs in a setting of estrogen-induced coagulation abnormalities and causes permanent destruction of renal function. Although neither the etiology nor pathogenesis of HUS is known, endemic distribution in some communities and familial aggregation suggest environmental or genetic alterations to the mechanisms of hemostasis. The occurrence of similar morphologic changes in a number of separate conditions indicates the existence of a variety of pathways for this pattern of renal damage and suggests that vascular spasm is implicated in the pathogenesis of the lesions.

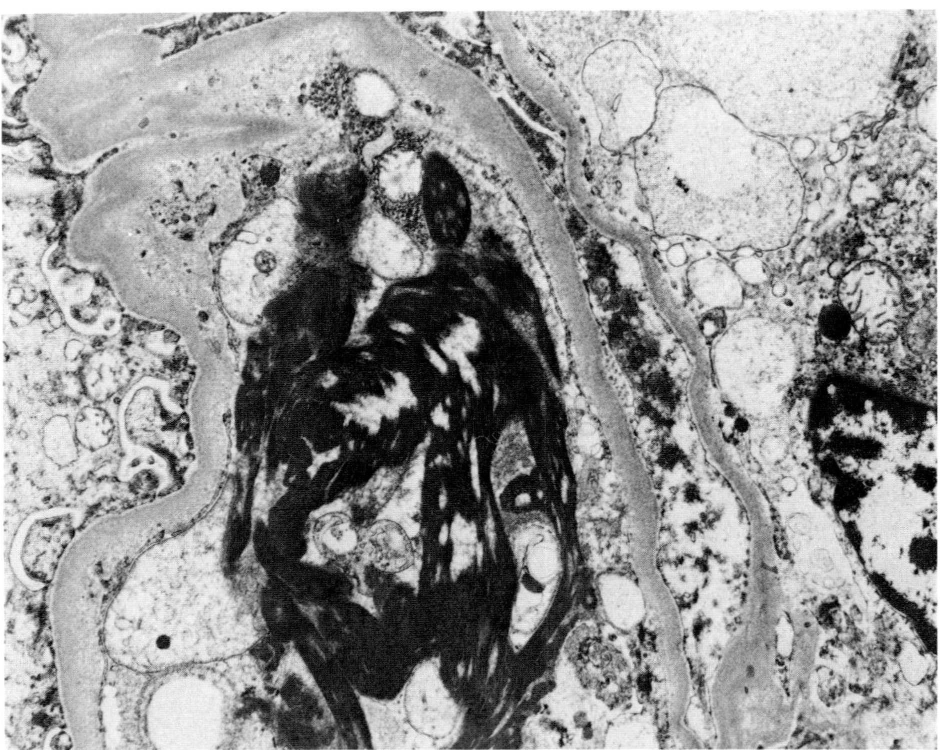

Figure 15-19. Electron micrograph of a portion of a glomerulus from a patient with disseminated intravascular coagulation. The capillary lumen is occluded by fibrin (×9,000).

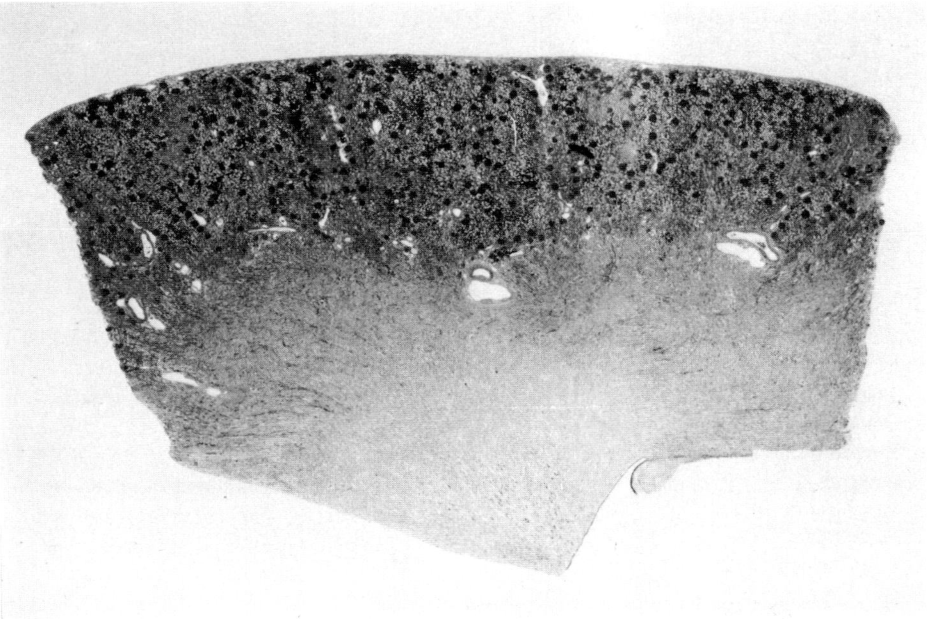

Figure 15-20. Low-power micrograph of a kidney from a patient who developed renal cortical necrosis secondary to gram-negative sepsis. Note that while the cortex is completely infarcted, the medulla is intact (H&E stain, ×8).

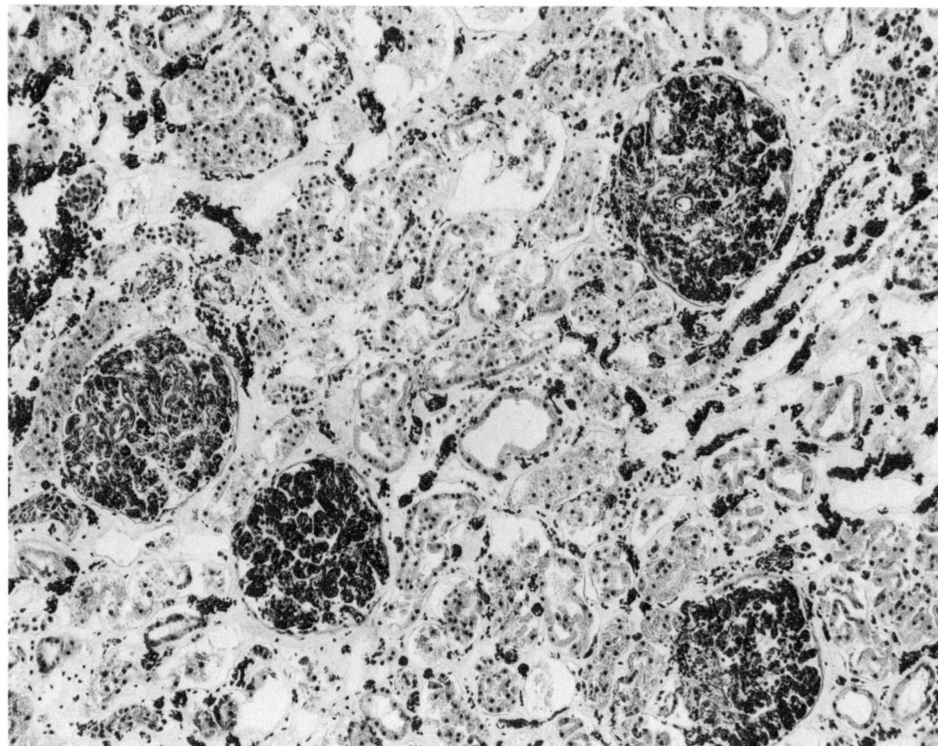

Figure 15-21. Higher magnification of the renal cortex of the same case as in Figure 15-20. The glomerular and peritubular capillaries are hyperemic and occluded by fibrin. The glomeruli show hemorrhagic infarction. The tubules are also necrotic and the interstitium appears edematous (H&E stain, ×120).

REFERENCES

1. Gasser C, Gautier E, Steck A, et al: Hamolytisch-uramische syndrome: bilaterale neirerindenneksosen bei akuten erwobenin hamolytischen-anamien. *Schweiz Med Wschr* 85:905, 1955.

2. Kaplan BS, Drummond KN: The hemolytic uremic syndrome is a syndrome. *N Engl J Med* 298:964, 1978.

3. Brain MC: Microangiopathic hemolytic anemia. *Annu Rev Med* 21:133, 1970.

4. Clarkson AR, Meadows R, Lawrence JR: Post-partum renal failure. The generalized Schwartzman reaction. *Aust Ann Med* 18:209, 1969.

5. Thomas L, Good RA: Studies on the generalized Schwartman reaction. I. General observations concerning the phenomenon. *J Exp Med* 96:605, 1962.

6. Kincaid-Smith P: Coagulation and renal disease. *Kidney Int* 2:183, 1972.

7. DeChadarevian J-P, Kaplan BS: The hemolytic uremic syndrome of childhood. *Perspectives Pediat Pathol* 4:465, 1978.

8. Gianantonio CA, Vitacco M, Mendilaharzu F, et al: The hemolytic-uremic syndrome. *Nephron* 11:174, 1973.

9. Habib R: Renal failure and vascular lesions, discussion, in Kincaid-Smith P, Mathew TH, Becker EL (eds): *Glomerulonephritis: Morphology, Natural History and Treatment.* New York, John Wiley & Sons, 1973, p 1084.

10. Clarkson AR, Lawrence JR, Meadows R, et al: The haemolytic uraemic syndrome in adults. *Quart J Med* 39:227, 1970.

11. Brown CB, Clarkson AR, Robson JS, et al: Haemolytic uraemic syndrome in women taking oral contraceptives. *Lancet* 1:1479, 1973.

12. Poller L: Oral contraceptives, blood clotting and thrombosis. *Br Med Bull* 34:151, 1978.

13. Wardle EN: Fibrin in renal disease: functional considerations. *Clin Nephrol* 2:85, 1974.

14. Colman RW, Robboy SJ, Minna JD: Disseminated intravascular coagulation (DIC): an approach. *Am J Med* 52:679, 1972.

15. Thorgeirsson G, Robertson AL: The vascular endothelium—pathologic significance; a review. *Am J Pathol* 93:801, 1978.

16. Wardle EN: Endotoxin and acute renal failure. *Nephron* 14:321, 1975.

17. Koster F, Levin J, Walker L, et al: Hemolytic-uremic syndrome after shigellosis: relation to endotoxinemia and circulating immune complexes. *N Engl J Med* 298:927, 1978.

18. Kim Y, Miller K, Michael AF: Breakdown products of C3 and factor B in hemolytic-uremic syndrome. *J Lab Clin Med* 89:845, 1977.

19. Bergstein JM, Michael AF: Generalized Schwartzman reaction in the rabbit: immunopathologic findings in the kidney. *Arch Pathol* 97:230, 1974.

20. Branson HE, Wyatt LL, Schmer G: Complement consumption in acute disseminated intravascular coagulation without antecedent immunopathology. *Am J Clin Pathol* 66:967, 1976.

21. Remuzzi G, Misiani R, Marchesi D, et al: Haemolytic-uraemic syndrome: deficiency of plasma factor(s) regulating prostacyclin activity? *Lancet* 2:871, 1978.

22. Upshaw JR: Congenital deficiency of a factor in normal plasma that reverses microangiopathic hemolysis and thrombocytopenia. *N Engl J Med* 298:1350, 1978.

23. van Wierengen PMV, Monnens LAH, Schretlen EDAM: Haemolytic-uraemic syndrome: epidemiological and clinical study. *Arch Dis Child* 49:432, 1974.

24. Barré P, Kaplan BS, de Chardarévian J-P, et al: Hemolytic uremic syndrome with hypocomplementemia, serum C3NeF and glomerular deposits of C3. *Arch Pathol Lab Med* 101:357, 1977.

25. Sun NCJ, Johnson WJ, Sung DW, et al: Idiopathic postpartum renal failure: review and case report of a successful renal transplantation. *Mayo Clin Proc* 50:395, 1975.

26. Vandewalle A, Kanfer A, Kourilsky O: Oliguric thrombotic microangiopathy during the fifth month of pregnancy. *Br Med J* 2:479, 1975.

27. Jackson B, Clarkson AR, Seymour AE: The haemolytic-uraemic syndrome and oral contraceptives. *Aust NZ J Med* 6:580, 1976.

28. Farr MJ, Roberts S, Morley AR, et al: The haemolytic uraemic syndrome—a family study. *Quart J Med* 44:161, 1975.

29. Grøttum KA, Flatmark A, Myhre E, et al: Immunological hereditary nephropathy. *Acta Med Scand* Suppl 571, 1974.

30. Kaplan BS, Chesney RW, Drummond KN: Hemolytic uremic syndrome in families. *N Engl J Med* 292:1090, 1975.

31. Kaplan BS: Hemolytic uremic syndrome with recurrent episodes: an important subset. *Clin Nephrol* 8:495, 1977.

32. Ponticelli C, Imbasciati E, Brancaccio D, et al: Acute renal failure in systemic lupus erythematosus. *Br Med J* 3:716, 1974.

33. Sachdev Y, Morley AR, Wilkinson R, et al: Addison's disease with renal microangiopathy and renal failure (a new syndrome). *Quart J Med* 46:151, 1977.

34. Dische FE, Culliford EJ, Parsons V: Haemolytic uraemic syndrome and idiopathic membranous glomerulonephritis. *Br Med J* 2:1112, 1978.

35. Bohle A, Helmchen U, Grund KE, et al: Malignant nephrosclerosis in patients with hemolytic uremic syndrome (primary malignant nephrosclerosis). *Current Topics Pathol* 65:81, 1977.

36. Vitsky BH, Suzuki Y, Strauss L, et al: The hemolytic-uraemic syndrome: a study of renal pathologic alterations. *Am J Pathol* 57:627, 1969.

37. Kincaid-Smith P: Participation of intravascular coagulation in the pathogenesis of glomerular and vascular lesions. *Kidney Int* 7:242, 1975.

38. Riella MC, George CRP, Hickman RO, et al: Renal microangiopathy of the hemolytic-uremic syndrome in childhood. *Nephron* 17:188, 1976.

39. Shigematsu H, Dikman SH, Churg J, et al: Mesangial involvement in hemolytic-uremic syndrome: a light and electron microscopic study. *Am J Pathol* 85:349, 1976.

40. McCoy RC, Abramowsky CR, Krueger R: The hemolytic uremic syndrome with positive immunofluorescence studies. *J Pediat* 85:170, 1974.

41. Dolislager D, Tune B: The hemolytic-uremic syndrome: spectrum of severity and significance of prodrome. *Am J Dis Child* 132:55, 1978.

42. Cossio PM, Laguens RP, Ratin DJ, et al: Persistent glomerulonephritis following the haemolytic-uraemic syndrome: immunopathological and morphological studies. *Clin Exp Immunol* 29:361, 1977.

43. Robson JS, Martin AM, Ruckley AV, et al: Irreversible post-partum renal failure: a new syndrome. *Quart J Med* 37:423, 1968.

44. Ponticelli C, Imbasciati E, Tarantino A, et al: Postpartum renal failure with microangiopathic haemolytic anaemia: long-term survival after anticoagulant therapy. *Nephron* 9:27, 1972.

45. Cerilli GJ, Nelsen C, Dorfman L: Renal homotransplantation in infants and children with the hemolytic-uremic syndrome. *Surgery* 71:66, 1972.

46. Folman R, Arbus GS, Churchill B, et al: Recurrence of the hemolytic uremic syndrome in a 3½ year old 4 months after second renal transplantation. *Clin Nephrol* 10:121, 1978.

46a. Peterson VP, Olsen TS, Kissmeyer-Nielsen F, et al: Late failure of human renal transplants: an analysis of transplant disease and graft failure among 125 recipients surviving for one to eight years. *Medicine* 54:45, 1975.

47. Amorosi EL, Ultmann JE: Thrombotic thrombocytopenic purpura: report of 16 cases and review of the literature. *Medicine (Balt)* 45:139, 1966.

48. Amorosi EL, Karpatkin S: Antiplatelet treatment of thrombotic thrombocytopenic purpura. *Ann Intern Med* 86:102, 1977.

49. Umlas J, Kaiser J: Thrombohemolytic thrombocytopenic purpura (TTP). *Am J Med* 49:723, 1970.

50. Feldman JD, Mardiney MR, Unanue ER, et al: The vascular pathology of thrombotic thrombocytopenic purpura: an immunohistochemical and ultrastructural study. *Lab Invest* 15:927, 1966.

51. Umlas J: Glomeruloid structures in thrombohemolytic thrombocytopenic purpura, glomerulonephritis and disseminated intravascular coagulation. *Human Pathol* 3:437, 1972.

52. Byrnes JJ, Khurana M: Treatment of thrombotic thrombocytopenic purpura with plasma. *N Engl J Med* 297:1386, 1977.

53. Robboy SJ, Colman RW, Minna JD: Pathology of disseminated intravascular coagulation (DIC): analysis of 26 cases. *Human Pathol* 3:327, 1972.

54. Sheehan HL, Lynch JB: *Pathology of toxaemia of pregnancy.* Edinburgh, London, Churchill Livingstone, 1973, p 189.

55. Kleinknecht D, Grünfeld J-P, Gomel PC, et al: Diagnostic procedures and long-term prognosis in bilateral renal cortical necrosis. *Kidney Int* 4:390, 1973.

56. Matlin RA, Gary NE: Acute cortical necrosis: case report and review of the literature. *Am J Med* 56:110, 1974.

16
Hypertension

Hypertension is both a product and a cause of renal disease. Like many of the clinical phenomena associated with renal disorders, hypertension is the single expression of many pathogenetic pathways. There is continuing controversy over the detailed mechanisms and individual significance of these pathways, but the effects of hypertension are not in doubt. Persistently increased arterial pressure causes vascular damage and ischemic tissue injury. Some degree of renal vascular disease is probably universal in patients with prolonged hypertension and, occasionally, may cause renal failure. The intense interest in renal function and morphology in hypertension is not, however, restricted necessarily to these tissue effects. The kidney plays a central role in the maintenance of normal blood pressure and may either cause or maintain an elevated pressure. Careful morphologic studies laid the framework for much of the current understanding of hypertensive vascular disease, and the pathologist still has much to contribute. By the study of serial renal biopsies in a variety of disorders, an appreciation of the vascular changes in developing and established hypertension can be developed. This experience can be of value when biopsy specimens are taken from hypertensive patients to establish either the cause or the tissue complications of the disease.

INCIDENCE

Hypertension is a disease of increasing age. Depending on the criteria used for diagnosis, hypertension has been discovered in 13–23% of surveyed populations (1), its incidence ranging from 3% in the fourth to more than 30% in the sixth decade (2). At all ages, more women then men are hypertensives (2), and the incidence is greatly increased among blacks (3). No definition has been universally accepted for hypertension, but a diastolic figure of 95 mm Hg has been suggested as an indication for therapy in men, with a slightly higher figure in women (4). Hypertension is severe in 16% of this population (1), depending on the criteria for diagnosis, but malignant hypertension, characterized by papilledema, is uncommon, with an incidence of only about 1% (5). There is, however, a continuous spectrum between the benign and malignant forms of hypertension.

PATHOGENESIS AND CLASSIFICATION

Blood pressure is the product of vascular tone and extracellular fluid volume. Vascular tone is influenced by both renal and systemic factors. The autonomic-vasoactive amine system is crucial to the maintenance of vascular reactivity and works in concert with both constrictor and dilator substances released in the kidney. The renin-angiotensin system plays a significant role in the adjustment of vascular tone and is intricately interwoven with the secretion of aldosterone, which controls sodium homeostasis and, thus, extracellular fluid volume (6). These constrictor effects are probably balanced by vasodilator mechanisms among which the secretion of prostaglandins from renomedullary interstitial cells is attracting increasing attention (7). This exquisitely controlled system, which includes many other mechanisms (8), may be interrupted at any point to produce hypertension. A great deal about the normal regulatory mechanism has been learned from the study of a number of uncommon but well-characterized diseases in which hypertension is the central feature. For example, renal artery stenosis is an important cause of clinical hypertension and has been one of the major experimental models used to study the interactions of the renin-angiotensin-aldosterone system (6). Similarly, endocrine tumors secreting vasoactive amines, aldosterone, or renin have allowed close scrutiny of the unopposed action of these hormones. These and other conditions caricature the normal physiologic control of blood pressure and are the most important causes of "secondary" hypertension (Table 16-1). The identification of "secondary" hypertension is important since successful treatment may eradicate the factors causing the disease and restore the blood pressure to normal.

Careful investigation of the majority of hypertensive patients, however, reveals no apparent cause (9). Whether this "essential" or idiopathic hypertension is mediated by one or many mechanisms is unknown. Mean blood pressure increases progressively with advancing age, and some have suggested that hypertension is not a disease but rather an exaggeration of this normal trend (4). Analysis of the changes in normal blood pressure is complicated by the enormous variations observed by continuous monitoring of both normotensive and hypertensive individuals (4). These variations sometimes coincide with external "stress" stimuli and may correspond to vasoconstriction mediated by the autonomic-vasoactive amine system. Studies of the renal circulation have confirmed the presence of an increase in both vascular tone and reactivity in hypertensive patients (10), and it has been suggested that either prolonged or repeated vasospasm might, in genetically predisposed people (11), eventually cause sufficient vascular damage to establish permanent hypertension (12). Various attempts to segregate groups within the general population of idiopathic hypertension have met with limited success. At present, the disease remains an amorphous and not clearly divisible clinical phenomenon. Whether several distinct diseases will eventually emerge from this mass or whether, instead, common pathways will be recognized is not yet clear.

Whatever its pathogenesis, hypertension causes a breakdown in the normal mechanisms governing vascular permeability. With increasing vascular pressure, progressively more severe structural changes develop in arterial walls as the result of insudation of plasma constituents. There is some argument over the contribution of such factors as renin and angiotensin to this augmented permea-

Table 16-1. A Simplified Classification of Hypertension

By degree
  Benign
  Malignant

By cause
  Idiopathic
  Secondary
    Renovascular
    Intrinsic renal disease
    Endocrine
      Primary aldosteronism
      Cushing's syndrome
      Pheochromocytoma
      Reninoma
    Coarctation of the aorta
    Hypertension of pregnancy

bility (13) but none about the critical importance of intravascular pressure. Direct examination of arterioles in experimental hypertension reveals a biphasic tonic response: an immediate, diffuse vasoconstriction followed by a delayed and patchy vasodilatation. In this second phase, the permeability of the dilated segments is increased, and plasma constituents accumulate in the walls (13). These experimental investigations confirm the preexisting suspicions that the hyaline in hypertensive and other vascular diseases merely represents inspissated plasma proteins (plasmatic vasculosis) (14). The controversy over the character and content of the various patterns of arteriolar hyalinosis, is, thus, no longer relevant. In almost all situations, hyaline is merely the static morphologic expression of increased permeability and its precise chemical nature simply reflects the severity or cause of this effect.

The character of the vascular deposits is altered by abrupt and intense elevation in blood pressure. In this situation, there is massive insudation across the wall with cellular damage and activation of the coagulation system, causing fibrin deposition. The pattern of fibrinoid "necrosis" is, in fact, an exaggeration of the hyalinizing process and does not imply vascular necrosis. In either this or the usual insudation pattern, the deposits are probably in a dynamic state of accretion and removal. Considerable degrees of repair may, therefore, occur, although fibrosis in the media and intima may distort the vessel and stenose the lumen. Prolonged hypertension leads in this way to tissue ischemia, which may, in the kidney, activate the juxtaglomerular apparatus and increase renin release. So ". . . a vicious cycle is, thereby, established which leads to a sustained elevation of the blood pressure and progressive renal destruction" (15).

CLINICAL MANIFESTATIONS AND PROGNOSIS

The development of significant renal disease is relatively rare in uncomplicated, benign hypertension, but varying degrees of renal function impairment and proteinuria may occur. The presence of large quantities of protein in the urine of such a patient should, however, suggest either previously unrecognized intrinsic disease or a superimposed glomerular lesion. In malignant hypertension, on the other hand, renal damage is common, and acute renal failure may even be the first indication of the hypertensive state (16). In this situation, a microangiopathic hemolytic state may be prominent, and it has been suggested that the fibrin products resulting from this state could propogate the vascular damage (17). Malignant hypertension has an organic renal basis in a significant proportion of cases (5), and the effects of this disease may be expressed in the urinary sediment. Proteinuria is often considerable, however, in apparently primary malignant hypertension and may be accompanied by numerous red cells.

Untreated hypertension shortens life, especially in males, and is a major cause of cardiac and cerebrovascular disease (4). This effect on life expectancy is a direct function of the degree of blood pressure elevation (4). Thus, patients with only minor hypertension may survive for many years, while few patients with untreated malignant hypertension survive for more than one year (5). Renal failure develops in more than half the patients with malignant hypertension and was a major cause of death before the advent of energetic and aggressive hypotensive therapy (5). With this therapy, the incidence of chronic renal failure has been substantially reduced, and considerable healing of the vascular lesions has been documented (4,18). In those patients developing chronic renal failure, transplantation has been successfully performed, but recurrent malignant hypertension has occasionally occurred (18a). Renal failure is very uncommon in benign hypertension, most patients dying of cardiac or cerebrovascular disease (2). Satisfactory reduction of blood pressure in benign hypertension diminishes many, but not all, of these complications (4), and there is some evidence for regression of the vascular lesions (19).

PATHOLOGIC CHARACTERISTICS

Benign Hypertension

Blood Vessels
Prolonged hypertension leads to diffuse thickening of all arterial walls by medial hypertrophy. This is associated, in arcuate and interlobular arteries, with intimal fibrosis and multilayered duplication of the internal elastic lamina (Fig. 16-1). Electron microscopy of these large vessels reveals hyperplasia and hypertrophy of the smooth muscle cells, with frequent cytoplasmic lipochrome granules and collagenous intimal thickening (Fig. 16-2). The fibrosis may become extensive enough to efface much of the muscular wall. The arterioles are deformed by cylinders of eosinophilic and PAS-positive hyalin, which cause mural thickening and luminal stenosis (Fig. 16-3). Ultrastructurally, hyalin is represented as granular and often variably electron-dense material, which frequently contains lipid droplets and cytoplasmic debris. Small hyalin deposits accumulate in a subendothelial location, but the larger masses extend throughout the wall (Fig. 16-4). The hyalinized arterioles usually react with immunofluorescent reagents for complement components, especially C3 and IgM (Fig. 16-3).

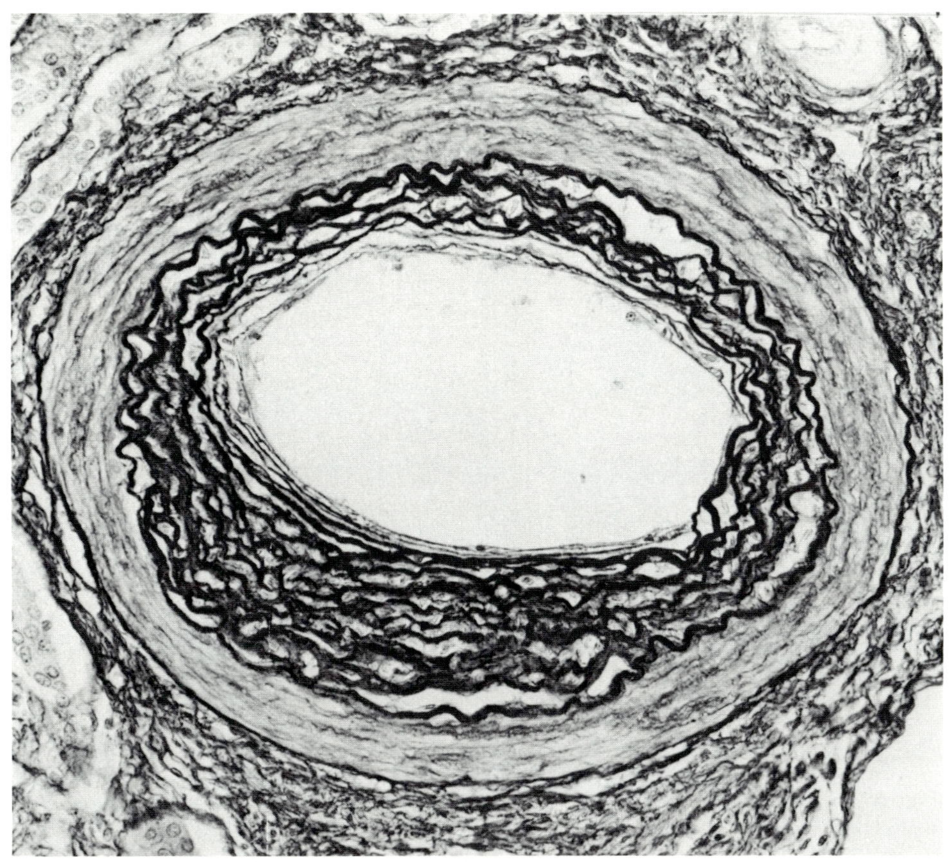

Figure 16-1. Arcuate artery with reduplication of the interna elastic lamina (Van Gieson stain, ×200).

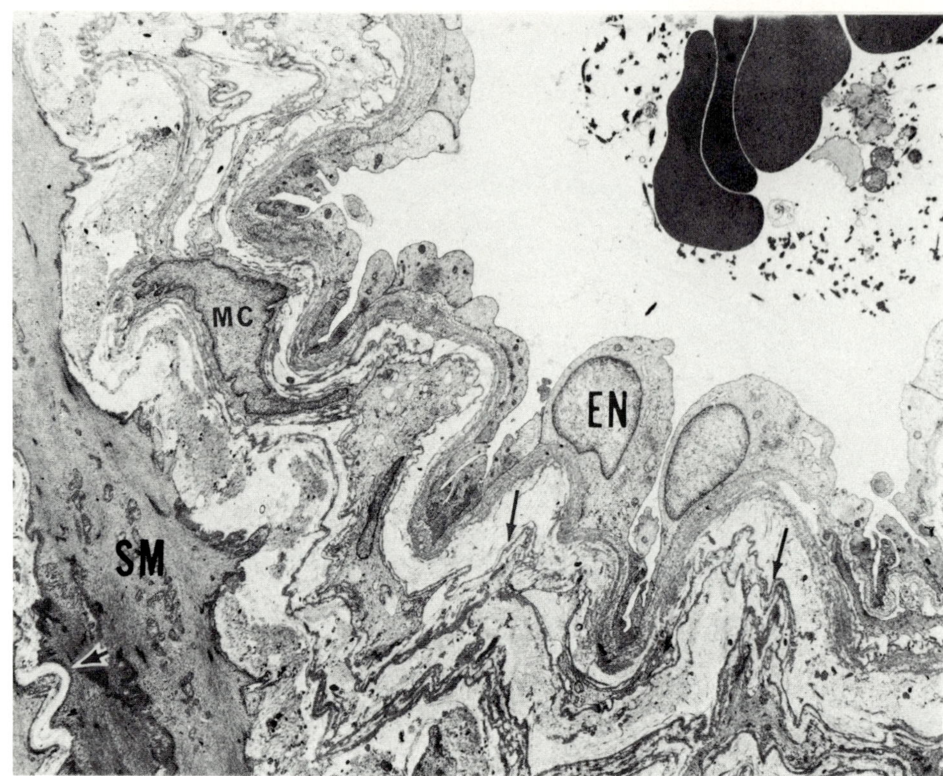

Figure 16-2. Electron micrograph of an interlobular artery. The intima consists of strands of basement membrane (arrows) and myointimal cells (MC). Portions of hypertrophied smooth muscle cells (SM) and elastic lamina (arrow head) are seen on the left. Red blood cells and small fibrin strands are present in the lumen. EN, endothelial cell (×5,000).

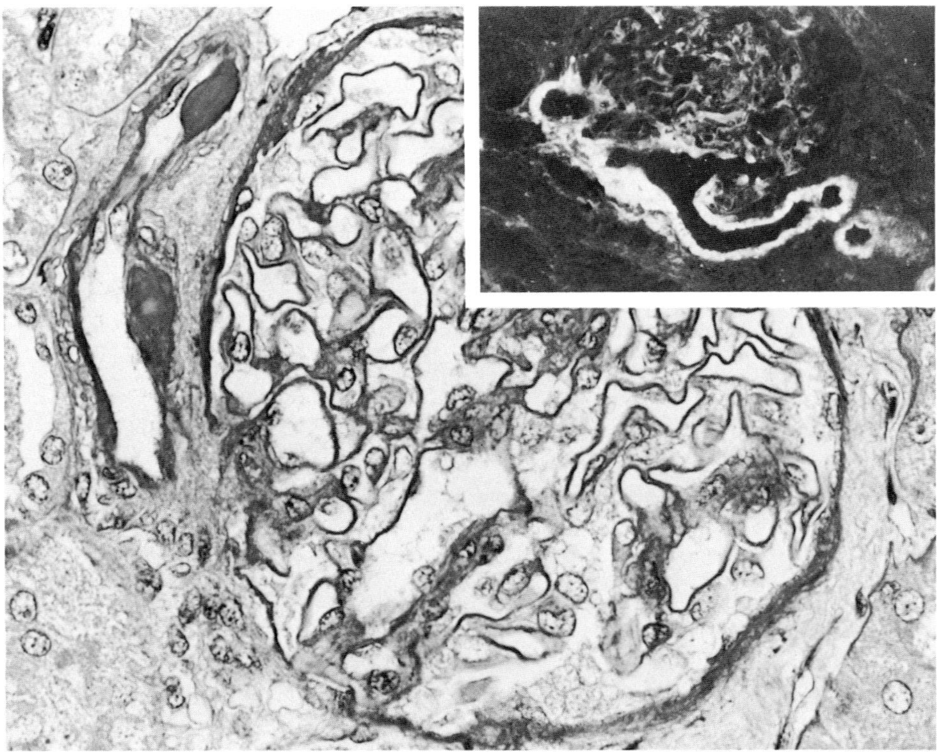

Figure 16-3. Afferent arteriole with subintimal homogenous hyaline material. Insert: immunofluorescent preparation showing reaction for C3 (H&E stain, ×650; insert, ×280).

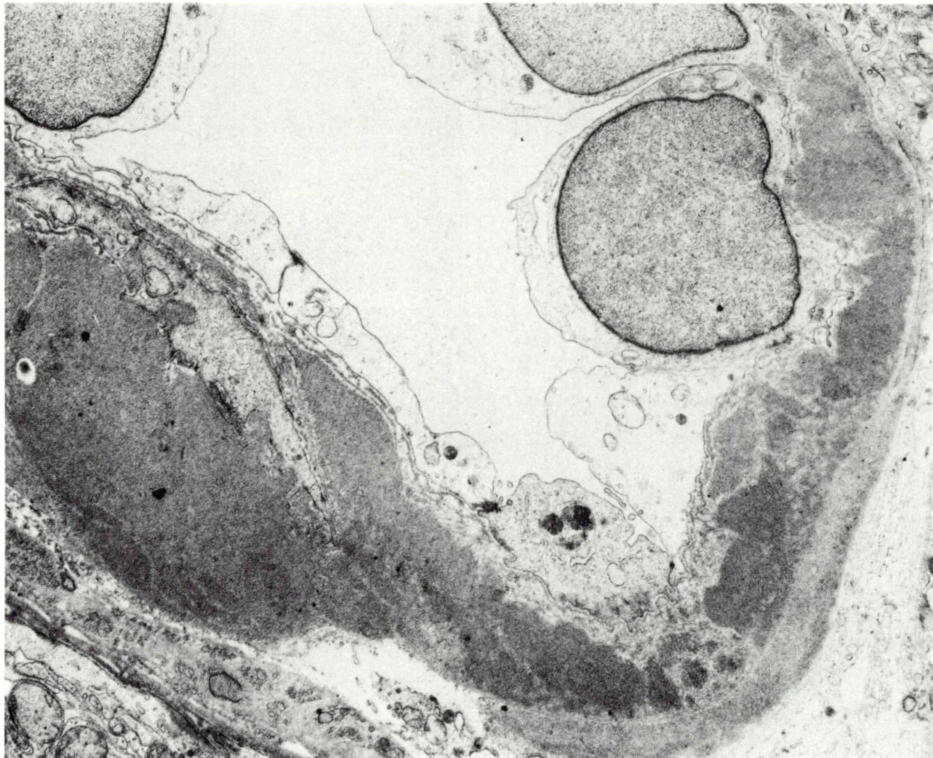

Figure 16-4. Electron micrograph of hyaline arteriole from a patient with hypertension showing subintimal electron-dense material (×8,100).

Glomeruli

A varying proportion of glomeruli shows the characteristic pattern of ischemic obsolescence with membrane wrinkling, disappearance of cells, and replacement of Bowman's space by PAS-negative material (20) (Fig. 16-5). Electron microscopy demonstrates that this material is collagen (21). The remaining glomeruli may appear normal or be enlarged, with mildly increased mesangial matrix (22) and thickening of the glomerular basement membrane (23), as a result of hypertrophy (Fig. 16-6). The pattern of obsolescence may, in some patients, be segmental so that segmental scars are distributed throughout the glomeruli. Immunofluorescence reactions are minimal, but the segmental scars may show nonspecific staining, and the arteriolar C3 reactions may frequently extend for variable distances from the hilum into the mesangium (Fig. 16-3).

Malignant Hypertension

Blood Vessels

The morphologic corollary of malignant hypertension was originally the pattern of fibrinoid "necrosis" (24). This pattern seems, however, to occur much less frequently than a decade or more ago (3), and "productive" lesions are now more common. These are characterized by profuse intimal thickening by myxoid and

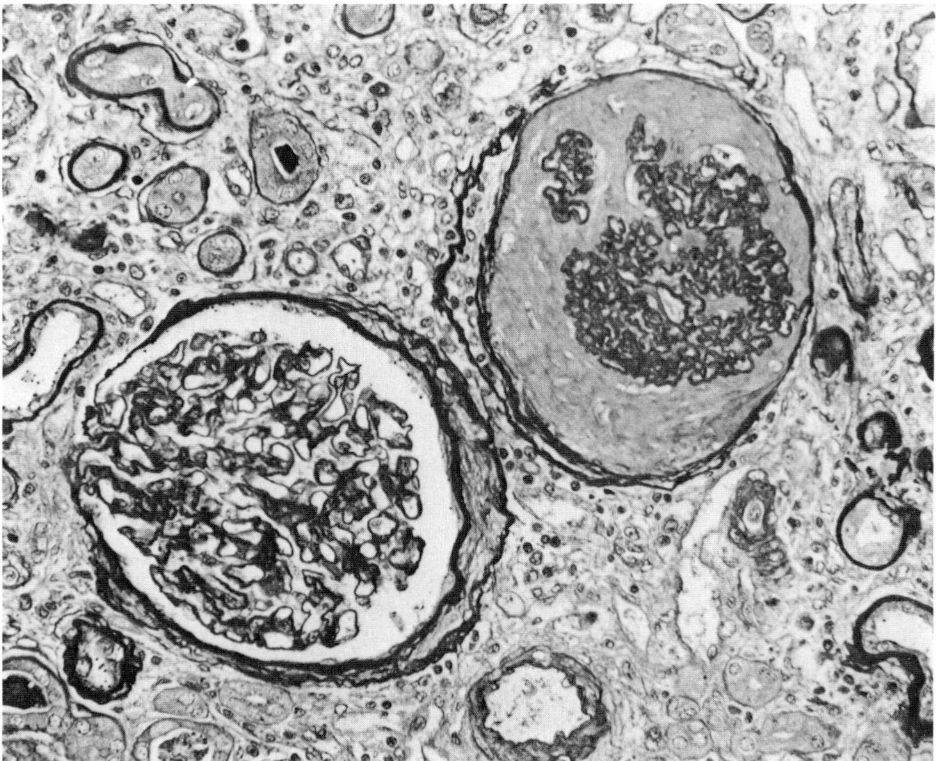

Figure 16-5. Two glomeruli showing early and advanced ischemic injury. The basement membrane of Bowman's capsule is laminated. The obsolescent glomerulus on the right has a wrinkled thickened basement membrane and shows replacement of Bowman's space by lightstaining collagenous material (PAS stain, ×300).

sparsely cellular connective tissue, which drastically reduces the lumen (25,26) (Fig. 16-7). With time, this acute change shows progressive scarring to produce a concentric "onion-skin" pattern of intimal fibrosis (Fig. 16-8). If there has been a preexisting benign phase, the intimal lesions may be superimposed upon medial hypertrophy but, in cases with acute and apparently spontaneous onset of malignant hypertension, the media may appear thinned and stretched over the exuberant intimal disease (Fig. 16-9). The productive changes are most pronounced in arcuate and interlobular arteries but extend into arterioles, where they may coexist with hyalinosis from longstanding hypertension. In all locations, electron microscopy reveals a similar pattern of proliferating myointimal cells in a thickened intima which is predominantly composed, in the early lesion, of amorphous material and, later, of collagen fibers (3,23).

When fibrinoid insudation is present, the picture in the arterioles is that of an acute pressure "burst" effect with abundant red cells admixed with fibrin in the wall and, usually, minimal associated inflammation (Figs. 16-10–16-12). Ultrastructurally, a number of phases and grades of severity are recognizable in the arteriolar lesions (23). Insudative deposition of plasma constituents is visible as the irregular accumulation of granular, electron-dense material with, in more

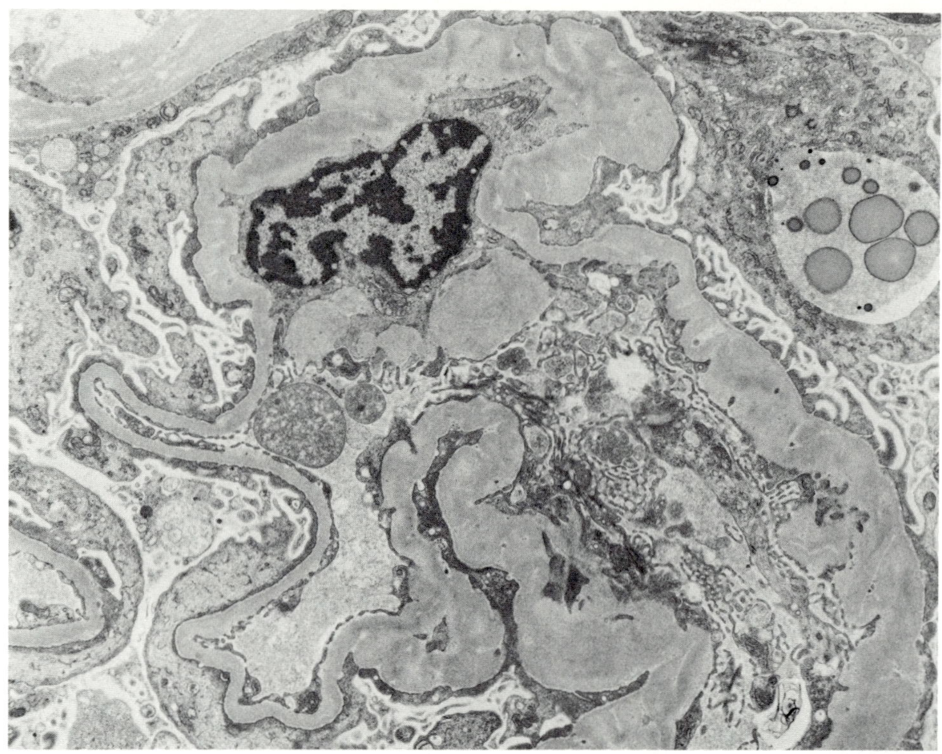

Figure 16-6. Portion of an ischemic glomerulus showing wrinkling and irregular thickening of the basement membrane (×9,000).

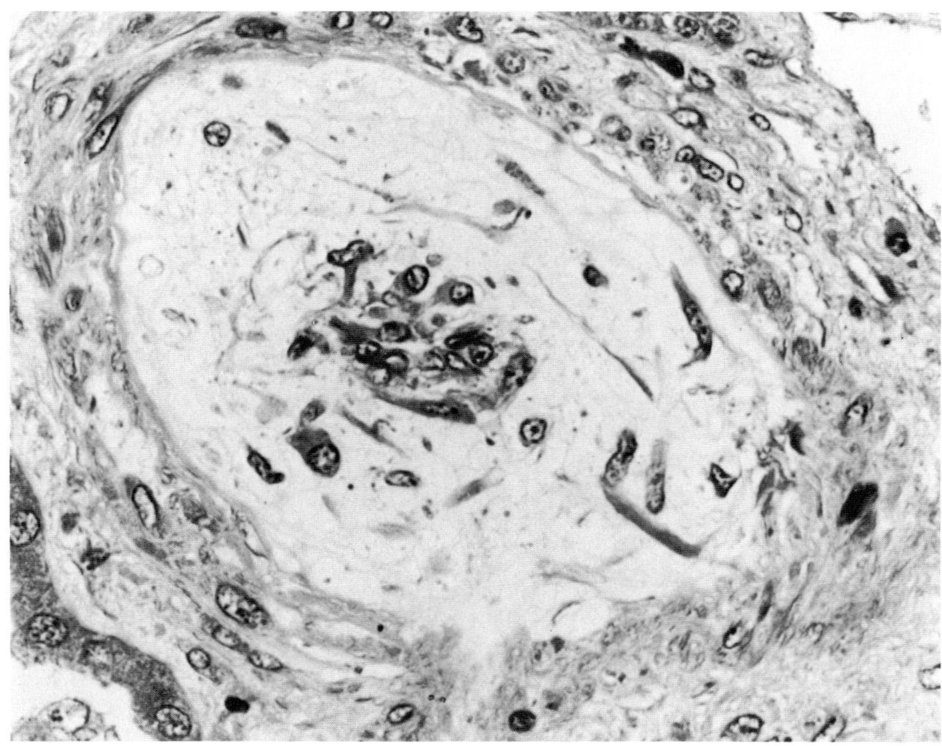

Figure 16-7. Malignant hypertension. Interlobular artery showing an accumulation of myxoidlike intimal tissue (H&E stain, ×280).

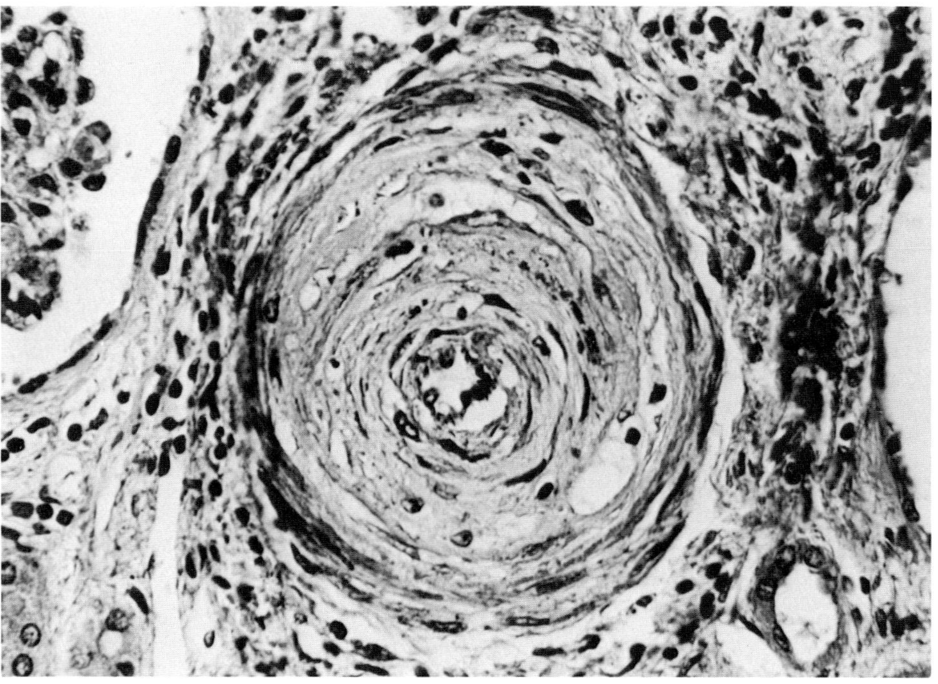

Figure 16-8. Onion bulb-like splitting of an interlobular artery in malignant hypertension. The arterial lumen is severely narrowed (H&E stain, ×245).

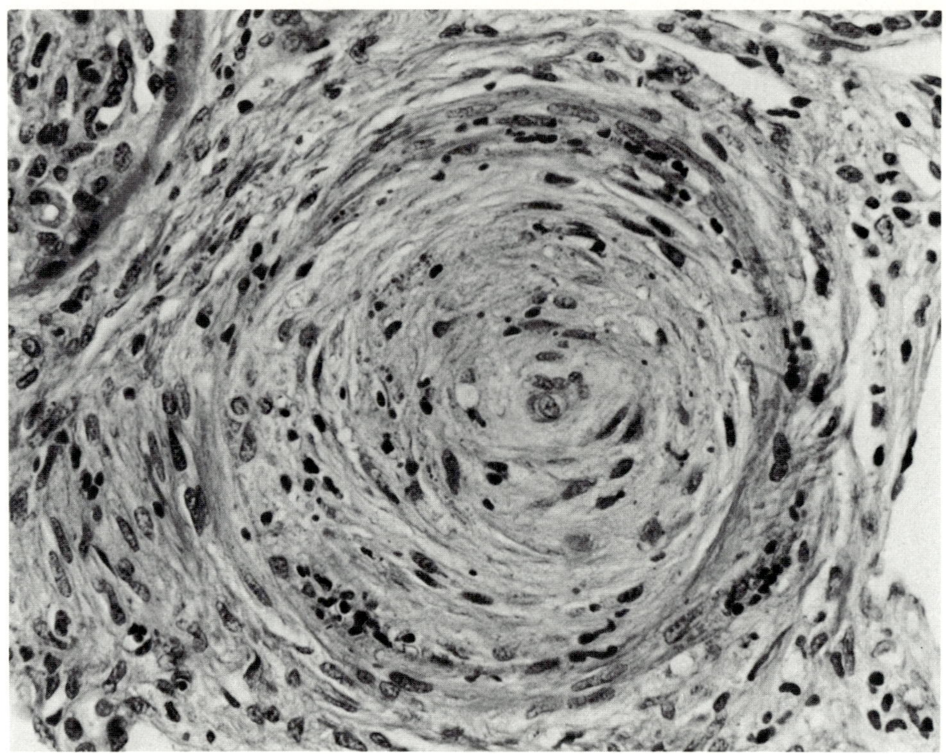

Figure 16-9. Malignant hypertension. Interlobular artery with thinning of the media and marked intimal hyperplasia with hemorrhage (H&E stain, ×320).

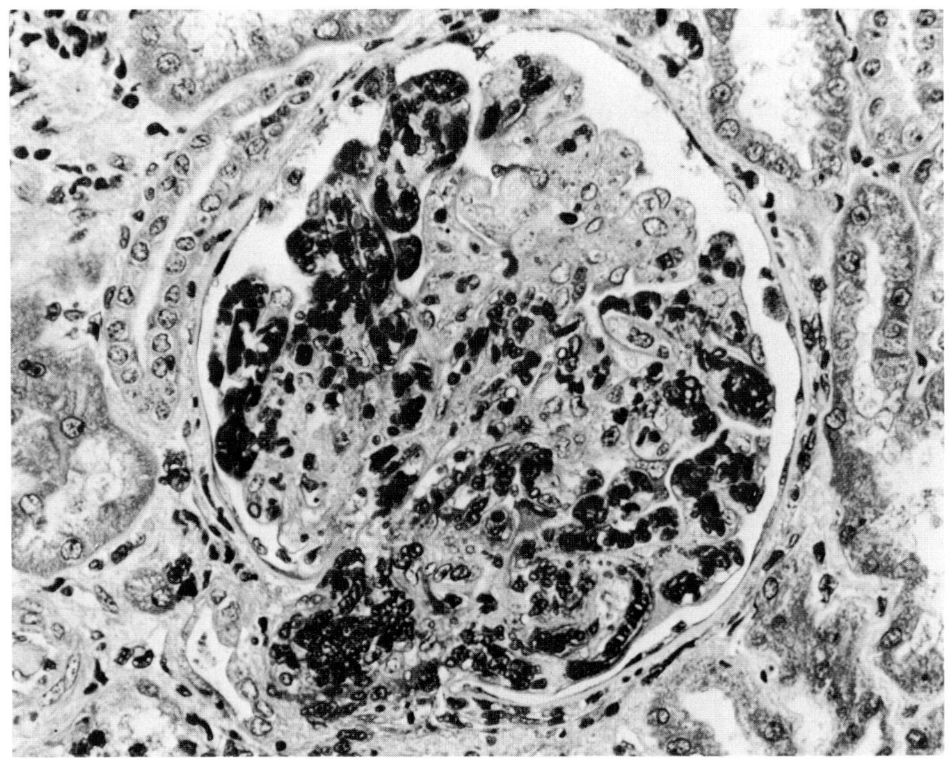

Figure 16-10. Extensive necrosis in a glomerulus from a patient with malignant hypertension. Fibrin is present in the afferent arteriole and glomerular capillaries (H&E stain, ×600).

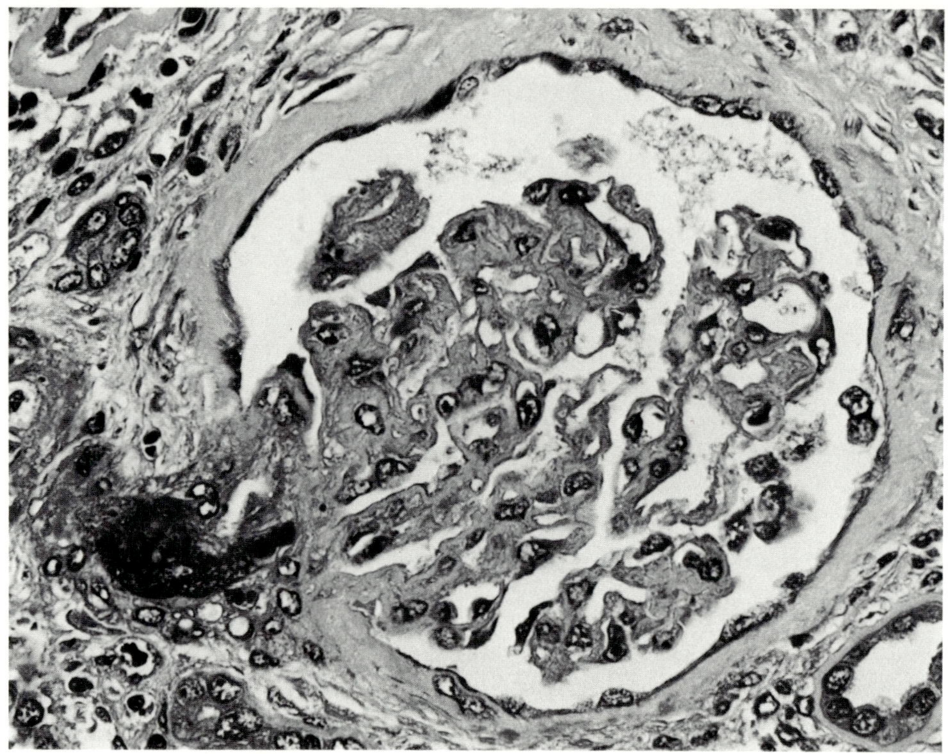

Figure 16-11. Malignant hypertension. Necrosis of the afferent areteriole with ischemic shrinkage of the tuft. (H&E stain, ×600).

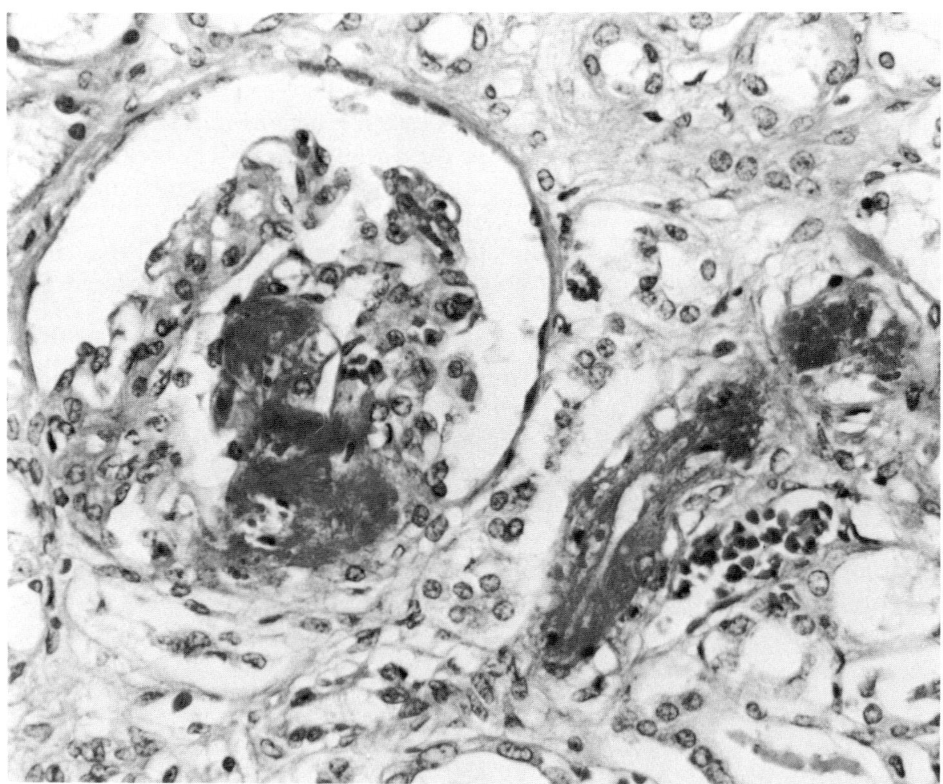

Figure 16-12. Malignant hypertension. Necrosis of the afferent arteriole and axial portion of the glomerular tuft (H&E stain, ×280).

severe lesions, abundant red cells and fibrin strands (Fig. 16-13). There may be death of individual cells, but extensive necrosis does not occur. Thrombosis may complete the arteriolar damage and, later, varying degrees of fibrosis, recanalization, and repair are visible. Immunofluorescent reactions mirror the massive insudation. In the acute stages, reactions for a wide variety of proteins may be seen, but the principal staining is for fibrin, IgM, and complement components (27) (Fig. 16-14). The early reports (28) of IgE in the vessel walls of malignant hypertension have not been substantiated, and there is no evidence that these reactions represent anything but a nonspecific trapping of plasma proteins.

Glomeruli

As with benign hypertension, two patterns of reaction occur. Many glomeruli show extensive ischemic wrinkling in an "accelerated obsolescence" pattern that differs from the usual pattern of obsolescence (23). Rather than progressive shrinkage to form a small knot of basement membrane, the wrinkling appears to be arrested and incomplete (Fig. 16-5). The endothelium often appears swollen in affected areas and may be separated from the membrane by accumulations of electron-lucent material (Fig. 16-15). These accumulations may be distributed over entire loops or form localized aggregates, which are sometimes associated

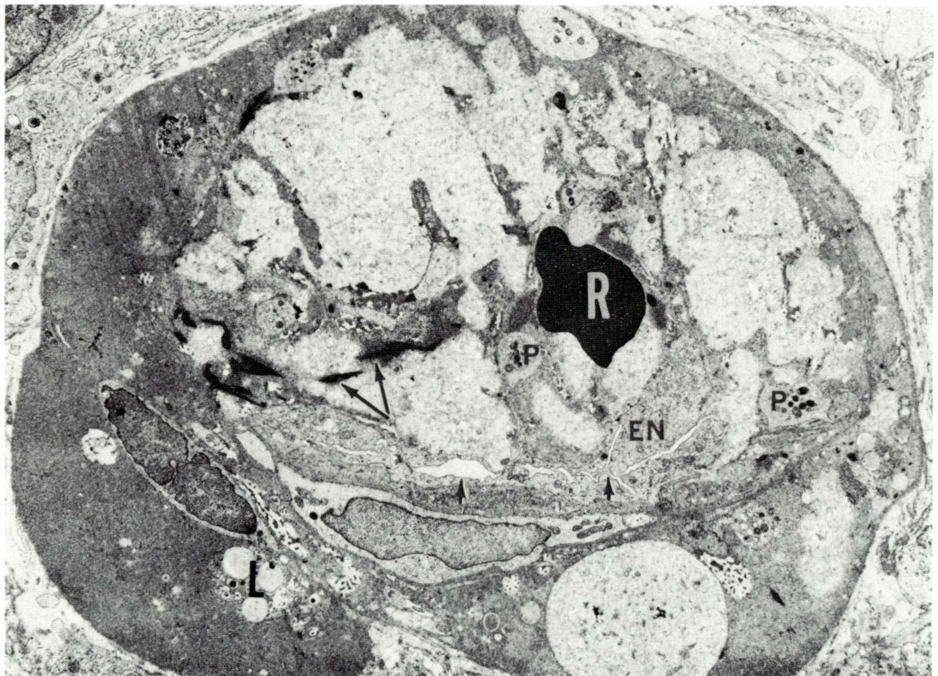

Figure 16-13. Electron micrograph of an afferent arteriole in malignant hypertension. There is accumulation of finely granular material of varying electron density in the subendothelial area and throughout the wall. Strands of fibrin (arrows), red blood cells (R), platelets (P), and lipid (L) are present at different levels of the vascular wall. The lumen is reduced to a narrow slitlike space (arrow heads). EN, endothelial cell (×5,500).

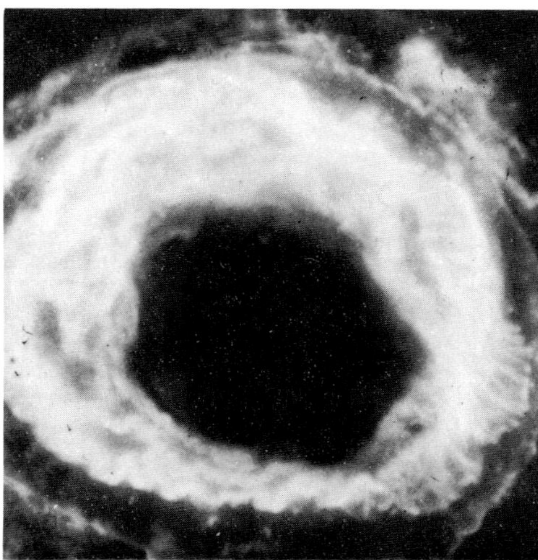

Figure 16-14. Malignant hypertension. Interlobular artery showing fluorescence with antifibrinogen serum (×350).

with endothelial disruption (23a). Replacement of this lucent deposit produces a corrugated and considerably thickened combined layer of new and old membrane. In addition to this diffuse pattern of ischemic damage, segmental lesions occur. These are either areas of apparent necrosis, in direct continuity with arteriolar lesions, or of proliferation (Fig. 16-12). The proliferative lesions may closely resemble segmental glomerulonephritis but are of a distinct "alterative" character (24). They are characterized by collapse of one or more loops with initial swelling and later proliferation of overlying epithelial cells to form small crescents. Ultrastructurally, these lesions may show collapse or there may be occlusion of loops by fibrin, platelets, red cells, and irregularly dense granular deposit (23) (Fig. 16-16). In some biopsy specimens, localized accentuation of the previously described diffuse ultrastructural changes produces intermediate patterns. Areas of subendothelial lucency merge into, or coexist with, larger foci of localized endothelial separation from the membrane by aggregates of fibrin, red cells, and granular material (23a) (Figs. 16-15, 16-16). These apparently intermediate stages suggest that the alterative changes result from direct capillary damage by elevated intraluminal pressure. The alterative changes gradually heal to form sclerotic segmental masses of collagen or matted membrane material with adhesions to Bowman's capsule and fibrocellular or fibrous crescents. As in the blood vessels, immunofluorescence microscopy may, occasionally, reveal a variety of reactions in the segmental lesions, most frequently fibrin, IgM, and complement components (Fig. 16-17).

DIFFERENTIAL DIAGNOSIS

The principal problem in the interpretation of benign hypertensive vascular disease is its differentiation from the normal changes occurring with increasing age. In arcuate and interlobular arteries, the distinction is essentially quantitative, the intimal changes being very similar but more impressive in hypertensive

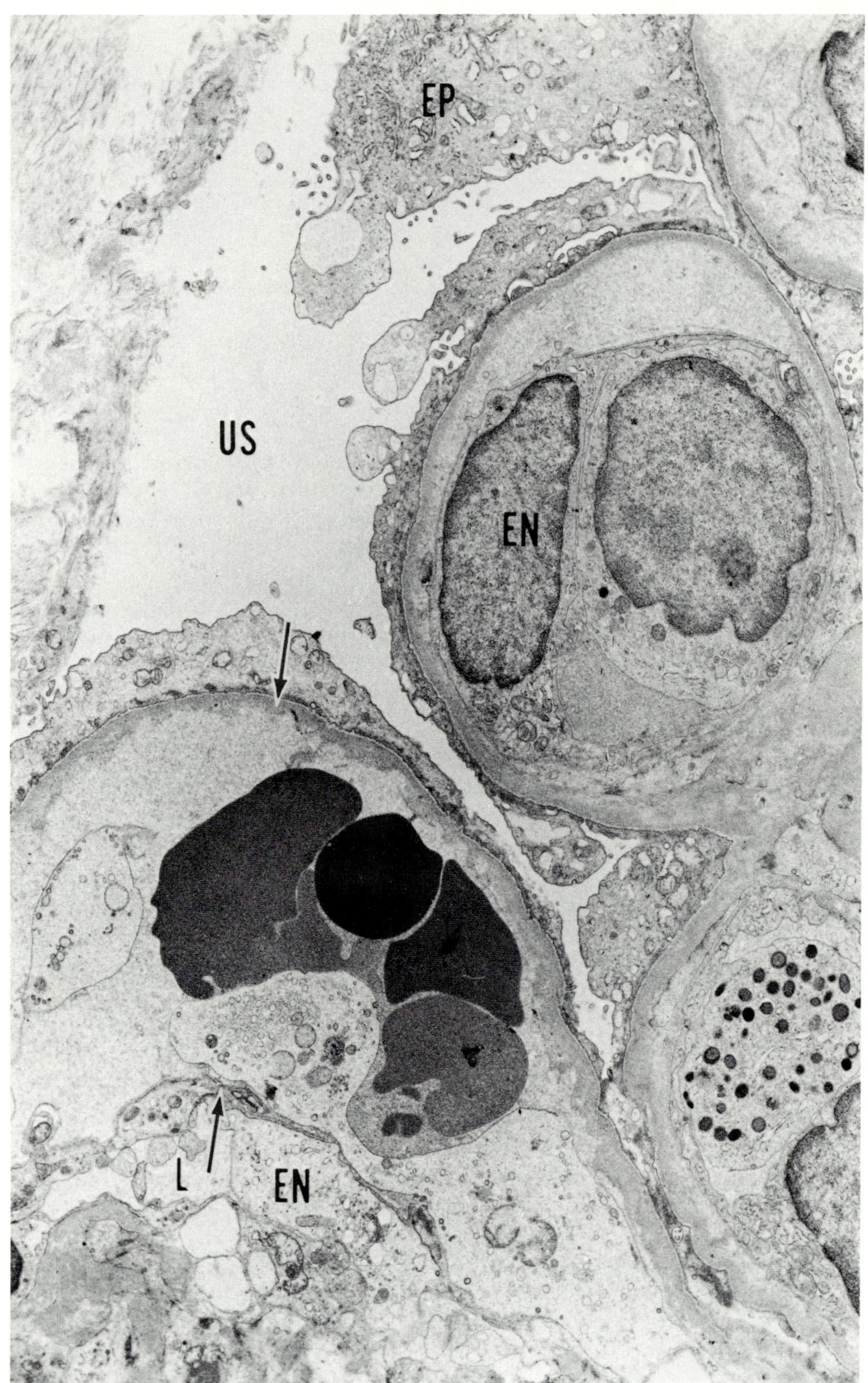

Figure 16-15. Portion of a glomerulus from a patient with malignant hypertension. The capillary walls show a wide electron-lucent zone in the endothelial side of the lamina densa (arrows), which contains finely electron-dense material, fragments of cell cytoplasm, and red blood cells. A few collagen fibrils are seen in the left upper corner. L, capillary lumen; EN, endothelial cell; EP, epithelial cell; US, urinary space (×7,500).

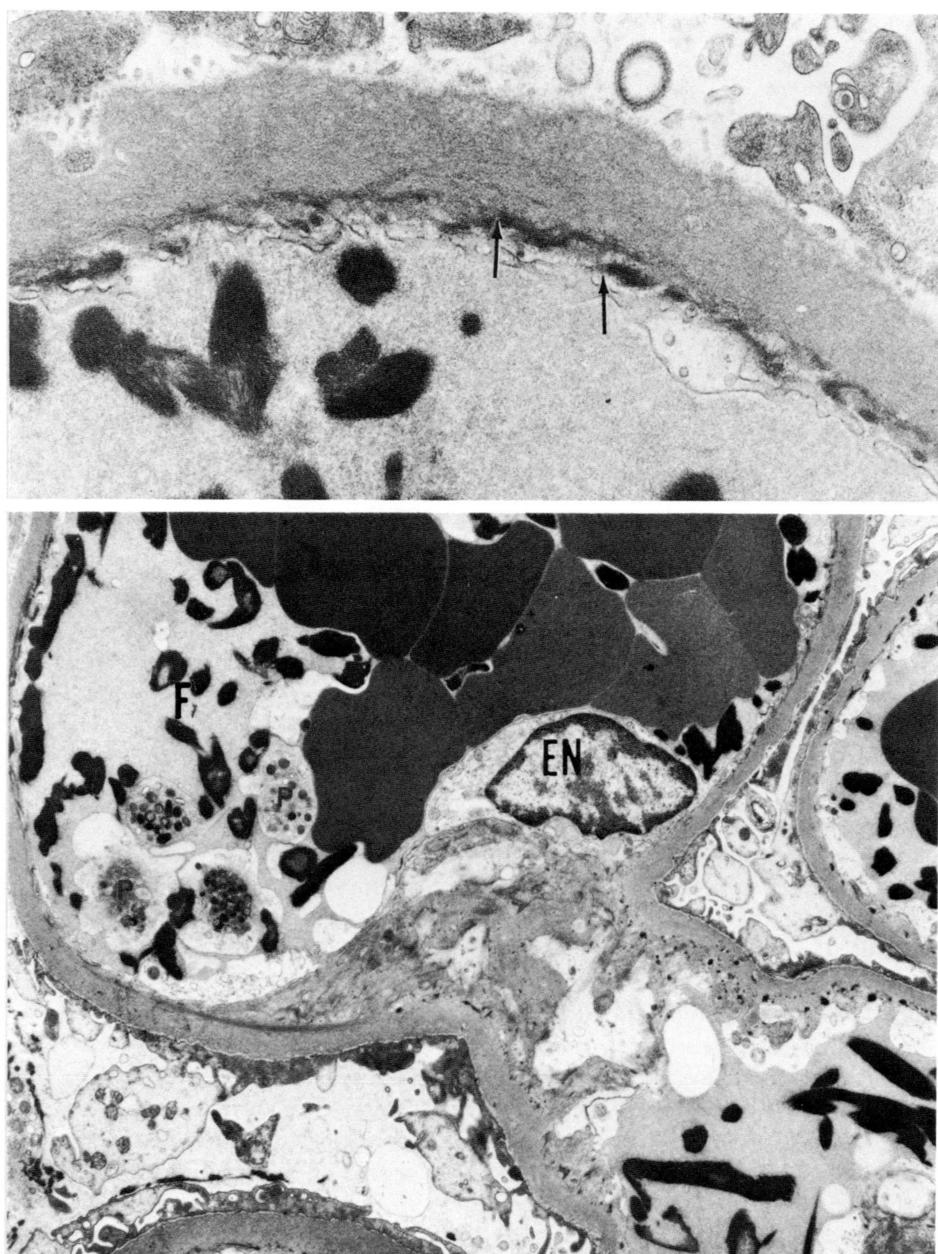

Figure 16-16. Numerous strands of fibrin (F) and platelets (P) in glomerular capillaries in malignant hypertension. Upper insert: higher-magnification electron micrograph demonstrating that while some of the fibrin strands are in the capillary lumen, others are in the subendothelial area (arrows). EN, endothelial cell (×8,000; insert, ×27,000).

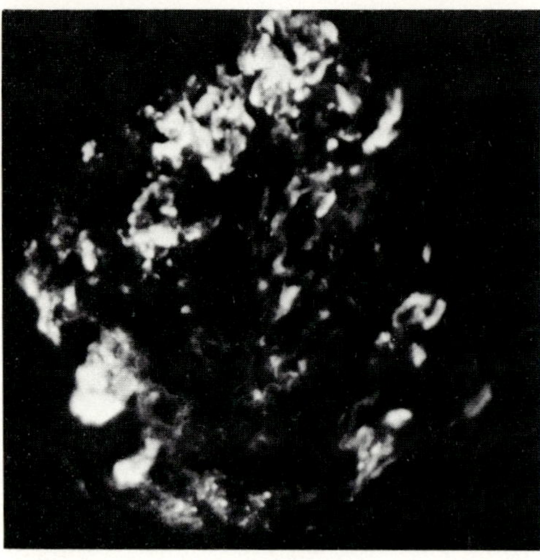

Figure 16-17. Immunofluorescence of malignant hypertension demonstrating segmental deposition of IgM (×320).

individuals. Arteriolar hyalinosis is highly suggestive of hypertension (29) in the absence of such diseases as diabetes mellitus, but there is not, in our experience, an absolute correlation between this appearance and blood pressure elevation. Nonetheless, in the assessment of renal biopsy specimens from patients with established hypertension, arteriolar hyalinosis can reasonably be accepted as a complication of the hypertensive state. The picture of malignant hypertension is, likewise, almost identical to that seen in scleroderma and the hemolytic uremic syndrome (30). There is usually no clinical difficulty in excluding scleroderma, but the presentations of malignant hypertension and the hemolytic uremic syndrome may be sufficiently similar to make absolute and universally accepted distinction between the two disorders almost impossible. In typical cases, the glomerular changes of the hemolytic uremic syndrome are characteristic enough to allow definite diagnosis. Occasionally, the necrotizing arteriolar lesions of malignant hypertension may be difficult to distinguish from necrotizing arteritis, but the absence of inflammation, distribution of lesions, and clinical features should allow differentiation. Finally, there may be great difficulty in deciding whether or not the glomerular changes in advanced and scarred malignant hypertension are secondary or the residua of intrinsic glomerular disease. The early "alterative" lesions are relatively characteristic, but the later sclerotic phase may very closely resemble that of advanced segmental glomerulonephritis with secondary hypertension. In such cases, immunofluorescence and electron microscopic data may be the only means of establishing a diagnosis of primary glomerulonephritis.

SECONDARY HYPERTENSION

The vascular effects of hypertension do not, in general, provide useful information about its cause. Detailed consideration of the various forms of secondary hypertension is beyond the scope of this text, but a few brief comments will be made about those conditions which particularly concern the kidney.

Renovascular Hypertension

Experimental production of hypertension by renal artery stenosis has been and remains the principal model for the study of the disease (31). In man, renal artery stenosis may be caused by atherosclerosis, dissection, or a variety of intimal, medial, or adventitial diseases that appear especially prone to affect renal arteries (32), although some also occur elsewhere (33). The pathogenesis of these peculiarly localized arterial diseases is unknown, but they may be bilateral and, by extension to intrarenal vessels, inoperable. Rarely, renal artery stenosis is produced by arterial involvement with neurofibromatosis (34), and stenotic changes in both major (35) and minor (36) renal arteries have been associated with oral contraceptive therapy. The affected kidney may show few changes but more often there is progressive tubular atrophy and glomerular coalescence in an "incomplete infarct" pattern (24). The arterial constriction protects the distal vessels from the effects of hypertension, but there is juxtaglomerular hyperplasia and increased renin secretion, which may be detected by differential sampling from the renal veins (6) (Figs. 16-18, 16-19). Quantitative assessment of juxtaglomerular hyperplasia is difficult in man, and the only real indication for percutaneous renal biopsy in these patients is to assess the degree of hypertensive vascular damage in the unprotected kidney (37). Treatment by nephrectomy, vascular repair, or autotransplantation cures or significantly improves the hypertension in a significant proportion of patients if proper selection procedures are used (38). Restoration of normal flow may cause striking enlargement of the affected kidney with reversal of the incomplete infarction pattern (39).

Radiation Nephritis

Severe hypertension may develop soon (40,41) or many years (42) after renal exposure to 2,300 or more rads of radiation within a four-week treatment period. Soon after irradiation there is a characteristic pattern of glomerular damage, caused by extensive subendothelial accumulation of lucent material, and arterioles show changes similar to those of malignant hypertension (40,41). Later, parenchymal atrophy develops, with extensive vascular thickening and juxtaglomerular hyperplasia, causing excessive renin release (42).

Chronic Renal Failure

Hypertension is common in chronic renal failure and may be very severe, especially when renal damage is the result of glomerular or vascular diseases (43). The pressure elevation may be dependent upon either excessive extracellular fluid volume or upon hyperreninemia (43), the latter probably related to juxtaglomerular hyperplasia (44). In extensively scarred kidneys, regardless of the cause of scarring, there is usually pronounced intimal thickening of larger arteries that is unrelated to hypertension and may represent a form of disuse atrophy (45,46).

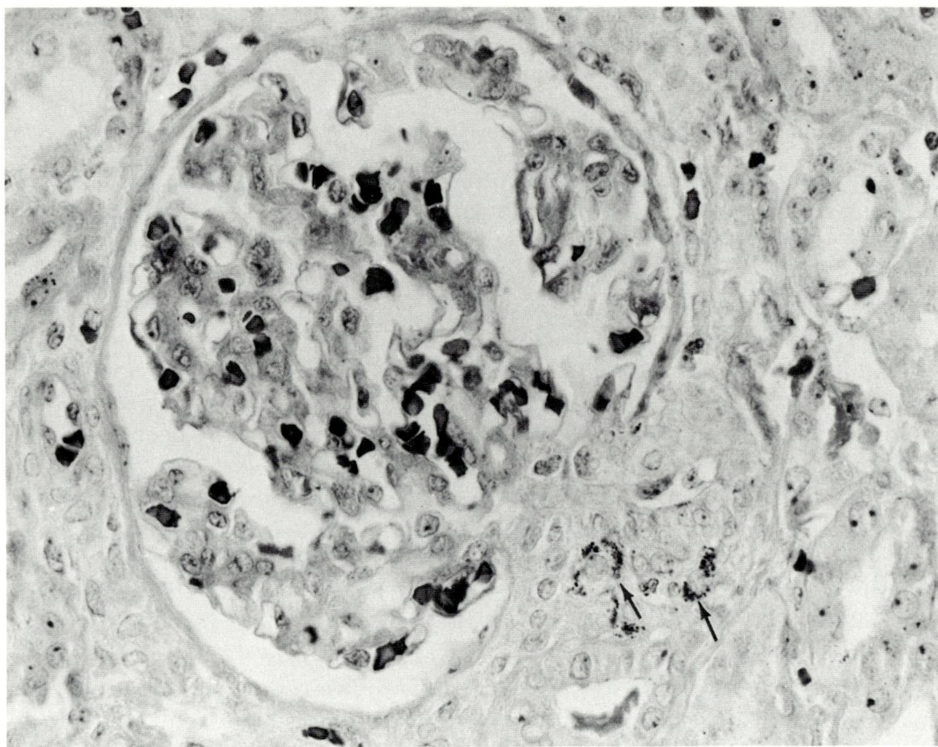

Figure 16-18. Hyperplastic juxtaglomerular apparatus from a patient with renal artery stenosis. Note renin granules (arrows) (Bowie's stain, ×600).

Adenoma of Juxtaglomerular Apparatus (Reninoma)

There are sparse, but steadily accumulating, reports of hypertension in young people caused by excessive renin secretion from tumors of the juxtaglomerular apparatus. The tumors have invariably been small and benign with a histologic pattern resembling hemangiopericytoma and abundant intracellular renin granules visible by electron microscopy (47). Accurate localization of the tumors is possible by segmental renal vein sampling, and preoperative diagnosis by needle biopsy is likely to be reported in the future.

SUMMARY

Hypertension may be caused by aberrations in many systems. The kidney is pivotal in the normal maintenance of most of these systems and renal disease is, therefore, an important cause of hypertension. Conversely, prolonged elevation of arterial blood pressure causes renal vascular damage with distal tissue effects that may propagate hypertension from other causes and can lead to renal failure. The vascular changes are the result of increased endothelial permeability, which allows transudation of plasma constituents. Inspissation of these constituents produces a variety of patterns, particularly in arterioles, which are

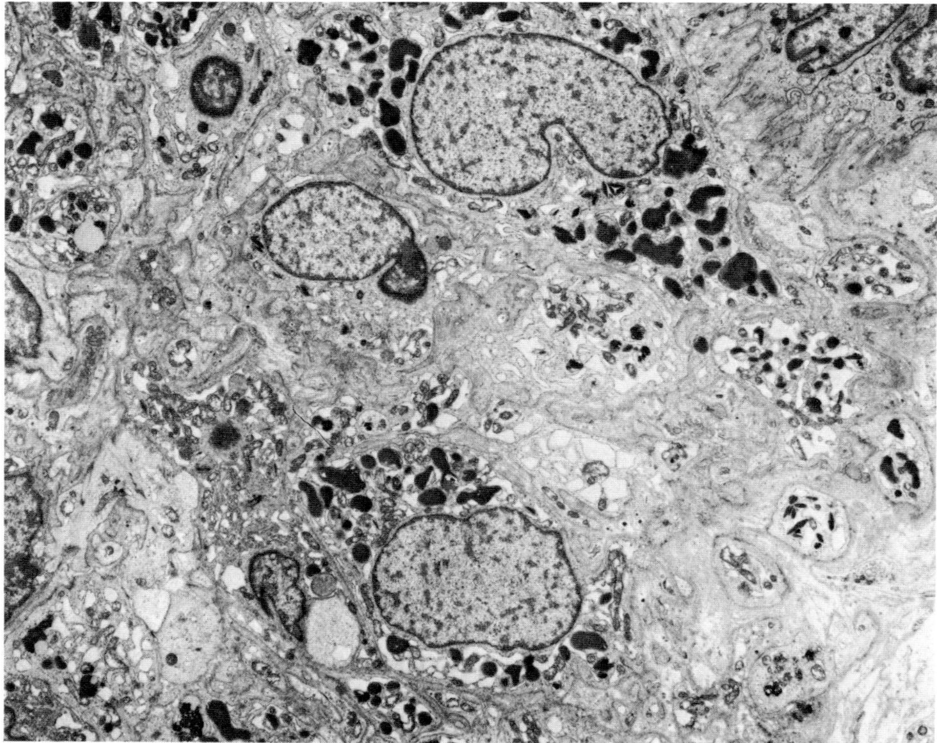

Figure 16-19. Electron micrograph of the juxtaglomerular apparatus from the same case as in Figure 16-18, showing granular cells containing numerous renin granules (×2,600).

characteristic of,but not diagnostic for, hypertensive vascular disease. Morphologic diagnosis may be straightforward in severe hypertension, but the vascular changes can be mimicked by several other diseases. Glomerular lesions occur in some hypertensive patients, and differentiation between chronic glomerulonephritis and hypertensive damage may be difficult when damage is advanced, with extensive scarring. The term *nephrosclerosis* has been used traditionally to encompass all of these changes but is better avoided and replaced by a more precise description of the lesions encountered.

REFERENCES

1. Wilber JA, Barrow JG: Hypertension—a community problem. *Am J Med* 52:653, 1972.
2. Fry J: Natural history of hypertension: a case for selective nontreatment. *Lancet* 2:431, 1974.
3. Pitcock JA, Johnson JG, Hatch FE, et al: Malignant hypertension in blacks: malignant intrarenal arterial disease as observed by light and electron microscopy. *Human Pathol* 7:333, 1976.
4. Pickering G: Hypertension: definitions, natural histories and consequences. *Am J Med* 52:570, 1972.
5. Kincaid-Smith P, McMichael J, Murphy EA: The clinical course and pathology of hypertension with papilloedema (malignant hypertension). *Quart J Med* 27:117, 1958.
6. Oparil S, Haber E: The renin-angiotensin system. *N Engl J Med* 291:389, 446, 1974.
7. Muirhead EE, Germain GS, Armstrong FB, et al: Endocrine-type antihypertensive function of renomedullary interstitial cells. *Kidney Int* 8:S-271, 1975.

8. Guyton AC, Coleman TG, Cowley AW Jr, et al: Arterial pressure regulation: overriding dominance of the kidneys in long-term regulation and in hypertension. *Am J Med* 52:584, 1972.

9. Tucker RM, Labarthe DR: Frequency of surgical treatment for hypertension in adults at the Mayo Clinic from 1973 through 1975. *Mayo Clin Proc* 52:549, 1977.

10. Hollenberg NK, Borucki LJ, Adams DF: The renal vasculature in early essential hypertension. *Medicine (Balt)* 57:167, 1978.

11. Platt R: Heredity in hypertension. *Lancet* 1:889, 1963.

12. Brown JJ, Lever AF, Robertson JIS, et al: Pathogenesis of essential hypertension, hypothesis. *Lancet* 1:1217, 1976.

13. Beilin LJ, Goldby FS, Möhring J: High arterial pressure versus humoral factors in the pathogenesis of the vascular lesions of malignant hypertension: the care for pressure alone and the care for humoral factors as well as pressure. *Clin Sci Molec Med* 52:111, 1977.

14. Lendrum AC: Deposition of plasmatic substances in vessel walls. *Path Microbiol* 30:681, 1967.

15. Wilson C, Byrom FB: The vicious circle in chronic Bright's disease. Experimental evidence from the hypertensive rat. *Quart J Med* 10:65, 1941.

16. Sevitt LH, Evans DJ, Wrong OM: Acute oliguric renal failure due to accelerated (malignant) hypertension. *Quart J Med* 40:127, 1971.

17. Gavras H, Brown WCB, Brown JJ, et al: Microangiopathic hemolytic anemia and the development of the malignant phase of hypertension. *Circ Res* 29 (suppl 11):127, 1971.

18. Woods JW, Blythe WB, Huffines WD: Management of malignant hypertension complicated by renal insufficiency: a follow-up study. *N Engl J Med* 241:10, 1974.

18a. Petersen VP, Olsen TS, Kissmeyer-Nielsen F, et al: Late failure of human renal transplants: an analysis of transplant disease and graft failure among 125 recipients surviving for one to eight years. *Medicine (Balt)* 54:45, 1975.

19. Tracy RE, Toca VT: Nephrosclerosis and blood pressure: II. Reversibility of proliferative arteriosclerosis. *Lab Invest* 30:30, 1974.

20. McManus JFA, Lupton CH Jr: Ischemic obsolescence of renal glomeruli: the natural history of the lesions and their relation to hypertension. *Lab Invest* 9:413, 1960.

21. Nagle RB, Kohnen PW, Bulger RE, et al: Ultrastructure of human renal obsolescent glomeruli. *Lab Invest* 21:519, 1969.

22. Hara M, Meyer D, Bohle A: The glomerular mesangium in hypertension: a morphometric comparison of nephrosclerosis with mesangioproliferative glomerulonephritis on renal biopsies. *Virchows Arch (A) Path Anat Histol* 368:275, 1975.

23. Jones DB: Arterial and glomerular lesions associated with severe hypertension: light and electron microscopic studies. *Lab Invest* 31:303, 1974.

23a. Shigematsu H, Dikman SH, Churg J, et al: Glomerular injury in malignant nephrosclerosis. *Nephron* 22:399, 1978.

24. Kimmelstiel P, Wilson C: Benign and malignant hypertension and nephrosclerosis: a clinical and pathologic study. *Am J Pathol* 12:45, 1936.

25. Sinclair RA, Antonovych TT, Mostofi FK: Renal proliferative arteriopathies and associated glomerular changes: a light and electron microscopic study. *Human Pathol* 7:565, 1976.

26. Kincaid-Smith P: Participation of intravascular coagulation in the pathogenesis of glomerular and vascular lesions. *Kidney Int* 7:242, 1975.

27. Hoyer JR, Michael AR, Hoyer LW: Immunofluorescent localization of antihemophilic factor antigen and fibrinogen in human renal diseases. *J Clin Invest* 53:1375, 1974.

28. Gerber MA, Paronetto F: New patterns of immunoglobulin deposition in the lesion of malignant nephrosclerosis, with special reference to IgE. *Am J Pathol* 65:535, 1971.

29. Allen AC: *The Kidney: Medical and Surgical Diseases,* ed 2. London, J A and Churchill Ltd, 1962, p 564.

30. Bohle A, Helmchen U, Grund KE, et al: Malignant nephrosclerosis in patients with hemolytic uremic syndrome (primary malignant nephrosclerosis). *Current Topics Pathol* 65:81, 1977.

31. Gordon DB: Some early investigations of experimental hypertension—an historical review. *Texas Rep Biol Med* 23:3, 1970.

32. Harrison EG Jr, McCormack LJ: Pathologic classification of renal arterial disease in renovascular hypertension. *Mayo Clin Proc* 46:161, 1971.

33. Claiborne TS: Fibromuscular hyperplasia: report of a case with involvement of multiple arteries. *Am J Med* 49:103, 1970.

34. Grad E, Rance CP: Bilateral renal artery stenosis in association with neurofibromatosis (Recklinghausen's disease): report of two cases. *J Pediat* 80:804, 1972.

35. Delin K, Aurell M, Claes G, et al: Multiple arterial occlusions and hypertension probably caused by an oral contraceptive: a patient in whom the development of renovascular hypertension has been followed. *Clin Nephrol* 6:453, 1976.

36. Irey NS, Norris HJ: Intimal vascular lesions associated with female reproduction steroids. *Arch Pathol* 96:227, 1973.

37. Vertes V, Grawel JA, Goldblatt H: Renal arteriography, separate renal function studies and renal biopsy in human hypertension: selection of patients for surgical treatment. *N Engl J Med* 270:656, 1964.

38. Maxwell MH: Cooperative study of renovascular hypertension: current status. *Kidney Int* 8:S-153, 1964.

39. Morgan TO: Renal artery surgery for renal failure and hypertension. *Kidney Int* 8:S-161, 1975.

40. Keane WF, Crosson JT, Staley NA, et al: Radiation-induced renal disease: a clinicopathologic study. *Am J Med* 60:127, 1976.

41. Kapur S, Chandra R, Antonovych T: Acute radiation nephritis: light and electron microscopic observations. *Arch Pathol Lab Med* 101;469, 1977.

42. Shapiro AT, Cavallo T, Cooper W, et al: Hypertension in radiation nephritis: report of a patient with unilateral disease, elevated renin activity levels, and reversal after unilateral nephrectomy. *Arch Intern Med* 137:848, 1977.

43. Weidmann P, Maxwell MH: The renin-angiotensin-aldosterone system in terminal renal failure. *Kidney Int* 8:S-219, 1975.

44. Cain H, Kraus B: The juxtaglomerular apparatus in malignant hypertension of man. *Virchows Arch A Path Anat Histol* 372:11, 1976.

45. Heptinstall RH: Pathology of end-stage kidney disease. *Am J Med* 44:656, 1968.

46. Tolnai G, Sarkar K, Jaworski ZF, et al: Obliterative intimal fibrosis in kidneys of dialyzed patients. *Canad Med Ass J* 100:116, 1969.

47. Bonnin JM, Cain MD, Jose JS, et al: Hypertension due to a renin-secreting tumor localized by segmental renal vein sampling. *Aust NZ J Med* 7:630, 1977.

17
Renal Disease in Pregnancy

The changes in renal physiology that accompany pregnancy may alter the manifestations of preexisting renal diseases. In particular, hypertension frequently complicates underlying glomerulonephritis, and there may be an increase in the degree of proteinuria. These exaggerations in the expressions of existing renal disorders have created difficulty in the definition of a specifically gestational disease, preeclampsia (PET). Because of clinical similarities between patients with chronic hypertension, glomerulonephritis, and PET there has been prolonged controversy over the incidence and prognosis of gestational hypertension (1). The demonstration of a characteristic glomerular lesion ("endotheliosis") by electron microscopy in patients with PET (2) has allowed careful prospective studies of the prevalence and behavior of the disease. This chapter outlines the methods for differentiating PET from other forms of gestational hypertension and briefly considers some of the other renal disorders that may occur during pregnancy.

CLASSIFICATION OF GESTATIONAL HYPERTENSION

The Terminology Committee of the American College of Obstetricians and Gynecologists has proposed a subdivision of gestational hypertension into four categories (3):

1. *Preeclampsia and Eclampsia.* PET is defined as hypertension with associated proteinuria or edema developing after the twentieth week of gestation; eclampsia describes the superimposition of convulsions upon this syndrome. In the third trimester, hypertension can be defined either as a sustained elevation of blood pressure over 140/85 mmHg or as an increase of over previous recorded pressures of 30 mmHg systolic or 15mmHg diastolic.

2. *Chronic Hypertension.* Established hypertension, whether primary or secondary, may be diagnosed before or early in pregnancy and continues after parturition.

3. *Chronic Hypertension with Superimposed PET.* The occurrence of the PET syndrome in a multiparous woman is suggestive of underlying chronic hypertension. The syndrome may be atypical with an accelerated pattern of increasing

316

blood pressure, oliguria, evidence of intravascular coagulation and, in some patients, the development of eclampsia. Whether or not the accelerated syndrome occurs, features of PET are likely to recur in each pregnancy of those women with chronic hypertension who show this tendency.

4. *Late or Transient Hypertension.* Transient blood pressure elevation, with or without other features of PET, may occur during consecutive pregnancies with no evidence of hypertension in between. The relationship of this clinical phenomenon to an underlying hypertensive diathesis in these women is unknown, and their long-term prognosis is not certain.

PREECLAMPSIA AND ECLAMPSIA

Incidence and Clinical Manifestations

PET is a disease of first pregnancies, 74% of cases occurring in primipara (4). The precise incidence of the disease is uncertain, because of differences in its definition, but 5–7% of first pregnancies in the United States may be affected (5). There is a clear familial tendency, although the genetic character of this is unknown (6), and PET occurs commonly in twin pregnancies (7) and in those complicated by hydatidiform mole or Rh incompatibility (8). The development of hypertension and proteinuria earlier than the twentieth week of pregnancy is a clear indication to consider either molar pregnancy or fetal hydrops (3). The onset is typically insidious with the gradual onset of edema, headaches, and visual symptoms. Although considerable emphasis was previously placed on excessive weight gain and edema, these features are now regarded as unrelated to the PET syndrome, and diagnosis requires the demonstration of hypertension and proteinuria (9). The proteinuria, which is usually of intermediate selectivity (10), is occasionally sufficient to cause the nephrotic syndrome, and PET is the major cause of the nephrotic syndrome during late pregnancy (11,12). Hypertension is usually moderate in degree but, especially in eclamptic patients, may be severe and progressive, requiring urgent therapeutic intervention.

Pathogenesis

Theories of the pathogenesis of PET abound, but no single mechanism is as yet established, and no completely satisfactory experimental model has been developed (13). The available evidence strongly favors an increase in systemic arterial reactivity with a continuous state of intravascular coagulation, each related to placental degeneration. Careful prospective studies suggest that hypertension develops earlier than previously accepted in patients with PET (14), and an exaggerated response to angiotensin can be demonstrated before the appearance of the typical clinical features (15). The pathogenesis of this altered vascular response is unknown, but the rapid resolution of hypertension after parturition strongly favors a central role for the uteroplacental unit. Renin and prostaglandins are concentrated in this region, and either augmented secretion or increased release could result from ischemia caused by the degenerative vascular changes that have been demonstrated in the placental bed early in pregnancy

(8,16). A range of coagulation abnormalities occurs in patients with PET, probably caused by thromboplastin release from the ischemic placenta (17–19). The vasospastic effects of persistent intravascular coagulation may contribute to the hypertension of PET, and mesangial uptake of fibrin products could produce the typical glomerular changes (18). There is good evidence for fibrin deposition in both the glomeruli (19) and liver (20) of patients with PET, and intravascular coagulation appears to be the major cause of many of the tissue complications of eclampsia (17).

Recently, there has been speculation that alterations in the immune relationship between mother and fetus may be implicated in the pathogenesis of PET. Immunofluorescence microscopy has demonstrated deposits of immunoglobulins and complement in glomeruli (21), liver (20), and placental bed (16,22), and circulating immune complexes have been detected in one study (23). Serum complement concentrations are, however, usually normal or even increased (21), and there is, as yet, insufficient evidence to support a humoral immune pathogenesis. Similarly, while occasional cases of striking genetic heterogeneity have suggested that genotypic differences between mother and child may stimulate immune reactions (24), studies of larger groups have not supported this concept (6,7). The special nature of the maternofetal homograft suggests, nonetheless, that immune factors are likely to contribute to PET, and further studies are necessary to elucidate the immune functions of pregnant women with and without the disease.

Pathologic Characteristics

There is general agreement about the typical renal changes of PET but continued uncertainty about the range and frequency of these changes. Prospective studies suggest that the lesion may be both minimal and irregularly distributed in some patients (25), but selective biopsy series, which necessarily sample only those patients with atypical or unusually severe disease, outline a more florid glomerular pattern. There is a rough correlation between the severity of the clinical syndrome and the morphologic changes and, since most biopsy specimens from laboratories not especially involved with prospective investigation will be from patients with severe disease, the emphasis here is upon the more florid morphologic features.

Light Microscopy

The glomeruli are enlarged and bloodless with thickened capillary walls and a characteristic pattern of longitudinal capillary collapse, producing cigar-shaped lobules (21,25,26). This collapse pattern is produced by intense cellular swelling, which is best seen in PAS- and PASM-stained sections and is associated with more or less widespread mesangial interposition but no significant increase in matrix (Fig. 17-1). The increase in capillary wall width is an effect of both the collapse and the interposition, wire loops and spikes being absent. Cellular swelling is usually regular throughout all glomeruli, but may be focally distributed in very mild disease, and sometimes has a multivesicular appearance, occasionally with scattered foam cells (Fig. 17-2). There is some controversy over the presence or absence of proliferation in the glomeruli of PET, but the most severe lesions

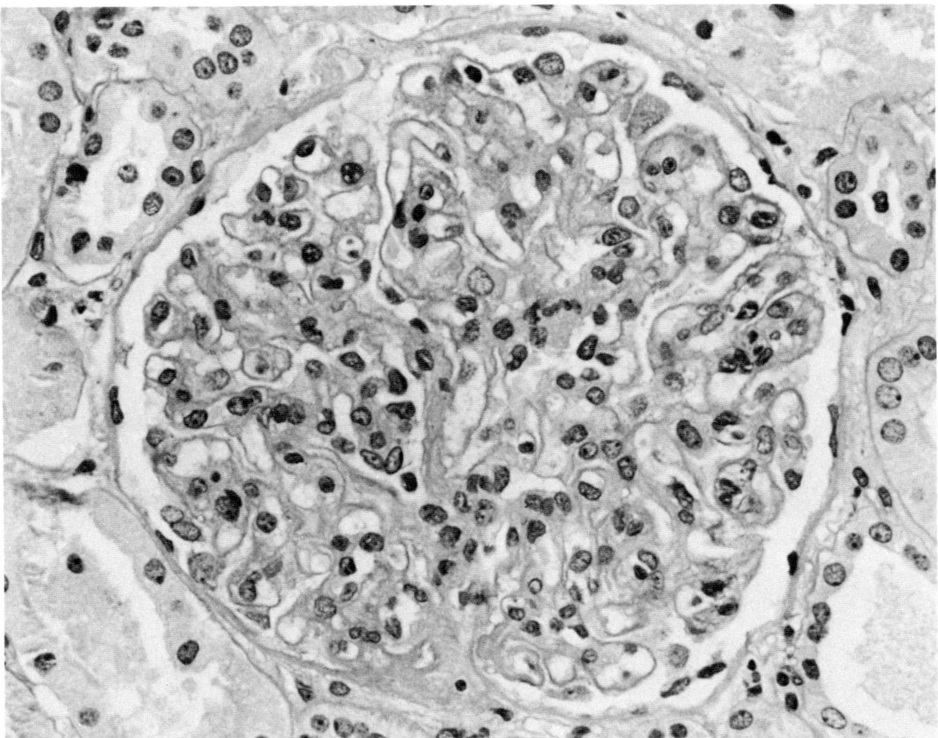

Figure 17-1. Preeclamptic nephropathy. The glomerulus is swollen and bloodless (PAS stain, ×500).

show undoubted hypercellularity and may mimic a proliferative glomerulonephritis. The swollen glomerular tufts sometimes pout into the proximal tubule, and there may be apparent enlargement of the juxtaglomerular apparatus, but no significant extraglomerular changes occur (Fig. 17-2). If vascular or other disease can be seen, the possibility of PET being superimposed on another disease must be seriously considered.

Electron Microscopy
There is striking mesangial cytoplasmic hypertrophy with minimal increase in matrix. Although these hypertrophic changes were originally considered to be endothelial ("endotheliosis"), it is now clear that the endothelial cells are much less affected than those in the mesangium (Fig. 17-3). These cells become considerably enlarged, with frequent and prominent organelles, and extend beneath the endothelium to produce the mesangial interposition seen by light microscopy (Fig. 17-4). While usually diffuse, the cellular changes in patients with very mild disease may be irregularly distributed, and their recognition may require careful examination of several glomeruli (25). There is frequently abundant lipid within these reactive cells, sometimes with cholesterol clefts (Figs. 17-5—17-7). Deposits are usually found in mesangial and subendothelial regions and have a characteristic mottled appearance (Fig. 17-6). Within each deposit, areas of relative

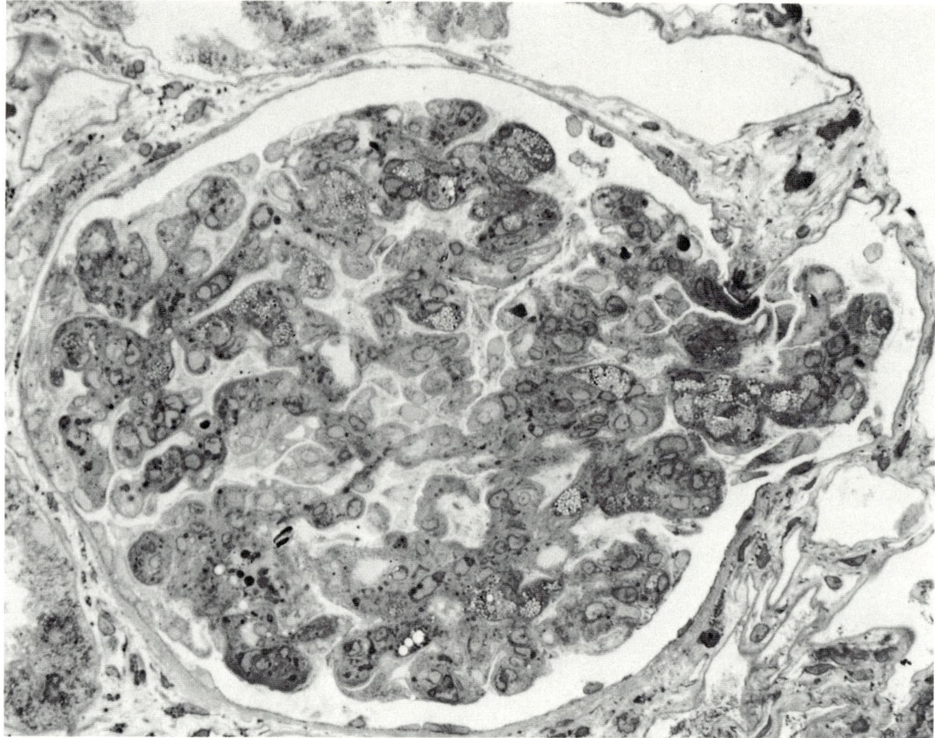

Figure 17-2. Glomerulus from a patient with severe preeclampsia. The capillary lumina are encroached upon by swollen endothelial and mesangial cells. Note prominent vacuolization of these cells and herniation of the tuft into the proximal tubule (plastic embedded toluidine blue stain, ×670).

lucency alternate with very dense areas, and there may be scattered fibrils or distinct tactoids of included fibrin (Fig. 17-8).

Immunofluorescence Microscopy

There is controversy about the immunofluorescent findings in PET, probably reflecting differences in the severity of the diseases studied by various groups. Most studies describe granular reactions for fibrin along capillary walls (19), and these have been associated with diffuse deposits of IgM and complement (21). Other workers, however, have found reactions for each of these reagents in less than half of the patients examined (25,27). When present, the reactions are finely granular and, although diffuse, may show some variation in intensity between individual loops (Fig. 17-9).

Evolution and Differential Diagnosis

Although there are few sequential biopsy studies of the glomerular lesions in PET, there is good evidence that the lesions resolve rapidly within a month of parturition. Biopsy specimens taken six months or more later show only mild,

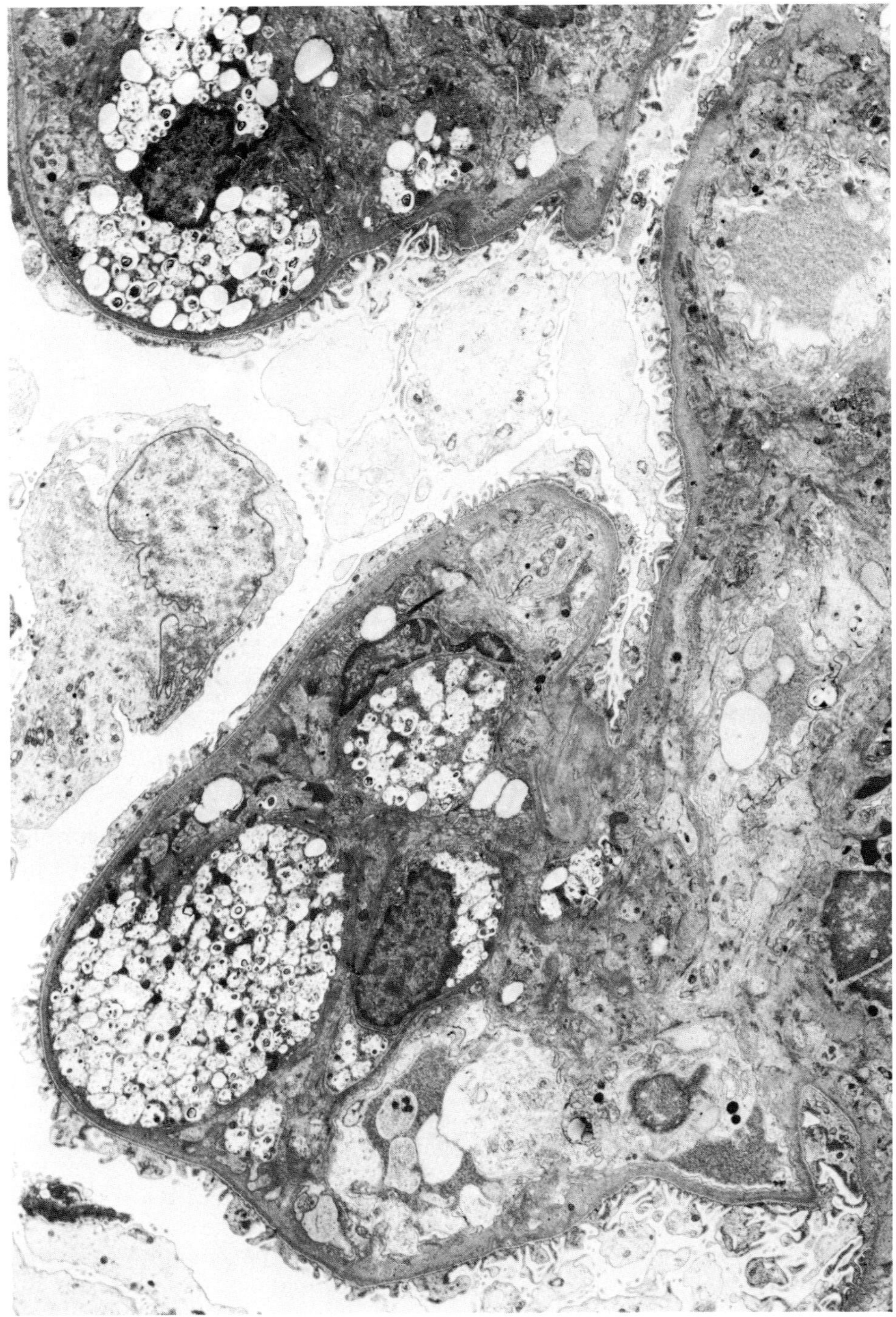

Figure 17-3. Electron micrograph of vacuolated areas as seen in Figure 17-2, showing mesangial prominence and containing numerous collections of lipid (×4,200).

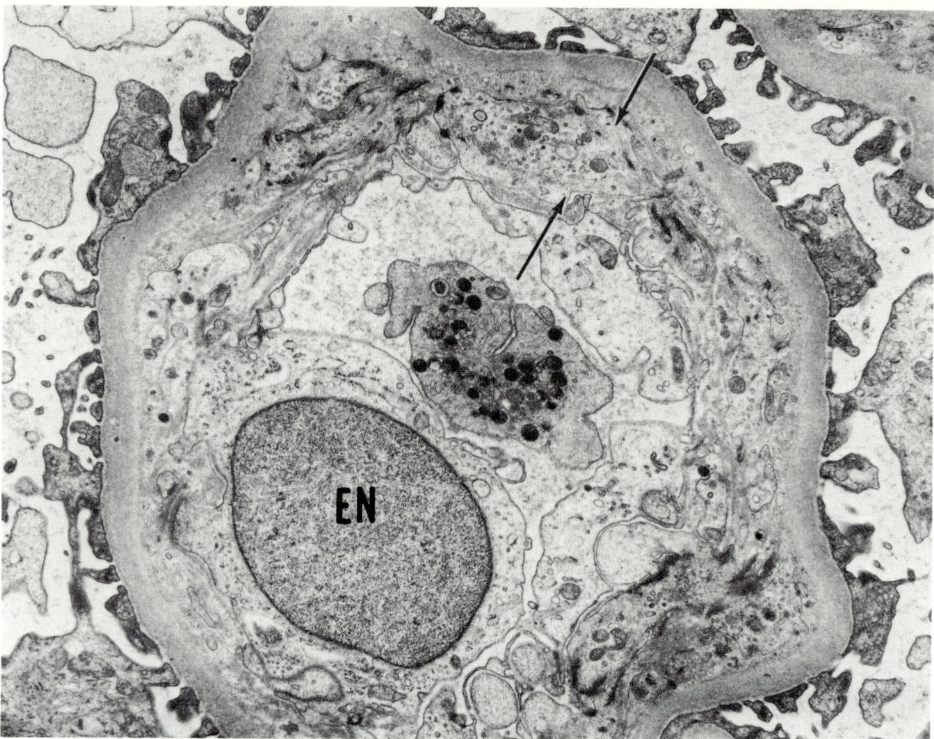

Figure 17-4. The capillary lumen, reduced by endothelial swelling and extensive mesangial interposition (arrows). EN, endothelial cell (×8,000).

residual mesangial proliferation (21). Rarely, reversible mesangial hypertrophy persists for some months postpartum, and such cases may be extremely difficult to distinguish from proliferative glomerulonephritis (21,28). A variety of glomerular disorders may be complicated during pregnancy by mesangial changes similar to those in PET, and specific diagnosis may, occasionally, be difficult if the biopsy specimen is taken before these changes regress. In typical cases, the PET lesion can be distinguished by the absence of excessive matrix and the mottled character of the deposits. On rare occasions, serial biopsies may be necessary to establish the nature of a particular glomerular lesion, but continuation of hypertension and proteinuria for more than one month after parturition is strong evidence against a diagnosis of PET.

Prognosis

The prolonged debate over the long-term outlook for patients with PET was largely due to the admixture of other causes for gestational hypertension. By examining a large group of patients with a more clearly defined clinical syndrome, eclampsia, Chesley et al. have demonstrated that the eventual prognosis differs little from that of women following normal pregnancies (29). Generally, both clinical and morphologic phenomena disappear within a month from parturition, and there is no increased risk of either chronic hypertension or other

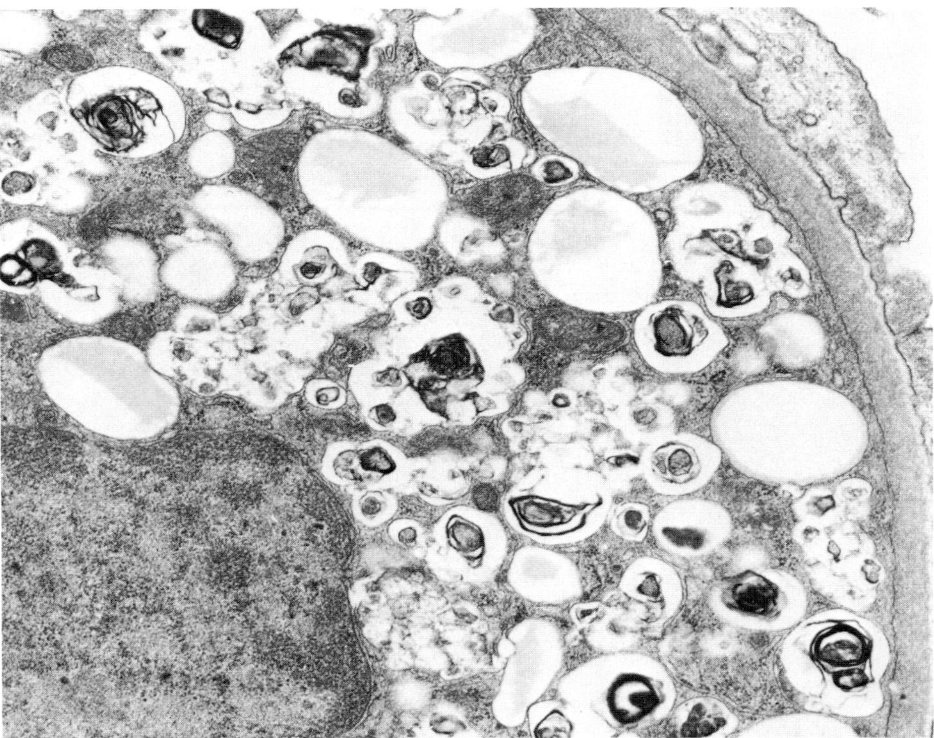

Figure 17-5. Higher magnification demonstrating membranous structures of different densities, some of which have the appearance of myelinlike figures (×21,000).

renal disease. Either hypertension or the complete PET syndrome may recur in the subsequent pregnancies of up to one-third of affected women but, even in this group, the long-term outlook appears to be favorable.

OTHER RENAL DISEASES IN PREGNANCY

A wide variety of renal diseases may be coincidentally associated with pregnancy, but a real association has been demonstrated only with renal cortical necrosis and with a form of the hemolytic-uremic syndrome that is discussed elsewhere (see p 286). Cortical necrosis, although extremely rare, is especially associated with pregnancy and has frequently followed acute placental separation. The condition has generally been attributed to a Schwartzman-like reaction with disseminated intravascular coagulation, but coagulopathic features cannot always be demonstrated and the precise pathogenesis is unknown (30,31). Renal failure in patients with cortical necrosis is usually irreversible, in contrast to the rapid recovery seen after other forms of acute renal failure associated with pregnancy, and the diagnosis should be considered when oliguria is unusually prolonged (32). Some forms of chronic glomerular disease, especially lupus glomerulonephritis and membranous nephropathy, may exacerbate or progress rapidly during pregnancy (33), and careful observation is always necessary if a pregnant

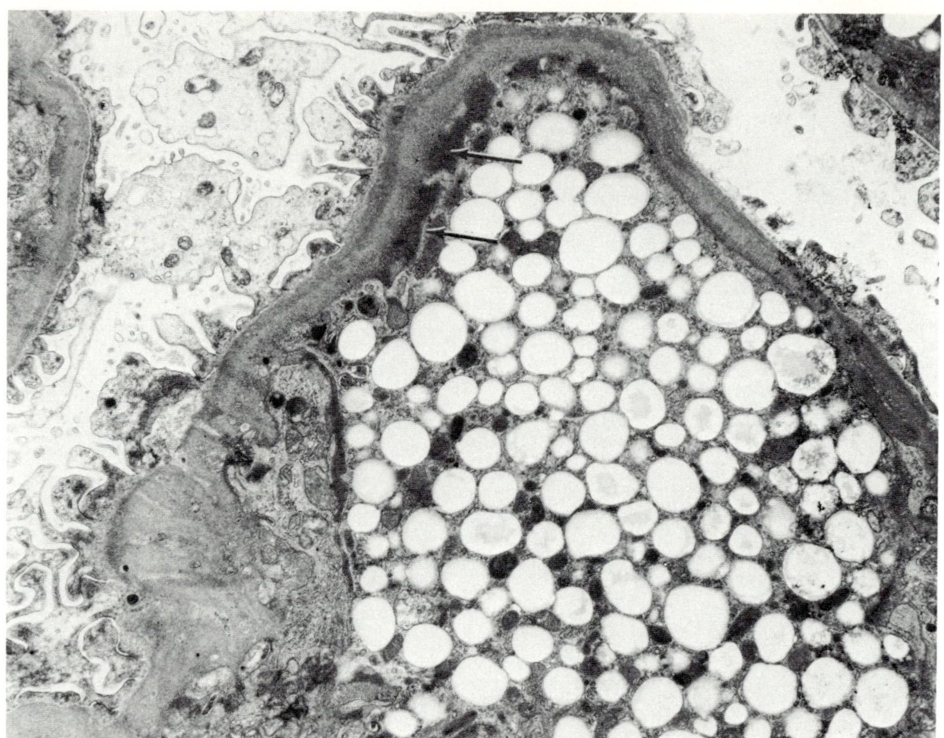

Figure 17-6. Numerous lipid-containing vacuoles in the swollen endothelial cell. Note the presence of electron-dense material in the subendothelial area (arrows) (×6,200).

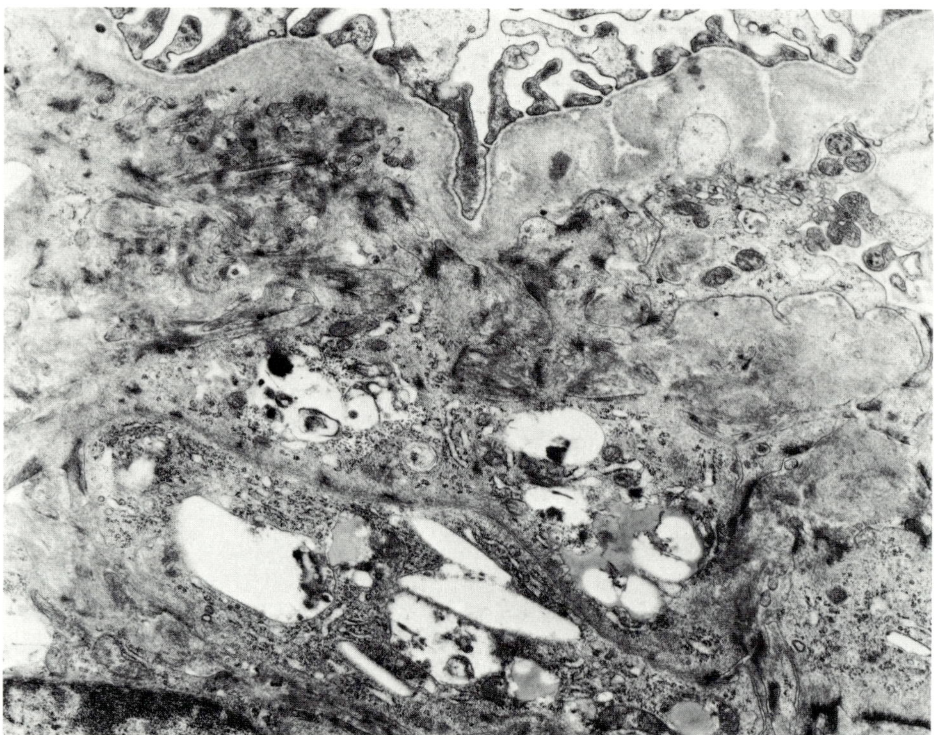

Figure 17-7. Electron micrograph demonstrating prominent mesangium and cholesterol clefts (×10,000).

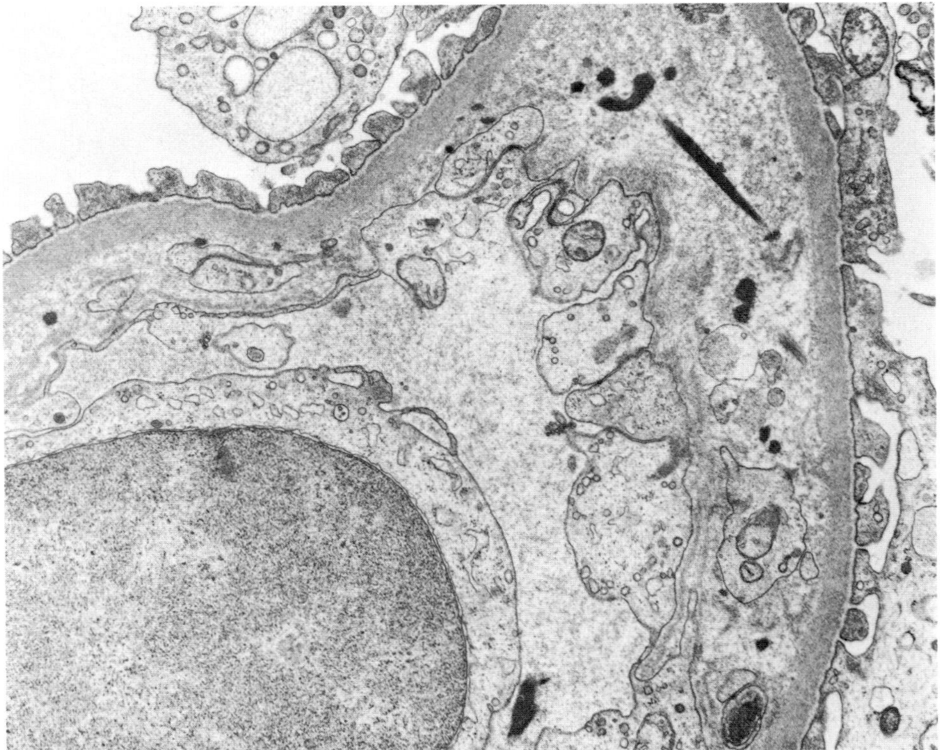

Figure 17-8. Translucent subendothelial zone containing loose electron-dense material and tactoids of fibrin ($\times$ 12,500).

patient has known renal disease. The majority of patients with known glomerular lesions, however, show no significant deterioration during pregnancy, providing that reasonable care is taken with management (34). There is a voluminous literature on the relationship between pregnancy and infectious renal disease, but the only significant difference from nonpregnant women appears to be a greater propensity for acute pyelonephritis in those pregnant women with documented urinary infection (32).

SUMMARY

Preeclampsia is one of several causes of hypertension during pregnancy. The pathogenesis of the condition is unknown, but there is evidence to suggest that altered vascular reactivity and persistent intravascular coagulation are implicated in the production of hypertension and glomerular disease. Each of these pathogenetic factors appears to be closely related to placental degeneration, possibly ischemic in nature, and the greatly increased incidence in first pregnancies suggests that disturbances in the maternofetal immune relationship may be involved. The glomerular lesion is characteristic, although there is uncertainty over the frequency and specificity of immunofluorescence reactions for fibrin, immunoglobulins, and complement. Mesangial cell hypertrophy causes reduc-

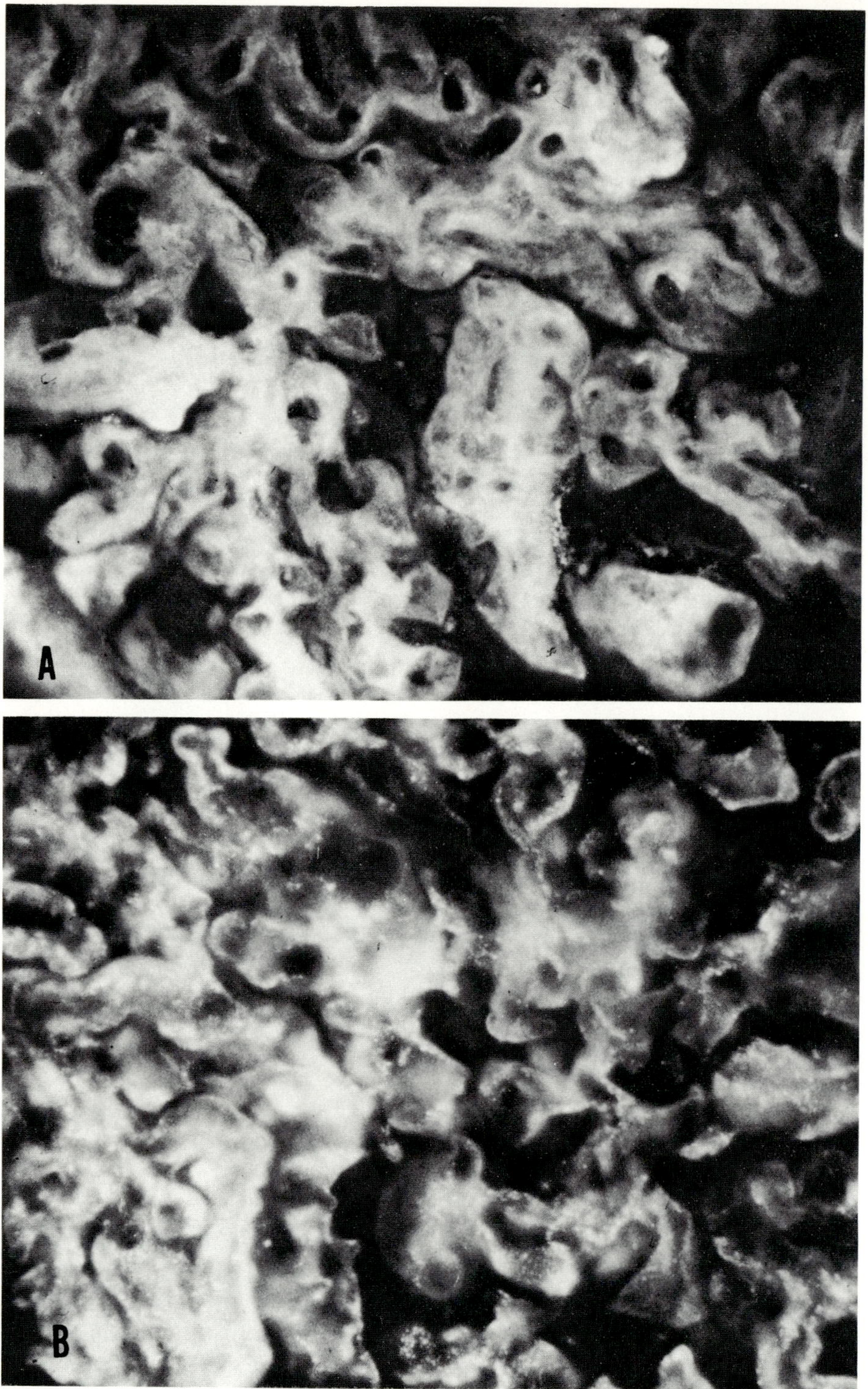

Figure 17-9. (*a*) Glomerulus from a patient with severe preeclamptic nephropathy, showing fluorescence with antiserum to fibrinogen. The distribution is along the inside of the loops. (*b*) Peripheral granular staining for IgM (×900).

tion in capillary vascularity and is associated with mottled deposits, which may contain recognizable fibrin. The clinical and morphologic features resolve rapidly after parturition, and there are no long-term sequelae, provided that the preeclamptic syndrome was not superimposed on preexisting hypertensive or glomerular disease. The glomerular changes in eclampsia are very similar though often more intense. Other renal diseases may mimic the preeclamptic syndrome and may occasionally become more aggressive during pregnancy. Careful clinical and morphological assessment is necessary in patients with preeclampsia or eclampsia to exclude the presence of other disease.

REFERENCES

1. Chesley LC: *Hypertensive Disorders in Pregnancy.* New York, Appleton Century Crofts, 1978.
2. Spargo B, McCartney CP, Winemiller R: Glomerular capillary endotheliosis in toxemia of pregnancy. *Arch Pathol* 68:593, 1959.
3. Lindheimer MD, Katz AI: *The Kidney Function and Disease in Pregnancy.* Philadelphia, Lea & Febiger, 1977, p 188.
4. Chesley LC: False steps in the study of preeclampsia, in Lindheimer MD, Katz AI, Zuspan FP (eds): *Hypertension in Pregnancy.* New York, John Wiley & Sons, 1976, p 1.
5. Ferris TF: Toxemia and hypertension, in Burrow GN, Ferris TF (eds): *Medical Complications During Pregnancy.* Philadelphia, W B Saunders Co, 1975, p 53.
6. Scott JS, Jenkins DM: Immunogenetic factors in aetiology of preeclampsia/eclampsia (gestosis). *J Med Genet* 13:200, 1976.
7. McFarlane A, Scott JS: Preeclampsia/eclampsia in twin pregnancies. *J Med Genet* 13:208, 1976.
8. Aber GM: Intrarenal vascular lesions associated with preeclampsia. *Nephron* 21:297, 1978.
9. Schewitz LJ: Hypertension and renal disease in pregnancy. *Med Clin N A* 55:47, 1971.
10. Robson JS: Proteinuria and the renal lesion in preeclampsia and abruptio placentae, in Lindheimer MD, Katz AI, Zuspan FD (eds): *Hypertension in Pregnancy.* New York, John Wiley & Sons, 1976, p 61.
11. Fisher KA, Ahuja S, Luger A, et al: Nephrotic proteinuria with pre-eclampsia. *Am J Obstet Gynecol* 129:643, 1977.
12. Weisman SA, Simon NM, Herdson PB, et al: Nephrotic syndrome in pregnancy. *Am J Obstet Gynecol* 117:867, 1973.
13. Ober WB: Experimental toxemia of pregnancy: review and speculation. *Pathol Annu* 12:383, 1977.
14. Gallery EDM, Ross M, Hunyor SN, et al: Predicting the development of pregnancy-associated hypertension: the place of standardized blood-pressure measurement. *Lancet* 1:1273, 1977.
15. Gant NF, Daley GF, Chand S, et al: A study of angiotensin. II. Pressor response throughout primigravid pregnancy. *J Clin Invest* 52:2682, 1973.
16. Robertson WB, Brosens I, Dixon G: Maternal uterine vascular lesions in the hypertensive vascular complications of pregnancy, in Lindheimer MD, Katz AI, Zuspan FP (eds): *Hypertension in Pregnancy.* New York, John Wiley & Sons, 1976, p 115.
17. McKay DG: Blood coagulation and toxemia of pregnancy, in Kincaid-Smith P, Mathew TH, Becker EL (eds): *Glomerulonephritis: Morphology, Natural History and Treatment.* New York, John Wiley & Sons, 1973, Vol II, p 963.
18. Wardle EN: Preeclamptic toxaemia: a reappraisal. *Nephron* 20:241, 1978.
19. Vassalli P, McCluskey RT: The pathogenetic role of the coagulation process in glomerular diseases of immunologic origin. *Adv Nephrol* 1:47, 1971.
20. Airas F, Mancilla-Jiminez R: Hepatic fibrinogen deposits in preeclampsia: immunofluorescent evidence. *N Engl J Med* 295:578, 1976.

21. Seymour AE, Petrucco OM, Clarkson AR, et al: Morphological and immunological evidence of coagulopathy in renal complications of pregnancy, in Lindheimer MD, Katz AI, Zuspan FD (eds): *Hypertension in Pregnancy*. New York, John Wiley & Sons, 1976, p 139.

22. Kitzmiller JL, Benirschke K: Immunofluorescent study of placental bed vessels in pre-eclampsia of pregnancy. *Am J Obstet Gynecol* 115:248, 1973.

23. Stirrat GM, Redman CWG, Levinsky RJ: Circulating immune complexes in preeclampsia. *Br Med J* 1:1450, 1978.

24. Need JA: Pre-eclampsia in pregnancies by different fathers: immunological studies. *Br Med J* 1:548, 1975.

25. Spargo BH, Lichtig C, Luger AM, et al: The renal lesion in pre-eclampsia, in Lindheimer MD, Katz AI, and Zuspan FP (eds): *Hypertension in Pregnancy*. New York, John Wiley & Sons, 1976, p 95.

26. Sheehan HL, Lynch JB: *Pathology of Toxemia of Pregnancy*. London, Churchill, Livingstone, 1973, p 53.

27. Kincaid-Smith P, Fairley KF: The differential diagnosis between preeclamptic toxemia and glomerulonephritis in patients with proteinuria during pregnancy, in Lindheimer MD, Katz AI, Zuspan FP (eds): *Hypertension in Pregnancy*. New York, John Wiley & Sons, 1976, p 157.

28. Kincaid-Smith P, Mathews DC: The similarity of lesions and underlying mechanism in pre-eclamptic toxemia and postpartum renal failure, in Kincaid-Smith P, Mathew TG, Becker EL (eds): *Glomerulonephritis: Morphology, Natural History and Treatment*. New York, John Wiley & Sons, 1973, Vol II, p 1013.

29. Chesley LC, Annitto JE, Cosgrove RA: The remote prognosis of eclamptic women. *Am J Obstet Gynecol* 124:446, 1976.

30. Matlin RA, Gary NE: Acute cortical necrosis: case report and review of the literature. *Am J Med* 56:110, 1974.

31. Kleinknecht D, Grunfeld J-P, Gomez PC, et al: Diagnostic procedures and long term prognosis in bilateral renal cortical necrosis. *Kidney Int* 4:390, 1973.

32. Zacur HA, Mitch WE: Renal disease in pregnancy. *Med Clin NA* 61:89, 1977.

33. Fairley KF, Whitworth JA, Kincaid-Smith P: Glomerulonephritis and pregnancy, in Kincaid-Smith P, Mathew TG, Becker EL (eds): *Glomerulonephritis: Morphology, Natural History and Treatment*. New York, John Wiley & Sons, 1973, Vol II, p 997.

34. Strauch BS, Hayslett JP: Kidney disease and pregnancy. *Br Med J* 4:578, 1974.

18
Diabetic Nephropathy

Diabetes mellitus is a clinicopathologic syndrome defined by sustained hyperglycemia. The hyperglycemia is an expression of relative or absolute insulin deficiency caused by a variety of mechanisms. Clarification of the patterns of genetic influence on the viral, autoimmune, and other factors causing pancreatic islet damage may allow the construction of workable pathogenetic classifications in the future (1). At present, however, the syndrome is divided chronologically into juvenile-onset and adult-onset varieties. While intermediate forms exist, this crude division separates two groups of diabetic patients with distinct therapeutic and prognostic characteristics. The systemic complications of the diabetic state are mediated by similar mechanisms regardless of the factors causing hyperglycemia. Among the most important mechanisms are diffuse disease of both large (macroangiopathy) and small (microangiopathy) blood vessels. Macroangiopathy is caused by atherosclerosis that is both premature and unduly severe in diabetics. Microangiopathy is characterized by widespread thickening of capillary basement membranes (BM) and damages tissues both by potentiating the ischemic complications of large vessel disease and by producing specific tissue effects.

Most areas of the kidney may be affected by diabetes. The major alterations are in glomeruli and arterioles, but a variety of tubulointerstitial changes occur. The term *diabetic glomerulosclerosis* embraces the glomerular changes considered to be an expression of the microangiopathy, together with localized lesions of different pathogenesis. As in systemic capillaries, glomerulosclerosis is caused by the progressive accumulation of BM material, causing both enlargement and increased weight of the glomeruli (2). The morphologic pattern is, however, modified by the occurrence of similar changes in the mesangium. Thus, the earliest glomerular lesions to be characterized were the mesangial nodules (3), which are still regarded as the most typical feature of diabetic nephropathy. There is, however, a morphologic continuum between predominant involvement of the peripheral BM (diffuse glomerulosclerosis) and principally mesangial disease (nodular glomerulosclerosis). Recognition of this continuum, which is most clearly demonstrated by electron microscopy, has caused many workers to discard the nodular and diffuse designations and, instead, to assess the degree of overall glomerular change (4,5). Paradoxically, the excessively thick BM is abnormally permeable to proteins. Protein leakage is manifest clinically as proteinuria and morphologically as localized protein collections. These collections, insudates, are analogous in both their morphology and pathogenesis to those occurring in the retina and also affect arterioles to cause the hyalinosis so typical of the disease. The degree of retinal microangiopathy is, in fact, a reasonably accurate guide to the severity of diabetic nephropathy. Many physicians are, therefore, reluctant to perform renal biopsies for the investigation of renal disease in diabetic patients unless retinopathy is minimal or there are other atypical features.

PATHOGENESIS OF MICROANGIOPATHY

The incidence and pathogenesis of microangiopathy are controversial (6). Studies from one group suggest that abnormally thick muscle capillary BM is found in the majority of newly diagnosed diabetics and that the abnormality is related to neither duration nor control of the diabetic state (7). Most workers, however, find a very low incidence of BM thickening in recently diagnosed diabetics and a progressively increasing width with disease duration (8). These divergent data probably reflect differences in the techniques of BM measurement (8,9). A direct relationship between BM thickening and the duration of hyperglycemia is supported by studies of experimental and human diabetic nephropathy. In experimental diabetic glomerulosclerosis, produced by Streptozocin, significant increases in glomerular BM width are directly correlated with hyperglycemia (10), and mesangial sclerosis is reversed by transplantation from diabetic to normoglycemic animals (11). Similarly, the glomerular BM width is normal soon after the onset of human juvenile diabetes but significantly increased several years later (12).

The mechanisms by which hyperglycemia causes BM thickening are, however, unknown, and the association seems unlikely to be direct (6,7). The static morphologic demonstration of a thickened BM could reflect alerations in synthesis, catabolism, or structure. Extensive biochemical analyses of glomerular BM have yielded conflicting data, which suggest, but do not yet prove, abnormalities in structure (13). In animal systems, there is evidence of increased anabolic enzyme activity and decreased catabolism in renal cortical slices (13), and a variety of mechanisms by which growth hormone (14) or chemical alterations (15) could modify BM synthesis have been suggested. There is also evidence for increased synthesis of glomerular basement membrane in experimental diabetes (15a), but no conclusive data have as yet appeared to confirm any of these mechanisms, and a number of studies suggest a major role for physical influences. Morphologic thickening of muscle capillary BM, similar to that occurring in diabetes, can be demonstrated in the dependent regions of normoglycemic people with increasing age and elevated venous pressure (8). Similar physical factors appear to influence glomerulosclerosis, since glomerular disease is worsened in experimental diabetes by uninephrectomy and ameliorated, both in animals and man, by renal artery stenosis (11). The mechanisms by which these physical factors influence BM status are unknown, but the effects of intravascular tension, increased permeability, and elevated viscosity (16) are being investigated (8). Any of these factors might damage the cells responsible for BM formation and, by cyclical cell death and renewal, might cause progressive accumulation of BM material.

Although the pathogenesis of diabetic microangiopathy remains unknown, there is considerable evidence to support a relationship with the hyperglycemic state. The central role of hyperglycemia is reinforced by the occurrence of microangiopathy in such "secondary" diabetic states as hemochromatosis (18) and chronic pancreatitis (19), but the possibility of a genetic diathesis to abnormal BM production cannot yet be excluded. Both renal disease and ischemic complications were recorded before the insulin era, and there is no evidence for a role of either insulin or antiinsulin antibodies in the production of abnormal BM (20). Microangiopathy is probably ubiquitous in patients who have had diabetes for some years, though its relationship to blood sugar control is controversial (7). The capillary changes magnify the circulatory effects of the macroangiopathy to produce premature and excessively frequent ischemic complications (21,22).

INCIDENCE OF DIABETIC NEPHROPATHY

Glomerulosclerosis is described in 8—48% of diabetic patients at autopsy (23), but the morphologic abnormalities are not necessarily correlated with clinical renal disease (4). Approximately 5—6% of diabetics in unselected autopsy (22,24) and prospective clinical (23) studies are found to die from renal failure, and insurance mortality statistics show a seventeen-fold excess of renal death compared to nondiabetics (23). In juvenile diabetics, renal failure accounts for half of these deaths, whereas ischemic complications of the macroangiopathy become more significant in older age groups (23). The incidence of renal involvement during life, as judged by the presence of proteinuria, is closely related to disease duration. Thus, only 2% of the juvenile diabetics examined less than 9 years after diagnosis have proteinuria, while protein is found in the urine of 63% after 35 years (23). For this reason, serious renal disease is rare in children (25). The prevalence of proteinuria in adult-onset diabetics is less well documented, figures of 5—38% being quoted (23), but there is some evidence that renal disease is neither as frequent nor as progressive in this group, especially if insulin therapy is not required (5). In both age groups, mortality is substantially greater in patients with proteinuria (23).

CLINICAL MANIFESTATIONS

Proteinuria is initially mild and intermittent and may remain static for many years without change in renal function (26). Initial presentation in renal failure without preceding proteinuria is uncommon and suggests the possibility of superimposed disease, such as acute glomerulonephritis (27). The urinary sediment is usually bland, though microscopic hematuria sometimes occurs, and the proteinuria is nonselective (4). The degree of proteinuria is closely correlated with the prognosis—patients excreting more than 3 gm per 24 hours usually progressing to renal failure within 6 years, whereas those with lesser amounts may show little change in renal function over long periods (4). The nephrotic syndrome is uncommon in the diabetic population overall but common in those with serious renal disease, and it is a grim prognostic sign (28). Spontaneous remission has only once been recorded in a patient with symptomatic diabetic glomerulosclerosis (29). Other causes for the nephrotic syndrome should, therefore, always be considered, since both membranous nephropathy (30,31) and corticosteroid-responsive epithelial cell disease (32,33) have been described in diabetics.

Varying degrees of chronic renal failure may appear within three (28) to five (23) years after proteinuria is first documented, but may, on the other hand, be delayed for many years (4,5). Once established, the progression of renal failure is often very rapid for reasons that are not clear (26). Irreversible acute renal failure occurs in some patients with impaired renal function after intravenous pyelography (34) and may, rarely, be caused by papillary necrosis (35). Hypertension is common once renal failure develops but is not otherwise significantly increased in the diabetic population (28). The major factor causing elevation of blood pressure appears to be fluid retention (28) and, perhaps for this reason, accelerated hypertension is rare in diabetics (23). Kidney size is usually increased in diabetic nephropathy (36), even in the presence of significant renal failure, but progressive contraction is usual in advanced azotemia. Throughout the course of diabetic nephropathy, there is often a close correlation between both morphologic and functional indices of glomerulosclerosis and retinal disease. Retinopathy may, however, be absent in patients with advanced renal failure or, conversely, severe in the face of mild and nonprogressive renal disease (4,28).

PATHOLOGIC CHARACTERISTICS

The changes of established diabetic glomerulosclerosis are readily recognizable by light microscopy. Early changes are, however, nonspecific and can be either missed or misinterpreted if light microscopy alone is available. Furthermore, a number of conditions closely mimic diabetic glomerulosclerosis and require electron and immunofluorescence microscopic examination for specific diagnosis. While most studies of the nature and evolution of diabetic glomerulosclerosis have depended on light microscopic criteria, it must be emphasized that reliance on these criteria is insufficient for specific diagnosis.

Light Microscopy

Glomerulosclerosis
The earliest detectable lesion of diabetic glomerulosclerosis is diffuse widening of mesangial areas by the accumulation of PAS-positive matrix (Figs. 18-1, 18-2). With progression, capillary basement membranes appear thickened and mesangia become increasingly prominent with, in some cases, a real or apparent increase in mesangial cellularity (37) (Fig. 18-3). The term *diffuse glomerulosclerosis* refers to this pattern of enlarged glomeruli with thickened membranes and excessive mesangial matrix. The diffuse pattern may occur alone or may be admixed with the characteristic picture of nodular glomerulosclerosis (38). The nodules appear as rounded and homogenous eosinophilic masses in centrolobular regions with either compression or, occasionally, aneurysmal dilatation of the surrounding capillaries (Figs. 18-4−18-6). One or many nodules may occur in

the same glomerulus, and careful examination often shows areas of nodular development in glomeruli showing, at first glance, only diffuse changes. While the nodules are typically homogenous, silver stains often reveal a highly characteristic pattern of concentric lamination (Fig. 18-5). Occasionally, nodular glomerulosclerosis may show striking hypercellularity and even mesangial interposition. There is no real doubt that both forms of glomerulosclerosis are part of the same evolving process, although the reasons for the differing patterns, often coexisting in the same biopsy specimen, are uncertain. Certainly, diffuse changes appear earliest, and are, therefore, the lesions most commonly described in autopsy studies (23). Nodular glomerulosclerosis is not, as originally suggested (3), invariably associated with the nephrotic syndrome, but is reasonably well correlated with severe renal dysfunction (4).

Insudative and Vascular Lesions

Localized accumulations of intensely eosinophilic material occur in various regions of the glomerulus, probably by insudation and inspissation of plasma proteins (39). These accumulations appear as rounded nodules situated either between Bowman's capsule and the parietal epithelium ("capsular drop") or in an apparent subendothelial location along capillary loops ("fibrin cap") (Figs. 18-1, 18-2, 18-7—18-9). Lipid globules and, occasionally, foam cells may be included in the lesions, which correlate closely with the severity of proteinuria (4). Insudative lesions are most common in advanced glomerulosclerosis but may occur at any stage and have been regarded as characteristic of diabetic renal disease (40). Very similar lesions occur, however, in a wide range of renal diseases and are occasionally seen in otherwise normal biopsy specimens from normoglycemic people. Vascular hyalinosis is, similarly, not in any way specific but occurs more extensively and at any earlier age in diabetics, with no relationship to hypertension (24). Extensive arteriolar hyalinosis is always a signal to suspect the presence of diabetes, and hyalinosis of both afferent and efferent arterioles is an almost specific feature of the disease (24). The hyalin lesions, as with the insudative, are almost certainly caused by plasma protein insudation (41) and may contain lipid globules or foam cells (Figs. 18-1, 18-9).

Crescents

Active epithelial crescents are rare in diabetic glomerulosclerosis, but areas of organizing epithelial proliferation are occasionally seen and have been correlated with an unusually aggressive clinical course (42) (Fig. 18-10).

Tubulointerstitial Lesions

Diffuse thickening of the tubular BM, similar to that seen in the glomerulus, is a common and characteristic feature of diabetic nephropathy (Figs. 18-7, 18-11). Tubulointerstitial scarring with infiltration by mononuclear inflammatory cells is common with advanced glomerulosclerosis and should not be misinterpreted as evidence of pyelonephritis (Fig. 18-12). The incidence of bacteriuria and pyelonephritis is controversial (23,28), and claims for an excessive incidence of infective renal scarring are not convincing. Glycogen vacuolation of proximal tubules ("glycogen nephrosis," Armanni-Ebstein lesion) correlates directly with uncontrolled hyperglycemia and is not commonly encountered in renal biopsy specimens.

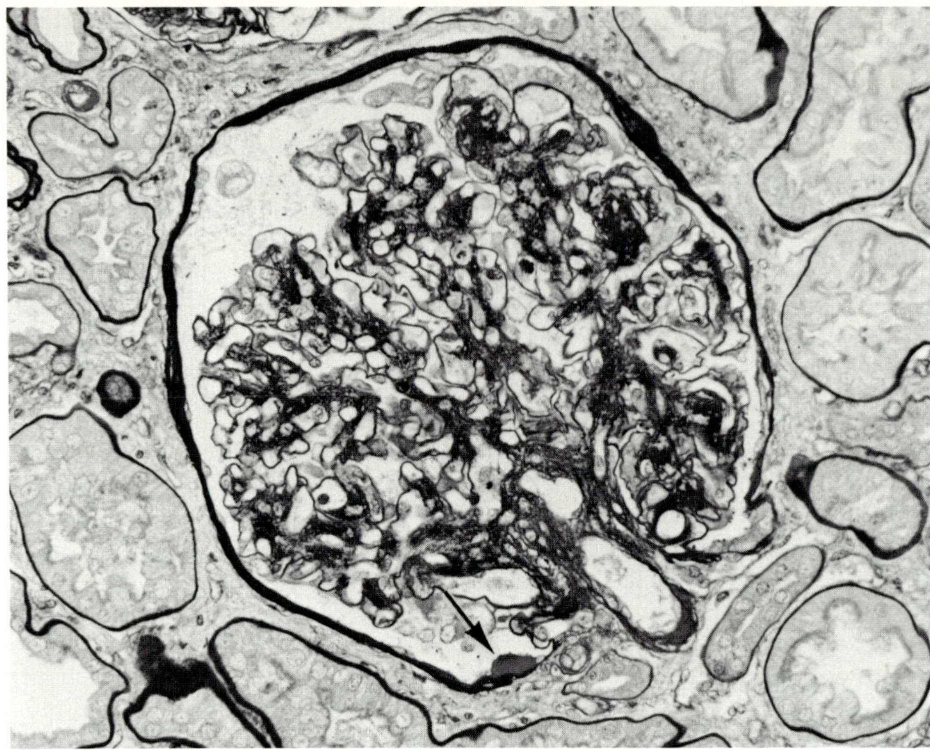

Figure 18-1. Enlarged glomerulus with diffuse increase of mesangial matrix in early diabetic glomerulosclerosis. Note insudative lesions ("capsular drops") (arrow) and hyalinization of the afferent arteriole (PAS stain, ×360).

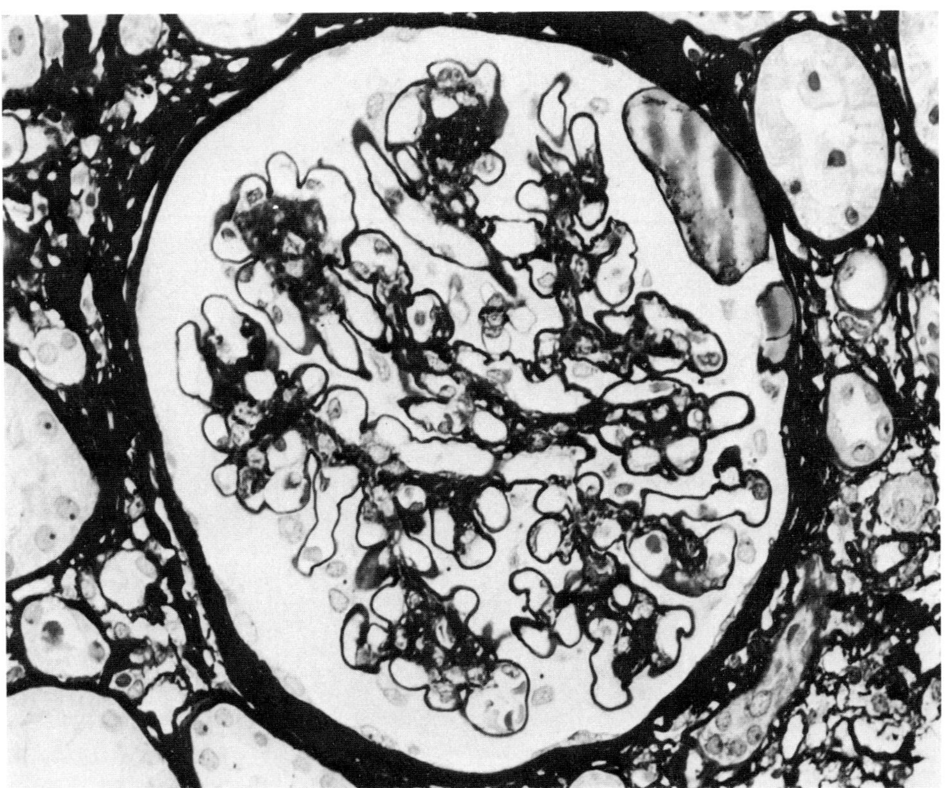

Figure 18-2. Silver preparation showing widening of the mesangium and thickening of the basement membrane in diffuse diabetic glomerulosclerosis. Large insudative lesions ("capsular drops") are present on the right upper portion of the glomerulus (PASM stain, ×440).

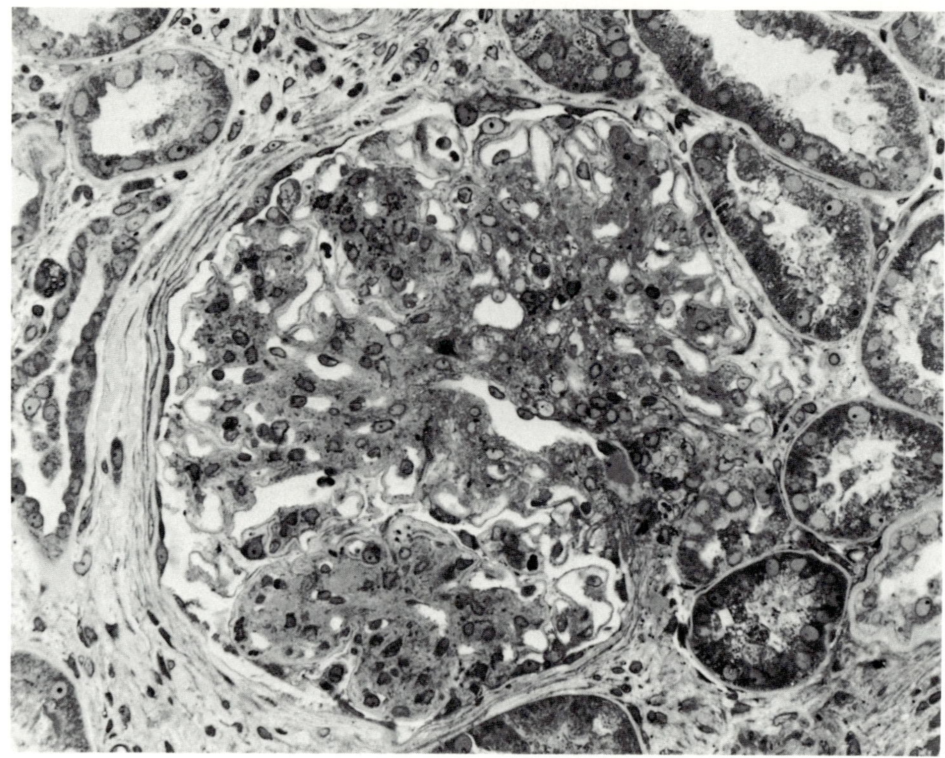

Figure 18-3. Diabetic glomerulosclerosis with glomerular enlargement and diffuse hypercellularity (plastic embedded toluidine blue stain, ×325).

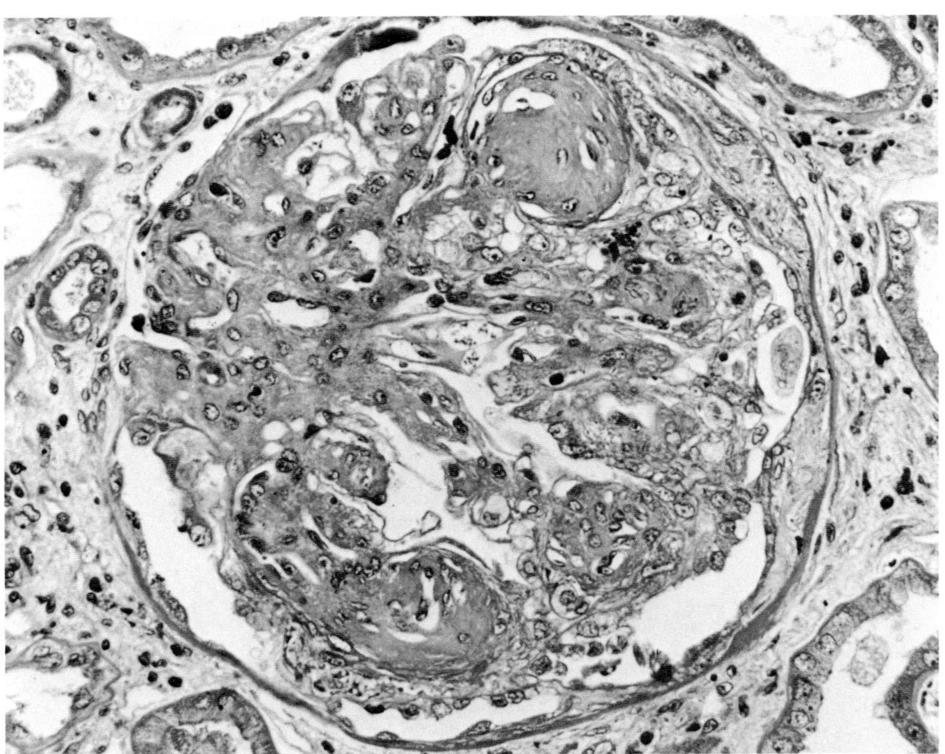

Figure 18-4. Nodules in nodular diabetic glomerulosclerosis (H&E stain, ×650).

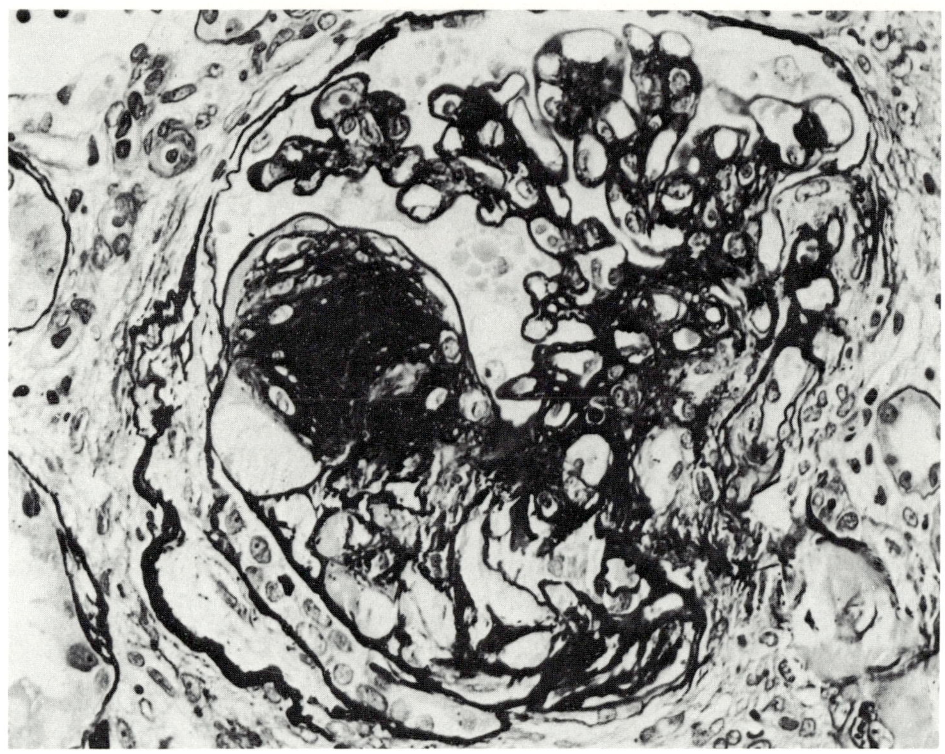

Figure 18-5. Nodular glomerulosclerosis with aneurysmal dilatation of surrounding capillaries. Note the laminated appearance of the sclerotic nodule (PASM stain, ×500).

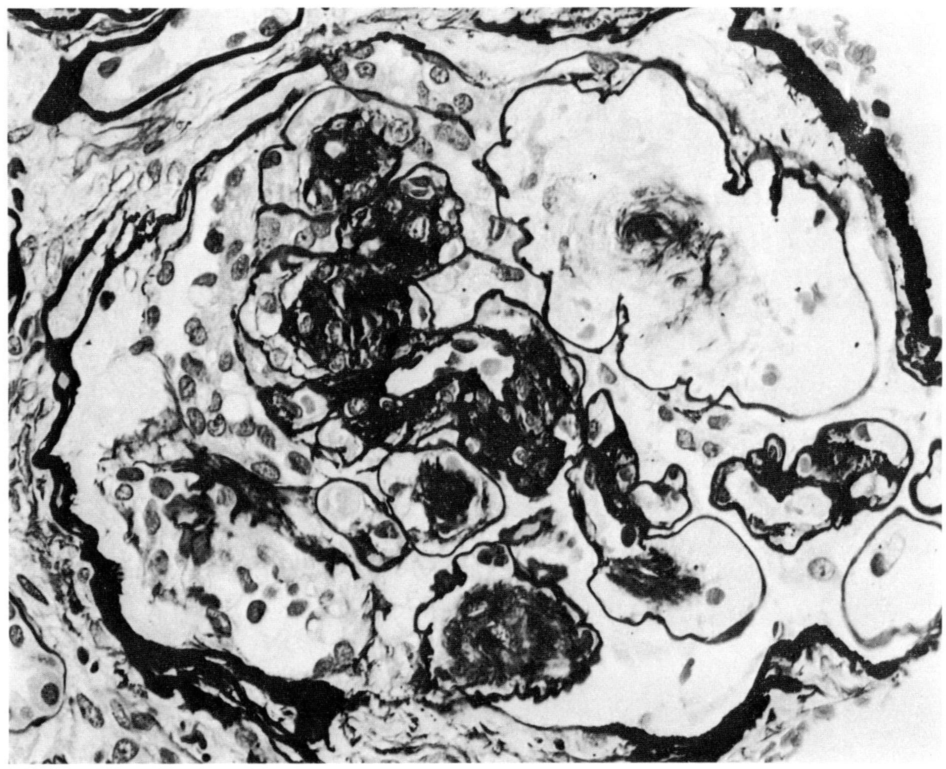

Figure 18-6. Pronounced aneurysmlike distention of the capillary loops in diabetic glomerulosclerosis (PASM stain, ×600).

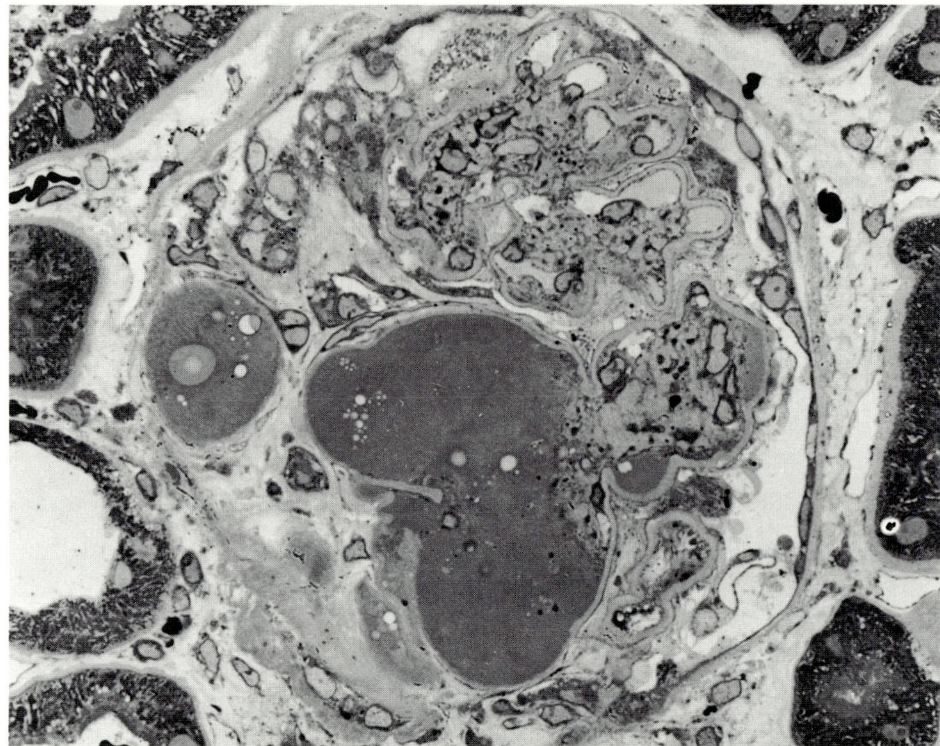

Figure 18-7. Diabetic glomerulosclerosis with well-developed intracapillary "fibrin caps" containing numerous vacuoles, partially filled by lipids. The glomerular and tubular basement membranes are markedly thickened (plastic embedded toluidine blue stain, ×600).

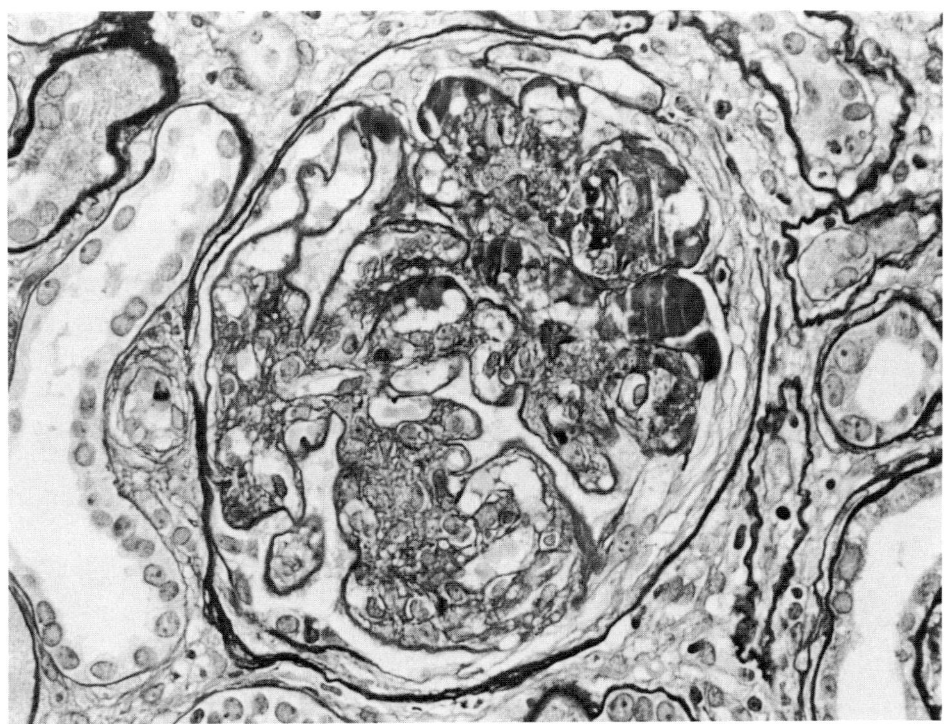

Figure 18-8. Numerous "fibrin caps" containing abundant lipid in advanced glomerulosclerosis (PAS stain, ×450).

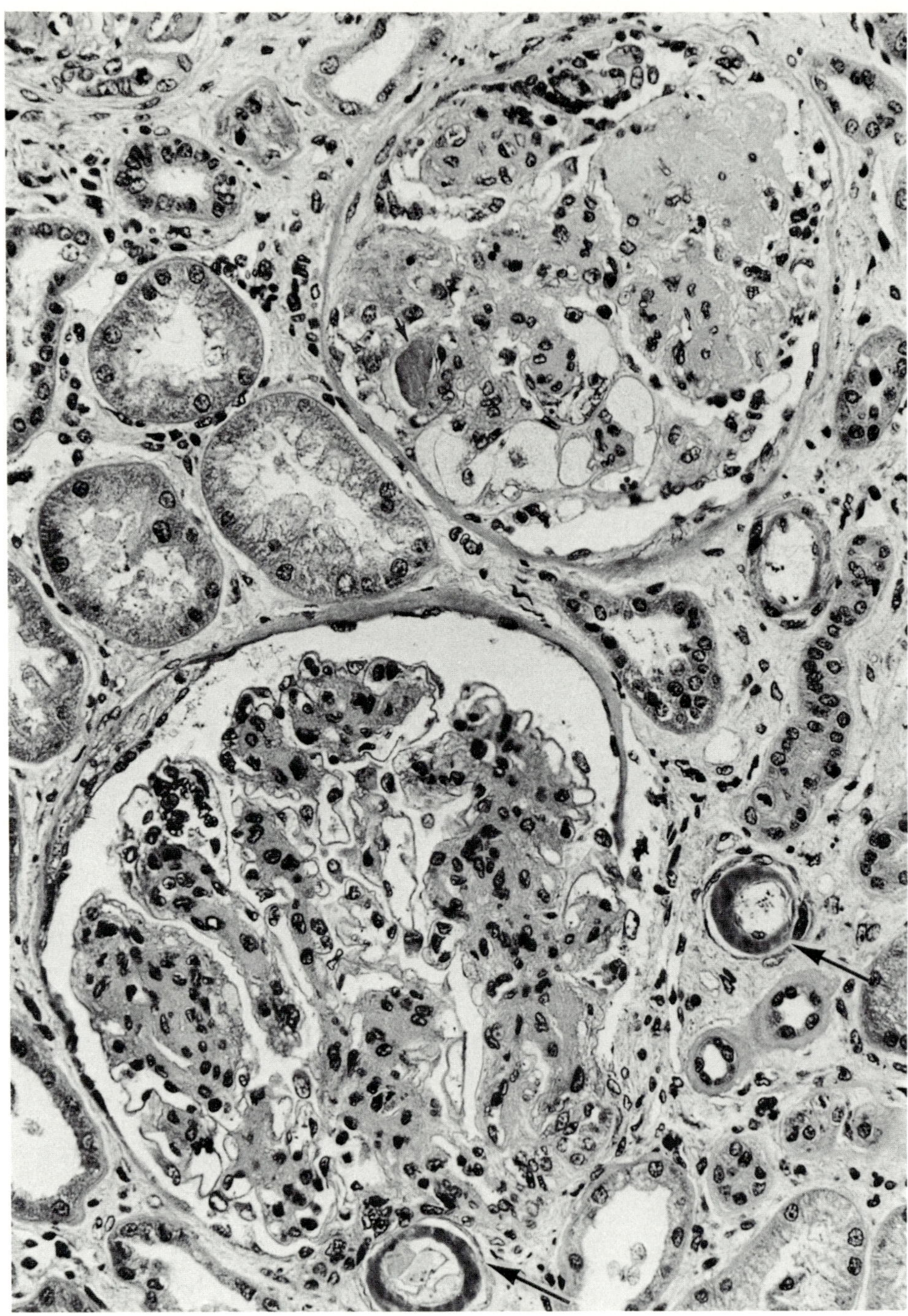

Figure 18-9. Diabetic glomerulosclerosis. Arteriolar and glomerular insudative lesions (arrows). Note numerous foam cells filled with lipids in the upper glomerulus as well as a "fibrin cap" (arrow head) (H&E stain, ×360).

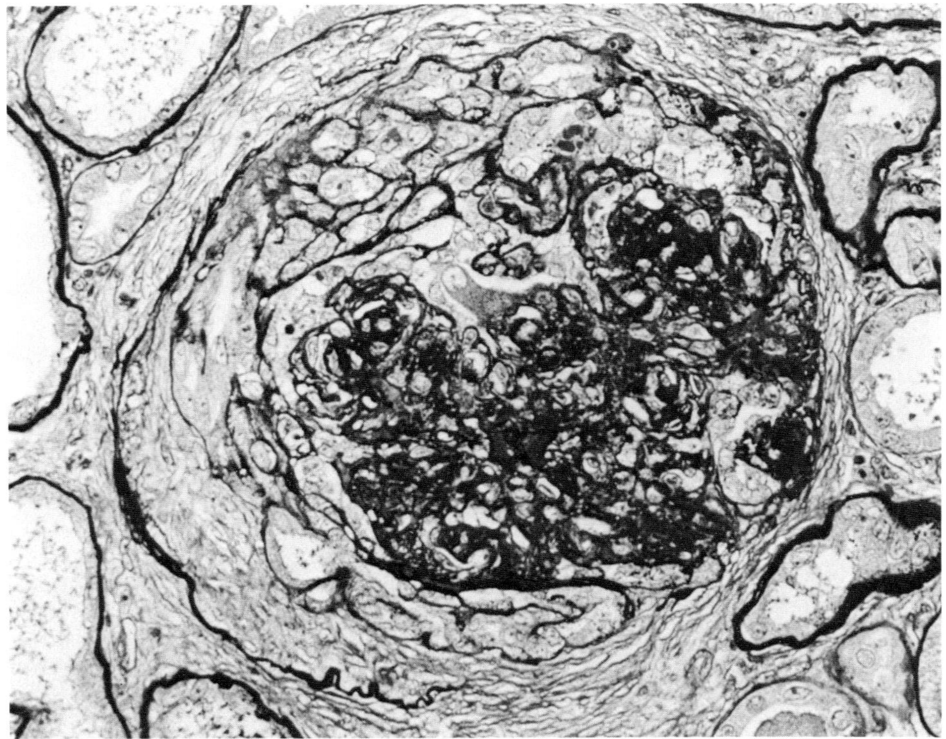

Figure 18-10. Glomerulus with diabetic glomerulosclerosis with fibroepithelial crescent (PAS stain, ×450).

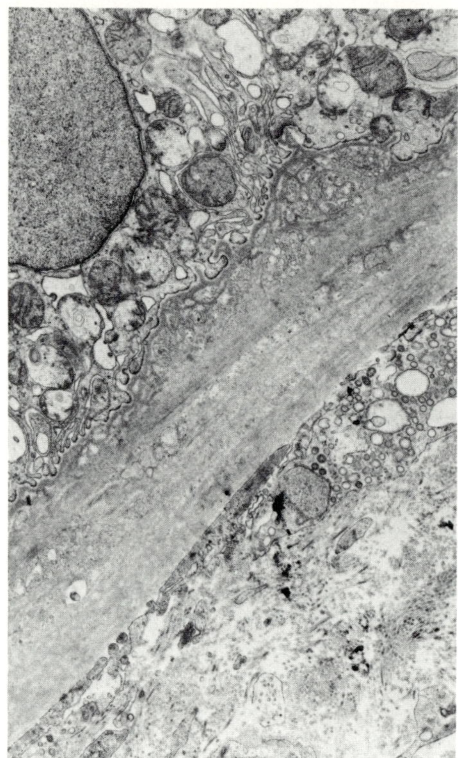

Figure 18-11. Tubular basement membrane showing marked thickening and lamellation (×2,500).

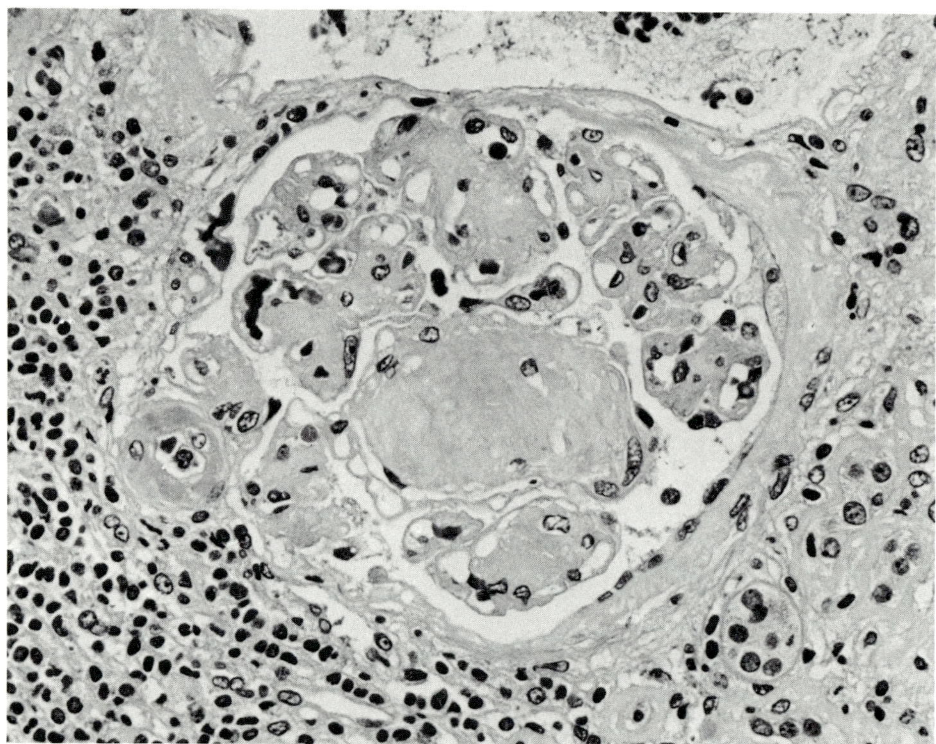

Figure 18-12. Advanced nodular glomerulosclerosis. There is prominent interstitial lymphocytic infiltrate and hyalinosis of the afferent arteriole (H&E stain, ×425).

344

Electron Microscopy

Measurement of glomerular BM width is the most satisfactory criterion for the detection of early diabetic glomerulosclerosis and for assessing its evolution (12). Indeed, ultrastructural evidence for BM widening can be seen long before light microscopic changes are visible. Mesangial matrix accumulates in parallel with the increase in BM width (43), and each of these changes progresses with the development of the glomerular disease, although either may become predominant (Fig. 18-13). In advanced disease, the membrane may reach many times its normal width and often has a prominent fibrillar pattern (38) (Figs. 18-14, 18-15). Mesangial matrix accumulates in an irregular pattern, with gradual replacement of mesangial cells, and frequently contains calcific foci, collagen fibers, lipid vacuoles, and cytoplasmic debris. The nodules may have an organized pattern of matrix bands arranged in a sandwichlike configuration, and nodules with this appearance can be detected in glomeruli showing, by light microscopy, only diffuse disease (44) (Fig. 18-16). Insudative lesions consist of granular, electron-dense masses that often contain lipid material and membranous debris (39) (Figs. 18-14, 18-17, 18-18). In tangential sections, these may be mistaken for mesangial or subendothelial deposits, but careful examination usually reveals their insudative character. Deposits are, in fact, rare in diabetic glomerulosclerosis and, if frequent or diffuse, suggest superimposed disease.

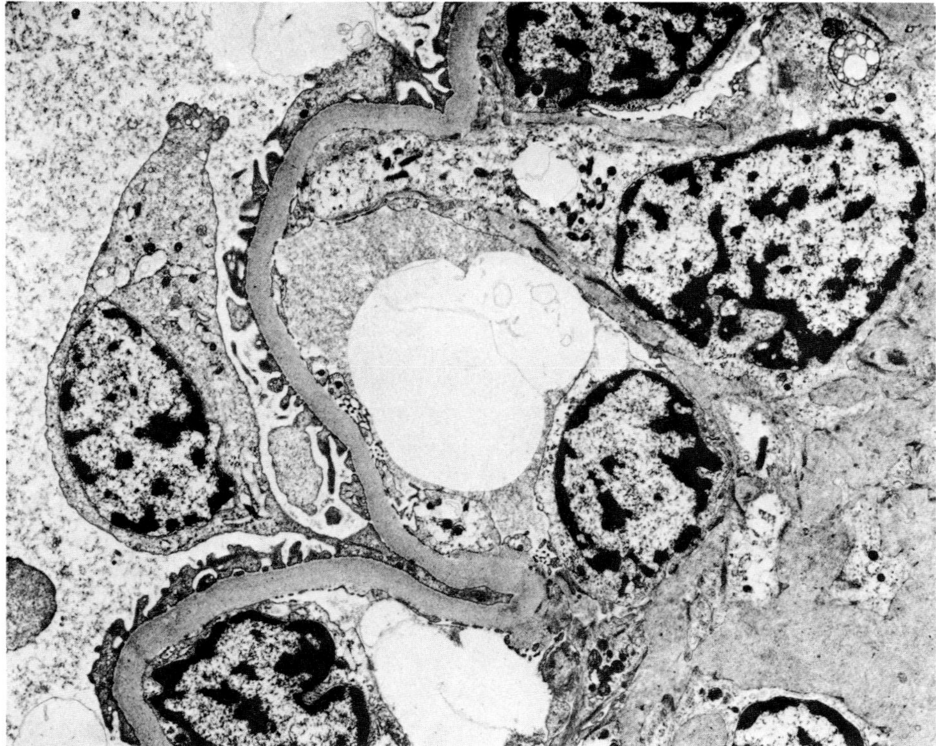

Figure 18-13. Diffuse thickening of the peripheral basement membrane and increase in mesangial matrix in diffuse diabetic glomerulosclerosis (×6,400).

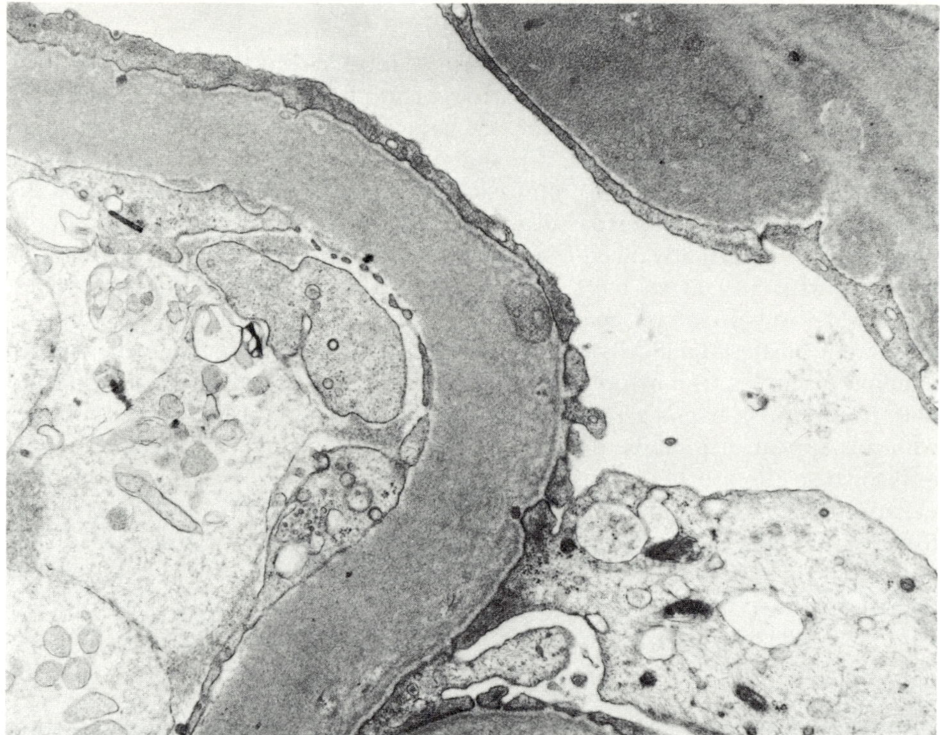

Figure 18-14. Electron micrograph showing the peripheral capillary basement membrane. The basement membrane is about five times the normal thickness. Note the finely granular electron-dense capsular drop within the basement membrane of Bowman's capsule (right upper corner) ($\times$ 14,800).

Areas of subepithelial "crater" formation containing striated membranous debris are common in diabetic glomerulosclerosis, but are quite nonspecific (45).

Immunofluorescence Microscopy

Diffuse, linear reactions for IgG along glomerular capillary (20), tubular, and Bowman's capsular (46) membranes are quite characteristic for diabetic glomerulosclerosis (Figs. 18-19, 18-20). Less intense and regular reactions may be seen in similar distributions for IgM, fibrin, and albumin, but staining for C3 is, if present, often granular. These linear reactions are unrelated to either the duration or the severity of glomerular lesions, and elution studies show no anti-BM antibodies (20,46). Insudative lesions may react with a variety of reagents, but most frequently contain IgM (46) (Fig. 18-21).

DIFFERENTIAL DIAGNOSIS

Although the fully developed lesion of nodular diabetic glomerulosclerosis is highly characteristic, no single morphologic feature is specific. A wide range of

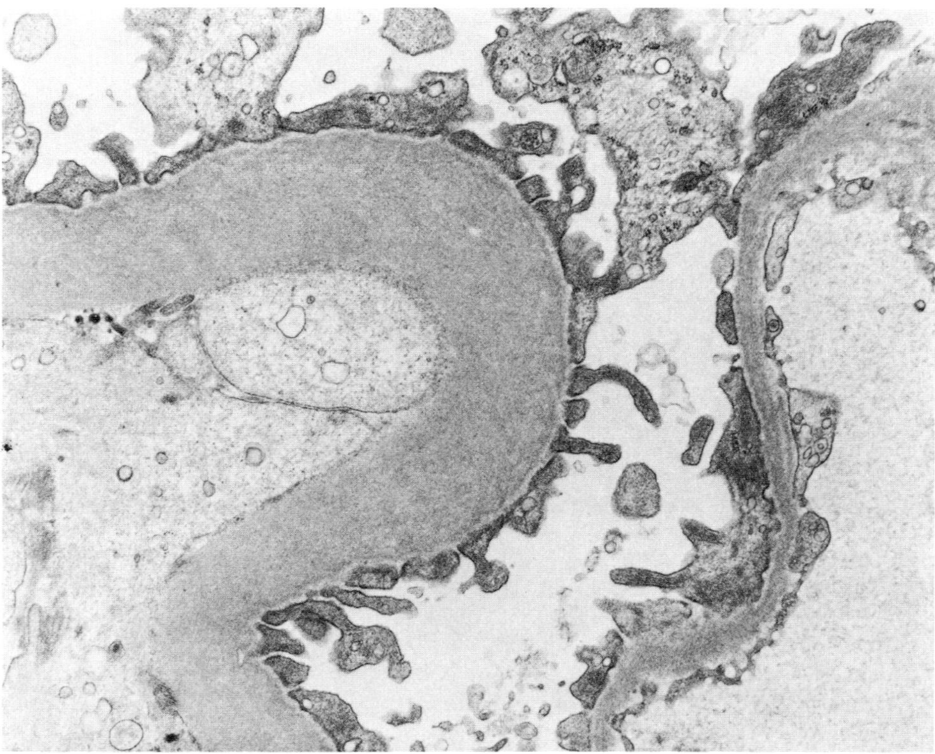

Figure 18-15. Electron micrograph showing pronounced thickening of the glomerular basement membrane, which can be contrasted with the membrane of an adjacent aneurysmally dilated capillary loop ($\times$18,000).

glomerular diseases may, therefore, mimic diabetic glomerulosclerosis more or less closely, and accurate diagnosis requires light, electron, and immunofluorescence microscopic examination. Insudative lesions and vascular hyalinosis are, as discussed, completely nonspecific. The pattern of diffuse glomerulosclerosis closely resembles the glomerular hypertrophy occurring in a number of disorders, especially hepatic glomerulosclerosis (47), some of which may show degrees of glomerular BM thickening. The mesangial proliferation in both diffuse and nodular glomerulosclerosis may suggest a diagnosis of either mesangial proliferative or mesangiocapillary glomerulonephritis, but the clinical, electron microscopic, and immunofluorescence data usually provide clear diagnostic distinction. On H&E sections alone, mesangial accumulation of amyloid may mimic the nodules of diabetic glomerulosclerosis, but confusion is unlikely if other stains and techniques are used. Glomerular nodules almost indistinguishable from diabetic glomerulosclerosis also occur rarely in multiple myeloma and the closely allied condition, kappa light chain nephropathy (48,49). In these conditions, ultrastructural examination demonstrates diffuse extension of granular dense material throughout the excessive mesangial matrix and the glomerular and tubular basement membranes. A number of the reported examples of diabetic glomerulosclerosis occurring in the absence of diabetes may represent misinterpretation of the appearances in some of these conditions. The presence of

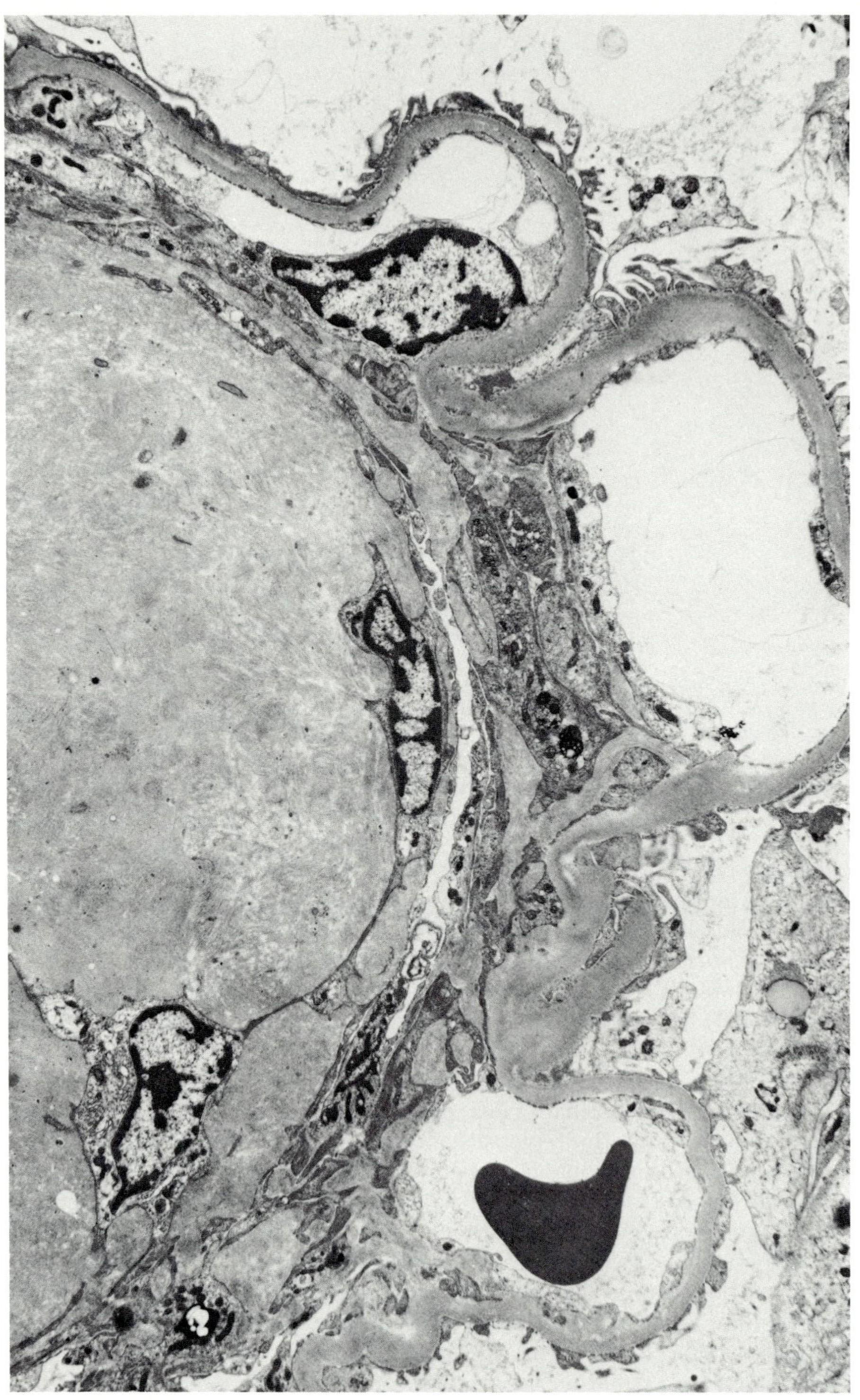

Figure 18-16. Electron micrograph of advanced nodular glomerulosclerosis. There is marked increase of fibrillar mesangial matrix. Some elongated mesangial cells are present at the periphery of the nodule (×5,500).

348

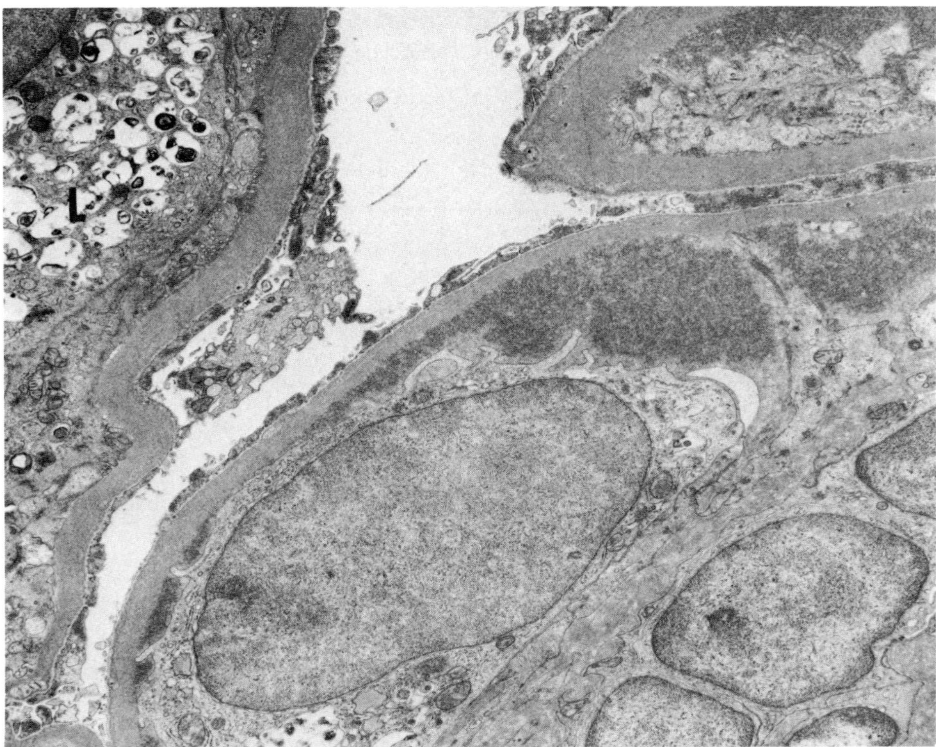

Figure 18-17. Electron micrograph demonstrating finely granular electron-dense in-sudative lesion located between the basement membrane and the endothelial cell cyto-plasm. An endothelial cell contains lipid (L) (×6,300).

abnormal insulin responses and muscle capillary BM thickening in some of these patients (50) suggests, however, that glomerulosclerosis may rarely develop in "prediabetic" states.

PROGNOSIS AND THERAPY

Established diabetic glomerulosclerosis is irreversible in man. Once proteinuria appears, the natural course is for inexorable progression into chronic renal failure. In adults, this progression may be very slow (4,5) and is often inter-rupted by fatal complications of the macroangiopathy (23). Chronic renal failure is, however, a major cause of death in juvenile-onset diabetes and is likely to develop within three to five years of the onset of proteinuria (23,28). There is controversy over the relationship between adequate control of the hyperglycemia and the course of renal disease (5,7).

There is no effective therapy for diabetic glomerulosclerosis, and hemodialysis is associated with a high incidence of mortality from infection and the complications of macroangiopathy (26,28). Transplantation remains, there-fore, the only hope for prolonging life and is best performed before advanced systemic disease contraindicates surgery. More than 100 patients with diabetic

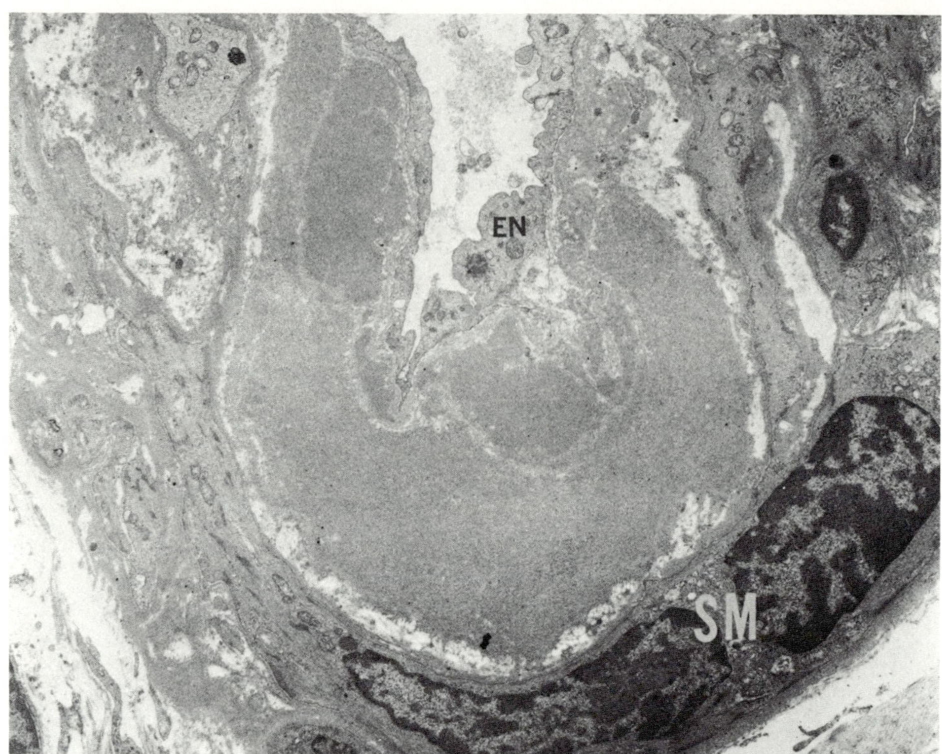

Figure 18-18. Cross section of small artery showing large insudative lesion between endothelium and media. EN, endothelium; SM, smooth muscle (×3,000).

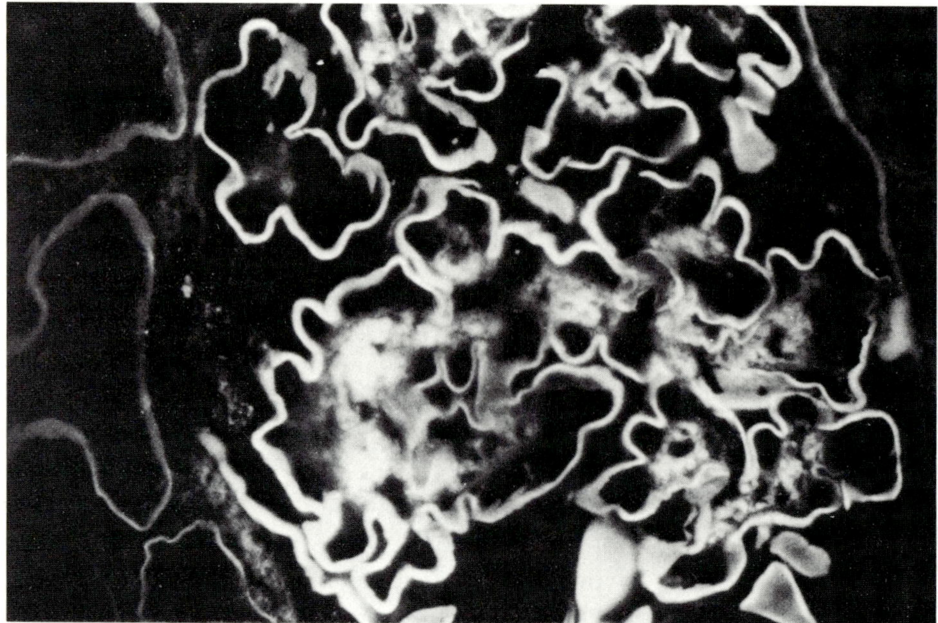

Figure 18-19. Diffuse glomerular sclerosis with linear staining along the glomerular basement membrane, Bowman's capsule, and tubules (left) (antihuman IgG, ×450).

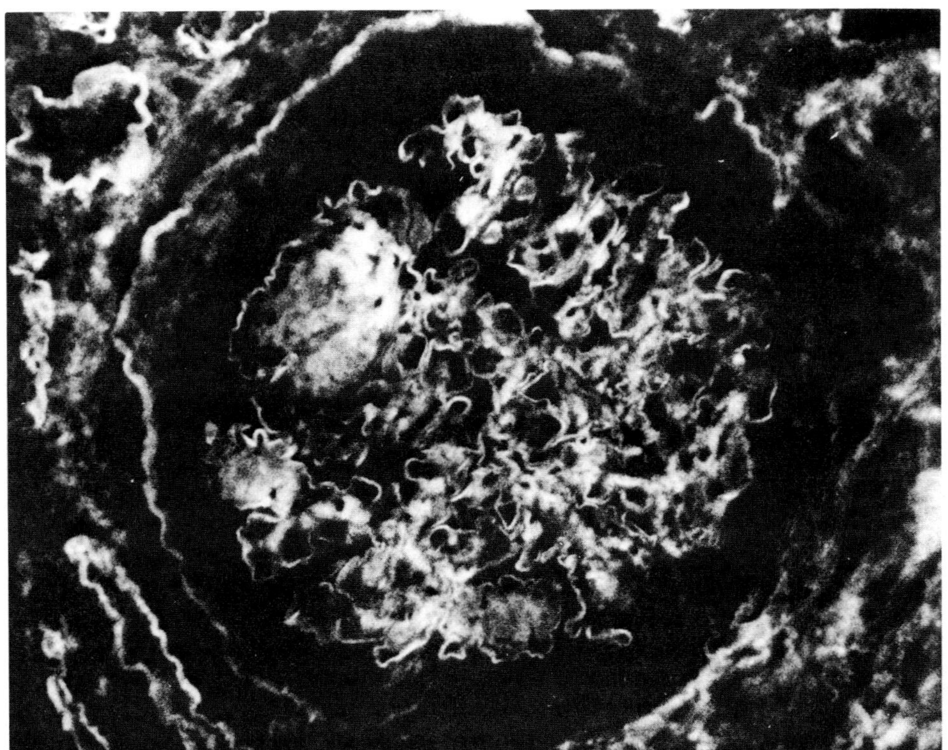

Figure 18-20. Nodular glomerulosclerosis with linear staining along the glomerular basement membrane and also in the middle of the nodules, Bowman's capsule, and tubules (antihuman IgG, ×450).

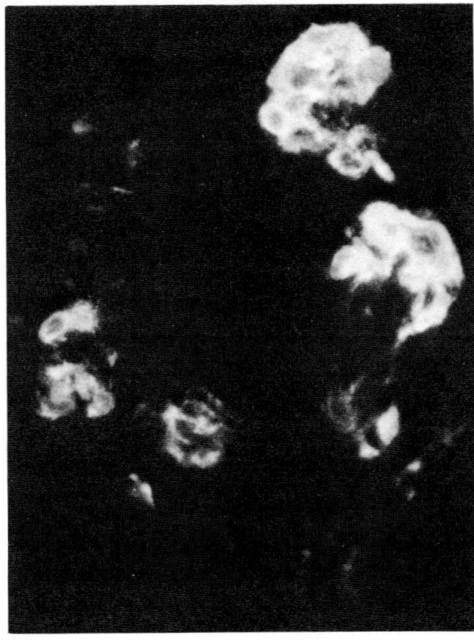

Figure 18-21. Segmental staining of glomerular insudative lesion (Antihuman IgM, ×350).

glomerulosclerosis have been treated by transplantation and, although successful engraftment with good renal function has occurred in some, both rejection and mortality are substantially more frequent than in nondiabetics (51,52). Recurrent nodular glomerulosclerosis has been reported in one patient, 4½ years after transplantation (53), and preliminary studies suggest a progressive increase in the glomerular BM width of the grafts (54). Less specific features suggesting recurrent disease, such as vascular hyalinosis (53) and linear tubular BM immunofluorescence (55), are also more common in kidneys transplanted into diabetics than into normoglycemic people. These phenomena cast some doubt on the value of transplantation in patients with diabetic glomerulosclerosis, but more experience will be necessary before firm conclusions can be drawn. A glomerular lesion resembling diabetic glomerulosclerosis has also been reported in one patient who did not exhibit biochemical features of diabetes until one month after the transplant was performed (56).

SUMMARY

Diabetic glomerulosclerosis is the major renal expression of a diffuse microangiopathy characterized by thickening of capillary basement membranes. The pathogenesis of this vascular lesion is presently unknown but it is almost certainly related, either directly or indirectly, to hyperglycemia. The glomerular lesion is caused by a progressive increase of BM material in capillary walls and in mesangia, causing enlargement and alterations in permeability. Glomeruli may be affected principally by peripheral BM thickening, producing diffuse glomerulosclerosis, or by mesangial sclerosis, producing nodular glomerulosclerosis. Rather than representing two distinct morphologic entities, these patterns are merely varying expressions of a single pathologic process that protein leakage may produce intensely eosinophilic insudative nodules, which are analogous in structure and formation to vascular hyalinosis and to retinal exudates. Proteinuria is the clinical expression of diabetic glomerulosclerosis, and an appearance of more than 3 gm per 24 hours is a clear prognostic sign of impending chronic renal failure. The morphologic diagnosis of diabetic glomerulosclerosis is seldom difficult in fully developed cases, but immunofglomerulosclerosis is seldom difficult in fully developed cases, but immunofluorescence and electron microscopy are required to exclude a number of other diseases that may produce almost identical appearances.

REFERENCES

1. Fajans SS, Cloutier MC, Crowther RL: The Banting Memorial Lecture 1978: clinical and etiologic heterogeneity of idiopathic diabetes mellitus. *Diabetes* 27:1112, 1978.

2. Butcher D, Kikkawa R, Klein L, et al: Size and weight of glomeruli isolated from human diabetic and nondiabetic kidneys. *J Lab Clin Med* 89:544, 1977.

3. Kimmelstiel P, Wilson C: Intercapillary lesions in the glomeruli of the kidney. *Am J Pathol* 12:83, 1936.

4. Watkins PJ, Blainey JD, Brewer DB, et al: The natural history of diabetic renal disease. A follow-up study of a series of renal biopsies. *Quart J Med* 41:437, 1972.

5. Takazakura E, Nakamoto Y, Hayakawa H, et al: Onset and progression of diabetic glomerulosclerosis: a prospective study based on renal biopsies. *Diabetes* 24:1, 1975.

6. Pathogenesis of diabetic microangiopathy, editorial. *Br Med J* 1:1555, 1977.

7. Siperstein MD, Foster DW, Knowles HC Jr, et al: Control of blood glucose and diabetic vascular disease. *N Engl J Med* 296:1060, 1977.

8. Williamson JR, Kilo C: Current status of capillary basement-membrane disease in diabetes mellitus. *Diabetes* 26:65, 1977.

9. Yodaiken RE, Pardo V: Diabetic capillaropathy. *Human Pathol* 6:455, 1975.

10. Fox CJ, Darby SC, Ireland JT, et al: Blood glucose control and glomerular capillary basement thickening in experimental diabetes. *Br Med J* 2:605, 1977.

11. Mauer SM, Steffes MW, Michael AF, et al: Studies of diabetic nephropathy in animals and man. *Diabetes* 25(suppl 2):850, 1976.

12. Osterby R: Morphometric studies of the peripheral basement membrane in early juvenile diabetes. I. Development of initial basement membrane thickening. *Diabetologia* 8:84, 1972.

13. Reddi AS: Diabetic microangiopathy. I. Current status of the chemistry and metabolism of the glomerular basement membrane. *Metabolism* 27:107, 1978.

14. Lundbaek K: Growth hormone's role in diabetic microangiopathy. *Diabetes* 25(suppl 2):845, 1976.

15. Levin NW, Cortes P, Silveira E, et al: Relation of renal growth to diabetic glomerulosclerosis. *Lancet* 1:1120, 1975.

15a. Brownlee R, Spiro RG: Glomerular basement membrane metabolism in the diabetic rat: *in vivo* studies. *Diabetes* 28:121, 1979.

16. Barnes AJ, Locke P, Scudder PR, et al: Is hyperviscosity a treatable component of diabetic microcirculatory disease? *Lancet* 2:789, 1977.

17. Vracko R: Basal lamina layering in diabetes mellitus: evidence for accelerated rate of cell death and cell regeneration. *Diabetes* 23:94, 1974.

18. Dymock IW, Cassar J, Pyke DA, et al: Observations on the pathogenesis, complications and treatment in 115 cases of haemochromatosis. *Am J Med* 52:203, 1972.

19. Wellman KF, Volk BW: Nodular intercapillary glomerulosclerosis in diabetes secondary to chronic calcific pancreatitis. *Diabetes* 25:713, 1976.

20. Westberg NG, Michael AF: Immunohistopathology of diabetic glomerulosclerosis. *Diabetes* 21:163, 1972.

21. Kessler II: Mortality experience of diabetic patients: a twenty-six year follow-up study. *Am J Med* 51:715, 1971.

22. Seymour A, Phear D: The causes of death in diabetes mellitus: a study of diabetic mortality in the Royal Adelaide Hospital from 1956 to 1960. *Med J Aust* 1:890, 1963.

23. Knowles HC Jr: Magnitude of the renal failure problem in diabetic patients. *Kidney Int* 6:S-2, 1974.

24. Bell ET: Renal vascular disease in diabetes mellitus. *Diabetes* 2:376, 1953.

25. Balodimos MC, Legg MA, Bradley RF: Diabetic glomerulosclerosis in children. *Diabetes* 20:622, 1971.

26. Watkins PJ, Parsons V, Bewick M: The prognosis and management of diabetic nephropathy. *Clin Nephrol* 7:243, 1977.

27. Aziz S, Cohen AH, Winer RL, et al: Diabetes mellitus with immune complex glomerulonephritis. *Nephron* 23:32, 1979.

28. Goldstein DA, Massry SG: Diabetic nephropathy: clinical course and effect of hemodialysis. *Nephron* 20:286, 1978.

29. Pabico RC, Panner BJ, McKenna BA, et al: Spontaneous remission of the nephrotic syndrome in diabetic nephropathy. *Am J Med* 59:434, 1975.

30. Ehrenreich T, Churg J: Pathology of membranous nephropathy. *Pathol Annu* 3:145, 1968.

31. Wehner H, Bohle A: The structure of the glomerular capillary basement membrane in diabetes mellitus with and without the nephrotic syndrome. *Virchows Arch A Path Anat Histol* 464:303, 1974.

32. Urizar RE, Schwartz A, Top F, et al: The nephrotic syndrome in children with diabetes mellitus of recent onset. *N Engl J Med* 281:173, 1969.

33. Brulles A, Caralps A, Vilardell M: Nephrotic syndrome with minimal glomerular lesions (lipoid nephrosis) in an adult diabetic patient. *Arch Pathol Lab Med* 101:270, 1977.

34. Harkonen S, Kjellstrand CM: Exacerbation of diabetic renal failure following intravenous pyelography. *Am J Med* 63:939, 1977.

35. Abdulhayoglu S, Marble A: Necrotizing renal papillitis (papillary necrosis) in diabetes mellitus. *Am J Med Sci* 248:623, 1964.

36. Kahn CB, Raman PG, Zic Z: Kidney size in diabetes mellitus. *Diabetes* 23:788, 1974.

37. Iidaka K, McCoy J, Kimmelstiel P: The glomerular mesangium. A quantitative analysis. *Lab Invest* 19:573, 1968.

38. Dachs S, Churg J, Mautner W, et al: Diabetic nephropathy. *Am J Pathol* 44:155, 1965.

39. Salinas-Madrigal L, Pirani CL, Pollak VE: Glomerular and vascular "insudative" lesions of diabetic nephropathy: Electron microscopic observations. *Am J Pathol* 59:369, 1970.

40. Kimmelstiel P: Diabetic nephropathy, in Mostofi EK, Smith DE (eds): *The Kidney*. Baltimore, Williams and Wilkins Co, 1966, p 226.

41. Lendrum AC: The hypertensive diabetic kidney as a model of the so-called collagen diseases. *Canad Med Ass J* 88:442, 1963.

42. Elfenbein IB, Reyes JW: Crescents in diabetic glomerulopathy. Incidence and clinical significance. *Lab Invest* 33:687, 1975.

43. Osterby R: A quantitative electron microscopic study of mesangial regions in glomeruli from patients with short-term juvenile diabetes mellitus. *Lab Invest* 29:99, 1973.

44. Seymour AE, Spargo BH, Penska R: Contributions of renal biopsy studies to the understanding of disease. *Am J Pathol* 65:550, 1971.

45. Bariety J, Callard R: Striated membranous structures in renal glomerular tufts: an electron microscopy study of 340 human renal biopsies. *Lab Invest* 32:636, 1975.

46. Miller K, Michael AF: Immunopathology of renal extracellular membranes in diabetes mellitus: specificity of tubular basement-membrane immunofluorescence. *Diabetes* 25:701, 1976.

47. Olsen S: Mesangial thickening and nodular glomerular sclerosis in diabetes mellitus and other diseases. *Acta Pathol Microbiol Scand (A)* 80(suppl 233):203, 1972.

48. Schubert GE, Adam A: Glomerular nodules and long-spacing collagen in kidneys of patients with multiple myeloma. *J Clin Pathol* 27:800, 1974.

49. Randall RE, Williamson WC, Mullinax F, et al: Manifestations of systemic light chain deposition. *Am J Med* 60:293, 1976.

50. Nash DA Jr, Rogers PW, Linglinais PC, et al: Diabetic glomerulosclerosis without glucose intolerance. *Am J Med* 59:191, 1975.

51. Barnes BA, Bergan JJ, Braun WE, et al: Renal transplantation in congenital and metabolic diseases. A report from the ASC/NIH Renal Transplant Registry. *JAMA* 323:148, 1975.

52. Kjellstrand CM, Shideman JR, Simmons RL, et al: Renal transplantation in insulin-dependent diabetic patients. *Kidney Int* 6:S-15, 1974.

53. Mauer SM, Barbosa J, Vernier RL, et al: Development of diabetic vascular lesions in normal kidneys transplanted into patients with diabetes mellitus. *N Engl J Med* 295:916, 1976.

54. Barbosa J, Burke B, Buselmeier TJ, et al: Neuropathy, retinopathy and biopsy findings in transplanted kidney in diabetic patients. *Kidney Int* 6:S-32, 1974.

55. Mauer SM, Miller K, Goetz FC, et al: Immunopathology of renal extracellular membranes in kidneys transplanted into patients with diabetes mellitus. *Diabetes* 25:709, 1976.

56. Doud R, Lee DBN, Waisman J, et al: Development of a lesion resembling diabetic nephropathy in a renal homograft. *Arch Intern Med* 137:945, 1977.

19
Amyloidosis

Amyloidosis is a clinicopathologic syndrome caused by tissue infiltration with eosinophilic scleroproteins. Progressive accumulation of these proteins causes obliteration of tissue structure and disturbed function. Because the chemical nature of the amyloid proteins was unknown until recent years, a bewildering variety of clinical and pathologic classifications have been proposed, largely based on tissue distribution and histochemistry. It is now becoming clear that amyloid is not one but a number of chemically distinct proteins having similar microscopic, histochemical, and diffraction properties. In the future, access to sophisticated analytical facilities will hopefully allow each of these protein types to be considered as a distinct entity, and the continued use of the existing classifications may become obsolete. For the moment, however, the techniques available in most laboratories do not provide reliable differentation between the varying amyloid types, and crude classification by clinical and morphologic criteria must continue.

Renal involvement occurs with most forms of amyloidosis. Glomeruli are most frequently and extensively involved, with consequent alterations in permeability, causing proteinuria, and vascularity, causing renal failure. Diagnosis is usually straightforward from the examination of renal biopsy tissue, but small quantities of amyloid may be overlooked by light microscopy, and ultrastructural examination is essential if the diagnosis is clinically suspected. Proteinuria may be the first clinical sign of systemic amyloidosis, and chronic renal failure is a common cause of death in these patients.

CLASSIFICATION AND PATHOGENESIS

Amyloid is conventionally defined as an eosinophilic amorphous material with a fibrillar ultrastructure and a β-pleated sheet configuration on x-ray diffraction analysis (1). A variety of cotton dyes, especially Congo red, are taken up by amyloid, and its organized substructure causes alteration in the path of polarized light to produce a characteristic apple-green color in Congo red-stained sections (2). This green birefringent property is the most reliable diagnostic feature by light microscopy, but it is not specific (3), and unequivocal diagnosis requires the ultrastructural demonstration of the specific fibrils. Although a variety of histochemical techniques and patterns of deposition, both light and microscopic, have been used to differentiate between the different classes of amyloid proteins, none has been shown to provide reliable results.

Classification of amyloid has relied for many years on the identification of associated diseases. Thus, systemic amyloidosis may be secondary to a variety of disorders, mainly "chronic inflammatory" in type, or may be apparently "primary." Alternatively, the propensity to develop amyloid deposits may be an inherited characteristic, or amyloid may occur sporadically as localized deposits with no tendency to systemic spread. These four groups form the basis for the conventional classifications into primary, secondary, heredofamilial, and localized types (1). The diseases associated with secondary amyloidosis include chronic suppuration (bronchiectasis, osteomyelitis, etc.), granulomatous infections (tuberculosis, leprosy, etc.), presumed "immune" disorders (rheumatoid arthritis and variants, ulcerative colitis, Crohn's disease, etc.), and a variety of malignancies (1,4). There is a tendency for secondary amyloidosis to involve parenchymal organs preferentially (liver, spleen, kidney, etc.) and for the primary form to affect the mesodermal tissues in particular (smooth and skeletal muscle, cardiovascular system, etc.), but there are so many exceptions to this trend that it is not diagnostically valuable (1).

Biochemical studies have recently defined three distinct proteins in the serum and deposits of patients with systemic amyloidosis (5−8). One of these, the AP protein, is present in both primary and secondary forms, while the other two are characteristic of each amyloid class. The AP protein is an α-globulin with a molecular weight of 200,000 daltons, which has a pentagonal structure and is the constituent of the pentagonal, doughnutlike bodies accompanying the fibrils in amyloid deposits (5). An apparent circulatory precursor, the SAP protein, is present in the serum of amyloidotic and (in minute quantities) normal people. This circulating protein is identical to a recently isolated subfraction of the first complement component (Clt) and closely resembles C-reactive protein. The AP protein cannot be identified in normal tissues, and its role in the production and/or deposition of amyloid fibrils is unknown.

The major constituent of the primary amyloid fibril is the variable portion of the immunoglobulin light chain, often with all or part of the constant segment (6,7). Although there is variation in the precise amino acid sequence between different patients with primary amyloid, the sequence is fixed in all deposits in each individual with the disease. There is, therefore, a monoclonal production of amyloid protein, corresponding to previous suspicions of an identity between primary amyloid and multiple myeloma. These suspicions were based on the demonstration of M spikes in the serum, sometimes with Bence-Jones proteins, and plasmacytosis in the bone marrows of these patients (9). In patients with multiple myeloma who develop amyloid, the chemical structure of the amyloid is identical to the light chain comprising the Bence-Jones protein (6). Myeloma and primary amyloidosis may, therefore, be regarded as points along a spectrum of B-cell neoplasia, the degrees of protein production and cell proliferation determining the pattern of clinical presentation (8). There is some evidence to suggest that only a portion of monoclonal light chains are capable of forming tissue deposits of amyloid. Thus, the ratio of kappa to lambda light chains in amyloid proteins is the reverse of that seen in paraproteinemias without amyloid (7), and Bence-Jones proteins from patients with myeloma and amyloidosis show a greater tendency to tissue binding than the proteins from myeloma patients without amyloidosis (10).

The fibrils in secondary and heredofamilial amyloidosis are composed of AA protein, a substance with a molecular weight of approximately 8,000 daltons that shares no chemical characteristics with any known immunoglobulin (5). An antigenically similar substance, the SAA protein, is present in the sera of these patients and may represent a circulating precursor of the tissue deposits. The biochemical structure of each protein is species-specific, but proteins with similar characteristics occur in the sera and deposits of animals with experimentally induced secondary amyloidosis (5). Although tissue AA protein cannot be identified in normal people, minute quantities of SAA are present in the normal population, and higher concentrations, approximating those of amyloidotic patients, occur in inflammatory and neoplastic diseases known to predispose to amyloidosis (5,11). In contrast to the central role of the B lymphocyte in primary amyloidosis, there is evidence for depression of T-lymphocyte function in experimental AA amyloidosis.

Localized amyloid deposits are probably of varying type. In one report of isolated pulmonary amyloidosis, for example, light chains were demonstrated in the plasma cells around the amyloid (12). In contrast, insulin and calcitonin have been identified in the amyloid contained in APUD tumors of the pancreas (13) and thyroid (14), respectively. Other examples of localized amyloid, including laryngeal masses and the cerebral plaques of Alzheimer's disease (1), are likely to have chemically distinct structures and separate mechanisms of production.

The pathway for final deposition of amyloid fibrils appears to be via cells of the reticuloendothelial system. Experimental studies of secondary amyloidosis demonstrate intracellular fibrils related to lysosomes (15), and lysosomal enzymes are capable of digesting light chains to form amyloid fibrils (6,7). Proteolytic digestion of SAA protein to form fibrils has not been demonstrated, but it is tempting to speculate that lysosomal digestion and processing of circulating proteins may be the mechanism for the production of both primary and secondary amyloidosis. The structure and histochemical properties long associated with amyloid, many of which are related to its β-pleated character, may depend as much on the process of deposition as the chemical structure. Future studies may reveal other common mechanisms for the deposition of these, at present, apparently distinct proteins, which Hobbs (8) has neatly divided into amyloid of types A (protein AA, secondary), B (light chain, B cell or primary) and C (localized types).

INCIDENCE

The frequency of renal amyloidosis depends both on the population under study and the methods used for diagnosis. Amyloid was demonstrated in 3% of one series of 1,500 renal biopsies (16) and in 0.4% of 20,000 consecutive autopsies performed at the Johns Hopkins Hospital (17). In the past, secondary amyloidosis was far more common than the primary form, and this distribution still applies in those parts of the world where leprosy and similar diseases remain endemic. The virtual eradication of mycobacterial and chronic suppurative infections in the western world has, however, caused a drastic reduction in the incidence of secondary amyloidosis with a concomitant increase in the proportion of primary disease. One recent study of 236 patients found only 19 (8%) with secondary amyloidosis, whereas 132 (56%) were regarded as primary and 61 (26%) were associated with multiple myeloma (18). Renal involvement was demonstrated by clinical criteria in 90% of this series and in 86% of another similar series, being the initial feature in 64% of the patients in the latter group (19). Most studies of renal amyloidosis, however, include more patients with secondary than with primary disease, suggesting that renal involvement is more likely in the secondary form. The heredofamilial syndromes tend to be defined by their anatomic distribution patterns of amyloid deposition and are generally so rare that incidence rates of renal involvement are meaningless (20). However, in the most common of these heredofamilial syndromes, that associated with familial Mediterranean fever, renal amyloid has been documented in approximately one-third of the patients (21,22).

CLINICAL MANIFESTATIONS

The age at onset of amyloidosis depends largely on its nature. Clearly, secondary disease may occur at any age according to the duration of the associated disease. In most series, however, the mean age at diagnosis has been between 55 and 61 years for primary amyloidosis and about 10 years younger in secondary disease (16,18,19). The disease is rare in children and usually related to chronic inflammation or heredofamilial disorders such as familial Mediterranean fever (23). There is a significant excess of males in many series, regardless of the cause or pattern of amyloidosis (16,18,19).

The principal renal manifestation of renal amyloidosis is altered glomerular permeability, producing nonselective proteinuria (1,16). This may be detected during the continuing care of a patient with one of the chronic diseases known to be associated with amyloidosis or may be a chance finding at routine physical examination. Proteinuria is frequently sufficient to cause the nephrotic syndrome at some stage during the clinical course, estimates of its frequency varying up to 60% (19). Conversely, from 3 to 12% of patients investigated for the nephrotic syndrome have been found to have amyloidosis (24). Microscopic hematuria may be found but, typically, the urinary sediment is bland (1). Early in the course of the disease, the kidneys may be either normal in size or enlarged; later there is progressive shrinkage with the onset of renal failure. The clinical combination of isolated proteinuria or the nephrotic syndrome with bilaterally enlarged kidneys is, however, suggestive of amyloidosis. Hypertension varies in frequency between different series but is probably less common than in other forms of chronic renal disease (25), except in some of the heredofamilial forms such as the Ostertag pattern (20). Many patients, in fact, suffer from debilitating postural hypotension (19), possibly secondary to amyloid infiltration of autonomic ganglia. An entirely separate clinical syndrome has occasionally been described in which amyloid infiltrates preferentially around medullary collecting tubules. When first seen, these patients had nephrogenic diabetes inspidus or other tubular syndromes (26,27). As already discussed, patients with primary and, to a lesser extent, secondary amyloidosis frequently have circulating paraproteins (9).

PATHOLOGIC CHARACTERISTICS

Light Microscopy

Amyloid affects all areas of the kidney but accumulates especially in the glomeruli. Deposition is initially mesangial, producing diffuse and hyaline widening of axial areas, but progressively spreads to replace capillary lumina (28) (Fig. 19-1). The pattern of deposition suggests a gradual obliteration of the filtering area by a large, insoluble, and nonfiltered molecular substance. With increasing deposition, the glomeruli become greatly enlarged, and the hyaline mesangial pattern is complicated by peripheral spread in either a nodular or diffuse pattern (Fig. 19-2). Mesangial nodules may sometimes closely resemble those of diabetic glomerulosclerosis but lack the laminated PASM-positive character of the diabetic lesion (Fig. 19-3). Diffuse spread through the glomerulus can produce a picture reminiscent of membranous nephropathy, and this resemblance may be heightened by the formation of frequent epimembranous spikes (29) (Fig. 19-4). A spicular pattern is, in fact, quite common in amylodotic glomeruli but is rarely diffuse, and the spicules lack the bulbous ends that are so typical of the spikes in membranous nephropathy. Giant cells are occasionally seen in relation to the amyloid deposits (30). Afferent arterioles and other blood vessels are commonly affected early in the disease, frequently in

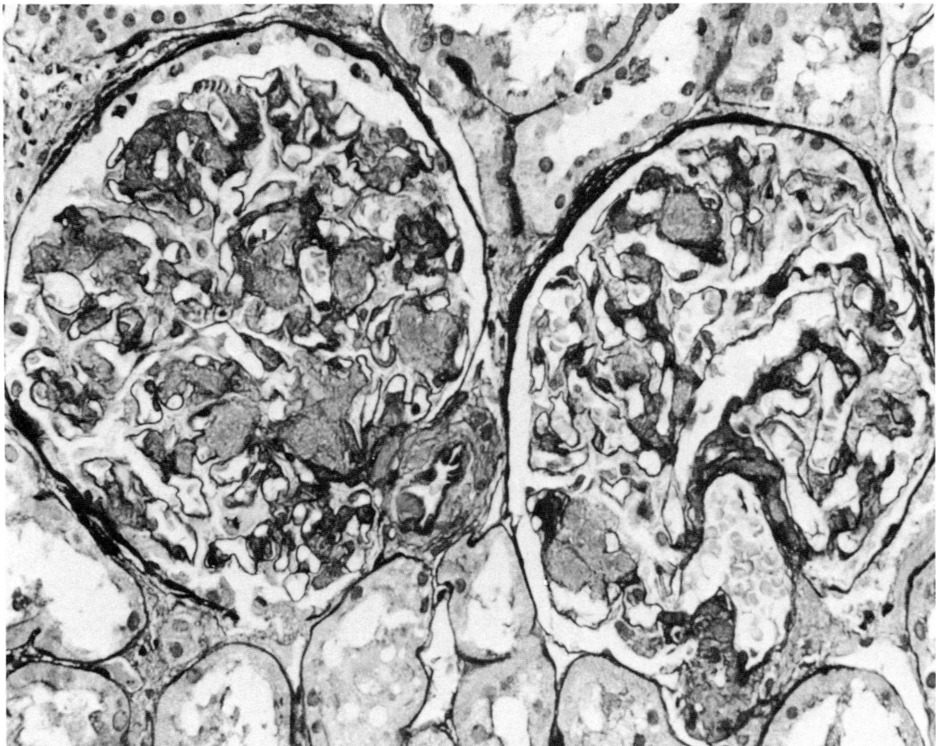

Figure 19-1. Glomerulus showing irregular mesangial deposits of amyloid (PAS stain, ×390).

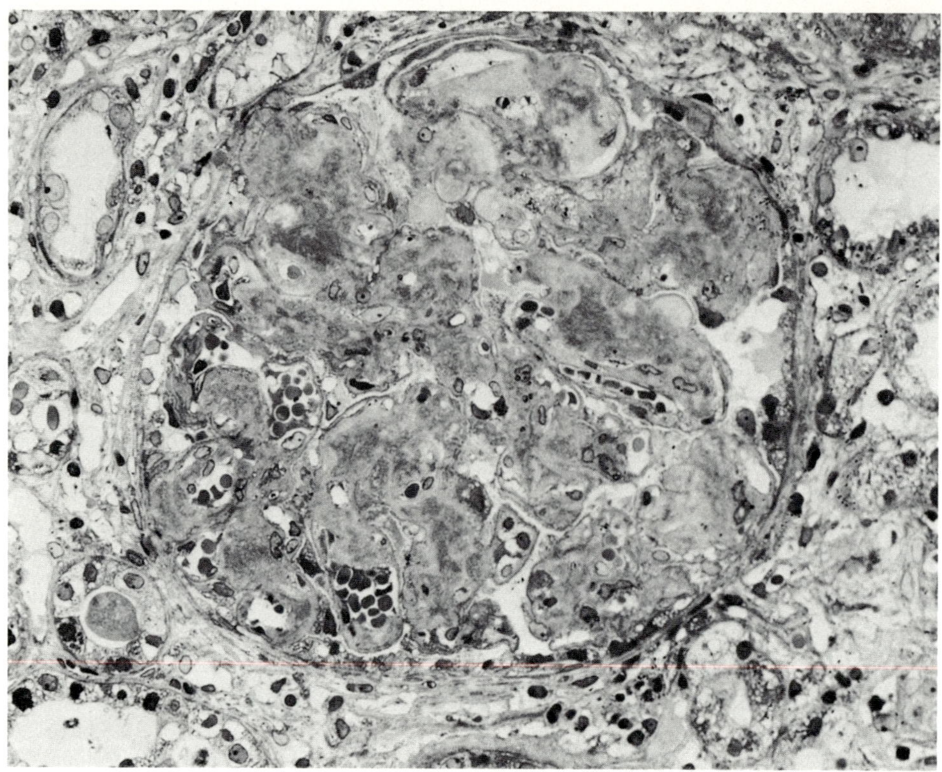

Figure 19-2. Advanced amyloidosis. The glomerulus is enlarged and diffusely infiltrated with amyloid (plastic embedded toluidine blue stain, ×400).

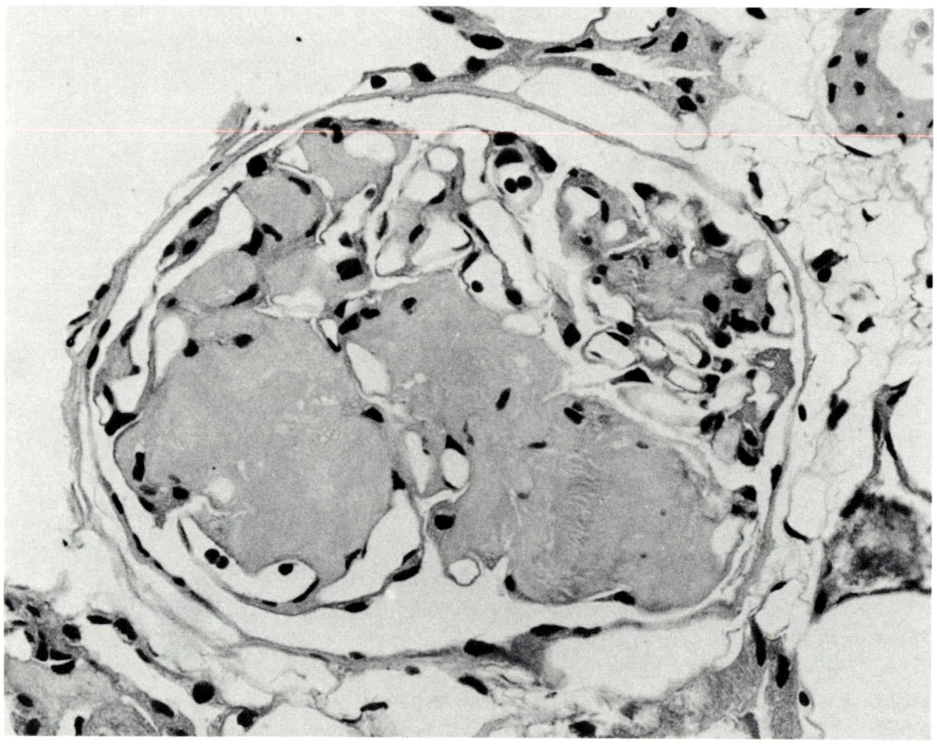

Figure 19-3. Nodular deposits of amyloid (H&E stain, ×550).

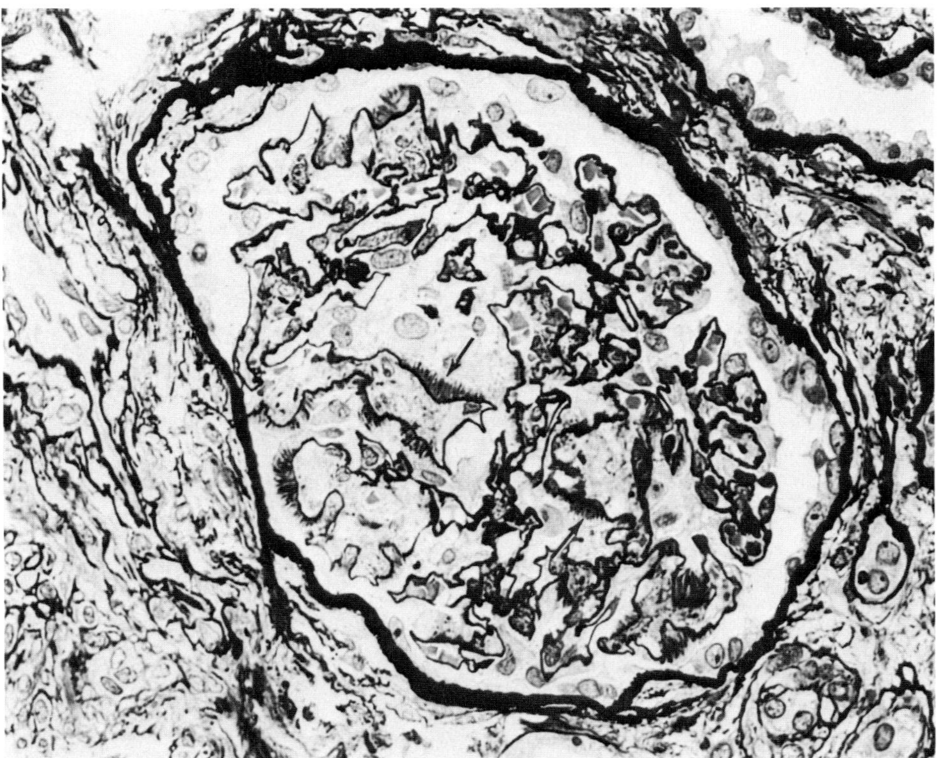

Figure 19-4. Amyloid deposits in peripheral capillary loops appearing as argyrophilic spikelike projections (arrows) (PASM stain, ×650).

direct continuity with the glomerular deposits (Fig. 19-5). The hyaline vascular involvement in biopsy tissue with only slight glomerular involvement may be misinterpreted unless special stains are used or electron microscopy demonstrates the fibrils.

With increasing deposition, glomerular structure is obliterated, and the glomeruli appear as large, hyaline balls with only fragments of the membrane skeleton being visible in PAS- and PASM-stained sections. Special stains may be difficult to interpret at this late stage since the typical reactions are often obscured. In parallel with glomerular obliteration, there is increasing tubular atrophy with interstitial scarring, and deposits of amyloid may become prominent in the interstitium. Casts may be present at all stages of the disease but become prominent and widespread with the onset of scarring. In most forms of amyloid, the casts are no different from those in other proteinuric conditions, being composed in large part of inspissated filtered proteins. In multiple myeloma, however, the casts frequently exhibit histochemical reactions for amyloid and have a fibrillar ultrastructure (8). The presence of amyloid material in the tubular casts of patients with myeloma is quite unrelated to the presence of glomerular amyloidosis, which is, in fact, relatively uncommon in this condition (1). Instead, the amyloid characteristics are probably produced via proteolytic precipitation of fibrils by the action of tubular lysosomal enzymes on Bence-Jones proteins (6).

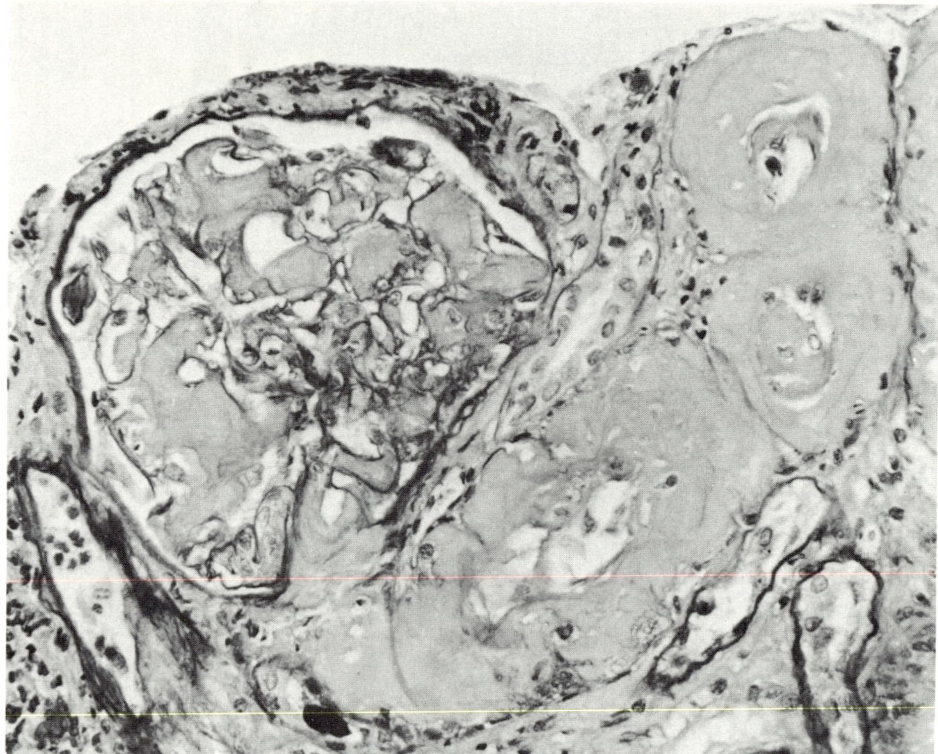

Figure 19-5. Vascular walls showing severe amyloid involvement. There is also prominent mesangial deposition of amyloid in the glomerulus (PAS stain, ×400).

Histochemistry

A wide variety of histochemical techniques have been suggested for the diagnosis
of amyloid (2). Generally, the most satisfactory of these for renal biopsy diagnosis are the thioflavine T and Congo red stains. Thioflavine T is extremely
sensitive but not absolutely specific, whereas the production of an apple-green
color by polarized light in Congo red-stained sections is accepted as the most
reliable light microscopic method of diagnosis (Figs. 19-6, 19-7). Each technique
requires the reaction of a critical quantity of amyloid with the reagent before
positive reactions can be produced. Small amounts of amyloid may, therefore, be
missed and, more important, neither technique is effective with very thin sections. The stains should always be performed on sections cut at more than 5 μ
and always with appropriate controls.

Electron Microscopy

Ultrastructural examination provides the only method presently available for
certain identification of amyloid and is mandatory for all biopsy specimens
where there is a clinical suspicion of the disease. The fibrils appear as randomly
arranged and apparently rigid, nonbranching rods, measuring 80−100 Å in
diameter and 300−10,000 Å in length. Sometimes a beaded structure, with

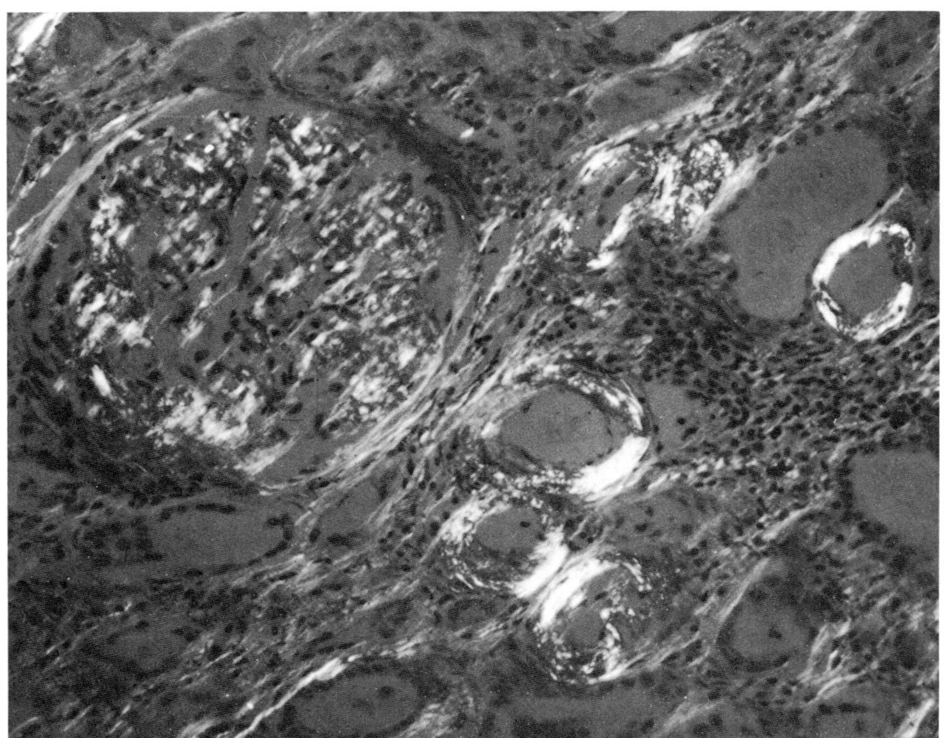

Figure 19-6. Deposits of amyloid exhibiting birefringence under polarized light (Congo red stain, ×250).

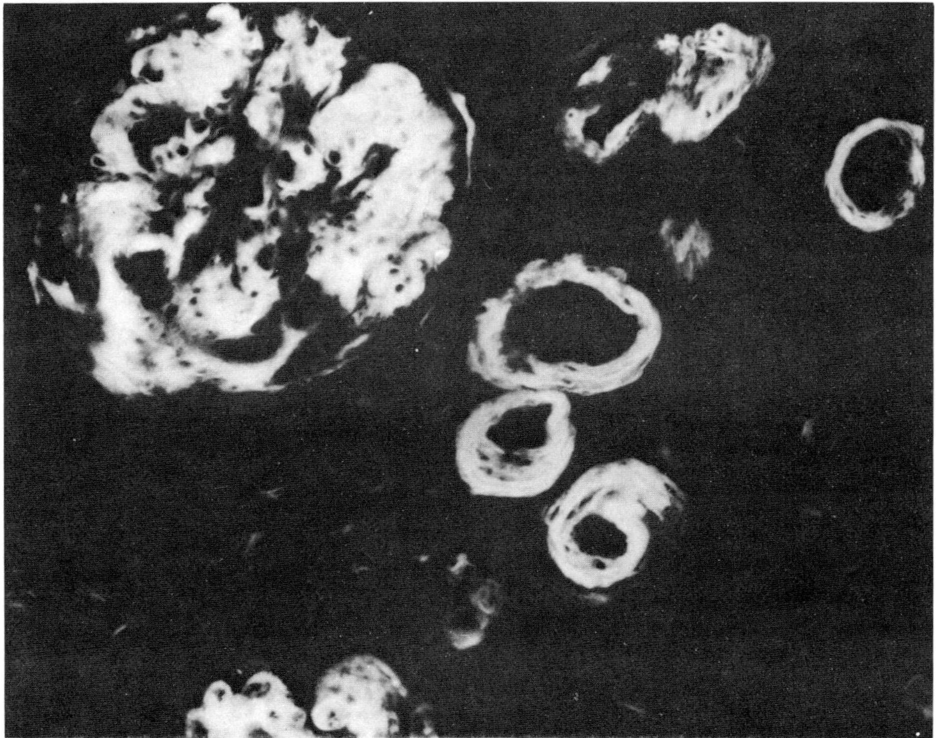

Figure 19-7. Fluorescence of amyloid under ultraviolet light (yellow in original preparation) (thioflavin T stain, ×250).

periodicity of 50 Å, can be detected (Fig. 19-8). Very high resolution examination reveals, in addition, pentagonal structures with a doughnut appearance (31,32), which represent the AP protein component. The fibrils are deposited first in mesangial regions, where they progressively permeate and replace the normal structure (33) (Fig. 19-9). From the mesangium, there is extension into subendothelial regions and through the overlying basement membrane. Characteristically, amyloid fibrils are unencumbered by any natural barrier and spread in continuity through all structures. Thus, the fibrils extend from mesangial and subendothelial regions into and through the basement membrane, which often has a thickened and frayed appearance (Fig. 19-10). Where amyloid penetrates the membrane, epithelial foot processes are obliterated, often separated from the membrane and sometimes apparently infiltrated by the extending fibrils. This process usually has the appearance of an infiltrating, irregular mass but may be manifest as parallel arrays of fibrils arranged perpendicular to the membrane in glomeruli showing a spicular pattern (29) (Fig. 19-11). There is a direct correlation between the extent of membrane involvement, with secondary epithelial changes, and the severity of proteinuria (33a). In doubtful cases, differentiation between amyloid fibrils and the fibrillar character of the mesangial matrix may be extremely difficult, requiring both careful measurement and experience. Usually, however, the diagnosis is relatively easy, providing enough glomeruli are examined. Amyloid fibrils are highly resistant to autolysis and to all forms of tissue processing. A confident ultrastructural diagnosis can, therefore, be made on autopsy tissue and on deparaffinized sections of renal biopsy specimens in those cases where no or inappropriate material is taken for electron microscopy.

Immunofluorescence Microscopy

Varying results have been reported with conventional antisera in glomerular amyloidosis, perhaps because amyloid is autofluorescent in ultraviolet light. The inclusion of an untreated section in the series examined by immunofluorescence will reveal a highly characteristic pattern of fluffy and poorly defined infiltration through the glomeruli. The positive reactions that have been reported (34) may be partially explained by exaggerated autofluorescence but probably also reflect nonspecific entrapment of a variety of proteins (Fig. 19-12). Sophisticated studies may, however, specifically detect the light chain (35), AA (36,37), and AP (38) components.

DIFFERENTIAL DIAGNOSIS

There is seldom any real difficulty in establishing a tissue diagnosis of amyloidosis when electron microscopy is available. The most common diagnostic problem is an inability to demonstrate the specific histochemical reactions in thin sections. At the light microscopic level, the other major difficulties in diagnosis are those biopsy specimens with minimal glomerular involvement, arteriolar deposits misinterpreted as "hyalin," and those in which a widespread spicular pattern raises the suspicion of membranous nephropathy. Each of these difficul-

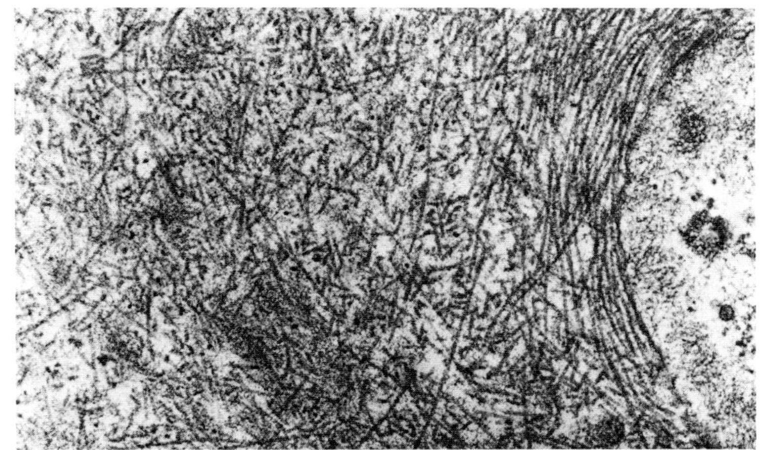

Figure 19-8. Amyloid fibrils (×65,000).

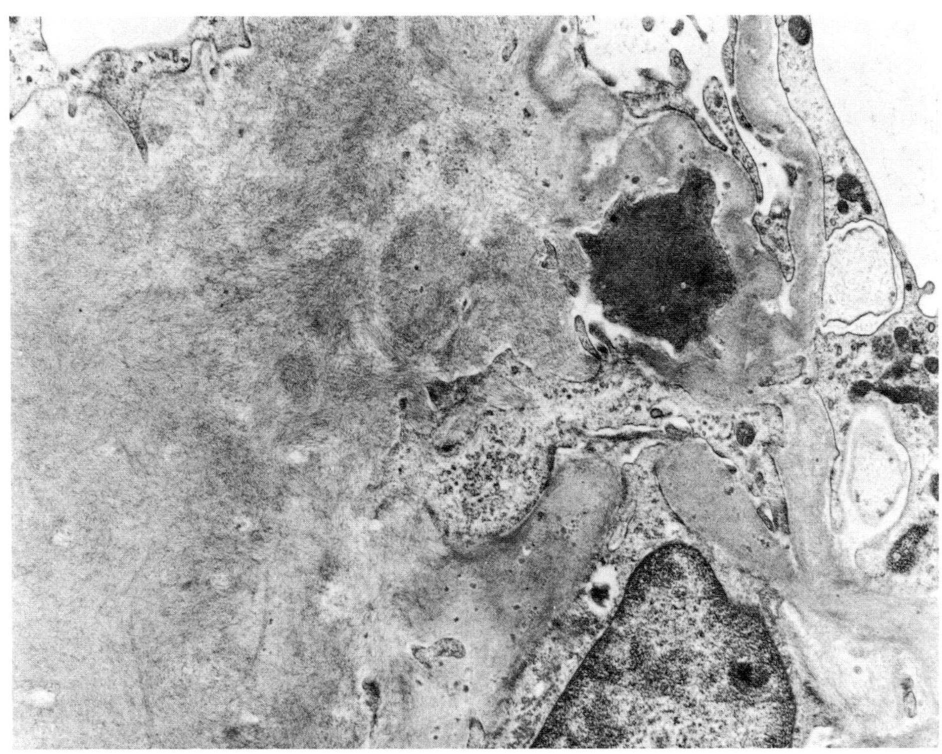

Figure 19-9. Mesangial deposits of amyloid (×12,900).

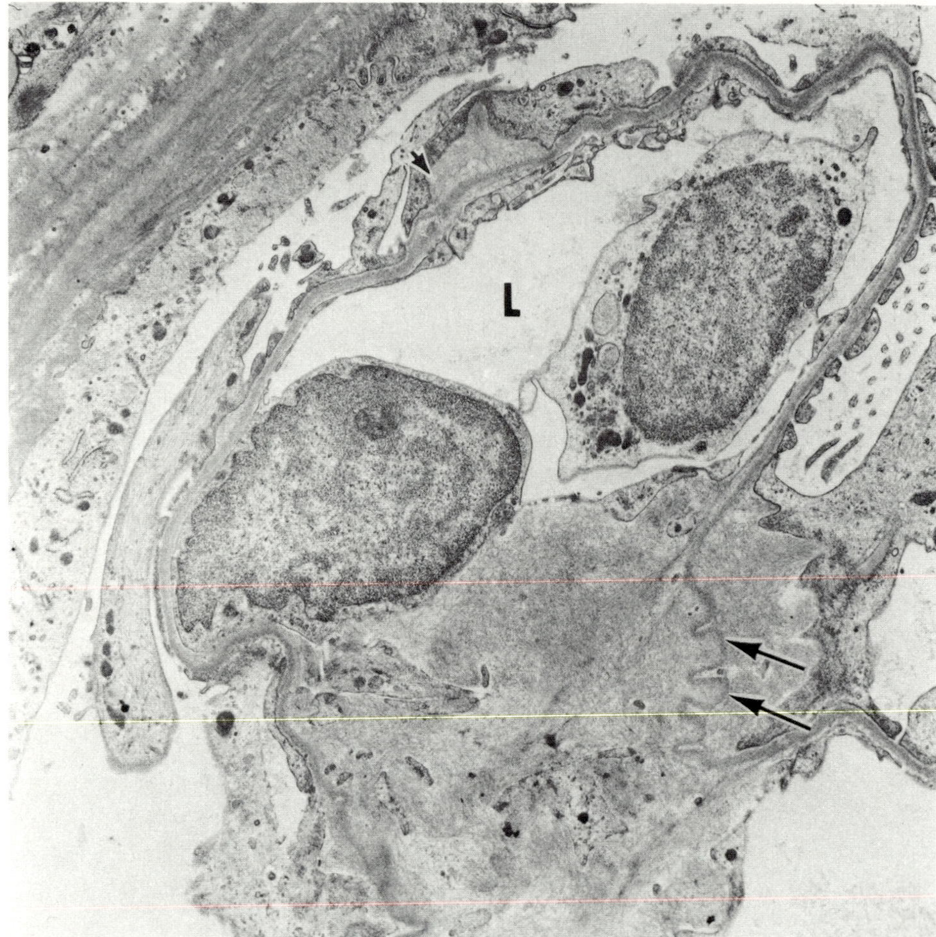

Figure 19-10. Mesangial and peripheral spicular subepithelial (arrow head) deposit of amyloid. The lamina densa is intact in spite of the large amounts of subepithelial and mesangial amyloid deposits (arrows). L, capillary lumen (×8,500).

ties is readily resolved by the ultrastructural demonstration of amyloid fibrils. Occasionally, amyloid is demonstrated by electron microscopy when there are no grounds for suspecting the diagnosis by light microscopy (8,39). There are rare examples of glomerular disease of uncertain type in which amyloid fibrils and apparent immune deposits coexist (40). The fibrillar structures often seen in the glomerular deposits of cryoglobulinemia are larger and the distinct light and immunofluorescent microscopic characteristics prevent confusion with amyloid (see p 375).

Vascular infiltration by amyloid creates a risk of uncontrollable hemorrhage with tissue biopsy. Many physicians, therefore, prefer to perform biopsies under direct observation in patients with suspected amyloidosis rather than risk the possibility of internal hemorrhage after needle biopsy. The usual sites for such open biopsies are the gingiva and rectum, each of which provides a high frequency of positive results with a low risk of hemorrhage (1,18). Recently, another

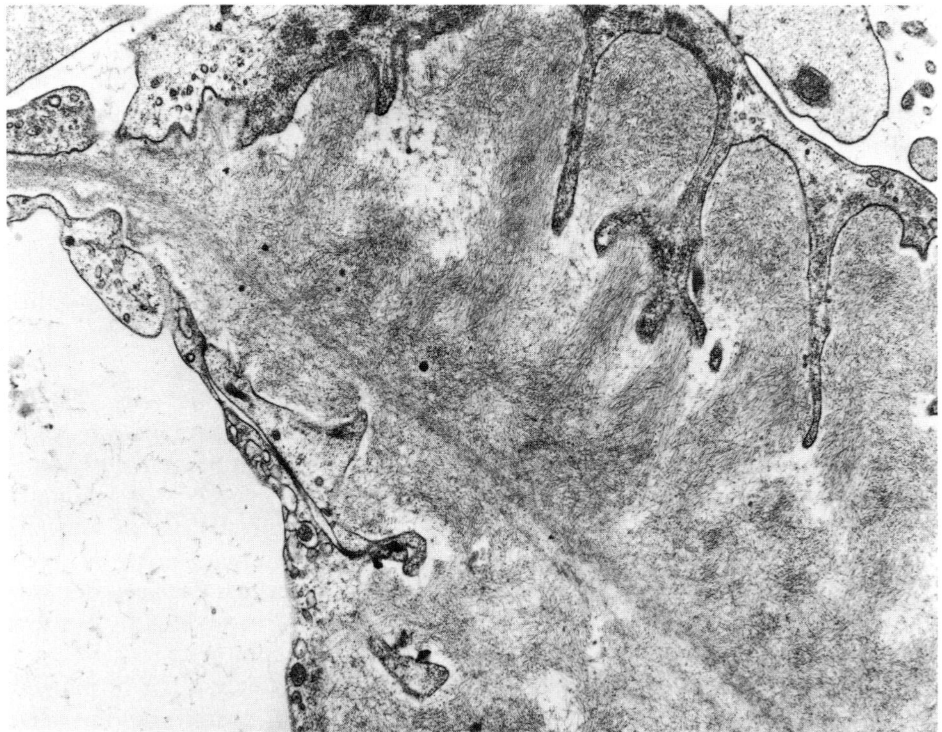

Figure 19-11. Intramembranous amyloid deposits. Some of the amyloid fibers are arranged in bundles perpendicular to the lamina densa (×15,200).

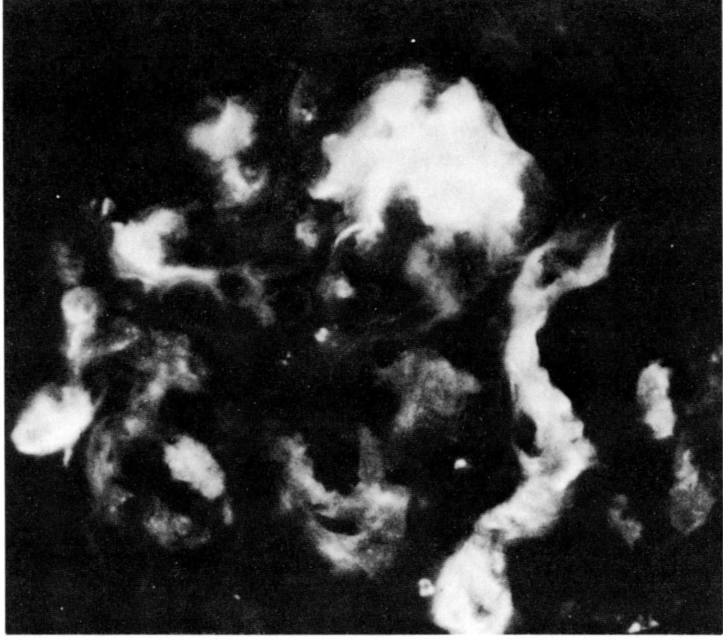

Figure 19-12. Glomerulus with irregular wide segmental deposits of amyloid (antihuman IgG, ×450).

noninvasive technique for the diagnosis of renal amyloidosis was suggested by the demonstration of amyloid fibrils in centrifuged urine (41), especially after a dose of dimethyl sulphoxide (42). Clearly, this technique would not be applicable in the presence of Bence-Jones proteinuria since proteolysis of these proteins is known to produce amyloid fibrils (6,43). Other studies of centrifuged urine have, however, shown amyloidlike fibrils in patients without evidence of either myeloma or amyloidosis and the value of this technique is at present uncertain (36,44,44a).

COURSE AND PROGNOSIS

The median survival after diagnosis of patients with amyloidosis is reported to be 14.7 months for systemic disease (18) and 31 months for predominantly renal (16) disease. Longer periods of survival occur, however, quite frequently, and may extend up to eight or more years (19). The usual course is of gradually increasing renal failure, frequently combined with manifestations of amyloid deposition elsewhere, especially cardiac failure (18). Renal failure may be accelerated by the superimposition of renal vein thrombosis, which has been demonstrated frequently in patients with familial Mediterranean fever (22) but less commonly in other forms (16).

The therapy of amyloidosis is still in its infancy. Hemodialysis has prolonged survival of patients with chronic renal failure for up to 63 months but has been complicated by a high mortality after the first year, largely attributable to cardiac and circulatory involvement (45). Transplantation was considered by many to be contraindicated in amyloidosis but has been used for a small number of patients after early reports of successful engraftment and survival (46). There is, as yet, insufficient evidence to fully evaluate the results in the few transplanted patients, but preliminary data suggest an unduly high mortality from infection (45), although prolonged survival has occasionally occurred (37). Recurrence in the graft has, however, been documented in patients with primary (47), secondary (45), and familial Mediterranean fever-related (37,48) amyloidosis so that the future of transplantation in the disease is uncertain. Amyloid deposits in other organs may become unusually extensive after transplantation, presumably because of the artificial prolongation of life (48).

Occasional examples of apparent regression of amyloid have been documented over many years (1) and have stimulated a search for more specific methods of therapy. Eradication of chronic septic foci has been associated with clinical improvement of secondary amyloidosis with, in some cases, persistence (49), but in others, reduction (16,50) in the renal deposits. In primary amyloidosis, attempts to modify the production of amyloidogenic light chains by intensive chemotherapy have been associated with sustained clinical improvement, but morphologic regression of renal deposits has not been demonstrated (8,51,52). In one of these patients, serial bone marrow examination revealed suggestive evidence for degradation of the amyloid deposits by macrophages (51). Macrophages have been implicated in both the degradation (53,54) and formation (15) of amyloid fibrils, and the effects of a number of drugs capable of altering macrophage function have, therefore, been studied. Corticosteroids are ineffective in amyloidosis (24), and amyloid deposits have been noted to progress in a patient treated with D-penicillamine (55). Colchicine, however, reduces the severity of experimental amyloidosis, and its administration has been associated with clinical improvement in a number of patients (56). Other therapeutic measures are likely to be studied in the future but, in spite of these sporadic successes, the outlook remains grim for patients with renal amyloidosis.

SUMMARY

Amyloidosis is a clinicopathologic syndrome probably comprising several distinct diseases. The kidney may be involved by two well-defined amyloid proteins: a portion of the immunoglobulin light chain in primary amyloidosis and AA protein in both the secondary and heredofamilial forms of the disease. The morphologic appearances of these apparently disparate proteins are identical, and reliable differentiation is not possible by conventional pathologic techniques. The histochemical features conventionally used to establish the diagnosis of amyloid are probably dependent upon a β-pleated arrangement within the fibrils, which may be an expression of enzymatic proteolysis of precursor proteins. This arrangement is not restricted to amyloid proteins, and false-positive histochemical reactions occur so that ultrastructural examination remains essential for specific diagnosis. In addition to the characteristic fibrils, electron microscopy demonstrates the presence of small pentagonal structures, composed of AP protein. Renal involvement is predominantly glomerular, causing proteinuria and, often, the nephrotic syndrome, and progresses over variable periods to chronic renal failure. In spite of a range of therapeutic measures, control or regression of amyloidosis is rare, and death eventually occurs from either azotemia or the involvement of other organs. Transplantation has been successful in a few patients, but recurrence of amyloid in the grafted kidneys has occasionally occurred. The most favorable results appear likely to be in those patients with amyloidosis secondary to chronic suppuration, in whom removal of the suppurative focus has been associated with clinical and morphologic improvement. The great advances in our understanding of the pathogenesis of amyloidosis have not, so far, led to effective therapy, but continued investigation may eventually enable control or cure of this group of diseases.

REFERENCES

1. Cohen AS: Amyloidosis. *N Engl J Med* 277:522,574,628, 1967.

2. Cooper JH: An evaluation of current methods for the diagnostic histochemistry of amyloid. *J Clin Pathol* 22:410, 1969.

3. Klatskin G: Nonspecific green birefringence in Congo red-stained tissues. *Am J Pathol* 56:1, 1969.

4. Brownstein MH, Helwig EB: Secondary systemic amyloidosis: analysis of systemic disorders. *South Med J* 64:491, 1971.

5. Cohen AS, Cathcart ES, Skinner M: Amyloidosis: current trends in its investigation. *Arthritis Rheum* 21:153, 1978.

6. Glenner GG, Terry WD, Isersky C: Amyloidosis: Its nature and pathogenesis. *Semin Hematol* 10:65, 1973.

7. Glenner GG, Page DL: Amyloid, amyloidosis and amyloidogenesis. *Int Rev Exp Pathol* 15:1, 1976.

8. Hobbs JR: An ABC of amyloid. *Proc Roy Soc Med* 66:705, 1973.

9. Isobe T, Osserman EF: Patterns of amyloidosis and their association with plasma cell dyscrasia, monoclonal immunoglobulins and Bence-Jones proteins. *N Engl J Med* 290:473, 1974.

10. Osserman EF, Takatsuk K, Talal N: The pathogenesis of "amyloidosis." *Semin Hematol* 1:3, 1964.

11. Rosenthal CJ, Franklin EC: Variation with age and disease of an amyloid A protein-related serum component. *J Clin Invest* 55:746, 1975.

12. Page DL, Isersky C, Harada M, et al: Immunoglobulin origin of localized nodular pulmonary amyloidosis. *Res Exp Med* 159:75, 1972.

13. Sletten K, Westermark P, Natvig JB: Characterization of amyloid fibril proteins from medullary carcinoma of the thyroid. *J Exp Med* 143:993, 1976.

14. Westermark P: Fine structure of islets of Langerhans in insular amyloidosis. *Virchows Arch A* 359:1, 1973.

15. Shirahama T, Cohen AS: Intralysosomal formation of amyloid fibrils. *Am J Pathol* 81:101, 1975.

16. Triger DR, Joekes AM: Renal amyloidosis—a fourteen year follow-up. *Quart J Med* 42:15, 1973.

17. Walker WG, Harvey AM, Yardley JH: Renal involvement in myeloma, amyloidosis, systemic lupus erythematosus and other disorders of connective tissue, in Strauss MB, Welt LG (eds): *Diseases of the Kidney* ed. 2. Boston, Little, Brown, and Co, 1971, p 825.

18. Kyle RA, Bayrd ED: Amyloidosis: Review of 236 cases. *Medicine (Balt)* 54:271, 1975.

19. Brandt DT, Cathcart ES, Cohen AS: A clinical analysis of the course and prognosis of forty-two patients with amyloidosis. *Am J Med* 44:955, 1968.

20. Alexander F, Atkins EL: Familial renal amyloidosis. Case reports, literature review and classification. *Am J Med* 59:121, 1975.

21. Sohar E, Gafni J, Pras M, et al: Familial Mediterranean fever. A survey of 470 cases and review of the literature. *Am J Med* 43:227, 1967.

22. Reuben A, Hirsch M, Berlyne GM: Renal vein thrombosis as the major cause of renal failure in familial Mediterranean fever. *Quart J Med* 46:243, 1977.

23. Strauss RG, Schubert WK, McAdams AJ: Amyloidosis in childhood. *J Pediat* 74:272, 1969.

24. Maxwell MH, Adams DA, Goldman R: Corticosteroid therapy of amyloid nephrotic syndrome. *Ann Intern Med* 60:539, 1964.

25. Bentwich Z, Rosenmann E, Eliakim M: Prevalence of hypertension in renal amyloidosis: correlation with clinical and histological parameters. *Am J Med Sci* 262:93, 1971.

26. Carone FA, Epstein FH: Nephrogenic diabetes insipidus caused by amyloid disease: evidence in man of the role of the collecting ducts in concentrating urine. *Am J Med* 29:539, 1960.

27. Luke RG, Allison ME, Davidson, JF, et al: Hyperkalemia and renal tubular acidosis due to renal amyloidosis. *Ann Intern Med* 70:1211, 1969.

28. Bell ET: Amyloid disease of the kidneys. *Am J Pathol* 9:185, 1933.

29. Ansell ID, Joekes AM: Spicular arrangement of amyloid in renal biopsy. *J Clin Pathol* 25:1056, 1972.

30. Weiss SW, Page DL: Amyloid nephropathy of Ostertag with special reference to renal glomerular giant cells. *Am J Pathol* 72:447, 1973.

31. Bladen HA, Nylen MU, Glenner GG: The ultrastructure of human amyloid as revealed by the negative staining technique. *J Ultrastruct Res* 14:449, 1966.

32. Shirahama T, Cohen AS: High resolution electron microscopic analysis of the amyloid fibril. *J Cell Biol* 33:679, 1967.

33. Jao W, Pirani CL: Renal amyloidosis: electron microscopic observations. *Acta Pathol Microbiol Scand (A)* 82(suppl 233):217, 1972.

33a. Gise H, Mikeler E, Gruber M, et al: Investigations on the cause of the nephrotic syndrome in renal amyloidosis: a discussion of electron microscopic findings. *Virchows Arch A Path Anat Histol* 379:131, 1978.

34. Bergstrand A, Bergström J, Bucht H, et al: Immunohistology in human amyloidosis. *Scand J Urol Nephrol* 5:51, 1971.

35. Isersky C, Page DL, Cuatrecasas P, et al: Murine amyloidosis: immunologic characterization of amyloid fibril protein. *J Histochem Cytochem* 19:1, 1971.

36. Shirahama AS, Skinner M, Cohen AS, et al: Uncertain value of urinary sediments in the diagnosis of amyloidosis. *N Engl J Med* 297:821, 1977.

37. Benson MD, Skinner M, Cohen AS: Amyloid deposition in a renal transplant in familial Mediterranean fever. *Ann Intern Med* 87:31, 1977.

38. Katz A, Weicker-Thorne J, Painter RH: The relationship of a serum protein, Clt, to a common non-fibrillar constituent of amyloid (P component) as revealed by immunohistochemical studies. *Am J Pathol* 88:679, 1977.

39. Jao W, Pollak VE, Norris SH, et al: Lipoid nephrosis: an approach to the clinicopathologic analysis and dismemberment of idiopathic nephrotic syndrome with minimal glomerular changes. *Medicine (Balt)* 52:445, 1973.

40. Rosemann E, Eliakim M: Nephrotic syndrome associated with amyloid-like glomerular deposits. *Nephron* 18:301, 1977.

41. Derosena R, Koss MN, Pirani CL: Demonstration of amyloid fibrils in urinary sediment. *N Engl J Med* 293:1131, 1975.

42. Ravid M, Kedar I, Sohar E: Effect of a single dose of dimethyl sulphoxide on renal amyloidosis. *Lancet* 1:730, 1977.

43. Linke RP: Urinary amyloid fibrils in the absence of amyloidosis. *Br Med J* 4:1259, 1976.

44. Orfila C, De Graeve P, Guilheim A, et al: Study of light-, electron- and immunofluorescence microscopy of urinary sediment in amyloidosis. *Virchows Arch A Path Anat Histol* 379:113, 1978.

44a. Shemer J, Messer GY, Pras M, et al: Amyloid in urinary sediments as a diagnostic technique. *Ann Intern Med* 90:61, 1979.

45. Jones NF: Renal amyloidosis: pathogenesis and therapy. *Clin Nephrol* 6:459, 1976.

46. Cohen AS, Bricetti AB, Barrington JT, et al: Renal transplantation in two cases of amyloidosis. *Lancet* 2:513, 1971.

47. Barnes BA, Bergan JJ, Braun WE, et al: Renal transplantation in congenital and metabolic diseases. A report from the ASC/NIH Renal Transplant Registry. *JAMA* 232:148, 1975.

48. Jones MB, Adams JM, Passer JA: Amyloidosis in a renal allograft in familial Mediterranean fever. *Ann Intern Med* 87:579, 1977.

49. Lowenstein J, Gallo G: Remission of the nephrotic syndrome in renal amyloidosis. *N Engl J Med* 282:128, 1970.

50. Dikman SH, Kahn T, Gribetz D, et al: Resolution of renal amyloidosis. *Am J Med* 63:430, 1977.

51. Cohen JH, Lessin LS, Hallal J, et al: Resolution of primary amyloidosis during chemotherapy: studies in a patient with nephrotic syndrome. *Ann Intern Med* 82:466, 1975.

52. Bradstock K, Clancy R, Uther J, et al: The successful treatment of primary amyloidosis with intermittent chemotherapy. *Aust NZ J Med* 8:176, 1978.

53. Wright JR, Ozdemir AI, Matsuzaki M, et al: Amyloid resorption: possible role of multinucleated giant cells. The apparent failure of penicillamine treatment. *Johns Hopkins Med J* 130:278, 1972.

54. Shirahama T, Cohen AS: Lysosomal breakdown of amyloid fibrils by macrophages. *Am J Pathol* 63:463, 1971.

55. Lake B, Andrews G: Rheumatoid arthritis with secondary amyloidosis and malabsorption syndrome. Effect of D-penicillamine. *Am J Med* 44:105, 1968.

56. Ravid M, Robson M, Kedar I: Prolonged colchicine treatment in four patients with amyloidosis. *Ann Intern Med* 87:568, 1977.

20
Paraproteinemia

For the purposes of this chapter paraproteins are defined as immunoglobulins that are either abnormally constituted or present in excessive concentration in blood or urine. Generally, paraproteins are of two types: monoclonal caricatures of all or part of the immunoglobulin molecule (M components) and abnormal mixtures of whole immunoglobulins. Either type may precipitate in the cold (cryoglobulins), and each implies a perversion of normal immunoglobulin synthesis. Monoclonal paraproteins are, by definition, the products of neoplastic clones of B lymphocytes or plasma cells. In some patients, the infiltrative characteristics of these clones cause the major clinical manifestations, as in myelomatosis, while, in others, the M component is the only indication of disease. In contrast, abnormal mixtures of immunoglobulins, principally characterized by cryoprecipitation, are usually not related to monoclonal B-cell neoplasia. The renal complications of paraproteinemia are diverse in both their morphology and pathogenesis (1). Glomerular deposits of paraprotein may cause capillary occlusion, either static or progressive, or be associated with complement activation and cellular proliferation. Alternatively, M components may be freely filtered to cause tubular lesions, with or without glomerular alterations. The frequency and type of each complication tends to be specific for its associated clinicopathologic entity, but intermediate forms occur and lesions typical of one disease may occasionally occur in another.

CYROGLOBULINEMIA

Cryoglobulins are defined by their capacity for in vitro precipitation at 4°C (2,3). This physical property is shared by two distinct groups of proteins: monoclonal M components and mixtures of immunoglobulin classes. Either form may be associated with a variety of other diseases, but cryoglobulinemia is an isolated abnormality in one-third of all patients (2). Monoclonal cryoglobulins, which represent one-third of the total, are most frequently of the IgM type and are expressions of B-cell neoplasia, whether overt or occult. The more common mixed cryoglobulins are, in contrast, immune complexes with a monoclonal or polyclonal component (usually IgM) attached to the antibody portion (usually IgG) of the complex (4). Because of this antiglobulin moiety, mixed cryoglobulins are almost always associated with demonstrable rheumatoid factor. Immune complexes in many glomerular and systemic diseases may evoke such an antiglobulin factor to be manifest as mixed cryoglobulins (3,5). Recent studies indicate that hepatitis B antigen (6) and DNA (7) may be included in a high proportion of apparently "primary" mixed cryoglobulins, possibly as the antigen, and isolated case studies have provided suggestive evidence of infectious antigen in the complexes (8). Thus, mixed cryoglobulinemia is merely a form of systemic immune complex disease with a relatively constant clinicopathologic pattern but, probably, many avenues of induction. The distinction between this and the monoclonal form of cryoglobulinemia is blurred by the demonstration of antibody activity in a number of M components (9), and immunopathologic evidence of immune complex glomerulonephritis in a number of patients with monclonal disease. The tissue effects of each cryoglobulinemic state are, therefore, similar, and are produced by varying combinations of mechanical vascular occlusion by protein precipitates and immune complex mediated inflammation.

Clinical Manifestations

Cryoglobulinemia occurs over a wide age range but is more common in the middle-aged and elderly, with more women in the mixed group (2,4). When first seen, patients typically have episodes of dependent purpura, which is often palpable and associated with ulceration, arthralgia, and Raynaud's phenomenon. Renal disease may be the reason the patient is first examined but usually develops after months or years of cutaneous symptoms (2). Glomerulonephritis occurs in 21% of all patients with cryoglobulinemia, more frequently in the mixed form, and may appear as either acute renal failure or a chronic nephropathy (2,10). The latter is typically manifested as proteinuria, sometimes severe enough to cause the nephrotic syndrome, with microscopic hematuria and varying degrees of azotemia. Hypocomplementemia is characteristic of renal involvement but may occur in its absence.

Pathologic Characteristics

Light Microscopy

The glomeruli in patients with acute renal failure show diffuse mesangial and endothelial proliferation with frequent polymorphs and massive deposits (10). There may be variation between glomeruli in the degree of proliferation and crescents are occasionally seen. The deposits appear as brightly eosinophilic thrombi that are PAS-positive, except in monoclonal IgG states, and are irregularly distributed (10). In chronic nephropathy, deposits are less extensive and are associated with persistent proliferation and increased matrix. Glomerular lesions may be either diffuse, often with a mesangiocapillary pattern, or focal and segmental, and crescents are not uncommon (10,11). Apparently typical membranous nephropathy has occasionally been associated with cryoglobulinemia (11). Glomerular thrombi are occasionally seen in chronic nephropathy, but the usual picture is of variably distributed wire loops, which may produce a picture reminiscent of lupus glomerulonephritis. Rarely, crystals have been demonstrated by light microscopy in mesangial and endothelial cells (12). Extraglomerular abnormalities are frequent in both the acute and chronic patterns. Interstitial inflammation roughly parallels the severity of glomerular disease, and either necrotizing arteritis or arterial thrombi may be seen (2,4,13).

Immunofluorescence Microscopy

The thrombi and wire loops show reactions for the appropriate cryoglobulin components (10). In mixed cryoglobulinemia, these localized reactions are almost always associated with granular reactions for immunoglobulins, C3 and early acting complement components in mesangia and along capillary walls, sometimes with extension to tubulointerstitial regions (10,14,15). Vascular reactions for immunoglobulins and complement have also been described in those patients with vasculitis (11,13). Monoclonal cryoglobulins may be present either alone (10) or in association with complement components, suggesting superimposed immune complex disease (11,16,17).

Electron Microscopy

Deposits are usually restricted to mesangia, subendothelial, and centrimembranous regions but may occasionally extend to subepithelial areas (11). Humps have been described (18) but have not been a feature of our cases. In approximately half of the biopsy specimens, the deposits have a highly characteristic organized structure which, in contrast to lupus, is always present throughout all deposited material. The nature of the cryoglobulin may be suspected from the pattern of organization, and comparative studies have shown similar configurations in both the tissue deposits and the cryoprecipitates (11). Mixed cryoglobulinemic deposits appear as duplicated cylinders, 250 Å in width, arranged in curved arrays and admixed with spoked annular configurations, 300 Å in diameter (Fig. 20-1). In contrast, monoclonal IgG and IgM deposits are fibrillar, with straight fibrils arranged in bundles 800 Å in width, and up to 1 μ in length (11,17). A peculiar pattern of dense and bandlike subendothelial deposits has occasionally been reported (13). Crystalline inclusions, with a structure similar to the extracellular deposits, may be seen in mesangial, endothelial, or epithelial cells, and in intraluminal monocytes (11,12,14,16,19).

Clinical Course and Prognosis

The glomerular lesions causing acute renal failure are potentially reversible and may completely resolve with plasmapheresis or only supportive therapy (2,10). In some patients, the initial damage is severe enough to cause extensive, permanent scarring, but repeat biopsy specimens in those patients who have recovered show only minor sclerosis with no deposits (10). The chronic nephropathy can progress relentlessly to renal failure. Corticosteroid and immunosuppressive therapy has been associated with improvement of both the immunologic abnormalities and renal function in patients with monoclonal (16) and mixed cryoglobulinemia (20), but the prognosis is generally poor (2).

MYELOMATOSIS

Myelomatosis is a malignant disease of plasma cells characterized by bone marrow infiltration and the production of M components. The serum concentration of the M components is closely correlated with the combined mass of the neoplastic plasma cells, and there is, as in all of these diseases, a spectrum of clinical

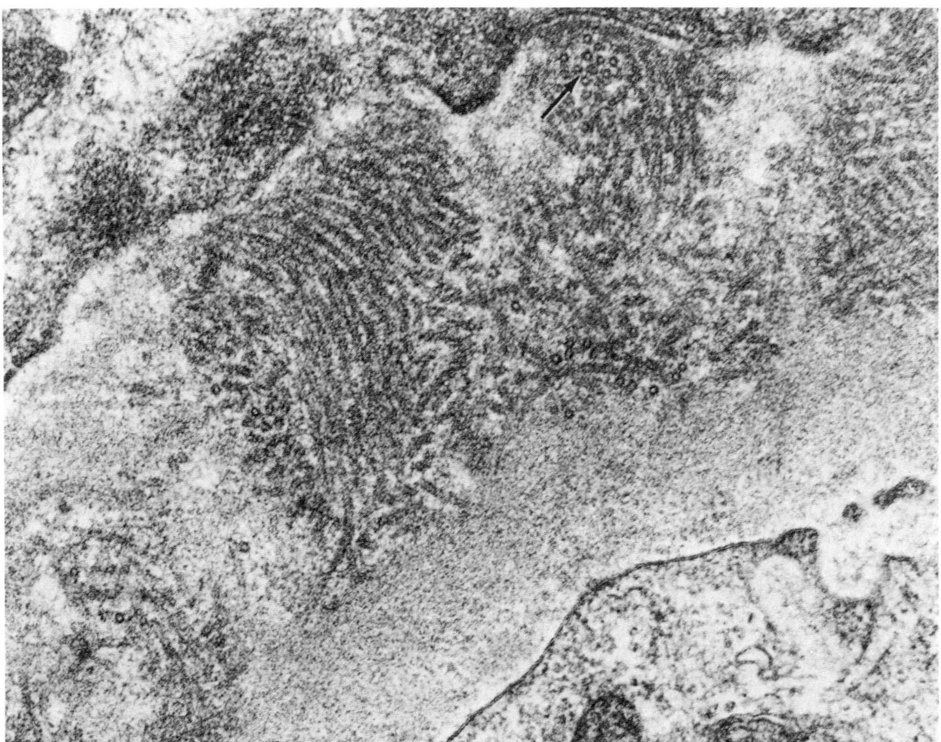

Figure 20-1. Renal biopsy specimen from a patient with IgG-IgM cryoglobulinemia. The deposits appear as annular structures in transverse sections (arrow) and cylinders in longitudinal sections (×48,000).

severity (21). Thus, while most patients with myelomatosis present with overt and extensive marrow infiltration, a few show only a circulating M component with no evidence of tissue involvement. A portion of this latter group develops typical myelomatosis up to eight years after symptoms first appear, but some die from the tissue effects of the M component or other causes before myelomatosis becomes overt (21). Complete absence of an M component is very rare (22). Either whole or incomplete immunoglobulin molecules may be produced and, with the exception of IgM, which is almost never seen in myelomatosis, the distribution of M types approximates the relative concentration of normal immunoglobulins (22,23). Light chains (Bence-Jones proteins, BJP) may be produced either alone or in combination with whole M components and are synthesized intact rather than representing breakdown products (24). BJP is present in up to 80% of all patients with myelomatosis and is the sole M component in 25% (light-chain myeloma) (22,25). Monoclonal BJP may be detected in the urine or serum of patients with neoplastic diseases other than myelomatosis and is occasionally found in the absence of overt neoplasia (24). The prognosis of myelomatosis is closely related to the M type, patients with IgD and light-chain myeloma having more extensive bone disease and an aggressive clinical course (23,25).

Clinical Manifestations

Myelomatosis occurs over a wide range but is most common in the seventh decade and is slightly more frequent in males (22). Appearance is usually with direct complications of bone marrow infiltration, causing bone pain, fractures, hypercalcemia, and anemia. Clinical evidence of renal disease is present in approximately 50% of patients during life and in 50–80% at autopsy (26). The range of renal complications is very wide, and the factors determining their occurrence are obscure. Most of the renal lesions to be discussed are quite rare, but acute renal failure is a major cause of morbidity and mortality.

Pathologic Characteristics

Amyloidosis

Amyloidosis occurs in about 7% of all patients with myelomatosis but is more common in the light-chain variety, especially of lambda type (22,25,27). The deposits are usually sporadic and clinically insignificant, usually in blood vessels and the interstitium, but may be the major cause of clinical symptoms (27,28). Giant cells may appear around the deposits (27). Histochemical reactions for amyloid are often present in the tubular casts, but there is no correlation between these reactions and tissue infiltration by amyloidosis (29). As is discussed elsewhere (see p 356), one type of amyloid is composed of precipitated light chains, and there is a spectrum of B-cell neoplasia ranging from apparently "primary" amyloidosis to amyloid occurring in myelomatosis with all points in between.

Glomerular Disease

A variety of minor glomerular lesions have been reported to be common in myelomatosis (28), but quantitative studies have revealed no abnormalities (30). Only a few cases of proliferative glomerulonephritis have been reported. These may represent secondary or incidental immune complex disease (31), with granular reactions for immunoglobulin and complement, or precipitation of cryoproteins analogous to that already discussed (32).

Nodular Glomerulosclerosis (Kappa Light-Chain Nephropathy)

A few patients with myelomatosis have glomerular lesions that by light microscopy are indistinguishable from diabetic glomerulosclerosis, usually in association with progressive azotemia (Figs. 20-2, 20-3). This lesion is extremely rare and has also been reported in one patient with monoclonal BJP, but no evidence of myelomatosis at autopsy (33). The glomeruli are enlarged with thickening of capillary walls by intensely PAS-positive material and nodular mesangial expansion by similar material admixed with excessive matrix. The degree of glomerular involvement may vary in the same biopsy specimen from mild mesangial expansion to the fully developed lesion and, although sporadic mesangial interposition may be seen, cellular proliferation is inconspicuous. Tubular basement membranes are thickened by similar PAS-positive material, deposited on the external aspect, and occasional casts with giant-cell reaction may be seen. His-

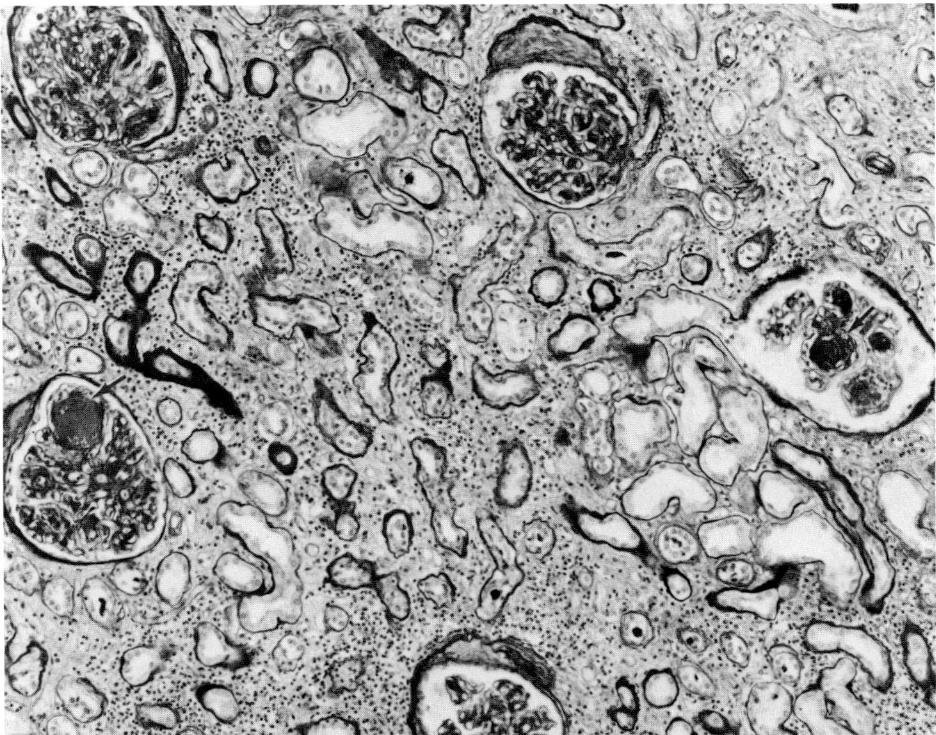

Figure 20-2. Renal biopsy specimen from a patient with myelomatosis showing mesangial nodules (arrows) and fibrous crescents. The tubules are atrophic and the interstitium is infiltrated by a moderate number of round cells (PAS stain, ×150).

tochemical stains for amyloid are negative. Immunofluorescence microscopy reveals diffuse deposition of kappa light chains in the regions outlined by the PAS-positive material, with abundant staining around blood vessels and in the interstitium (Fig. 20-4). Similar deposition was demonstrated in many extrarenal tissues of some patients at autopsy (33). The deposits are represented ultrastructurally by a remarkably uniform dense transformation of glomerular and tubular basement membranes, and of mesangial matrix (Figs. 20-5–20-7). This transformation differs from dense deposit disease, from which it must be differentiated, by being distributed principally along the outer aspect of the membranes and having a distinctly granular character. Similar material is also present in and around blood vessels, where it may be extensive enough to mimic amyloid deposits (Fig. 20-8). A peculiar form of collagen has been described in several patients (34), but has not been seen in our patients. The renal lesion appears to be the product of kappa light-chain deposition, which may be associated with myelomatosis of IgA (34), IgE (35), or light-chain (36) type, and with IgG (19) or BJP (33) monoclonal gammopathy. Similar light microscopic lesions have been reported with macroglobulinemia (28), and there is one report of a similar ultrastructural pattern in two patients with no apparent immunoglobulin abnormality (36).

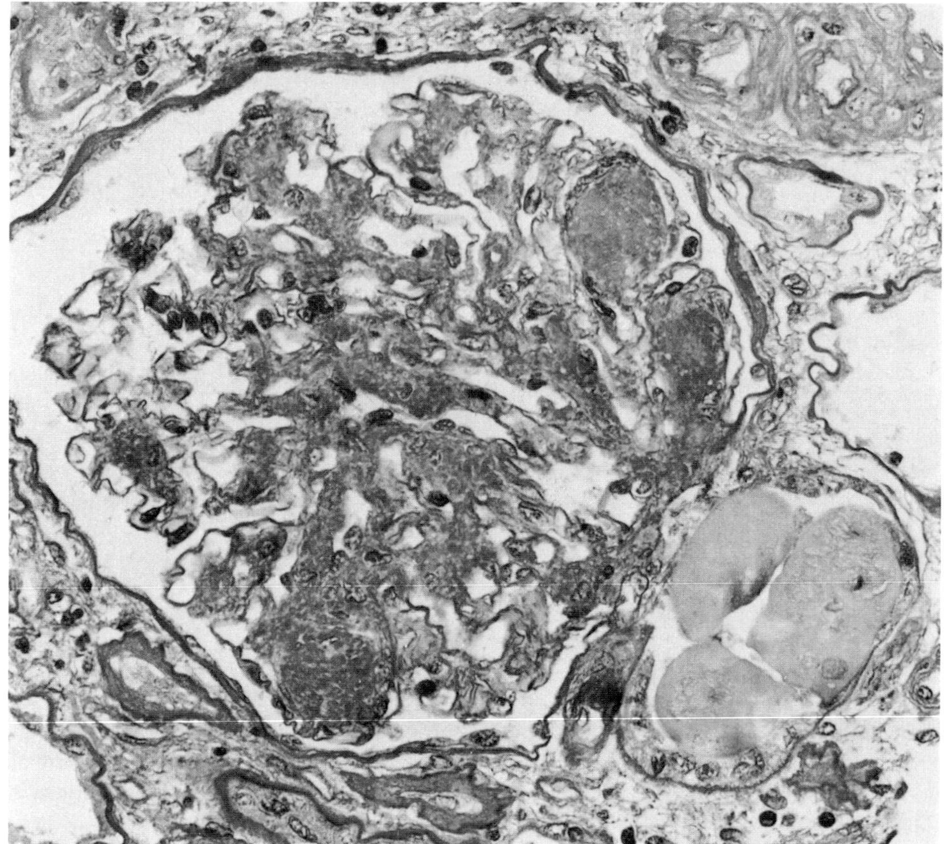

Figure 20-3. Glomerulus with mesangial expansion and nodular sclerosis. The tubular basement membranes are thickened and a distal tubule contains proteinaceous cast (PAS stain, ×610).

Tubulointerstitial Disease

The principal extraglomerular abnormality in patients with myelomatosis is usually tubular occlusion by typical casts. Nephrocalcinosis may, however, be prominent, and isolated examples of neoplastic infiltration and acute pyelonephritis may be seen (26,27) (Fig. 20-9).

Casts: "Myeloma Kidney."   The BJP filtered by the glomeruli is normally reabsorbed and metabolized by proximal tubular cells (37,38). Overwhelming of proximal tubular capacity allows the BJP to reach the distal nephron, where precipitation to form casts is favored by the increased concentration and lowered pH of the tubular fluid (26). Although there has been some disagreement over the content of myeloma casts, experimental infusion of BJP into mice has produced an appearance identical to that occurring in man (38). In both human and experimental disease, the casts are found in the distal convoluted tubules, ascending Henle's loops, and collecting ducts (27,38). These are dilated and distended by dense, refractile casts, which often appear fractured in various planes

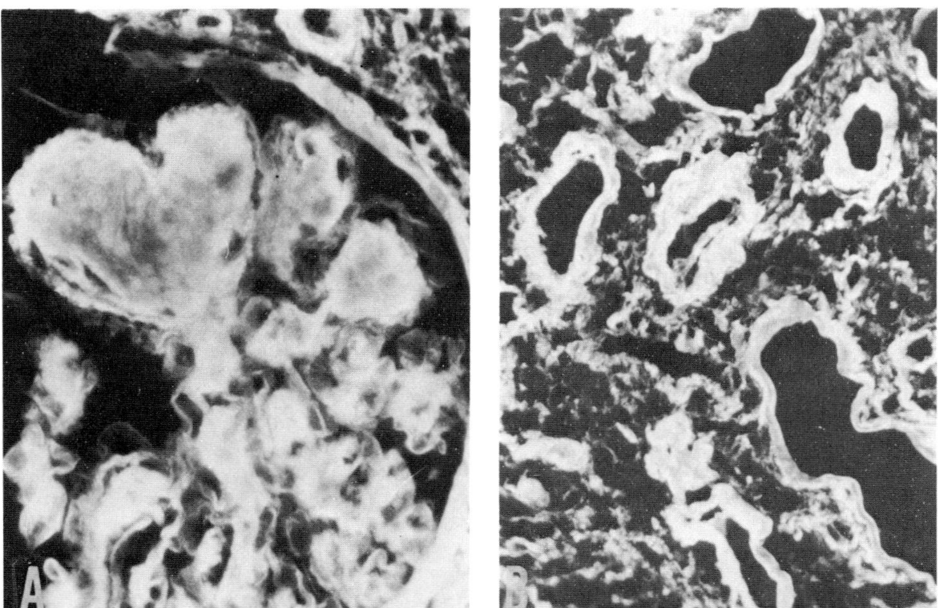

Figure 20-4. (*a*) Kappa light-chain deposits in the mesangium as well as along glomerular capillary walls and Bowman's capsule (*b*) There is strong fluorescence along the tubular basement membranes, vascular walls, and interstitium (antikappa light chain, ×350).

and are usually intensely eosinophilic and PAS-positive but may show irregular basophilia because of included calcium. The tubular epithelium is alternately flattened and distorted by syncytial giant cells surrounding the cast material with, in some cases, a mononuclear or polymorphonuclear reaction in the adjacent interstitium (Fig. 20-10). The origin of these giant cells is uncertain, both tubular and histiocytic features having been demonstrated in ultrastructural studies (38,39). The casts frequently exhibit the staining reactions of amyloid, essentially with thioflavin T, and have a fibrillar ultrastructure (29). These reactions probably reflect the presence of BJP, which can be demonstrated by immunofluorescence (40), and the reported variability in histochemical reactions for amyloid is likely to be the result of dilution of BJP by other proteins (38). Dense casts form in the distal nephron in many proteinuric states, but can usually be differentiated by their granular character and the lack of giant-cell reaction. Casts with features very similar to those of myelomatosis have been reported in association with BJP excretion in malignant lymphoma (41) and rifampicin therapy (42), and with mucoprotein precipitation in a patient with carcinoma of the pancreas (43).

Fanconi Syndrome.   Some degree of distal tubular dysfunction is common in patients with myelomatosis, defects in acidification and concentration being most frequent (44). Occasionally, the complete Fanconi syndrome occurs, indicating diffuse proximal tubular damage (45,46). The distal tubular defects are almost always associated with BJP excretion, of either kappa or lambda type (44), while the Fanconi syndrome occurs only with kappa BJP (45). Features of the Fanconi

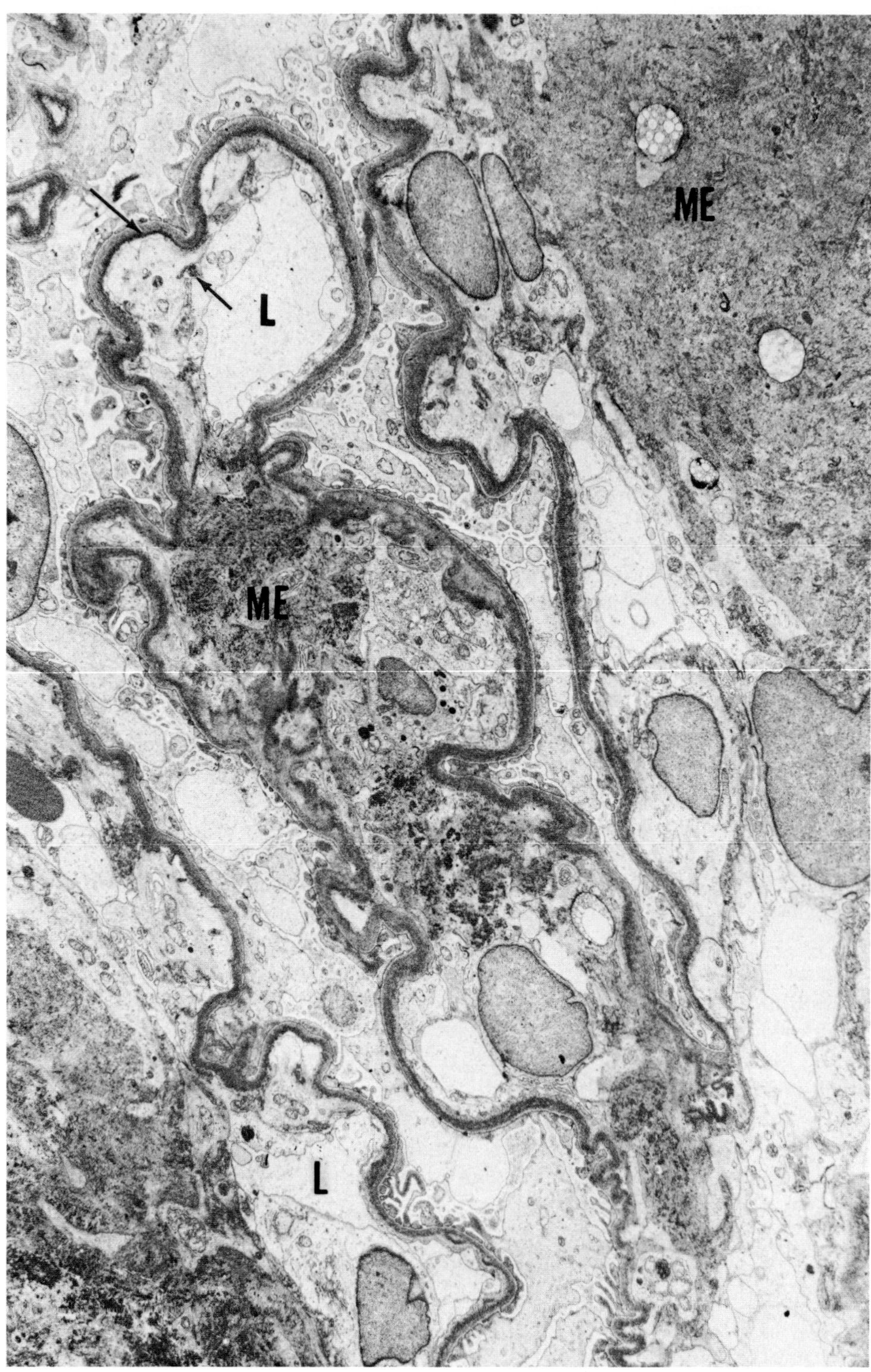

Figure 20-5. Electron micrograph showing mesangial and intramembranous deposition of electron-dense material. In some loops there is peripheral mesangial expansion (arrows). L, capillary lumen; ME, mesangium (×6,000).

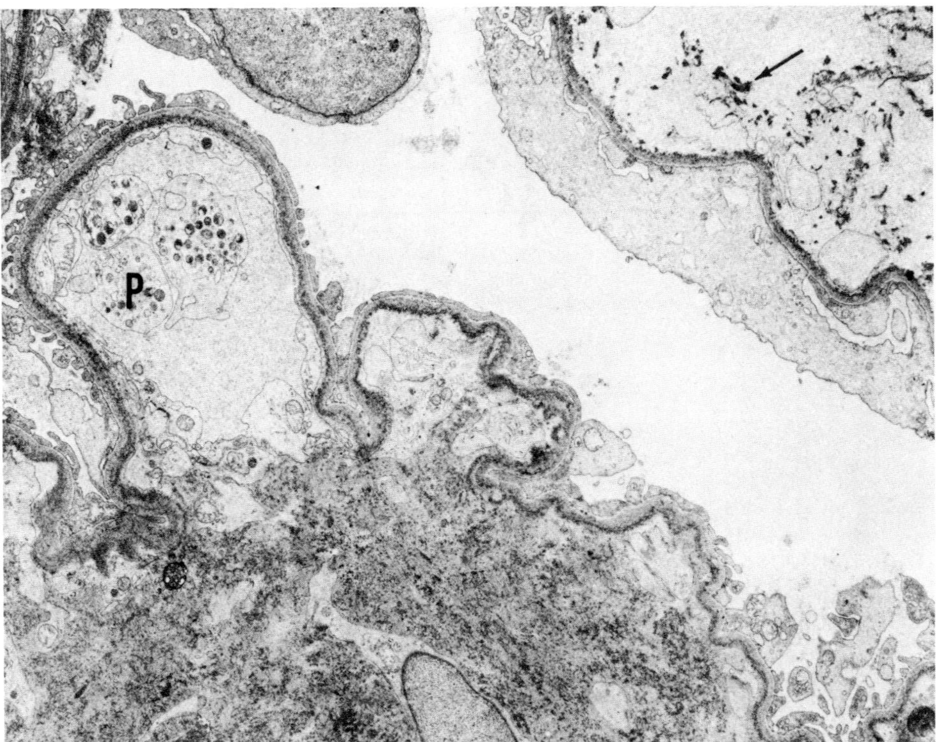

Figure 20-6. Electron micrograph illustrating the granular appearance of the material deposited in the mesangium and within the basement membrane. The capillary lumina contain platelets (P) and tactoids of fibrin (arrow). The loop on the right upper corner appears denuded of endothelium (×5,600).

syndrome may be discovered during investigation of a patient with myelomatosis but usually occur on the background of a monoclonal gammopathy characterized only by kappa BJP in the urine (45,46). The gammopathy may develop into either myelomatosis or amyloidosis, but this progression may be delayed for more than 16 years. Renal biopsy specimens in these cases reveal diffuse proximal tubular damage with focal scarring and crystals in tubular cells, but no myeloma casts. The functional defects are probably produced by direct tubular damage, since BJP is toxic to tubular cells in vitro (47), and similar morphologic changes have been produced by the experimental infusion of kappa BJP into rats (48).

Crystals

Crystalline structures are present in the kidneys of about 5% of patients with myelomatosis (27) (Fig. 20-11). They are most frequently seen in proximal tubular cells or lumina and are weakly eosinophilic or basophilic, PAS-negative, and refractile needle or rodlike structures measuring $0.5-2\times80\ \mu$ (27). Occasionally, similar crystals may be present in distal tubular casts, and both glomerular and interstitial involvement has been recorded (27,49). Ultrastructurally, the crystals have a fibrillar or lattice configuration with a periodicity of $85-105$ Å (45) (Fig. 20-12). The presence of similar crystals in neoplastic plasma cells suggests that

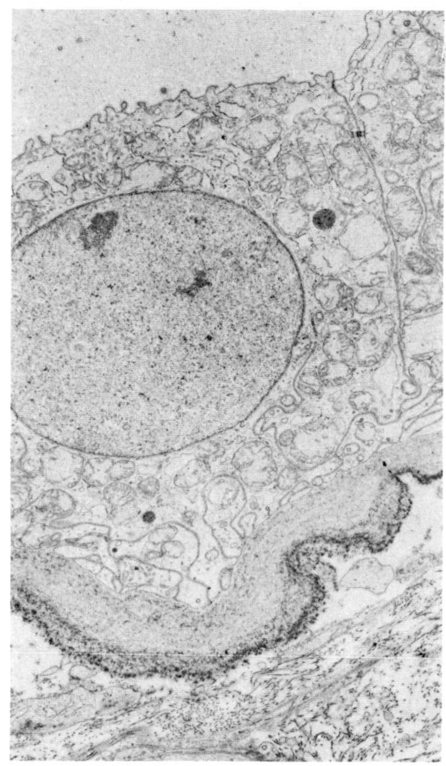

Figure 20-7. Electron micrograph illustrating the finely granular electron-dense material along the outer aspect of the tubular basement membrane (×5,500).

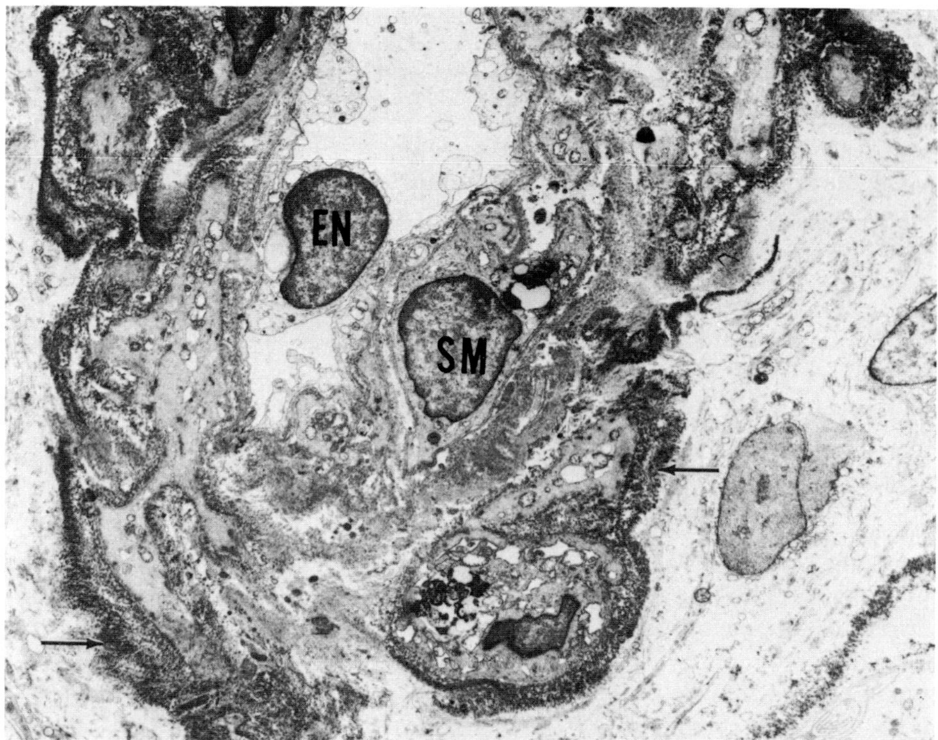

Figure 20-8. Electron micrograph of a blood vessel showing deposition of electron dense material (arrows). EN, endothelial cell; SM, smooth muscle (×6,000).

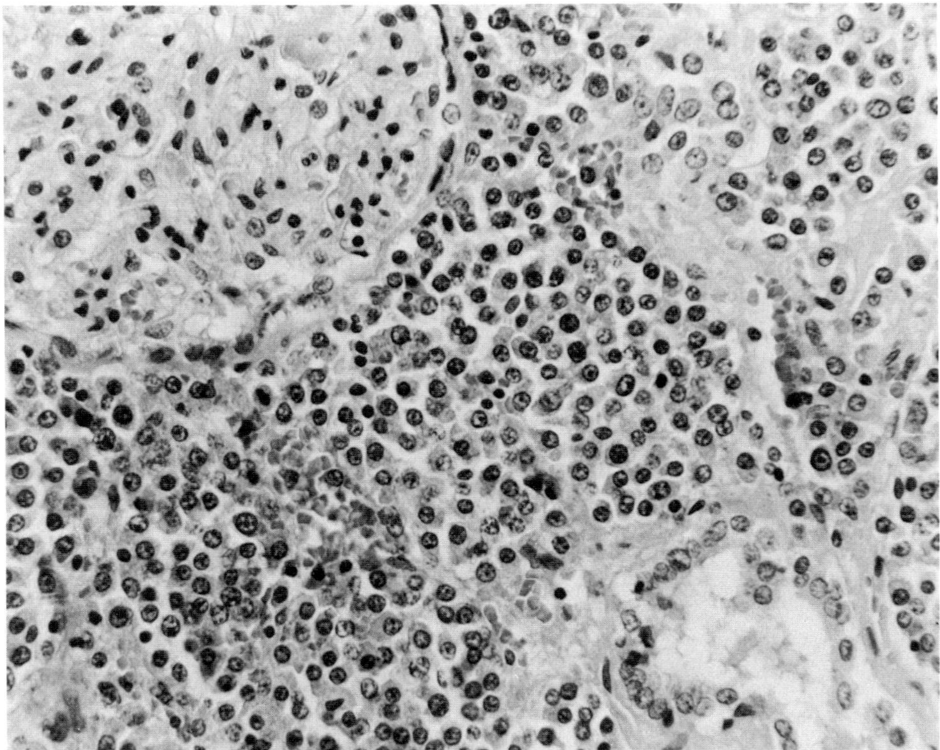

Figure 20-9. Plasma cell infiltration in the renal cortex from a patient with multiple myeloma (H&E stain, ×300).

they consist of BJP aggregates, and this has been proved by the formation of similar structures in the kidneys of animals injected with BJP (49) and by immunofluorescence studies in two of our patients (Fig. 20-13).

Acute Renal Failure in Myelomatosis

Acute renal failure develops in 7% of patients with myelomatosis and is the cause of death in 14% (22,50). Occasionally, acute renal failure is the initial manifestation of the disease, myelomatosis being first suggested by the renal biopsy pattern, but renal decompensation usually occurs months or years (average 15.6 months) after diagnosis (50). Individual cases may show a clear correlation between the acute renal failure and episodes of hypercalcemia, hyperuricemia, increased serum viscosity, urinary tract infection or neoplastic infiltration, but no single cause can be isolated in the majority (26). Similarly, there are numerous case reports of an association between acute renal failure and intravenous urography in patients with myelomatosis, but this complication is quite rare in prospective studies (50,51). The abrupt reduction in renal function is generally considered to be an effect of widespread tubular obstruction by the characteristic dense casts, but careful morphologic studies have shown a poor correlation between "myeloma kidney" and azotemia (27,40,44). Instead, the usual finding is extensive tubulointerstitial damage with no or relatively few typical casts. This has led to the suspicion that the myeloma cast may be a secondary development,

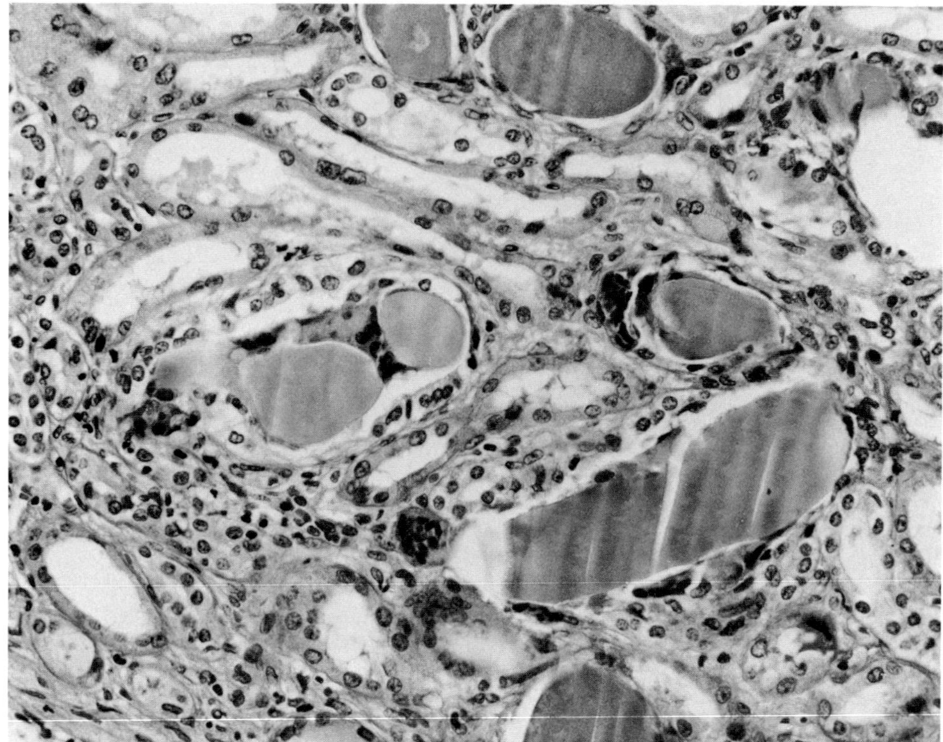

Figure 20-10. Large laminated tubular casts surrounded by multinucleated giant cells (H&E stain, ×400).

caused by sluggish tubular flow, rather than the major functional abnormality (44). Experimental studies of cast formation suggest, however, that cast formation precedes renal decompensation and that combinations of tubular blockade and cellular damage by the BJP are the mechanisms of acute renal failure (25,26,44,50), suggesting that the many other nephrotoxic factors present in patients with myelomatosis may be potentiated by the effects of BJP on tubular cells, whether or not casts are formed. Intravascular coagulation has been suggested as one especially effective mechanism of renal damage (52), but we have not been impressed by evidence of coagulation in our material. Whatever its pathogenesis, the prognosis of acute renal failure in patients with myelomatosis is poor, less than 20% of patients surviving in one collated series (50), unless specific and reversible factors can be identified (26).

Macroglobulinemia (Waldenström's Disease)

Macroglobulinemia is usually an indolent disorder associated with malignant lymphoma of well-differentiated lymphocytic type (53,54). There is, however, a spectrum of disease ranging from apparently benign monoclonal gammopathy, without identifiable underlying neoplasia, to rapidly progressive disease associated with a variety of nonlymphoid tumors (53). Regardless of its

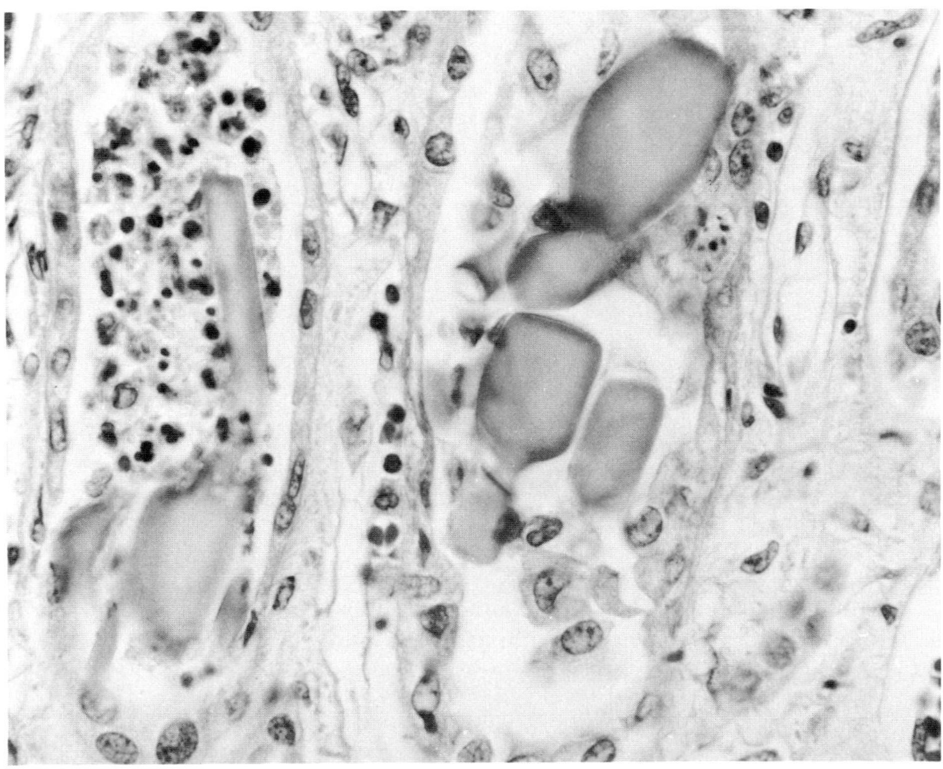

Figure 20-11. Intratubular refractile crystaloid casts in a patient with multiple myeloma (H&E stain, ×657).

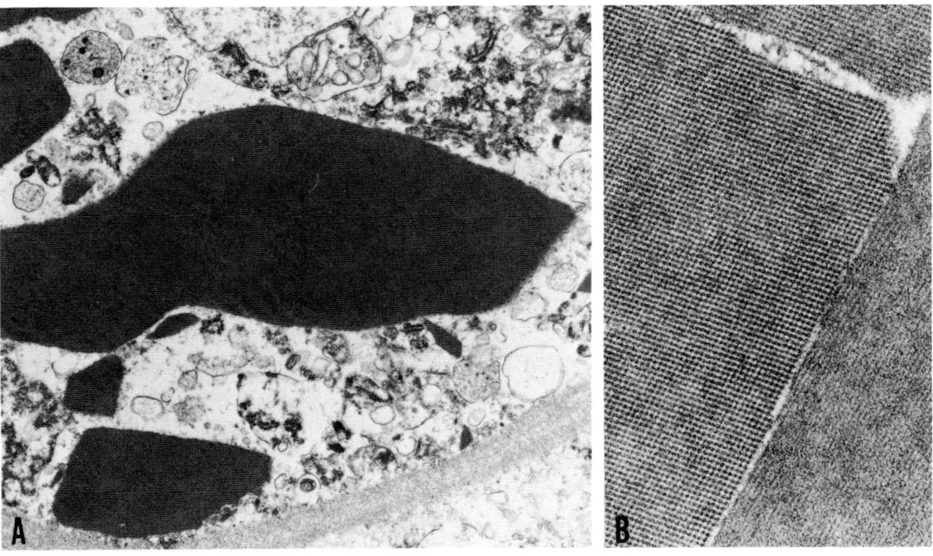

Figure 20-12. (*a*) An electron micrograph of a tubule of the same case as in Figure 20-11, showing intracytoplasmic crystals. (*b*) Higher magnification illustrating the latticelike configuration of the crystals (*a*, ×12,000; *b*, ×745,000).

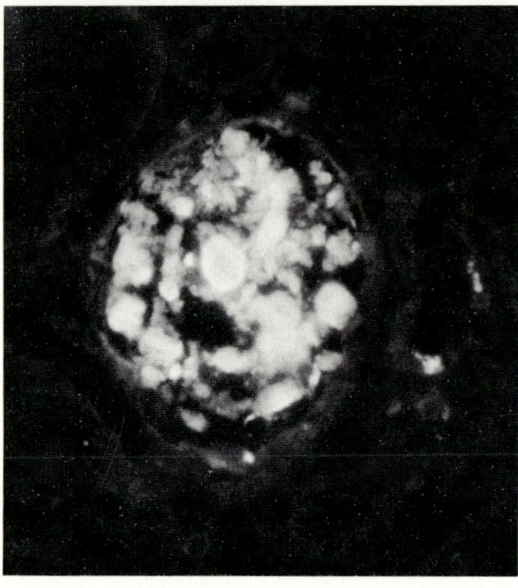

Figure 20-13. Immunofluorescence preparation of the tubular casts of the same case as in Figure 20-11 (Antilambda light chain, ×400).

background, macroglobulinemia is characterized by a high serum concentration of monoclonal IgM, which causes marked elevation of viscosity and may be associated with BJP in the urine.

Clinical Manifestations

Macroglobulinemia is a disease of the elderly, with a maximal incidence in the sixth and seventh decades, and occurs slightly more frequently in men (53). When first seen, the patient. may have either the tissue effects of malignant lymphoma, such as lymphadenopathy or hepatosplenomegaly, or the complications of hyperviscosity, including purpura and altered vision. Renal disease is quite uncommon. Proteinuria develops in approximately one-third of patients, occasionally with the nephrotic syndrome, and acute renal failure has been reported (19,55).

Pathologic Characteristics

A range of morphologic lesions has been described in macroglobulinemia, and the relationship between structure and function is not always clear, especially in acute renal failure. The usual morphologic pattern, and that which is best correlated with proteinuria, is partial or complete occlusion of glomerular capillaries by PAS-positive deposits or "thrombi" (10,55) (Fig. 20-14). These deposits may be relatively inconspicuous or may replace many capillary lumina, but they are not associated with significant proliferation. Similar "thrombi" may be seen in extraglomerular blood vessels, but intratubular casts are uncommon. Immunofluorescence microscopy confirms the presence of monoclonal IgM in the "thrombi," showing either diffuse or peripheral patterns of staining, without complement or other immunoglobulins (Fig. 20-15). There is no evidence to suggest that this pattern of glomerular disease is capable of progressing to chronic renal failure. Other patterns of glomerular disease, including membranous nephropathy and proliferative glomerulonephritis with features suggesting immune complex deposition, have been described in patients with

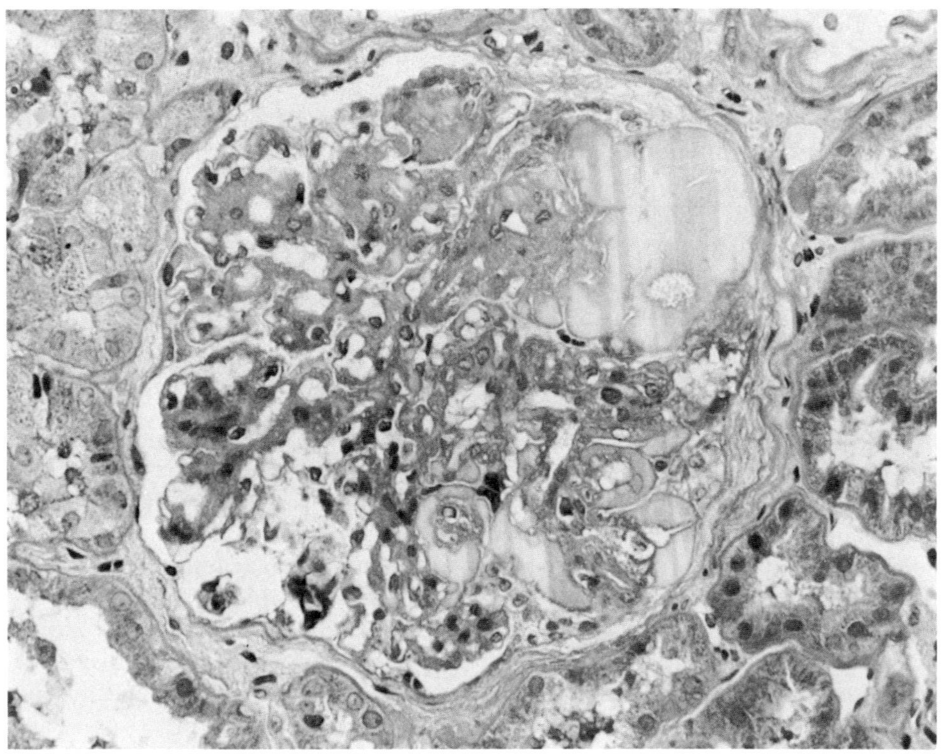

Figure 20-14. Renal biopsy specimen from a patient with Waldenström's macroglobulinemia. Some glomerular capillaries are occluded by proteinaceous thrombi. The mesangium is prominent but not hypercellular (H&E stain, ×450).

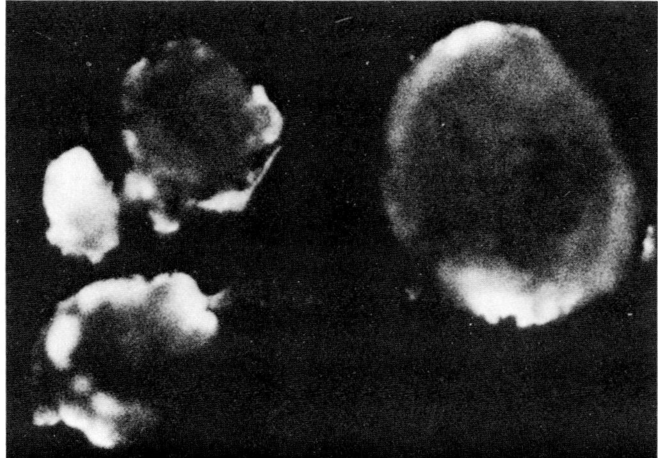

Figure 20-15. Glomerulus from the same case as in Figure 20-14, showing intracapillary deposition of IgM (×600).

macroglobulinemia, but appear to be very rare (19,56,57). Several studies have described nodular glomerulosclerosis suggestive of kappa light-chain deposition but have not been reported in sufficient detail for definitive assessment (19,28,57). Amyloidosis occurs in approximately 5% of patients with macroglobulinemia (53) and may be extensive, but it is usually focally distributed in only minor amounts (19). Finally, invasion of the interstitium by neoplastic lymphocytes is commonly seen in autopsy studies, and may occasionally be massive enough during life to cause acute renal failure (19,55,58).

SUMMARY

The paraproteinemias are characterized by excessive quantities of either normal or abnormal immunoglobulins in serum or urine. The most common paraprotein is a mixture of immunoglobulin classes which precipitates in the cold to form a mixed cryoglobulin. The mixed cryoglobulinemias are, in fact, a heterogeneous group of chronic immune complex diseases, which may be complicated by either acute or chronic glomerulonephritis. The glomerular lesions are characterized by large subendothelial or intraluminal deposits, which correspond to the circulating cryoglobulins and often have a characteristic ultrastructural pattern of curved cylindrical arrays. Cryoglobulins with monoclonal characteristics are associated with similar glomerular lesions but may have a distinctive ultrastructural pattern of straight fibrils in the deposits. Monoclonal paraproteins are also characteristic of B-cell neoplasms such as macroglobulinemia and myelomatosis. The large IgM molecules of macroglobulinemia may be precipitated in glomerular capillaries to form deposits, but are rarely associated with either glomerular proliferation or tubular lesions. In contrast, glomerular disease is quite rare in myelomatosis, and the usual clinical complications are caused by the effects of immunoglobulin fragments, light chains or Bence-Jones proteins, on tubules. Most commonly, these cause progressive renal failure—often with characteristic casts—but a few patients develop proximal tubular damage with a Fanconi syndrome. Occasionally, light chains may accumulate in glomeruli, to cause nodular glomerulosclerosis, or may precipitate to form amyloid deposits. The activity of the B-cell clone varies widely, and any of these manifestations may occur without identifiable neoplastic disease. Although there are common morphologic features between the renal complications of the paraproteinemias, pathogenetic studies in the future are likely to provide evidence of many different mechanisms of both paraprotein production and tissue damage.

REFERENCES

1. Beaufils M, Morel-Maroger L: Pathogenesis of renal disease in monoclonal gammopathies: current concepts. *Nephron* 20:125, 1978.
2. Brouet J-C, Clauvel J-P, Danon F, et al: Biologic and clinical significance of cryoglobulins: a report of 86 cases. *Am J Med* 57:775, 1974.
3. Cream JJ: Immune complexes in cryoprecipitates. *Ann Rheum Dis* 36(suppl 2): 45, 1977.
4. Meltzer M, Franklin EC, Elias K, et al: Cryoglobulinemia—a clinical and laboratory study: II. Cryoglobulins with rheumatoid factor activity. *Am J Med* 40:837, 1966.
5. Adam C, Morel-Maroger L, Richet G: Cryoglobulins in glomerulonephritis not related to systemic disease. *Kidney Int* 3:334, 1973.

6. Levo Y, Gorevic PD, Kassab HJ, et al: Association between hepatitis B virus and essential mixed cryoglobulinemia. *N Engl J Med* 296:1501, 1977.

7. Roberts JL, Lewis EJ: Identification of antinative DNA antibodies in cryoglobulinemic states. *Am J Med* 65:437, 1978.

8. Gamble CN, Ruggles SW: The immunopathogenesis of glomerulonephritis associated with mixed cryoglobulinemia. *N Engl J Med* 299:81, 1978.

9. Franklin EC: Cryoglobulinemia. *Am J Med Sci* 262:50, 1971.

10. Morel-Maroger L, Verroust P: Glomerular lesions in dysproteinemias. *Kidney Int* 5:249, 1974.

11. Feiner H, Gallo G: Ultrastructure in glomerulonephritis associated with cryoglobulinemia: a report of six cases and review of the literature. *Am J Pathol* 88:145, 1977.

12. Porush JG, Grishman E, Alter AA, et al: Paraproteinemia and cryoglobulinemia associated with atypical glomerulonephritis and the nephrotic syndrome. *Am J Med* 47:957, 1969.

13. Bartlow BG, Oyama JH, Ing TS, et al: Glomerular ultrastructural abnormalities in a patient with mixed IgG-IgM essential cryoglobulinemic glomerulonephritis. *Nephron* 14:309, 1975.

14. Monga G, Mazzucco G, Coppo R, et al: Glomerular findings in mixed IgG-IgM cryoglobulinemia: light, electron microscopic, immunofluorescence and histochemical correlations. *Virchows Arch B Cell Pathol* 20:185, 1976.

15. Lehmann DH, Wilson CB, Dixon FJ: Extraglomerular immunoglobulin deposits in human nephritis. *Am J Med* 58:765, 1975.

16. Bengtsson U, Larsson O, Lindstedt G, et al: Monoclonal IgG cryoglobulinemia with secondary development of glomerulonephritis and nephrotic syndrome. *Quart J Med* 44:491, 1975.

17. Avasthi PS, Erickson DG, Williams RC Jr, et al: Benign monoclonal gammaglobulinemia and glomerulonephritis. *Am J Med* 62:324, 1977.

18. Törnröth T, Skrifvars B: Ultrastructural changes in acute nonstreptococcal glomerulonephritis associated with mixed cryoglobulinemia. *Exp Mol Pathol* 19:160, 1973.

19. Verroust P, Mery J-P, Morel-Maroger L, et al: Glomerular lesions in monoclonal gammopathies and mixed essential cryoglobulinemias IgG-IgM. *Adv Nephrol* 1:161, 1971.

20. Mathison DA, Condemi JJ, Leddy JP: Purpura, arthralgia, and IgM-IgG cryoglobulinemia with rheumatoid factor activity: response to cyclophosphamide and splenectomy. *Ann Intern Med* 74:383, 1971.

21. Hobbs JR: Immunocytoma o' mice an' men. *Br Med J* 2:67, 1971.

22. Kyle RA: Multiple myeloma: review of 869 cases. *Mayo Clin Proc* 50:29, 1975.

23. Pruzanski W: Clinical manifestations of multiple myeloma: relation to class and type of M component. *Canad Med Ass J* 114:896, 1976.

24. Solomon A: Bence-Jones proteins and light chains of immunoglobulins. *N Engl J Med* 294:17, 1976.

25. Stone MJ, Frenkel EP: The clinical spectrum of light chain myeloma: a study of 35 patients with special reference to the occurrence of amyloidosis. *Am J Med* 58:601, 1975.

26. Martinez-Maldonado M, Yium J, Suki WN, et al: Renal complications in multiple myeloma: pathophysiology and some aspects of clinical management. *J Chron Dis* 24:221, 1971.

27. Schubert GE, Veigel J, Lennert K: Structure and function of the kidney in multiple myeloma. *Virchows Arch Abt A Path Anat* 355:135, 1972.

28. Zlotnick A, Rosenmann E: Renal pathologic findings associated with monoclonal gammopathies. *Arch Intern Med* 135:40, 1975.

29. Limas C, Wright JR, Matsuzaki M, et al: Amyloidosis and multiple myeloma: a reevaluation using a control population. *Am J Med* 54:166, 1973.

30. Wehner H, Feurer F, Wehner I: Histometrical glomerular studies on the kidneys in multiple myeloma and in acute membranous glomerulonephritis (lipoid nephrosis). *Pathol Europ* 6:422, 1971.

31. Case records of the Massachusetts General Hospital. *N Engl J Med* 297:266, 1971.

32. Schuurmans Stekhoven JH, van Haelst JGM: Unusual findings in the human renal glomerulus in multiple myeloma: a light and electron microscopic study. *Virchows Arch B Cell Pathol* 9:311, 1971.

33. Randall RE, Williamson WC Jr, Mullinax F, et al: Manifestations of systemic light chain deposition. *Am J Med* 60:293, 1976.

34. Schubert GE, Adam A: Glomerular nodules and long-spacing collagen in kidneys of patients with multiple myeloma. *J Clin Pathol* 27:800, 1974.

35. Vladutiu AO, Kohli RK, Prezyna AP: Monclonal IgE with renal failure. *Am J Med* 61:957, 1976.

36. King JT, Valenzuela R, McCormock LJ, et al: Granular dense deposit disease. *Lab Invest* 39:591, 1978.

37. Wochner RD, Strober W, Waldman TA: The role of the kidney in the catabolism of Bence-Jones proteins and immunoglobulin fragments. *J Exp Med* 126:207, 1967.

38. Koss MN, Pirani CL, Osserman EF: Experimental Bence-Jones cast nephropathy. *Lab Invest* 34:579, 1976.

39. Factor SM, Winn RB, Biempica L: The histiocytic origin of the multinucleated giant cells in myeloma kidney. *Human Pathol* 9:114, 1978.

40. Levi DR, Williams RC, Lindstrom FD: Immunofluorescent studies of the myeloma kidney with special reference to light chain disease. *Am J Med* 44:922, 1968.

41. Burke JF Jr, Flis R, Lasker N, et al: Malignant lymphona with "myeloma kidney" acute renal failure. *Am J Med* 60:1055, 1976.

42. Warrington RJ, Hogg GR, Paraskevas F, et al: Insidious rifampin-associated renal failure with light-chain proteinuria. *Arch Intern Med* 137:927, 1977.

43. Hobbs JR, Evans DJ, Wrong OM: Renal tubular obstruction by mucoproteins from adenocarcinoma of the pancreas. *Br Med J* 2:87, 1974.

44. De Fronzo RA, Cooke CR, Wright JR, et al: Renal function in patients with multiple myeloma. *Medicine (Balt)* 57:151, 1978.

45. Maldonado JE, Velosa JA, Kyle RA, et al: Fanconi syndrome in adults: a manifestation of a latent form of myeloma. *Am J Med* 58:354, 1975.

46. Smithline N, Kissane JR, Cohen JJ: Light-chain nephropathy: renal tubular dysfunction associated with light-chain proteinuria. *N Engl J Med* 294:71, 1976.

47. Pruess HG, Weiss RF, Iammaniro RM, et al: Effects on rat kidney slice function in vitro of proteins from the urines of patients with myelomatosis and nephrosis. *Clin Sci Molec Med* 46:283, 1974.

48. Clyne DH, Brendstrup L, First MR, et al: Renal effects of intraperitoneal kappa chain injection: indication of crystals in renal tubular cells. *Lab Invest* 31:131, 1974.

49. Sickel GW: Crystalline glomerular deposits in multiple myeloma. *Am J Med* 27:354, 1959.

50. De Fronzo RA, Humphrey RL, Wright JR, et al: Acute renal failure in multiple myeloma. *Medicine (Balt)* 54:209, 1975.

51. Myers GH Jr, Whitten DM: Acute renal failure after excretory urography in multiple myeloma. *Am J Roentgen Rad Ther Nucl Med* 113:583, 1971.

52. Ward AM, Preston FE: The kidney and intravascular coagulation in myelomatosis. *Br Med J* 2:529, 1974.

53. MacKenzie MR, Fundenberg HH: Macroglobulinemia: an analysis of forty patients. *Blood* 39:874, 1972.

54. Pangalis GA, Nathwani BN, Rappaport H: Malignant lymphoma, well differentiated lymphocytic: its relationship with chronic lymphocytic leukemia and macroglobulinemia of Waldenström. *Cancer* 39:999, 1977.

55. Morel-Maroger L, Basch A, Danon F, et al: Pathology of the kidney in Waldenström's macroglobulinemia: study of sixteen cases. *N Engl J Med* 283:123, 1970.

56. Lin JH, Orofino D, Sherlock J, et al: Waldenström's macroglobulinemia, mesangiocapillary glomerulonephritis, angiitis and myositis. *Nephron* 10:262, 1973.

57. Martelo OJ, Schultz DR Jr, Pardo V, et al: Immunologically-mediated renal disease in Waldenström's macroglobulinemia. *Am J Med* 58:567, 1975.

58. Grossman ME, Bia MJ, Goldwein MJ, et al: Giant kidneys in Waldenström's macroglobulinemia. *Arch Intern Med* 137:1613, 1977.

21
Hereditary and Congenital Glomerular Diseases

The familial occurrence of renal disease has been recognized for many years, but not so well appreciated has been the heterogeneity of these familial renal syndromes (1). A wide range of cystic, tubulointerstitial, and glomerular disorders are known to occur with excessive frequency within family or population groups. Even when the best characterized of these disorders are excluded, familial aggregation can still be demonstrated in groups of patients with chronic renal failure (2). Recently, some progress has been made in the identification of specifically glomerular hereditary diseases by other than crude clinical criteria. Thus, a variety of glomerular diseases occurring in family and population groups have been attributed to particular environmental factors (3) or to inherited immune defects affecting, for example, the complement pathway (4). These diseases occur with undue frequency because of modification of host responses, and are not necessarily morphologically specific. In contrast, in recent studies several disparate disorders have been identified in which the glomerular diseases are direct expressions of inherited traits with relatively specific morphologic features. The pathologist plays a central role in the diagnostic and prognostic assessment of these diseases.

HEREDITARY GLOMERULONEPHRITIS (ALPORT'S DISEASE)

Alport (5) defined the clinical combination of deafness and familial, progressive renal damage in the disease that now bears his name. The disease has traditionally been defined by Alport's criteria, but expression of either the renal or auditory phenomena may be variable within families, and the occurrence of spontaneous mutations means that cases will be encountered without a family history. The deafness is bilateral, neurosensory, and predominantly high-tone in type, but has not been satisfactorily explained by morphologic studies (6–8). A relatively small proportion of patients with Alport's disease may show a range of other associated abnormalities, including ocular changes (most frequently affecting the lens), alterations in amino acid homeostasis, platelet disorders, and a variety of neurologic phenomena (1,6,7,9,10).

Pathogenesis

That Alport's disease is an inherited disorder is known, but neither the precise mode of inheritance nor the mechanism of tissue damage is certain. There is general agreement that the disease is transmitted as a dominant characteristic, but the variability of its expression in male and female progeny has caused controversy (9). In some series, renal disease has been inherited only from females (11,12), whereas, in others, paternal inheritance has been demonstrated but with relatively infrequent expression in the male offspring (13). The data have been variously interpreted as indicating sex linkage (12), prejudiced intrauterine survival of males inheriting the gene from affected fathers (13), or abnormal gene segregation (14). Definitive assessment of these various mechanisms must await further studies of well-characterized families, and it is possible that more than one syndrome will emerge. The gene, if only one is implicated, is probably present in approximately 106×10^6 births, has a relatively high frequency of new mutations, and is distributed worldwide (14). No satisfactory mechanism for the tissue effects of Alport's disease is known, but genetically controlled disturbances of basement membrane formation in the glomerulus, inner ear, and lens capsule have been suggested (15).

Clinical Manifestations

The sexual inequality in the transmission of Alport's disease is matched by a bias in its expression. In most families, renal disease appears earlier and is more severe in males. Appearance may be in infancy or may be delayed, especially in females, until adulthood, but is most commonly in the first decade (6,7,10,11). Typically, the first notice of the disease is an episode of macroscopic hematuria, often occurring after exercise or an upper respiratory infection. The most reliable indication of renal involvement, in the assessment of families with the disease, is microscopic hematuria (12). Proteinuria is generally mild, but may become sufficiently severe in advanced disease to cause the nephrotic syndrome (16,17). Deafness occurs in a varying proportion of patients in different series, is usually noted in late childhood or early adolescence, and is more common in males with significant renal disease (16). Either deafness or renal disease, or both, may skip generations (16, 18), and the frequency of new mutations means that a significant number of patients presenting with the disease have no family history. Ocular involvement is generally uncommon, but usually occurs in patients with severe deafness and renal disease (19).

Pathologic Characteristics

Light Microscopy

In young children, renal biopsy specimens usually show no abnormalities, although increased numbers of "immature" glomeruli may be seen (15,17) (Fig. 21-1). With increasing age, the mesangia show a mild and irregular excess in matrix, with areas of segmental proliferation, and the capillary walls may appear thickened and irregular (Fig. 21-2). These may be the only changes detectable in

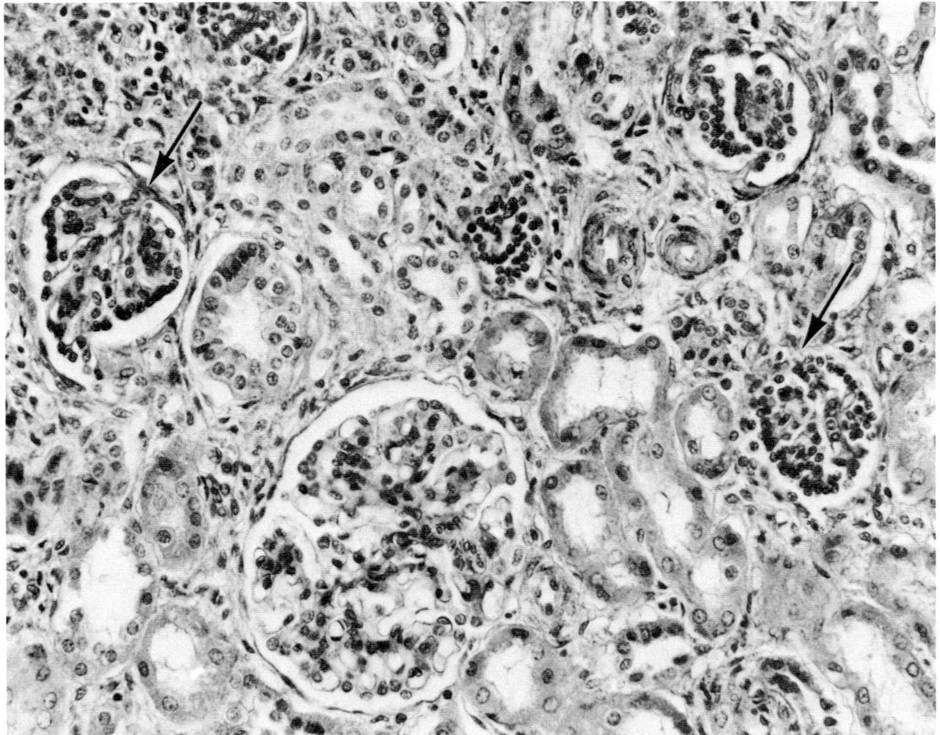

Figure 21-1. Fetallike glomeruli (arrows) in hereditary nephritis (H&E stain, ×385).

females with static disease, but in severely affected males, there is progressive glomerular damage. Advancing glomerular disease is characterized by increasing mesangial enlargement, segmental and global sclerosis, and organizing epithelial crescents (Figs. 21-3, 21-4). Tubulointerstitial changes appear relatively early and are not easily explicable from the extent of glomerular damage. Irregular areas of nonspecific scarring are frequent, and groups of interstitial foam cells occur along the corticomedullary junction, as stripes in the outer medulla and irregularly throughout the cortex (20) (Figs. 21-2, 21-3). The lipid in these cells has been identified as cholesterol ester, and is no different to that in the foam cells seen in other disorders (21).

Electron Microscopy

Glomerular basement membrane changes are the earliest and most specific features of Alport's disease, appearing as early as 2 years of age (8,22) and being demonstrable in the absence of light microscopic abnormalities. The membrane is irregular in contour, width, and density. Areas of marked thickening alternate with zones of extreme attenuation and of normal width, with irregularities on both internal and external aspects (8,23,24). The most specific appearance, however, is a diffuse alteration in density caused by splitting or fraying of the membrane with multiple, interwoven lamellae (11,25). The lamellae are 300–1000 Å in width and enclose electron-lucent areas containing finely granular material,

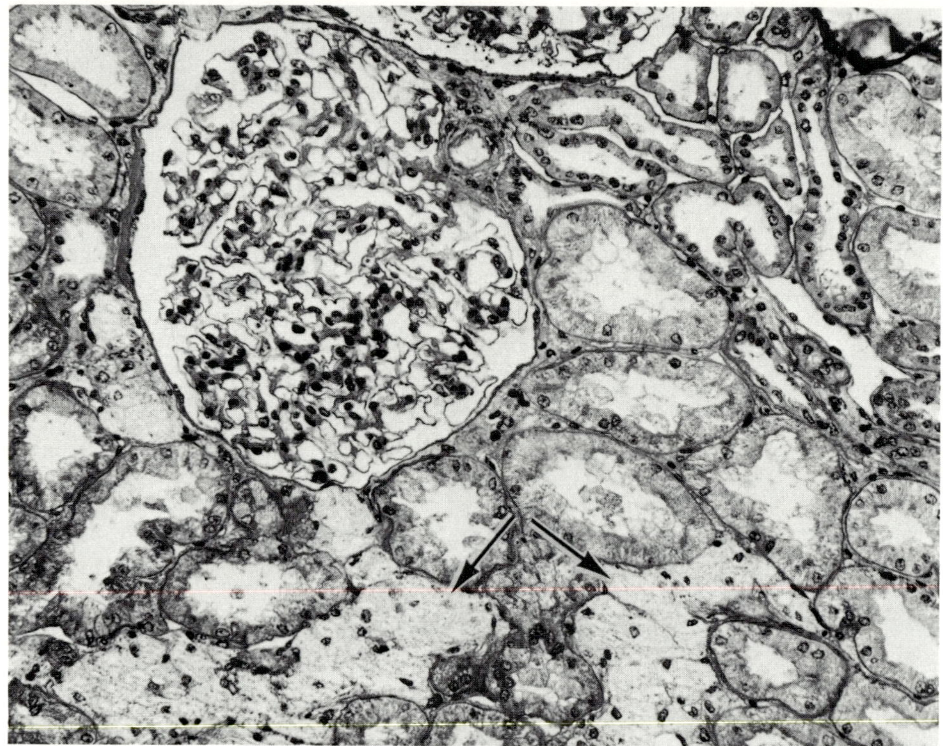

Figure 21-2. Biopsy specimen from a patient with hereditary nephritis, demonstrating a glomerulus with mild mesangial hypercellularity and clusters of tubular foam cells (arrows) (PAS stain, ×310).

coarse particles, and irregularly rounded bodies 200–900 Å in diameter (17,24) (Fig. 21-5). These bodies are also found in the adjacent, normally dense basement membrane, and may be difficult to distinguish from cytoplasmic invaginations (24,25). Some of the ultrastructural features may, indeed, reflect an abnormally irregular membrane with trapped and degenerate cytoplasmic organelles. Epithelial foot processes are often obliterated over wide areas (20), but other cell components appear normal. The glomerular changes are restricted to the basement membrane and do not affect mesangial matrix, which is often increased but not otherwise altered. In established disease, membrane changes are diffusely distributed throughout all glomeruli, but mild or early involvement may affect only a minority of capillary loops (17). Similar lamellation is present in tubular basement membranes (1), but changes of this type are so common in adult biopsy specimens that they are of limited diagnostic significance (22).

Immunofluorescence Microscopy
There is no evidence of participation of immunologic mechanisms in the production of glomerular lesions. Diffuse immunofluorescent reactions have been described in only one patient with coexistent IgA nephropathy (26). In other reports, either no reactions or only segmental and nonspecific reactions have been described (8,17).

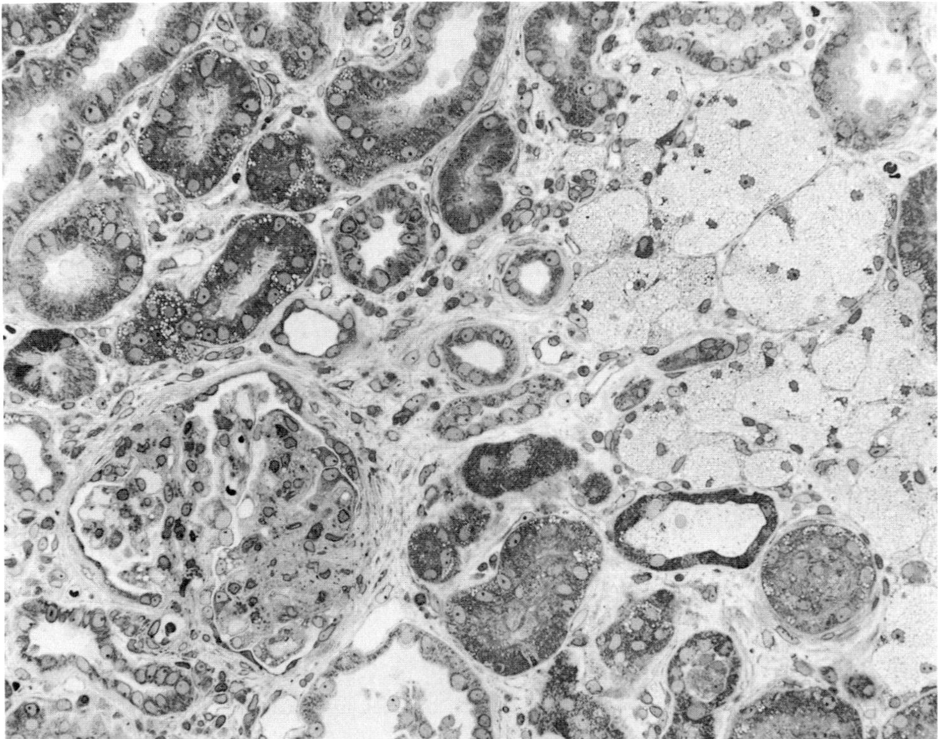

Figure 21-3. Advanced hereditary nephritis showing a glomerulus with segmental glomerulosclerosis and prominent tubular and interstitial foam cells (plastic embedded toluidine blue stain, ×310).

Differential Diagnosis

The light microscopic changes are entirely nonspecific, and morphologic diagnosis relies absolutely on demonstration of the ultrastructural changes. In particular, the demonstration of the interstitial foam cells in a renal biopsy specimen has no diagnostic value (27). The membrane changes seen by electron microscopy are unfortunately not universal in Alport's disease, and their absence does not, paradoxically, exclude this diagnosis (25), although they may indicate patients with progressive disease. Generally, however, all affected members of a family with the disease will show a similar pattern (25). Thus, the absence of membrane changes in a patient whose relatives have shown typical membrane lamellation is good evidence against Alport's disease. In the members of one family, however, the ultrastructural lesions developed during the course of the disease and were absent in biopsy specimens taken from family members younger than 14 years (28). Isolated areas of lamellation and irregular density are commonly found in biopsy specimens showing minimal other changes, and lesions very similar to those of Alport's disease occur in a wide variety of disorders, particularly those associated with deposits (24). Before making an ultrastructural diagnosis of Alport's disease, therefore, it is prudent to require definite and more than occasional areas of lamellation, especially if there is no family history (22).

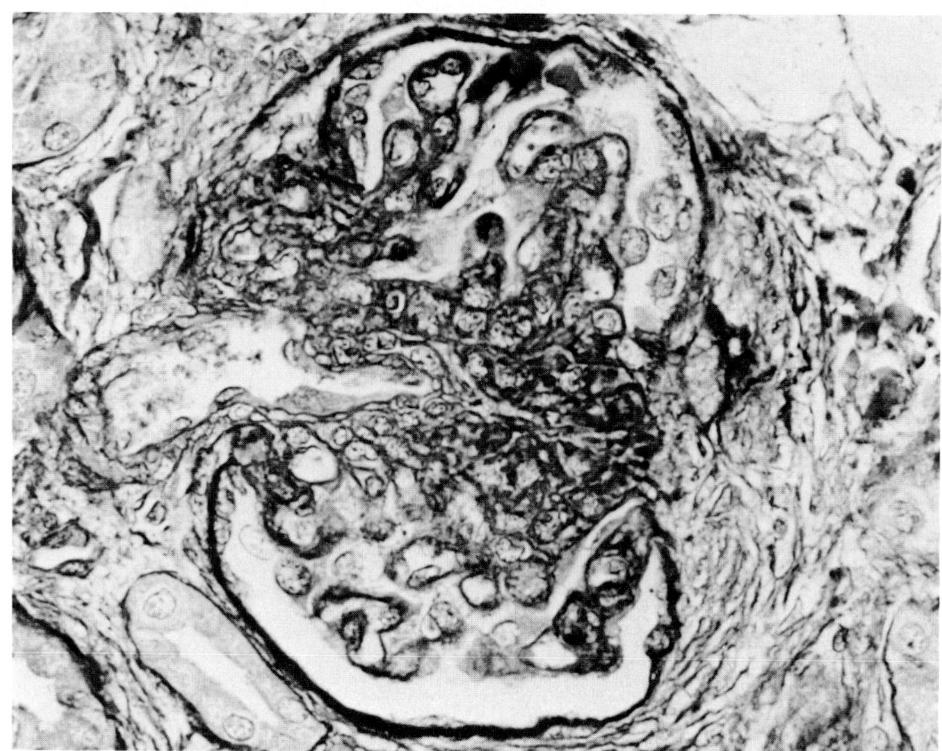

Figure 21-4. Glomerulus with adhesions and sclerosis in a biopsy specimen from a patient with advanced hereditary nephritis (PAS stain, ×800).

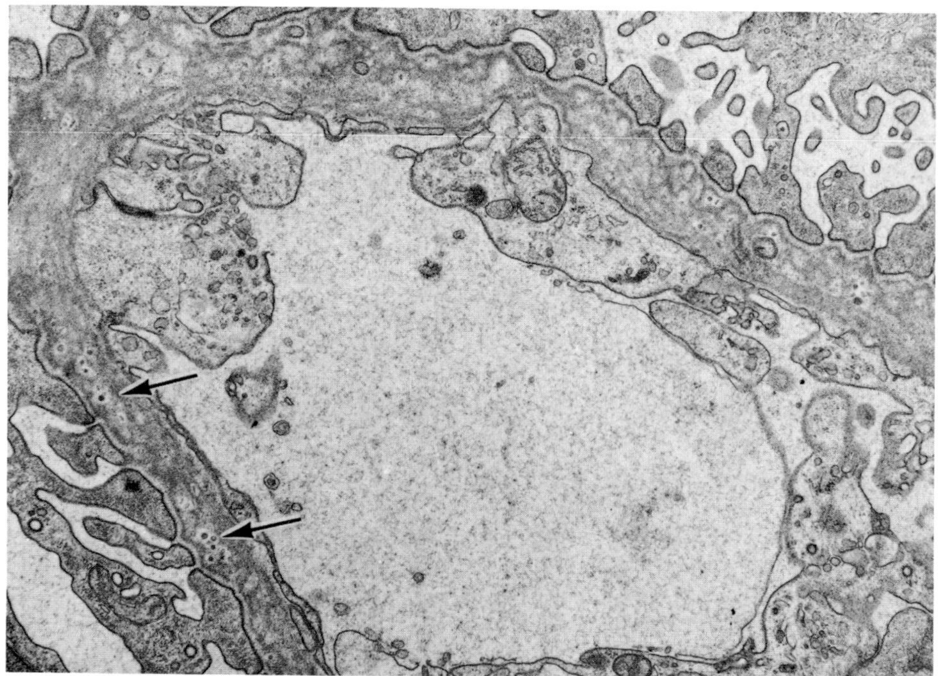

Figure 21-5. Glomerular capillary loop showing diffuse thickening of the basement membrane. The lamina densa is split into multiple interwoven lamellae and contains small round granules surrounded by clear halos (arrows) (×14,000).

396

Prognosis

The majority of males with Alport's disease progress relentlessly into chronic renal failure by the age of 20 years (6,7,12). Renal failure develops in females in some kinships (7,16), but affected women generally have a normal life expectancy. There is no specific treatment for any of the manifestations of Alport's disease. Successful transplantation has now been reported in a number of patients without recurrence of the membrane lesions, except in one very doubtful case (29), even though some patients received kidneys from related donors (30).

BENIGN FAMILIAL HEMATURIA

Macroscopic or microscopic hematuria may occur in a familial pattern without progression to renal failure or other associated abnormalities (11,31,32). The syndrome of benign familial hematuria is usually transmitted as a dominant characteristic (31,32), and affects both sexes with equal frequency and intensity. Appearance may be with either recurrent macroscopic hematuria or as an incidental finding of red blood cells in the urinary sediment. Proteinuria is usually minimal or absent. No progression to renal failure has been recorded in several studies (31,32), but azotemia has occurred in an apparently similar clinical disorder (26). Whether this syndrome will remain distinct or will merge into the milder end of the Alport spectrum is not yet certain.

Pathologic Characteristics

There are no light microscopic changes and immunofluorescence studies are invariably negative. The syndrome has been defined by the ultrastructural demonstration of extreme attenuation of the glomerular basement membrane with focal gaps, which may represent the sites of erythrocyte efflux (24,32). Although this appearance is highly characteristic, it must be remembered that capillary dilatation from any cause can attenuate the membrane and, possibly for this reason, thin membranes are occasionally seen in hematuric patients without family history. The membrane thinning in this syndrome is usually described as uniform, but focal irregularities and lamellation may occur (22,24) (Figs. 21-6, 21-7).

NAIL-PATELLA SYNDROME

The nail-patella syndrome (onycho-osteodysplasia) is a rare skeletal disorder transmitted as an autosomal dominant with strong linkage to the ABO blood group locus (34). Among the many bony abnormalities characterizing the syndrome are fingernail changes, absence or subluxation of the patella, iliac spurs, and subluxation of the radial head (34).

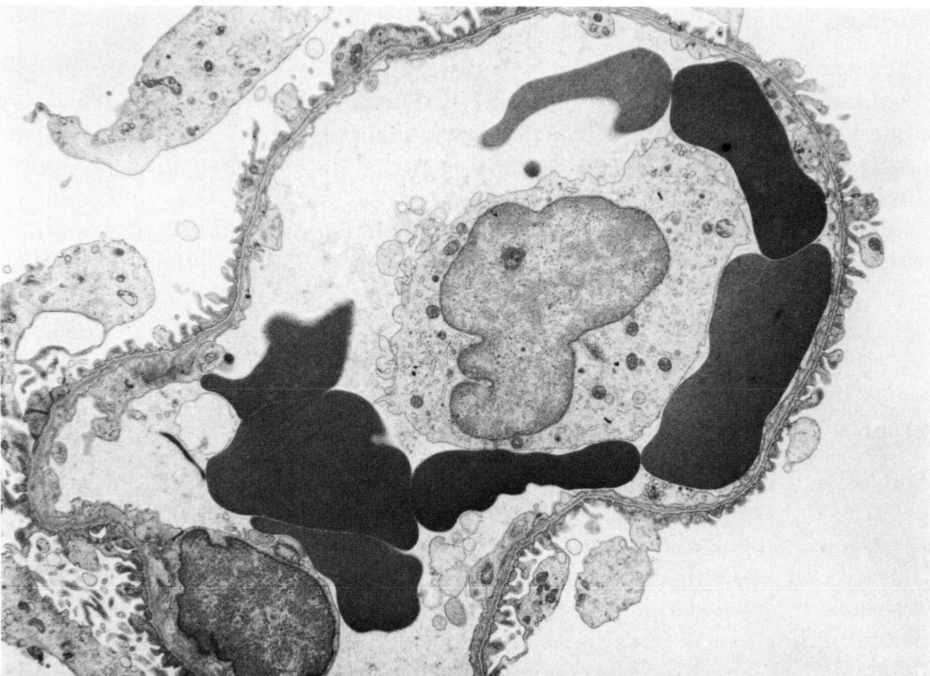

Figure 21-6. Capillary loop showing marked uniform thinning of the basement membrane in benign familial hematuria (×4,200).

Clinical Manifestations and Prognosis

The principal indication of renal damage is proteinuria, which may be sufficient to cause the nephrotic syndrome (34). Although all patients with skeletal abnormalities probably have abnormal glomeruli, proteinuria occurs in only 30−50%, and progressive renal disease has not been documented in its absence. Proteinuria appears in infancy and may remain static for up to 25 years before renal failure develops in the second to fourth decades (33,36). The proportion of patients progressing to renal failure has not been established but is probably less than 10% (33). No evidence of recurrent disease has been demonstrated in transplanted kidneys (37). One patient with this syndrome has developed anti-GBM disease (38), and we have seen another with superimposed IgA nephropathy.

Pathologic Characteristics

Light Microscopy
There are few changes early in the disease, although irregular thickening of the glomerular basement membrane may be seen (35,36,39). The later stages are characterized by nonspecific glomerular and tubulointerstitial scarring.

Electron Microscopy
The glomerular basement membrane is irregularly thickened and contains numerous lucent areas, within which are bundles of collagen fibers (33,35,36,39)

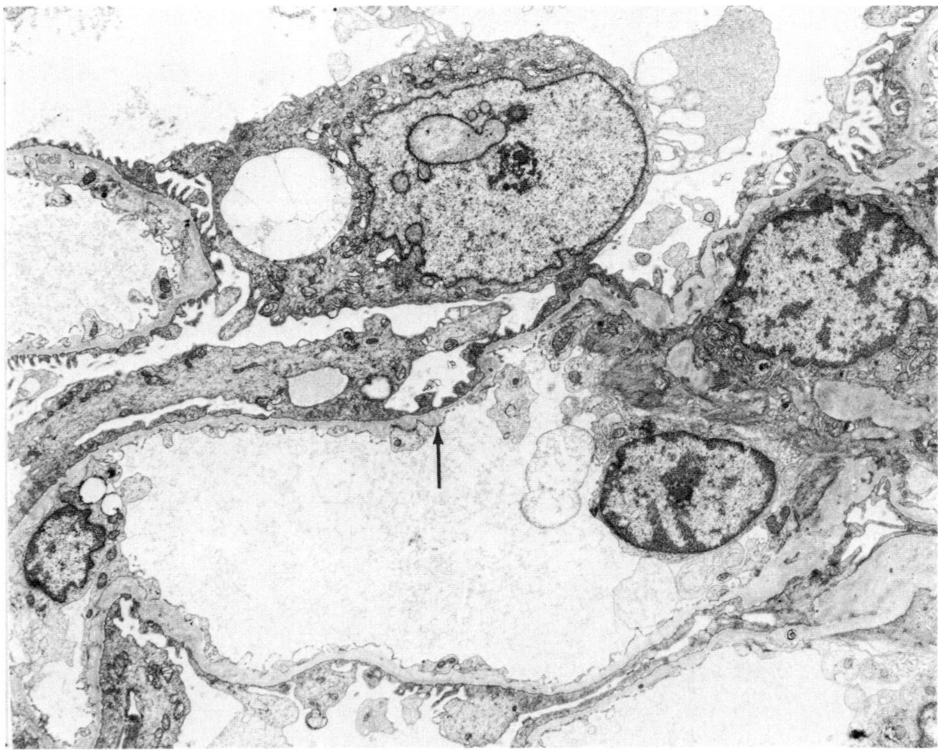

Figure 21-7. Biopsy specimen from a patient with benign familial hematuria. The basement membrane is markedly attenuated. The lamina rara interna is slightly irregular (arrow). The mesangial matrix is moderately increased and the foot processes are focally obliterated (×4,300).

(Fig. 21-8). The lucent areas impart a "moth-eaten" appearance to the membrane, and careful study—in some cases even needing special stains (35)—may be required to demonstrate the fibers. The changes may be irregularly distributed throughout glomeruli or interspersed with segments of normal membrane, and need to be differentiated from the membrane fibrosis occurring in healed segmental inflammation. The diagnosis should, therefore, only be considered when collagen fibers are found in distinct lamellae away from areas of scarring. The ultrastructural abnormalities are present in all patients with the skeletal syndrome, regardless of the presence or absence of proteinuria (33), and occasional patients may have significant renal disease with only subtle bony changes.

Immunofluorescence Microscopy
No specific reactions have been reported with the uncomplicated disease, although minor staining may be seen (33,36).

CONGENITAL NEPHROTIC SYNDROME

The nephrotic syndrome is rare in infancy and may be caused by a variety of diseases. Only 37 of 1,000 children with the nephrotic syndrome were less than 1

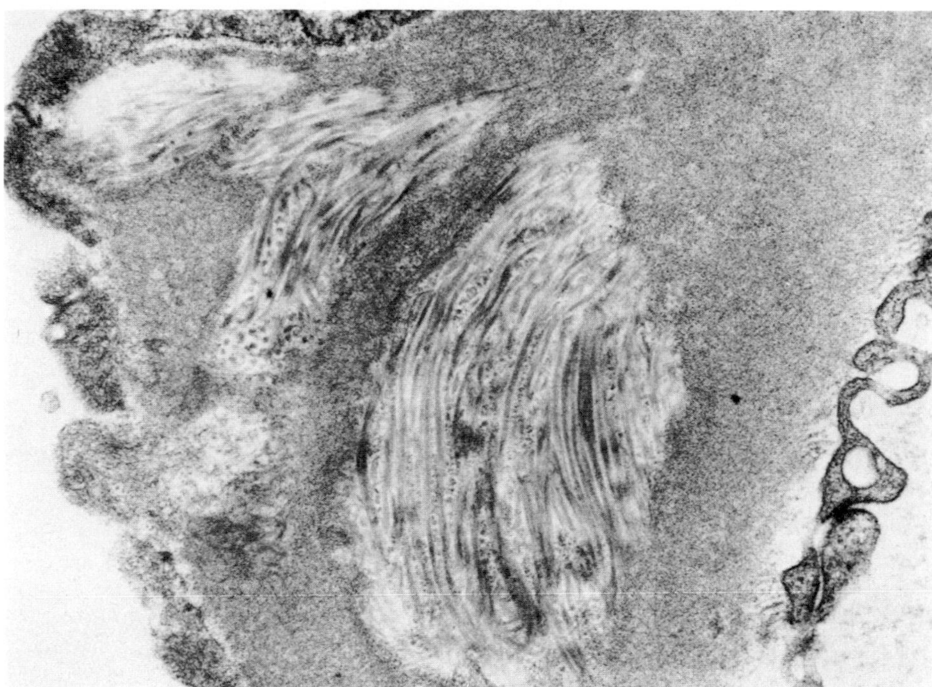

Figure 21-8. Collagenlike fibers within the basement membrane in nail-patella syndrome (×35,000).

year of age at diagnosis in one series (40). Within this small group are two general categories: first, a collection of disorders that occur at all ages but may occasionally present in early life, and second, disorders restricted to infancy. The first group embraces epithelial cell disease, focal glomerulosclerosis, membranous nephropathy, and a range of other, very rare, disorders (40). The second group includes two distinct infantile diseases with differing clinical and morphologic features but equally disastrous prognoses: congenital nephrotic syndrome of Finnish type and diffuse mesangial sclerosis. Differentiation between all these conditions can be achieved only by renal biopsy.

CONGENITAL NEPHROTIC SYNDROME OF FINNISH TYPE (CNF)

Although CNF occurs in many countries and in a variety of ethnic groups (41), it was first reported and remains most common in Finland (42). This is probably because the autosomal recessive gene carrying the condition is more likely to be expressed in a small and stable community where consanguineous marriage is more frequent (42). In Finland, CNF affects 1 in 8,200 births (43), but in other countries the incidence is extremely low (40). The pathogenesis of the disease is completely unknown, although there is some evidence for a biochemical abnormality in the glomerular basement membrane (44).

Clinical Manifestations and Prognosis

The manifestations of CNF are truly congenital. Affected children are usually premature, have abnormal placentae, and develop edema in the first week of life (42). Edema or abdominal distension may actually be present at birth and almost never develops after the age of 3 months. There is good evidence for renal malfunction in utero, and antenatal diagnosis of CNF has been achieved by the demonstration of elevated concentrations of alpha-fetoprotein in amniotic fluid or maternal serum (45). The proteinuria is initially highly selective, but becomes nonselective with advancing glomerular damage, and the nephrotic syndrome is completely resistant to corticosteroid therapy (46). Death is inevitable and, although mild azotemia may develop, is never from renal failure, but rather is caused by systemic infection or electrolyte disorders (40,42,43). Thrombosis of renal or other large veins commonly complicates the nephrotic state (40,45). The nephrotic features disappear completely after bilateral nephrectomy, indicating that the lesion is peculiarly renal, but transplantation has rarely been successful (43,47).

Pathologic Characteristics

Biopsy specimens taken early in the disease show few notable abnormalities by light microscopy but, ultrastructurally, there is diffuse obliteration of epithelial foot processes (Fig. 21-9). Frequently, two populations of glomeruli can be seen. The majority are normal in size, with diffuse or irregular mesangial sclerosis and proliferation, while the remainder are small and "immature," with dilatation of Bowman's space (40,42). Immunofluorescent studies are uniformly negative (42). Later, there is progressive glomerular obsolescence, often in an irregular pattern with adhesions and segmental sclerosis, with concomitant tubulointerstitial scarring. Dilatation of proximal convoluted tubules, initially at the corticomedullary junction, but later throughout the cortex, may produce a microcystic appearance is approximately 75% of cases (42) (Fig. 21-10). This appearance is, however, neither constant nor specific and is absent in biopsy specimens taken early in the disease. Differential diagnosis from epithelial cell disease is impossible on morphologic grounds early in the course of the disease and close clinical consultation is essential for accurate diagnosis in the infantile nephrotic syndrome.

DIFFUSE MESANGIAL SCLEROSIS

A small proportion of patients with the congenital nephrotic syndrome have a peculiar and highly characteristic morphologic pattern of diffuse mesangial sclerosis without cellular proliferation (40). This appearance requires differentiation from mesangial proliferative glomerulonephritis occurring in the neonatal period (41), since the prognosis of the two conditions is quite distinct. Infants with diffuse mesangial sclerosis usually develop the nephrotic syndrome within the first few months of life, but manifestation may occasionally be delayed for up to 2 years. The prognosis is as disastrous as that in CNF, but in contrast to the usual maintenance of normal renal function in that condition, progression to

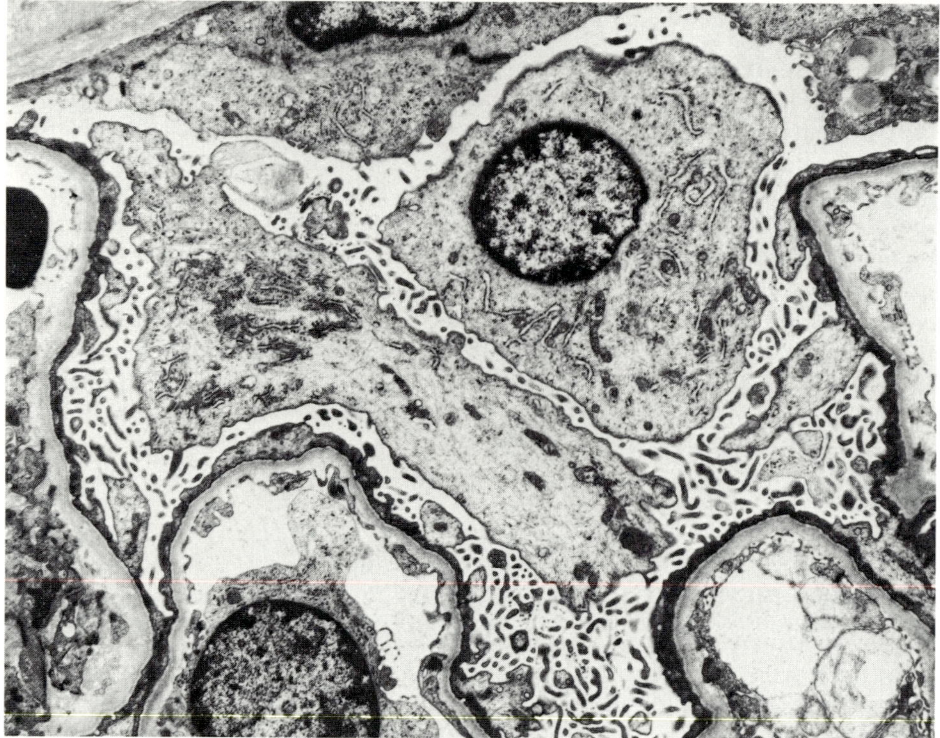

Figure 21-9. Electron micrography from a patient with congenital nephrotic syndrome (Finnish type) demonstrating extensive foot process obliteration and microvillous hyperplasia (×7,000).

azotemia is inevitable. Death always occurs before the age of 3 years. There is a striking increase in mesangial matrix, which may, initially, be focal, but later becomes diffuse and progressively transforms the glomeruli into shrunken, PAS-positive balls (40). No tendency to a segmental pattern is seen and neither endocapillary nor extracapillary proliferation can be detected. In the later stages, tubulointerstitial scarring is widespread, and there may be a microcystic cortical pattern like that in CNF. Ultrastructural and immunofluorescence studies have not been reported. The condition appears to be familial, but too few patients have been studied to determine its pattern of inheritance. No evidence of recurrence has been seen in transplants performed on a few patients who may have had this condition (47).

FABRY'S DISEASE

Fabry's disease is a recessive and X-linked disorder in which deficiency of the α-galactosidase enzyme leads to systemic accumulation of trihexosyl ceramide (48,49). Progressive lysosomal storage of this glycosphingolipid causes a characteristic, albeit protean, clinical syndrome of punctate angiokeratotic skin lesions, renal disease, and recurrent "shooting" pains in the lower limbs. The syndrome

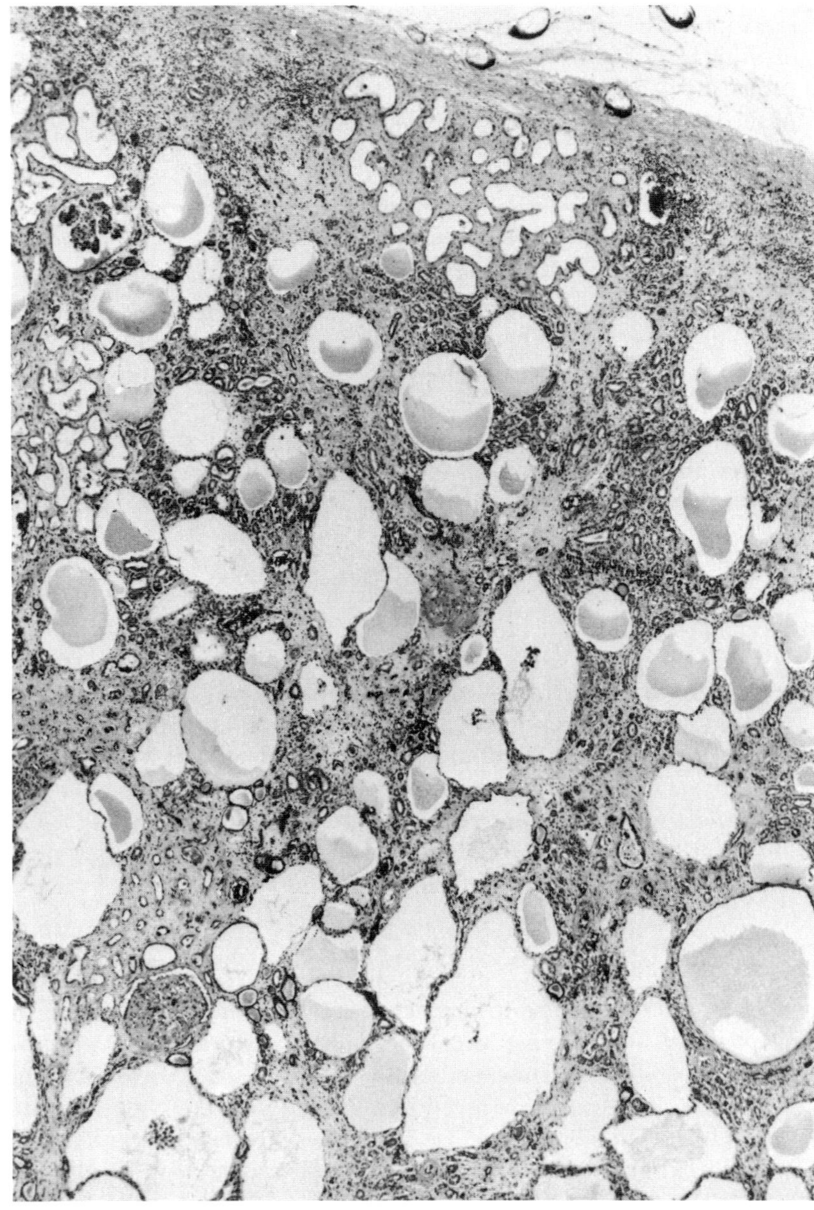

Figure 21-10. Microcystic dilatation of proximal tubules and marked interstitial scarring in a 1-year-old child with congenital nephrotic syndrome (Finnish type). A glomerulus in the left upper corner shows dilatation of Bowman's capsule (H&E stain, ×42).

may be incomplete, skin lesions, in particular, sometimes being absent (50), and a variety of organic or psychiatric disorders may be considered before the diagnosis is established (51). Biochemical analysis of α-galactosidase activity in cells, urine, or serum allows specific diagnosis of the disease and the detection of heterozygous females (52).

Clinical Manifestations and Prognosis

Renal failure is the major cause of death in hemizygous males with Fabry's disease, usually occurring in the third or fourth decades, but is unusual in heterozygous females (48). The initial manifestation of renal involvement is usually proteinuria, but progression into azotemia may occur before renal damage is suspected. There is no effective therapy for the disease. An early report suggested that renal transplantation might provide a source for the missing enzyme (51). Subsequent studies have not confirmed this suggestion (53), although glycosphingolipid has apparently not accumulated in the grafts (54).

Pathologic Characteristics

Light Microscopy

In hemizygotes, there is massive microvacuolar accumulation in visceral epithelial cells, producing a glomerular honeycomb appearance (48). Lesser degrees of storage may be detected elsewhere in the glomerulus, and there is prominent vacuolation in distal convoluted tubules and loops of Henle as well as in arteries. The vacuoles in each of these locations are PAS-negative (48,55). Similar, but less extensive, changes are seen in heterozygotic females. With increasing age, there is segmental and global sclerosis of glomeruli with interstitial scarring and a characteristic nodular pattern of arteriolar hyalinosis (48).

Electron Microscopy

There is massive accumulation of osmiophilic inclusions, measuring $0.3-10~\mu$ in diameter, in all cell types. The principal areas of accumulation are the visceral epithelial cells, which are greatly enlarged and packed with the typical bodies. These bodies are either membrane-bound or free in the cytoplasm and are round or ovoid with a concentric myelinlike structure of laminated membranes (48,55) (Fig. 21-11). Smaller numbers of inclusions affect other glomerular cells, occur in tubules, interstitial cells, and arteries and may be demonstrated in cells collected from the urine.

Differential Diagnosis

The ultrastructural pattern is almost diagnostic of Fabry's disease, but biochemical studies are required for unequivocal identification. Occasional myelinlike bodies may be seen in the visceral epithelium in a variety of conditions and have no significance. The demonstration of foam cells by light microscopy alone is in no way diagnostic of Fabry's disease. Intracapillary foam cells are commonly seen accompanying the hyperlipidemia in many glomerular disorders (56), but may also be seen in lipid storage diseases of Gaucher and Niemann-Pick types (57).

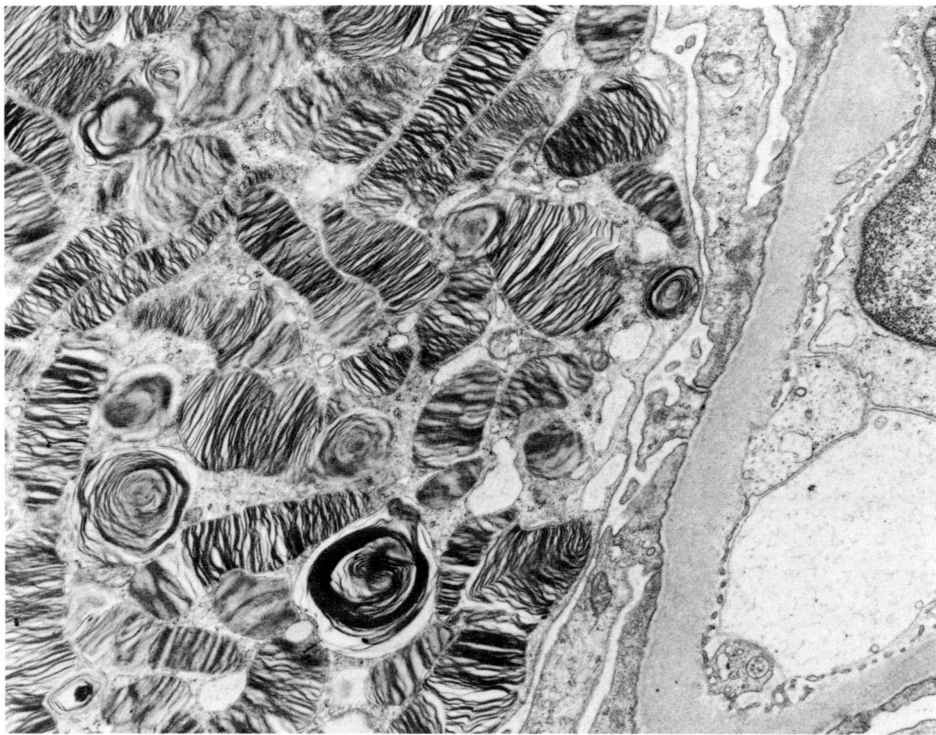

Figure 21-11. Electron micrograph of a glomerulus from a patient with Fabry's disease demonstrating numerous laminated inclusions in the epithelial cell cytoplasm (×12,600).

Microvacuolar transformation of visceral epithelium, closely resembling that in Fabry's disease, is described in mucopolysaccharidoses (57,58). The demonstration of glomerular foam cells is, therefore, usually of no great diagnostic significance. If the foam cells are unusually extensive, and especially if they are epithelial, a storage disease may be suspected. Ultrastructural demonstration of the pattern of the inclusions may provide a guide to the type of enzyme defect, but biochemical analysis of tissue or blood is always required for specific diagnosis.

SUMMARY

Familial renal disease is relatively frequent, but may be an expression of common environmental factors or abnormalities in handling systemic immune insults rather than a sign of an inherited renal defect. There are, however, several diseases in which genetic disorders affect the kidneys in specific morphologic patterns. Careful morphologic examination can diagnose many of these diseases, and may provide important prognostic information as well as guiding the physician in genetic counseling. Although these diseases have well-defined patterns of inheritance, spontaneous mutations, and other factors may lead to biopsy before a familial syndrome is expected. The pathologist is thus continually in a position in which the possibility of familial renal disease must be considered. While each of the disorders considered in this chapter have highly characteristic morphologic patterns, some of these patterns merge with those occurring in sporadic renal disease. Furthermore, the patterns may in some cases be subtle and not present in each glomerulus. Detailed light and electron microscopic examination is, therefore, required whenever a familial renal disease is suspected.

REFERENCES

1. Bernstein J: The pathology of the hereditary nephritides, in Strauss J (ed): *Pediatric Nephrology*, New York, Stratton Intercontinental Medical Book Corp, 1976, Vol 2, p. 301.

2. Johnstone SM: The familial occurrence of chronic renal disease. *Nephron* 9:371, 1972.

3. Queiroz FP, Brito E, Martinelli R: Influence of regional factors in the distribution of the histologic patterns of glomerulopathies in the nephrotic syndrome. *Nephron* 14:466, 1975.

4. Peters DK, Williams DW: Complement and mesangiocapillary glomerulonephritis: role of complement deficiency in the pathogenesis of nephritis. *Nephron* 13:189, 1974.

5. Alport AC: Hereditary familial congenital haemorrhagic nephritis. *Br Med J* 1:504, 1927.

6. Purriel P, Drets M, Pascale E, et al: Familial hereditary nephropathy (Alport's syndrome). *Am J Med* 49:753, 1970.

7. Chazan JA, Zacks J, Cohen JJ, et al: Hereditary nephritis. Clinical spectrum and mode of inheritance in five new kindreds. *Am J Med* 50:764, 1971.

8. Spear GS: Pathology of the kidney in Alport's syndrome. *Pathol Annu* 9:93, 1974.

9. Iversen UM: Hereditary nephropathy with hearing loss: "Alport's syndrome." *Acta Paediat Scand Suppl* 245:7, 1974.

10. Epstein CJ, Sahud MA, Piel CF, et al: Hereditary macrothrombocytopenia, nephritis and deafness. *Am J Med* 52:299, 1972.

11. Grüfeld I-P, Bois EP, Hinglais N: Progressive and nonprogressive hereditary chronic nephritis. *Kidney Int* 4:216, 1973.

12. O'Neill WM, Atkin CL, Bloomer A: Hereditary nephritis: a re-examination of its clinical and genetic features. *Ann Intern Med* 88:176, 1978.

13. Preus M, Fraser FC: Genetics of hereditary nephropathy with deafness (Alport's disease). *Clin Genet* 2:331, 1971.

14. Shaw RF, Kallen RJ: Population genetics of Alport's syndrome: hypothesis of abnormal segregation and the necessary existence of mutation. *Nephron* 16:427, 1976.

15. Antonovych TT, Deasy PF, Tina LU, et al: Hereditary nephritis. Early clinical, functional and morphological studies. *Pediat Res* 3:545, 1969.

16. Kaufman DB, McIntosh RM, Smith FG Jr, et al: Diffuse familial nephropathy. A clinicopathological study. *J Pediat* 77:37, 1970.

17. Gaboardi F, Edefonti A, Imbasciati E, et al: Alport's syndrome (progressive hereditary nephritis). *Clin Nephrol* 2:143, 1974.

18. Ferguson AC, Rance CP: Hereditary nephropathy with nerve deafness (Alport's syndrome). *Am J Dis Child* 124:84, 1972.

19. Crawford MD, Toghill PJ: Alport's syndrome of hereditary nephritis and deafness. *Quart J Med* 37:563, 1968.

20. Sherman RL, Churg J, Yudis M: Hereditary nephritis with a characteristic renal lesion. *Am J Med* 56:44, 1974.

21. Neustein HB, O'Brien JS, Rosser RJ, et al: Chronic nephritis and renal foam cells: Cholesterol ester storage. *Arch Pathol* 93:503, 1973.

22. Kohaut EC, Singer DB, Nevels BK, et al: The specificity of split renal membranes in hereditary nephritis. *Arch Pathol Lab Med* 100:475, 1976.

23. Rumpelt HJ, Langer KH, Schärer K, et al: Split and extremely thin glomerular basement mem-

branes in hereditary nephropathy (Alport's syndrome). *Virchows Arch A Path Anat Histol* 364:225, 1974.

24. Hill GS, Jenis EH, Goodloe S Jr: The nonspecificity of the ultrastructural alterations in hereditary nephritis with additional observations on benign familial hematuria. *Lab Invest* 31:516, 1974.

25. Churg J, Sherman RL: Pathologic characteristics of hereditary nephritis. *Arch Pathol* 95:374, 1973.

26. Sessa A, Cioffi A, Conte F, et al: Hereditary nephropathy with nerve deafness (Alport's syndrome): electron microscopy studies on the renal glomerulus. *Nephron* 13:404, 1974.

27. Sanerkin NG: On the nature of "interstitial foam cells" in chronic glomerulonephritis. *J Pathol Bact* 86:135, 1963.

28. Beathard GA, Granholm NA: Development of the characteristic ultrastructural lesion of hereditary nephritis during the course of the disease. *Am J Med* 62:751, 1977.

29. Mathew TH, Mathews DC, Hobbs JR, et al: Glomerular lesions after renal transplantation. *Am J Med* 59:117, 1975.

30. Barnes BA, Bergan JJ, Braun WE, et al: Renal transplantation in congenital and metabolic diseases. A report from the ASC/NIH Renal Transplant Registry. *JAMA* 232:148, 1975.

31. McConville JM, McAdams AJ: Familial and nonfamilial benign hematuria. *J Pediat* 69:207, 1966.

32. Rogers PW, Kurtzman NA, Bunn SM Jr, et al: Familial benign essential hematuria. *Arch Intern Med* 131:257, 1973.

33. Bennett WM, Musgrave JE, Campbell RA, et al: The nephropathy of the nail-patella syndrome. *Am J Med* 54:305, 1973.

34. Valdueza AF: The nail-patella syndrome: a report of three families. *J Bone Joint Surg* 55B:145, 1973.

35. Morita T, Laughlin LO, Kawano K, et al: nail-patella syndrome: light and electron microscopic studies of the kidneys. *Arch Intern Med* 131:271, 1973.

36. Hoyer JR, Michael AF, Vernier RL: Renal disease in nail-patella syndrome: clinical and morphologic studies. *Kidney Int* 2:231, 1972.

37. Uranga VM, Simmons RL, Hoyer JR, et al: Renal transplantation for the nail-patella syndrome. *Am J Surg* 125:777, 1973.

38. Curtis JJ, Bhathena D, Leach RP, et al: Goodpasture's syndrome in a patient with the nail-patella syndrome. *Am J Med* 61:401, 1976.

39. Ben-Bassat M, Cohen L, Rosenfeld J: The glomerular basement membrane in the nail-patella syndrome. *Arch Pathol* 92:350, 1971.

40. Habib R, Bois E: Congenital and Infantile nephrotic syndrome, in Strauss J (ed): *Pediatric Nephrology*, vol 2, New York, Stratton Intercontinental Medical Book Corp, 1976, p 335.

41. George CRP, Hickman RO, Striker GE: Infantile nephrotic syndrome. *Clin Nephrol* 5:20, 1976.

42. Hallman N, Norio R, Rapola J: Congenital nephrotic syndrome. *Nephron* 11:101, 1973.

43. Huttunen N-P: Congenital nephrotic syndrome of Finnish type: study of 75 patients. *Arch Dis Child* 51:344, 1976.

44. Mahieu P, Monnens L, van Haelst U: Chemical properties of glomerular basement membrane in congenital nephrotic syndrome. *Clin Nephrol* 5:135, 1976.

45. Seppala M, Aula P, Rapola J, et al: Congenital nephrotic syndrome: prenatal diagnosis and genetic counselling by estimation of amniotic fluid and maternal serum alpha-fetoprotein. *Lancet* 2:123, 1976.

46. Huttunen N-P, Savilahti E, Rapola J: Selectivity of proteinuria in congenital nephrotic syndrome of the Finnish type. *Kidney Int* 8:255, 1975.

47. Hoyer JR, Kjellstrand CM, Simmons RL, et al: Successful transplantation in 3 children with congenital nephrotic syndrome. *Lancet* 1:1410, 1973.

48. Gubler M-C, Lenoir G, Grunfeld J-P, et al: Early renal changes in hemizygous and heterozygous patients with Fabry's disease. *Kidney Int* 13:223, 1978.

49. Pabico RC, Atanacio BC, McKenna BA, et al: Renal pathologic lesions and functional alterations in a man with Fabry's disease. *Am J Med* 55:415, 1973.

50. Clarke JTR, Knaack J, Crawhall JC, et al: Ceramide trihexosidosis (Fabry's disease) without skin lesions. *N Engl J Med* 284:233, 1971.

51. Philippart M, Franklin SS, Gordon A: Reversal of an inborn sphingolipidosis (Fabry's disease) by kidney transplantation. *Ann Intern Med* 77:195, 1972.

52. Desnick RJ, Allen KY, Desnick SJ, et al: Fabry's disease: enzymatic diagnosis of hemizygotes and heterozygotes. *J Lab Clin Med* 81:157, 1973.

53. Spence MW, MacKinnon KE, Burgess JK, et al: Failure to correct the metabolic defect by renal allotransplantation in Fabry's disease. *Ann Intern Med* 84:13, 1976.

54. Bühler FR, Thiel G, Dubach UC: Kidney transplantation in Fabry's disease. *Br Med J* 2:28, 1973.

55. Savi M, Olivetti G, Neri TM, et al: Clinical, histopathological and biochemical findings in Fabry's disease: A case report and family study. *Arch Pathol Lab Med* 101:536, 1977.

56. McKenzie IFR, Kincaid-Smith P: Foam cells in the renal glomerulus. *J Pathol* 97:151, 1969.

57. Rosenman E, Aviram A: Glomerular involvement in storage diseases. *J Pathol* 111:61, 1973.

58. Scott CD, Lagunoff D, Pritzl P: A mucopolysaccharide storage disease with involvement of the renal glomerular epithelium. *Am J Med* 54:549, 1973.

22
Interstitial Nephritis

Interstitial inflammation is a feature of many renal diseases. Usually, the interstitial changes appear to be secondary to damage elsewhere and are relegated to a position of minor importance in biopsy interpretation. There is, however, abundant evidence for an influence of interstitial disease on renal function. Several studies of patients with glomerulonephritis have shown that the degree of renal dysfunction is better correlated with the interstitial than the glomerular changes (1–3). Significant renal failure may, indeed, accompany disease confined to the interstitium. This chapter reviews a number of conditions in which isolated interstitial disease affects renal function. No attempt is made to present an encyclopedic description of all interstitial disorders. Rather, those conditions are discussed in which *diffuse* interstitial changes are associated with transient or permanent renal failure likely to be an indication for renal biopsy. Clearly, this approach groups together a series of diseases that share no common factors other than their localization at the time of biopsy. For this reason, a morphologic rather than a pathogenetic approach is used (Table 22-1). Although the descriptive term *interstitial nephritis* is morphologically appropriate for all situations in which the renal interstitium contains inflammatory cells, this discussion is restricted to conditions in which changes in other nephron components are absent or minimal.

IMMUNOLOGIC MECHANISMS OF INTERSTITIAL DAMAGE

Recently, there has been intense interest in immune interstitial disorders. This interest was stimulated by the demonstration of interstitial immunofluorescent

Table 22-1. Morphologic Classification of Interstitial Disease

Predominantly polymorphonuclear

Predominantly mononuclear
    With significant numbers of eosinophils
    With few or no eosinophils
    With frequent foam cells
    Granulomatous
    Malacoplakia

Predominantly mononuclear with scarring

reactions in a number of human diseases (4) and by the development of several experimental models (5,6). The relevance of these models to disease in man is, as yet, uncertain, but continued investigation is likely to elucidate the mechanisms by which interstitial damage occurs.

Immune Complex Interstitial Disease

Experimental interstitial nephritis mediated by immune complexes has been studied using both endogenous and exogenous antigens. Repeated injections of both cortical extracts and bovine serum albumin produce interstitial inflammation with granular immunofluorescence for IgG and C3 along tubular basement membranes and in the interstitium (5,6). Apparently, primary interstitial nephritis mediated by immune complexes is extremely rare in humans, but interstitial deposits are frequently seen accompanying the glomerular lesions of cryoglobulinemia and lupus nephritis (6).

Antitubular Basement Membrane (Anti-TBM) Disease

Linear reactions along the TBM occur most often in anti-GBM disease (4,7). Anti-TBM antibodies are demonstrable in these patients and probably contribute to the interstitial changes (7). Interstitial nephritis with anti-TBM antibodies has also been reported in a few patients following presumed immune complex mediated glomerulonephritis, possibly following tubular damage secondary to glomerular disease with release of TBM antigens (6). Rare examples of anti-TBM disease have been recorded in transplanted kidneys (5,7a) and in association with methicillin-induced interstitial nephritis (see below). Only one patient has, so far, been reported with isolated and apparently spontaneous anti-TBM nephritis, characterized by a Fanconi-like tubular syndrome (8). These human examples share features with a number of recently developed experimental models produced by the injection into rats of either cortical suspensions or purified TBM antigens (5,6). In some of the models, glomerulonephritis of either immune complex or anti-GBM type has occurred, but tubulointerstitial disease has been predominant, and circulating anti/TBM antibodies have been demonstrated.

Cytotoxic Damage to Tubular Cells

There is some evidence for direct cellular damage by circulating antibodies in Heymann's experimental nephritis, but none for this action in human membranous nephropathy (5). Antibodies to tubular cells have been demonstrated in a few patients with hyperglobulinemia and renal tubular acidosis (see below).

Cell-Mediated Interstitial Disease

Mononuclear cells are the predominant component of the inflammatory infiltrate in most forms of human and experimental interstitial nephritis. No clear evidence for the participation of cell-mediated immune mechanisms has, however, been demonstrated in these conditions (5,6).

MORPHOLOGIC PATTERNS OF INTERSTITIAL NEPHRITIS

Predominantly Polymorphonuclear Interstitial Nephritis

Acute Pyelonephritis
There is usually no clinical difficulty in establishing a clinical diagnosis of acute pyelonephritis, but occasional patients may not exhibit the characteristic diagnostic features. Unexplained acute renal failure may be the indication of acute pyelonephritis in such patients, and a tissue diagnosis may be achieved before other features are recognized. This sequence of events is most likely to occur in very young, very old, or debilitated patients. Appropriate antibiotic therapy is usually curative, but significant renal scarring may ensue (9).

Pathology.   The tubules are separated by intense edema within which are numerous polymorphs admixed with lesser numbers of mononuclear cells (Fig. 22-1). Microorganisms may be seen in appropriately stained sections. The inflammation may involve glomeruli, tubules, and blood vessels, but the principal changes are interstitial.

Septicemia and Pyemia
Small collections of polymorphs develop in the renal cortex in systemic pyogenic infections and may be encountered in renal biopsies performed to investigate bacterial endocarditis or unexplained renal failure.

Predominantly Mononuclear Interstitial Nephritis with Significant Numbers of Eosinophils

The presence of numerous eosinophils in an interstitial inflammatory infiltrate is highly suggestive of drug-induced acute interstitial nephritis. The drugs concerned are most frequently of the penicillin family, but a large number of therapeutic agents have been implicated (Table 22-2). Occasionally, acute interstitial nephritis is an unexpected finding in a biopsy performed to investigate deteriorating renal function, as in the reported cases complicating diuretic therapy in the nephrotic syndrome (10). Typically, however, there is a systemic syndrome with fever, skin rash, and eosinophilia preceding the onset of acute renal failure, which may develop in the face of a normal or even increased urinary output. This syndrome develops after a latent period of five days to five weeks from exposure to the drug (11). Proteinuria is usually minimal, reflecting the absence of glomerular damage, but there may be an active urinary sediment in which eosinophils are identifiable. The renal and systemic phenomena remit spontaneously after cessation of the drug, but recovery may be prolonged and dialysis or, in severe cases, corticosteroid therapy may be required. Providing that the nature of the disease is recognized promptly, the vast majority of the patients regain normal renal function, and the few reports of residual renal failure do not provide satisfactory details of renal function before the onset of the disease (12,13).

Pathologic Characteristics
The appearances are essentially similar in all reported cases. Focally distributed throughout the cortex are areas of congestion with interstitial edema and an

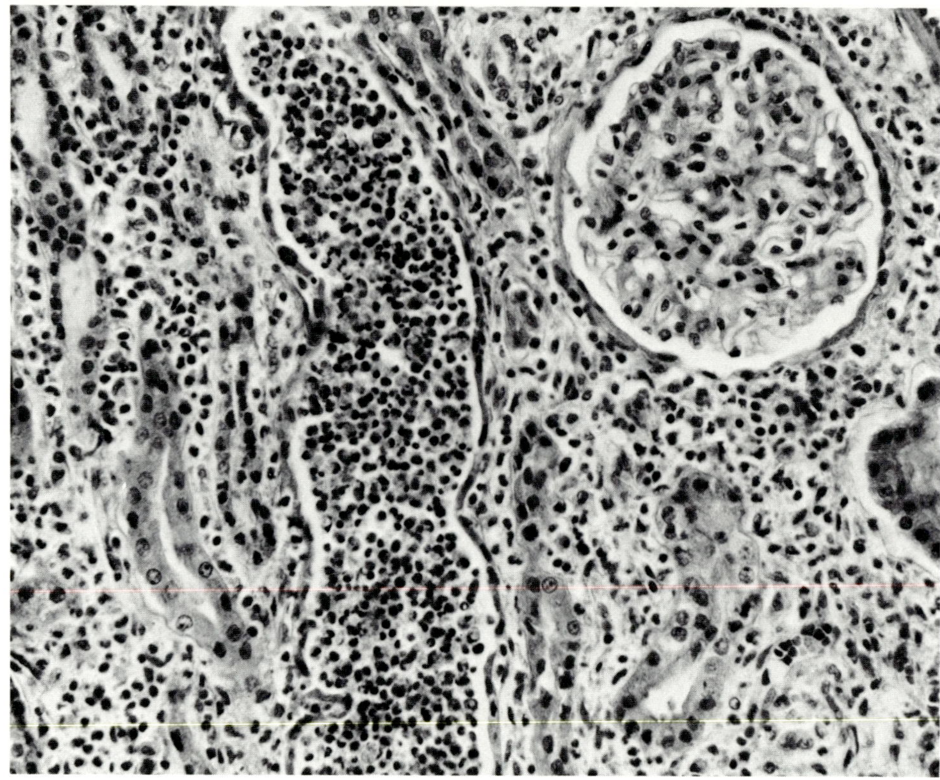

Figure 22-1. Acute pyelonephritis. The tubule shown in the center of the picture contains polymorphonuclear leukocytes, and the interstitium is heavily infiltrated by acute inflammatory cells mixed with a lesser number of mononuclear cells (H&E stain, ×320).

Table 22-2. Drugs Implicated in Acute Eosinophilic Interstitial Nephritis

Antibacterial agents
Penicillin and analogues: penicillin (18)[a] methicillin (19), ampicillin (19), oxacillin (19), nafcillin (19), cloxacillin (20)
Sulphonamides (21)[a]
Cephalothin (22) and cephalosporin (19)
Rifampicin (23)
Tetracyclines (23a)

Diuretics
Thiazides and furosemide (10)

Others
Allopurinal (24), azathioprine (25), Dilantin (14), phenazone (26), phenindione (27), phenobarbital (16), phenylbutazone (28).

[a]Arteritis and glomerulonephritis have been reported in a few patients with disease related to penicillin (29) and sulfonamides (30).

412

intense inflammatory infiltrate. While eosinophils are prominent, they rarely comprise more than 15% of the infiltrate, the remainder of the cells being immunoblasts, lymphocytes, plasma cells, and histiocytes (Fig. 22-2). Aside from a few cases related to penicillin and sulfonamides (see Table 22-2), the glomeruli and blood vessels appear normal. Immunofluorescence studies are usually negative, although there are occasional reports of linear IgG staining (see below) and convincing ultrastructural deposits have not been documented (Fig. 22-3).

The pathogenesis of drug-induced interstitial nephritis is unknown, but its relative rarity supports a hypersensitivity basis. Although a few patients have shown lymphocyte reactivity to the drugs involved (14), convincing evidence of cell-mediated mechanisms has not appeared (6). Several recent reports have described linear TBM immunofluorescence for IgG and C3 with circulating anti-TBM antibodies in patients with methicillin-induced interstitial nephritis (6) (Fig. 22-3). Methicillin-derived antigens were found along the TBM in one of these patients, raising the possibility of antibodies formed against a hapten conjugate of the drug with the TBM (6). These findings are, however, exceptional, and it is likely that the antibodies are a secondary response to tubular damage mediated by other mechanisms. In addition, the significance of finding methicillin-derived antigens is reduced by the demonstration at autopsy of an-

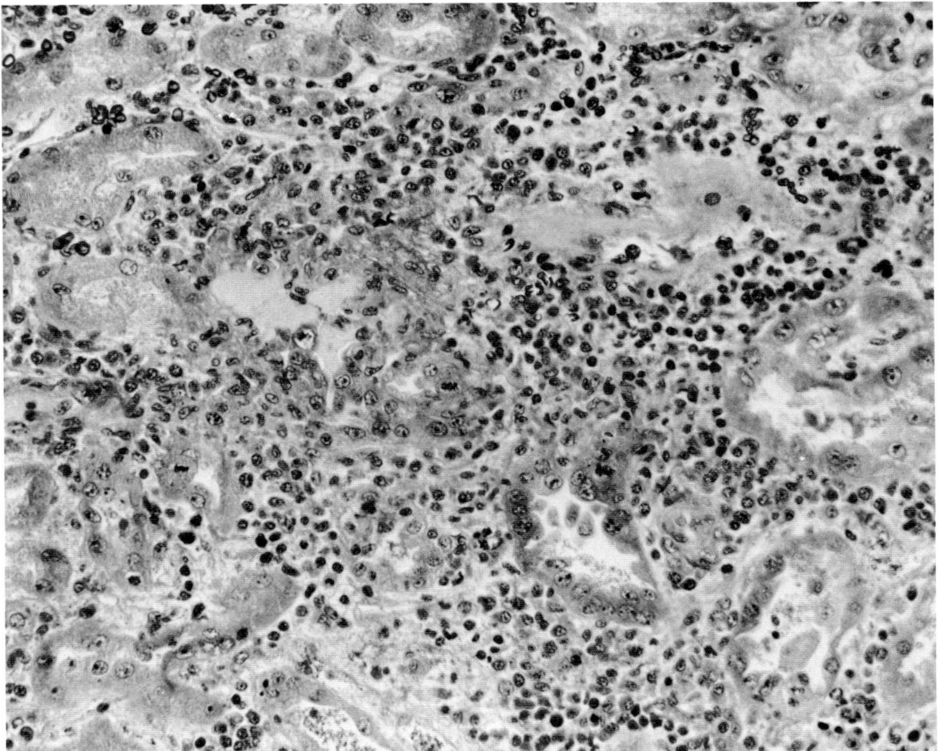

Figure 22-2. Renal biopsy specimen from a patient who developed acute renal failure following therapy with methicillin. Interstitial infiltrate present consists predominantly of lymphocytes, plasma cells, and eosinophils (H&E stain, ×325).

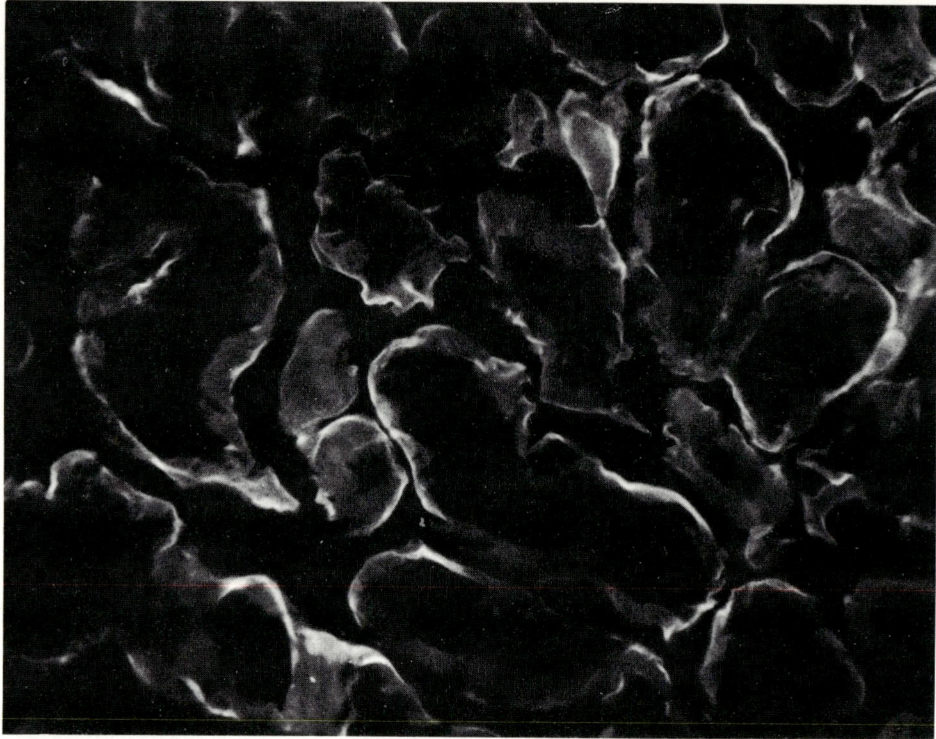

Figure 22-3. Same case as shown in Figure 22-2, demonstrating linear fluorescence along tubular basement membranes. Circulating anti-TBM antibodies were detected in the patient's serum by indirect immunofluorescence (antihuman IgG, ×500).

tibodies to penicillin along the TBM in the normal kidneys of several patients given penicillin shortly before death (6). Circulating levels of IgE are increased in parallel with the activity of the disease in most patients (15), suggesting participation of reaginic antibody, and this immunoglobulin has been demonstrated in plasma cells within the inflammatory infiltrate (16). Finally, in some patients with this morphologic pattern of interstitial nephritis, there is no identifiable drug or other cause for the disease. One report describes two apparently unrelated patients with a systemic syndrome of eosinophilic interstitial nephritis, uveitis, and granulomata in lymph nodes and bone marrow for which no cause could be found (17).

Predominantly Mononuclear Interstitial Nephritis with Few or No Eosinophils

Focal or diffuse infiltration of the unscarred kidney by mononuclear inflammatory cells occur in many diseases (Table 22-3). Fortunately, the clinical features of these diseases usually allow a confident diagnosis before the biopsy specimen is taken. Occasionally, however, the cause of renal deterioration may be obscure, and the pathologist is asked to provide a differential diagnosis. Unfortunately, the morphologic appearances in this group of diseases may be very similar, and a specific diagnosis is often not possible on morphologic grounds alone.

Table 22-3. Causes of Mononuclear Renal Infiltrates

Infections
Acute renal failure
Transplant rejection
Systemic lupus erythematosus
Accompanying glomerulonephritis
Lymphoma, leukemia
Hyperglobulinemia

Infections

The concept of acute interstitial nephritis was first established in 1898 by Councilman, who described interstitial changes in a range of fatal infectious diseases (31). Following the virtual disappearance from the western world of scarlet fever and diphtheria, the most common causes of systemic infective interstitial nephritis (32), this picture is now rarely seen in either biopsy or autopsy material. Acute interstitial nephritis has rarely been described in brucellosis (33), legionnaire's disease (34), and toxoplasmosis (35), but is probably quite common in infectious mononucleosis (36). Presently, the most common systemic infection causing interstitial nephritis is probably leptospirosis. Renal involvement may occur with all *leptospira* serotypes and is almost certainly present in all patients with the disease (37). Recovery is always complete, although dialysis may be required, and usually occurs without the need for specific antileptospiral therapy.

Pathologic Characteristics.   Patchy accumulation of mononuclear inflammatory cells occurs within edematous areas, distorting the tubular pattern (37). The remainder of the tubules often appear normal, and the morphologic appearances may appear insufficient for the degree of observed renal failure.

Acute Renal Failure

The pathogenesis of the acute renal failure occurring in hypovolemic states remains controversial. Studies of various experimental models have suggested two principal alternate theories: tubular necrosis with leakage into the interstitium (38), and altered cortical bloodflow, or "vasomotor nephropathy" (39). The subject is too complex for discussion in this chapter, but it is likely that combinations of these two pathways are involved, possibly with a deficiency of the vasodilatory substance normally produced in the medulla (38,39).

Pathologic Characteristics.   Renal biopsy specimens from patients with established acute, oligemic renal failure frequently show no or only minimal alterations. As a term, then, *acute tubular necrosis* is not appropriate and is to be condemned as a generic name for this syndrome. When changes are found, they consist of focal interstitial edema with distal tubular dilatation and, often, frequent eosinophilic and basophilic casts. The glomeruli are normal. Sporadic collections of mononuclear inflammatory cells are sometimes seen but are less prominent than those occurring in the other conditions described in this chapter (40).

Transplant Rejection

Even the least cooperative renal unit is unlikely to provide the pathologist with a biopsy specimen from a transplanted patient without appropriate information. However, cellular rejection is an archetypal example of acute interstitial nephritis, and seems likely to provide much information in the future about the mechanisms of the disease in other situations. The morphologic appearances of transplant rejection are described in Chapter 23.

Systemic Lupus Erythematosus

Interstitial inflammation is a common accompanying feature of lupus glomerulonephritis. Indeed, tubulointerstitial deposits are regularly found by both immunofluorescence and electron microscopy (4,41) (Figs. 22-4, 22-5). The interstitial component almost certainly contributes to renal functional impairment, and the combined lesion is very similar to that produced by repeated injections of exogenous antigen into experimental animals (41). Rarely, functional impairment in lupus patients has been caused by progressive interstitial immune complex disease without significant associated glomerulonephritis (42).

Accompanying Glomerulonephritis

The presence of significant interstitial inflammation in a biopsy specimen showing glomerulonephritis always raises the question of either lupus (see above) or anti-GBM (7) glomerulonephritis. Interstitial changes are, however, common to a wide range of glomerulonephritides and probably contribute to functional derangement (1–3). There is usually no diagnostic problem in these cases but, occasionally, the glomerular lesions may not be obvious on casual inspection.

Lymphoma and Leukemia

Infiltrates of neoplastic cells are commonly found post mortem in the kidneys of patients with all forms of lymphoma (43) and leukemia (44). These infiltrates usually cause little functional abnormality, but acute renal failure caused by massive renal infiltration has been reported in malignant lymphoma of lymphocytic (45), histiocytic (45), and Burkitt (46) types, in Waldenström's macroglobulinemia (47), and in acute lymphoblastic leukemia (48). We have seen a similar situation in a patient with chronic lymphocytic leukemia. The diagnosis of lymphoma is usually established before acute renal failure occurs but, occasionally, the renal biopsy appearance is the first indication of malignant disease (45). In all patients, aggressive chemotherapy has been effective in reducing the neoplastic infiltrate and improving renal function but there is a high mortality from other systemic involvement and/or the side effects of therapy.

Pathologic Characteristics.   The renal parenchyma is suffused by neoplastic cells with distortion but relative sparing of the normal structures. The pleomorphic appearance of the infiltrate readily allows diagnosis in most cases but, in well-differentiated tumors, the clue to the neoplastic nature of the infiltrate lies only in the monotonous cell type and the absence of the usual admixture of histiocytes and plasma cells (Fig. 22-6). Infiltration is usually diffuse but may be nodular or irregular and may involve only one kidney (47).

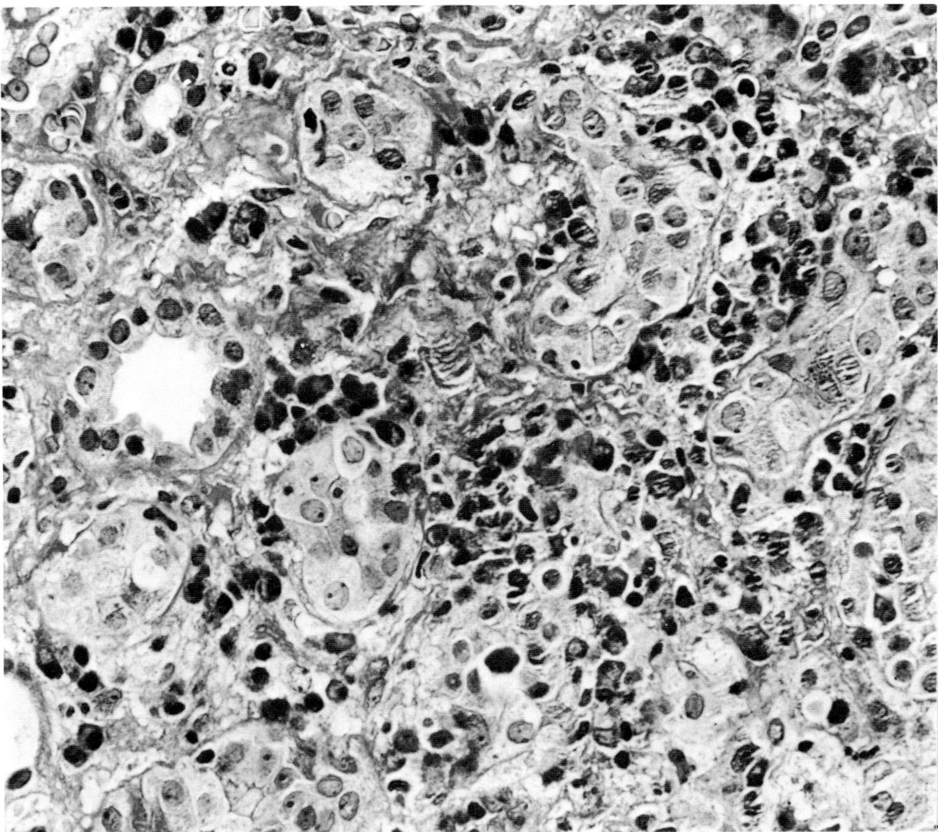

Figure 22-4. Renal biopsy specimen from a patient with active lupus nephritis showing interstitial nephritis. The interstitial infiltrate is mainly composed of plasma cells and lymphocytes (H&E stain, ×480).

Hyperglobulinemia

Focal mononuclear inflammatory infiltration of the renal cortex, with or without scarring, has been associated with renal tubular acidosis in a number of diverse conditions characterized by hyperglobulinemia. These conditions have included Sjögren's syndrome (49), fibrosing alveolitis (50), and various forms of chronic thyroid and liver disease (50). In some of these patients, immunofluorescent deposits in tubular cells were noted (49), and other studies have shown circulating antibodies (51) or lymphocyte cytotoxicity (52) against tubular cells.

Predominantly Mononuclear Interstitial Nephritis with Frequent Foam Cells

Isolated foam cells are found frequently in biopsy specimens from patients with chronic proteinuria and may be prominent in hereditary glomerulonephritis. Masses of interstitial foam cells occur in an uncommon variant of chronic renal suppuration, xanthogranulomatous interstitial nephritis. This condition may occur at all ages and usually manifests with fever, unilateral loin pain, and a flank

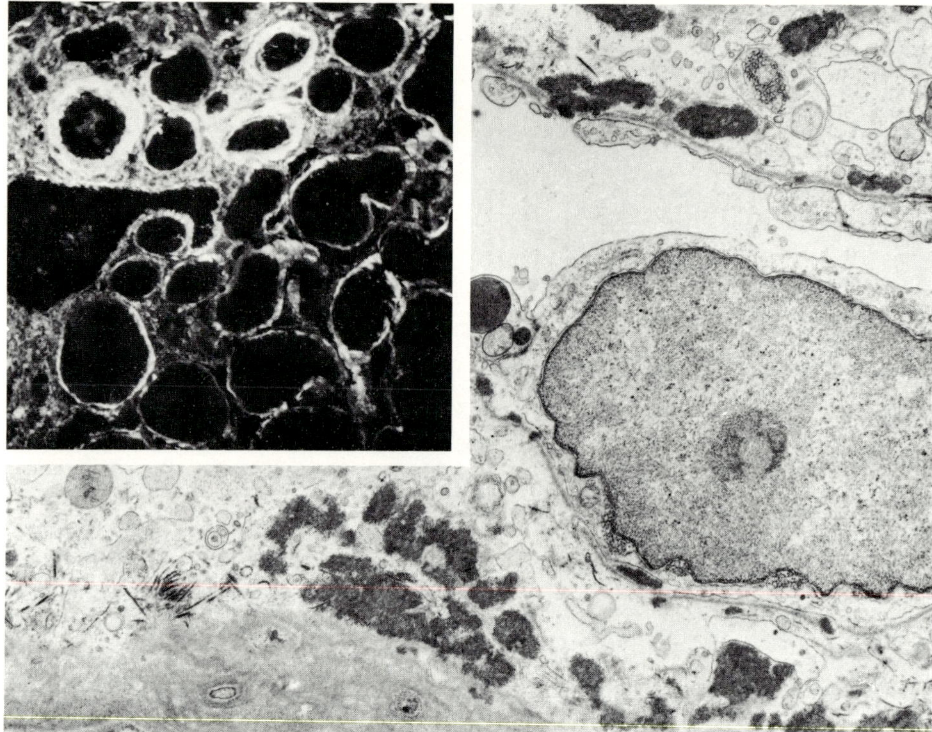

Figure 22-5. Same case as shown in Figure 22-4. Electron micrograph demonstrating deposits around the basement membrane of tubules and interstitial capillaries as well as in the interstitial tissues (×6,000). Insert: strosng granular fluorescence along tubular basement membranes, blood vessel walls, and interstitium (antihuman IgG, ×335).

mass (53). There may be a localized intrarenal mass, often a chronic abscess cavity containing calculi, or diffuse replacement of the entire kidney by firm, yellow tissue. Microscopically, this infiltrate consists of foam cells arranged in irregular sheets or groups with variable associated inflammation of polymorphonuclear and mononuclear types and scattered multinucleate giant cells (Fig. 22-7). In some areas, the picture may resemble malokoplakia, which is probably a closely related condition, but the major differential diagnosis is from clear cell adenocarcinoma of the kidney cortex (53). In small biopsy samples this may be extremely difficult, but extensive associated inflammation and the absence of nuclear pleomorphism or mitotic figures suggest the benign condition. Xanthogranulomatous interstitial nephritis is invariably unilateral and is cured by nephrectomy. The same morphologic pattern can be produced in experimental animals, and the reason for its rarity in man is unknown, there being no evidence of a particular association with any infecting organism or of an associated metabolic defect.

Granulomatous Interstitial Nephritis

Granulomatous interstitial nephritis is rare and, when encountered, is highly suggestive of sarcoidosis (Fig. 22-8). Although granulomata are found post-

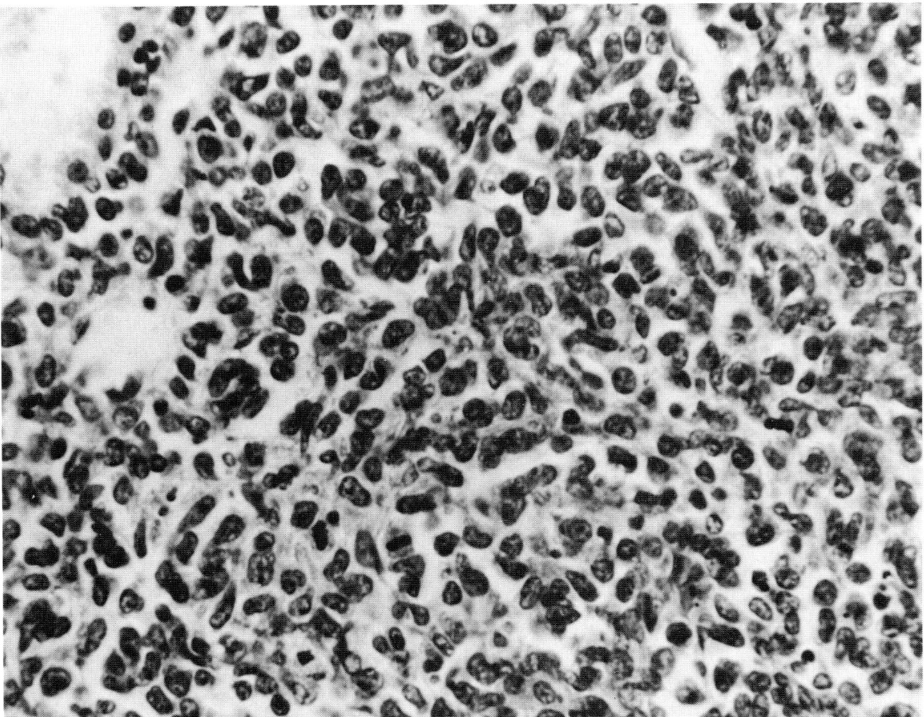

Figure 22-6. Monomorphic infiltrate in malignant lymphoma, poorly differentiated lymphocytic type (H&E stain, ×435).

mortem in the kidneys of 20% of patients with sarcoidosis (54), clinical renal abnormalities are rare in the disease and are most often caused by nephrocalcinosis (55). There are, however, rare reports of acute renal failure caused by diffuse infiltration by sarcoidlike granulomata. In some of these reports, the diagnosis of sarcoidosis was well established (56) but, in others, extrarenal granulomata were either absent or sparse (57). A number of the latter cases may represent systemic or principally renal granulomatous reactions to drugs, such as methicillin (58a), sulfonamides (30), or narcotics (58a), or to other agents. Whatever the cause, granulomatous interstitial nephritis responds rapidly to corticosteroid therapy and does not leave impaired renal function.

Malakoplakia

Malakoplakia is characterized by the accumulation within various tissues, most commonly the urinary bladder, of large mononuclear cells with abundant cytoplasm containing large and laminated phagolysosomes. These phagolysosomes show progressive mineralization to form the characteristic Michaelis-Gutmann bodies. The pathogenesis of these cellular accumulations is unknown, but there is suggestive evidence of a defect in lysosomal function which is correctable with cholinergic antagonists (59). Renal involvement by malakoplakia is rare and usually develops in the context of acute or chronic urinary infection (60) but occa-

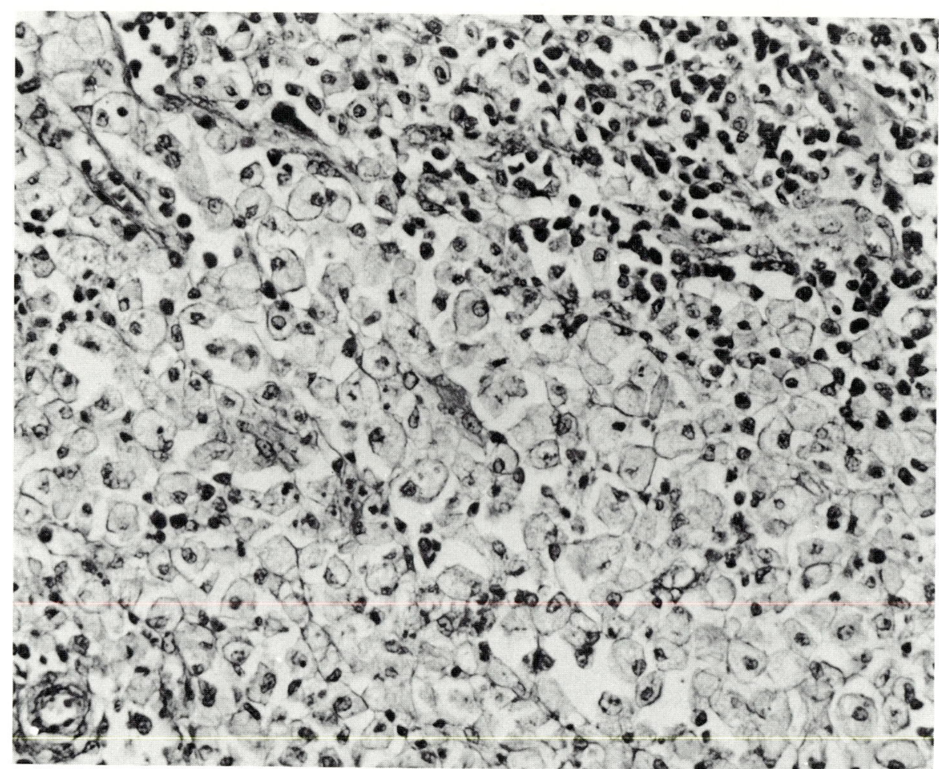

Figure 22-7. Foam cells in xanthogranulomatous interstitial nephritis (H&E stain, ×380).

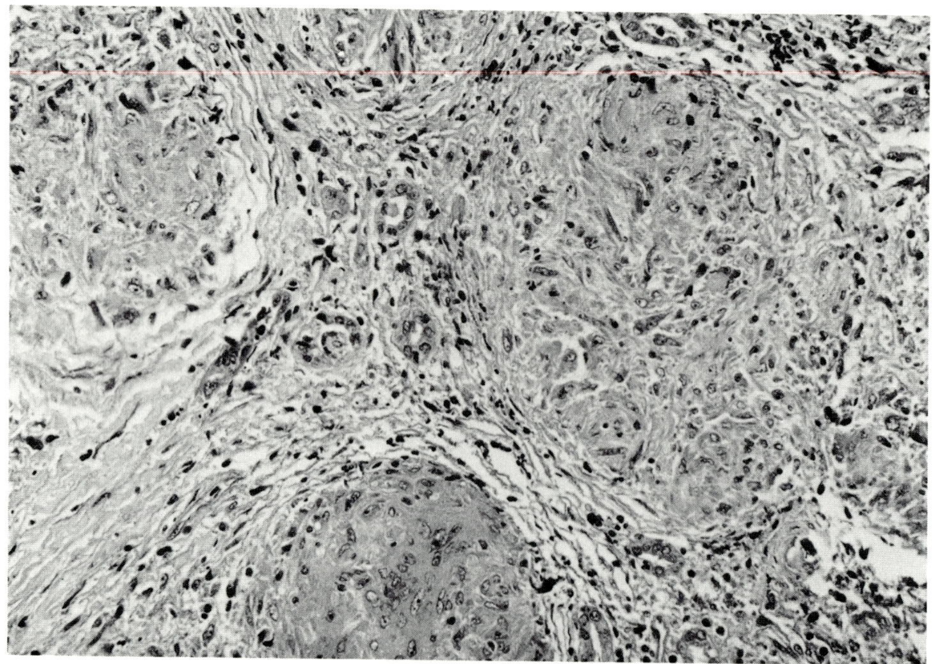

Figure 22-8. Interstitial granulomata in sarcoidosis (H&E stain, ×300).

420

sionally it appears with other manifestations such as nonspecific malaise (61) or a hemolytic-uremic syndrome (62). There have been rare reports of the disease in transplanted kidneys (63). The diagnosis is usually made at nephrectomy or autopsy but has been occasionally established in biopsy tissue (61,62). There is only fragmentary information about the natural history of the disease, but recovery has followed intensive antibiotic therapy (61,62).

Pathologic Characteristics

Sheets of large mononuclear cells separate and replace tubules in either a nodular or diffuse pattern (Figs. 22-9, 22-10). The cells have abundant, granular cytoplasm, and small, regular nuclei. Lesser numbers of mononuclear and polymorphonuclear cells may accompany this infiltrate, and abscesses have been described in some cases. Ultrastructurally, the cells contain large and numerous phagolysosomes with included membranous debris (Fig. 22-11). These bodies show all degrees of mineralization up to the formation of Michaelis-Gutmann bodies, which appear laminated and basophilic by light microscopy (Fig. 22-10). Several cases have been separately characterized, because of the absence of Michaelis-Gutmann bodies by light microscopy, as "megalocytic interstitial nephritis" (64). In fact, however, these bodies may be visible only by electron microscopy in some cases (60), and the separation is not justified.

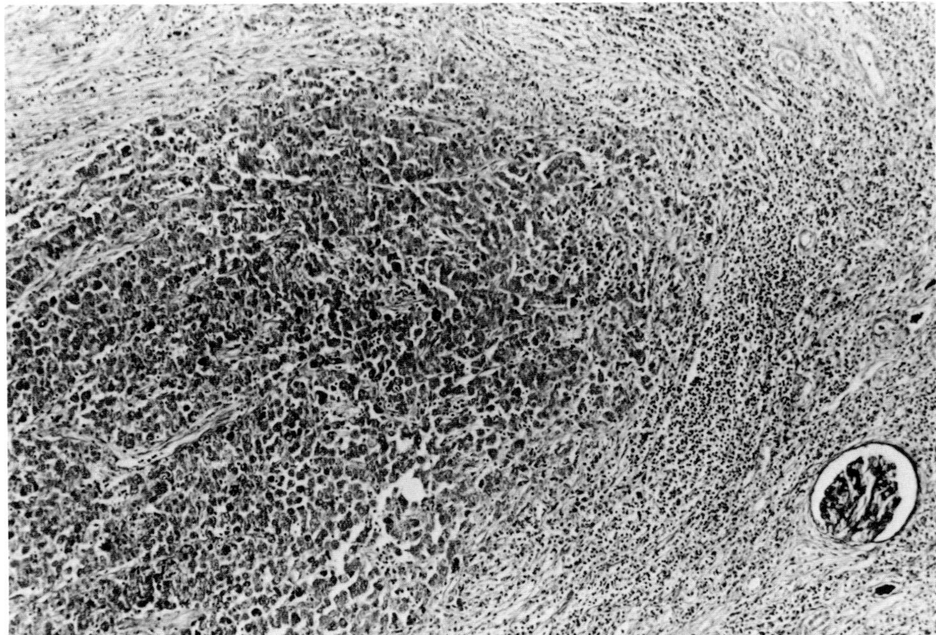

Figure 22-9. Nephrectomy specimen from a patient with malakoplakia. The interstitium is infiltrated by mononuclear cells with abundant cytoplasm accompanied by lymphotytes (PAS stain, ×75).

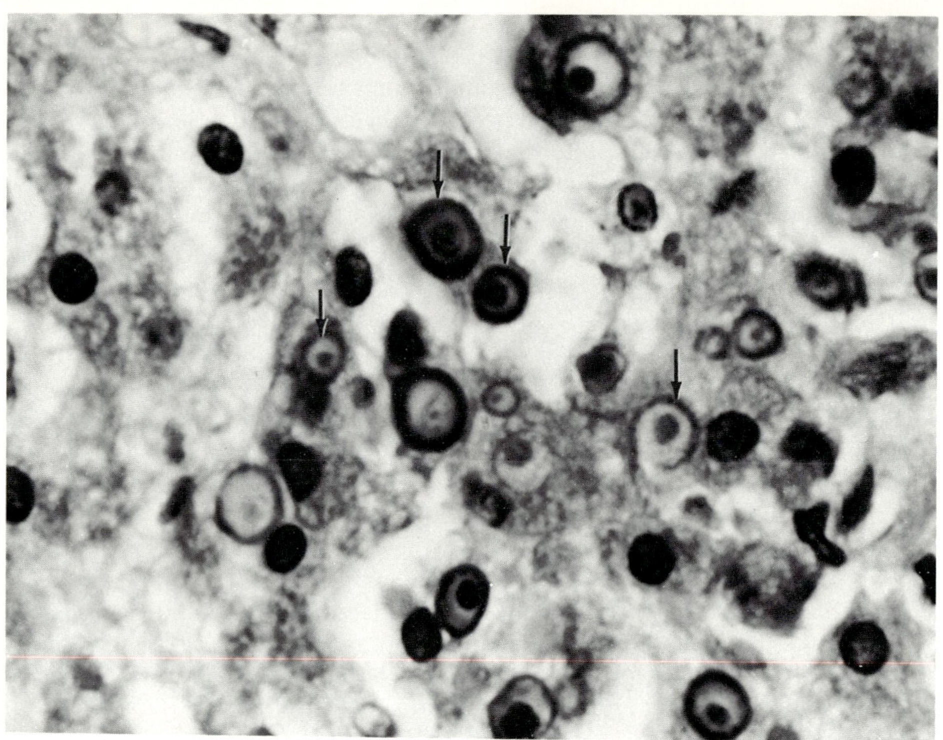

Figure 22-10. Michaelis-Gutmann bodies in macrophages (arrows) (PAS stain, ×970).

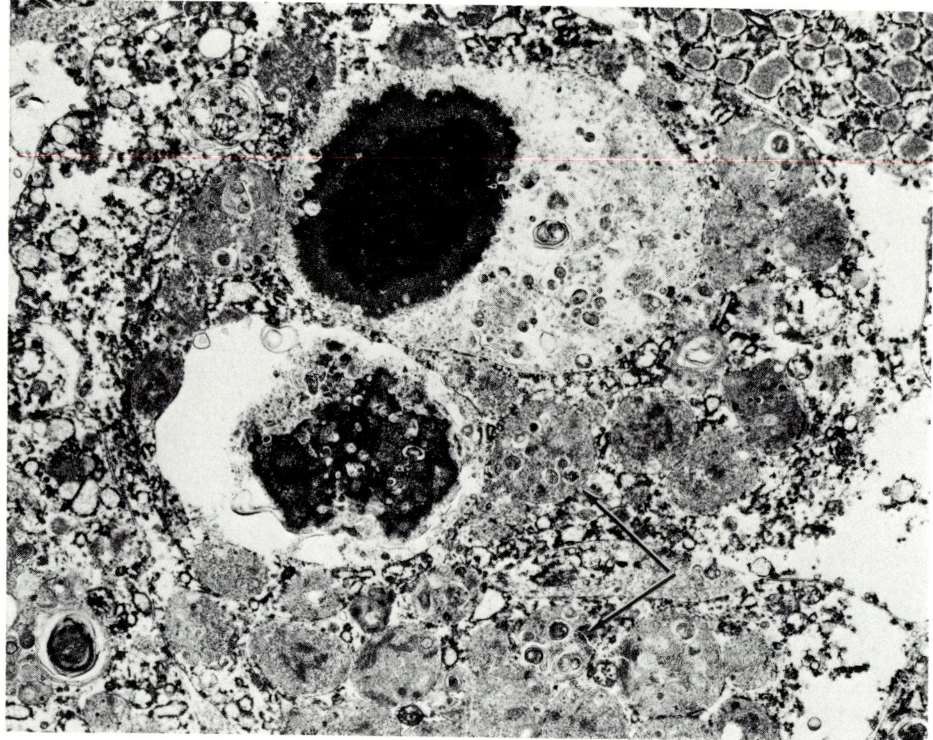

Figure 22-11. Electron micrograph showing numerous phagolysosomes (arrows) and Michaelis-Gutmann bodies with deposits of calcium in the central cores (×6,800).

Mononuclear Interstitial Nephritis with Scarring
(Chronic Interstitial Nephritis)

Renal scarring from any cause is associated with patchy or diffuse mononuclear inflammation (Figs. 22-12, 22-13). The significance of these cells in the scarring process is uncertain since, ultrastructurally, they usually lack the cytoplasmic characteristics of active cells. Occasional renal biopsy specimens taken for tubular syndromes or unexplained azotemia show only this pattern, with no apparent cause. The use of the term *chronic interstitial nephritis* to classify such biopsy tissue is arguable. This term implies a primary and progressive renal disorder with an established natural history. In fact, further studies of patients with this biopsy appearance usually demonstrate a cause for the cortical damage. In one study of 101 patients with "chronic interstitial nephritis," no explanation could be found in only 11 patients (65). The most common primary disorders implicated in this study were anatomic genitourinary abnormalities, analgesic nephropathy, hyperuricemia, nephrosclerosis, and renal calculi. An unqualified diagnosis of "chronic interstitial nephritis" in such cases may, therefore, be actually misleading to the physician managing the patient. With further study, it is likely that syndromes of progressive inflammatory and fibrosing interstitial disease will be defined. The rare examples of apparently primary immune complex and anti-TBM interstitial nephritis have already been discussed, and only occasional other

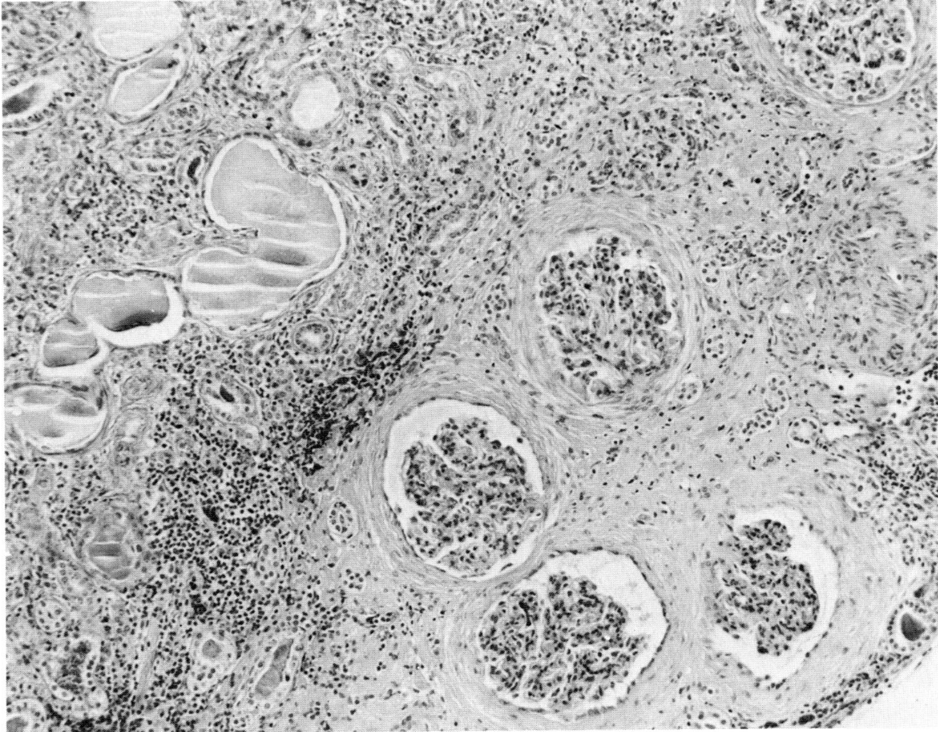

Figure 22-12. Nephrectomy specimen from a patient with obstructive hydronephrosis. There is interstitial scarring with periglomerular fibrosis and mononuclear inflammatory cell infiltration. The tubules are atrophic and contain hyaline casts (H&E stain, × 160).

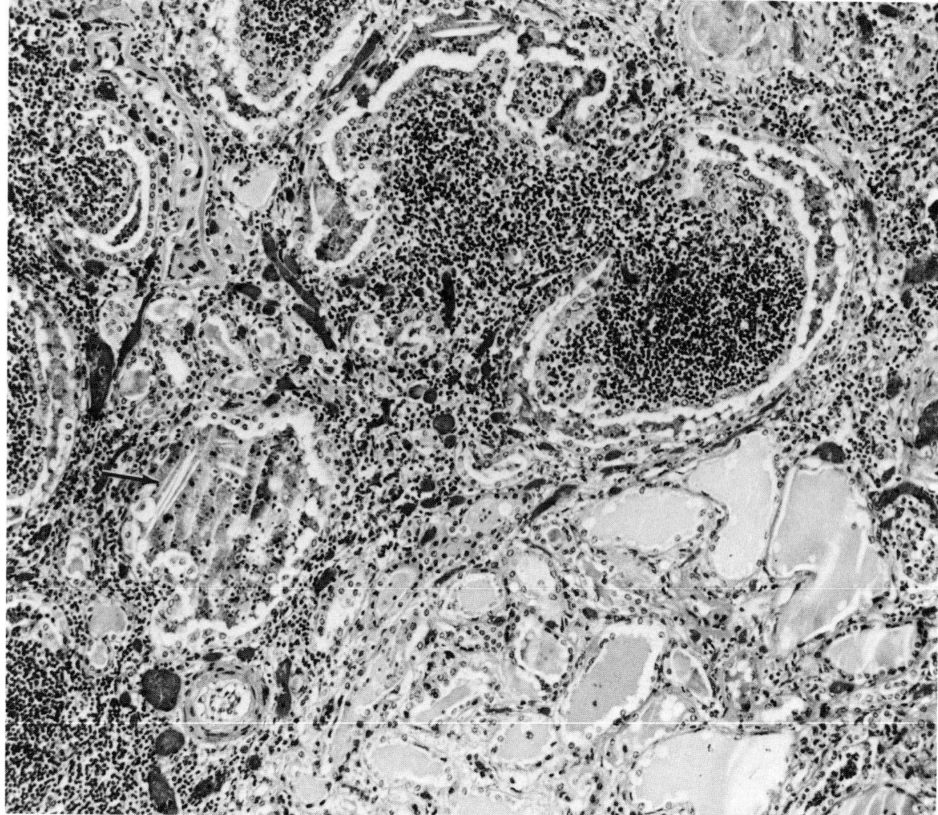

Figure 22-13. Lymphoid follicle formation in a nephrectomy specimen from a patient with renal calculi and recurrent urinary tract infections. The tubules are dilated and contain proteinaceous material or granular casts with cholesterol clefts (arrow) (H&E stain, ×130).

causes for principally cortical disease have been reported (58a). Most often the tubulointerstitial changes will be secondary to diseases in the medulla (such as analgesic nephropathy), in the renal vessels, or in the pelvis or outflow tract, which are not diagnosable from the biopsy tissue. The responsibility of the pathologist is, then, to describe the changes and suggest a differential diagnosis for further investigation. There are, however, two chronic tubulointerstitial syndromes in which the pathologist may suspect the diagnosis even though the appearances are morphologically nonspecific.

Balkan Nephropathy

In several restricted areas of the Danube basin there is a high incidence of progressive renal failure among middle-aged people, especially in women (66). No satisfactory cause has been isolated for either the renal damage or the high incidence of urothelial tumors affecting these patients. Although the morphologic features are nonspecific, the disease may be suspected when middle-aged patients who originally came from endemic areas have azotemia and whose biopsy specimens show cortical atrophy and fibrosis.

Pathologic Characteristics.   There is progressive wasting of tubules occurring symmetrically in each kidney and leaving extensive interstitial fibrosis with residual mummified glomeruli and isolated, hypertrophied nephrons. Interstitial inflammation is rarely conspicuous.

Juvenile Nephronophthisis (Medullary Cystic Disease)

Studies from America (67) and Europe (68) separately described a familial syndrome of progressive renal failure in children and adults characterized by polyuria, salt wasting, and minimal proteinuria. In each study, the principal morphologic abnormality was extensive tubular atrophy, but the additional finding of medullary cysts was given different emphasis by the two groups. Thus the terms *medullary cystic disease* (67) and *juvenile nephronophthisis* (68) have since been applied, although morphologic studies have suggested that the two diseases may be identical (69). In spite of this morphologic identity, genetic analysis indicates the presence of at least two distinct groups within the syndrome (70). One group is manifest in early childhood or adolescence and is inherited as an autosomal recessive, while the other affects young adults and has an autosomal dominant pattern of inheritance. A minority of patients have no family history and may represent new mutations. Aside from the age at presentation and the pattern of inheritance, all groups appear to be clinically and morphologically inseparable. There is, as yet, no uniform nomenclature for the syndrome components, but the use of one accepted diagnostic term, with separation into childhood and adult forms, appears long overdue (71). Of the two terms commonly used, nephronophthisis is more appropriate, since the medullary cysts are variably expressed even in single kindreds (72) and are often not included in biopsy samples. Furthermore, medullary cysts occur in a variety of unrelated renal diseases (73), and the use of terms emphasizing the cystic or spongelike nature of the medulla can only lead to etymologic confusion.

In all forms of the disease, its clinical appearance shows an insidious onset of chronic renal failure, often manifested by complications such as anemia, bone pain, or salt wasting. Investigation reveals a bland urinary sediment with minimal proteinuria, fixed and low specific gravity and, frequently, excessive sodium excretion. Hypertension is often absent. Once established, the disease is relentlessly progressive. Although the possibility of a circulating toxic factor has been suggested to explain the morphologic changes, no such factor has been demonstrated and recurrence in kidney transplants has not been documented (70).

Pathologic Characteristics.   The kidneys are symmetrically reduced in size by wasting (phthisis) of cortical tubules. In biopsy specimens, there is extensive tubular atrophy with coalescence of normal or obsolescent glomeruli, and minimal vascular changes. The typical cysts, which are confined to distal convoluted and collecting tubules (74), are best seen in deep wedge biopsy specimens and are frequently not included in specimens obtained by percutaneous biopsy (Figs. 22-14, 22-15). Small cortical cysts are formed by dilatation of atretic tubules in this and a variety of other chronic renal diseases and should not be mistaken for the cysts of this condition, which are characteristically located around the corticomedullary junction. Although a number of supposedly characteristic light

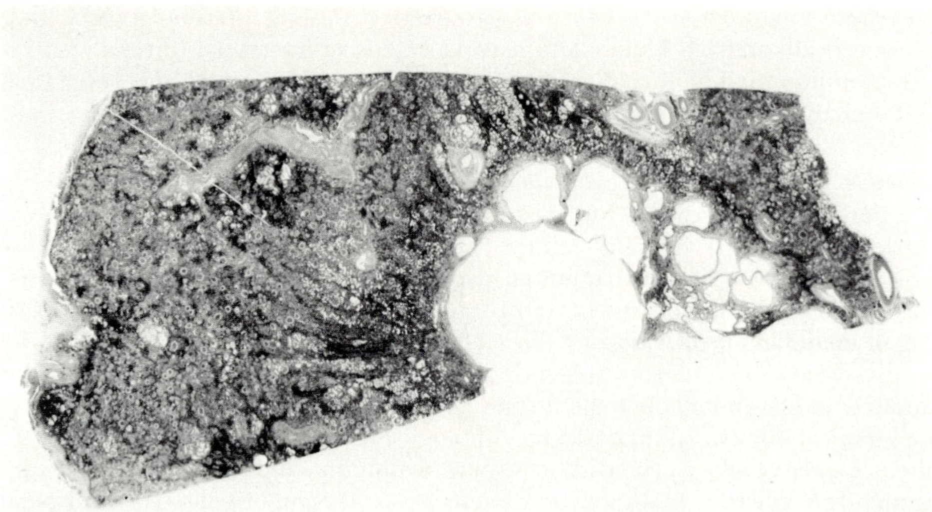

Figure 22-14. Medullary cystic disease (juvenile nephronophthisis). Low-power photograph of a kidney section showing large medullary cysts, dilated tubules in the corticomedullary area, and diffuse interstitial scarring (H&E stain, ×7).

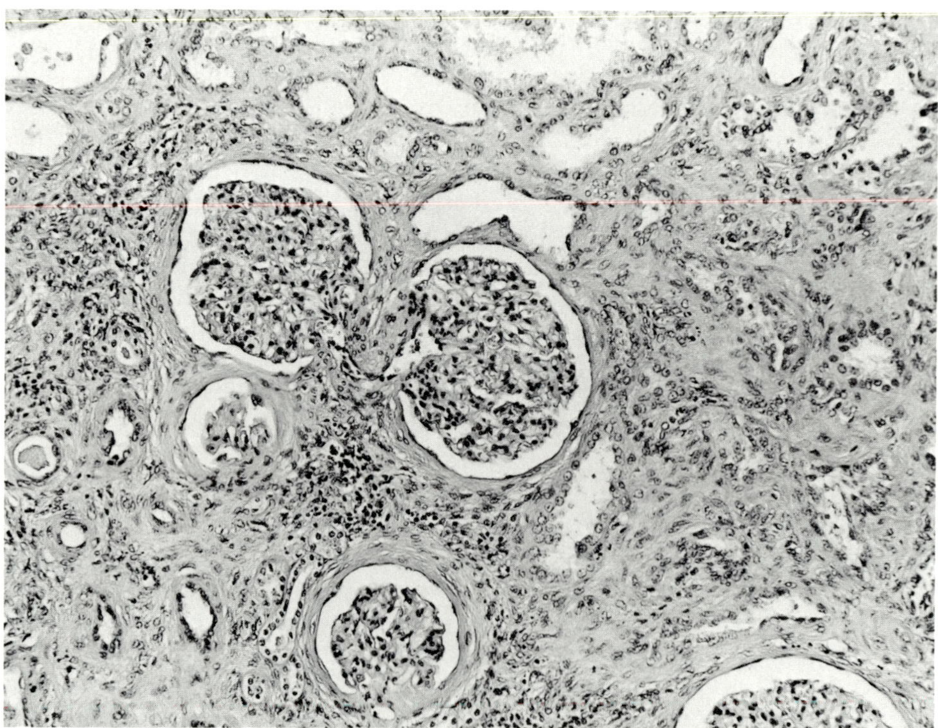

Figure 22-15. Photomicrograph of the cortex from the same case as in Figure 22-14, showing dilated and atrophic tubules, interstitial fibrosis with mononuclear cell infiltration, and periglomerular fibrosis (H&E stain, ×165).

426

(74) and electron microscopic (75) features have been described, the diagnosis rests more upon recognition of the clinicopathologic syndrome than upon specific morphology.

SUMMARY

The renal interstitium may be involved in a variety of inflammatory disorders, some of which are localized principally or entirely in this region. Current knowledge does not allow categorization of these diseases beyond separation by morphologic criteria, and the mechanisms by which inflammation is localized are largely unknown. However, categorization by analysis of the cell types in the inflammatory exudate allows the recognition of a number of apparently distinct disease entities. In the absence of significant scarring, most of these diseases appear to be self-limiting with either specific therapy or removal of the inciting agent. Interstitial changes are important in the determination of renal function and are worthy of notice in assessing renal biopsy specimens in which the glomeruli or blood vessels appear to be principally involved. Further study of the mechanisms by which interstitial changes occur is thus likely to contribute to our understanding of renal pathophysiology.

REFERENCES

1. Risdon RA, Sloper JC, De Wardener HE: Relationship between renal function and histologic changes found in renal biopsy specimens from patients with persistent glomerular nephritis. *Lancet* 2:363, 1968.

2. Bohle A, Grund KE, Mackensen S, et al: Correlations between renal interstitium and level of serum creatinine: morphometric investigations of biopsies in perimembranous glomerulonephritis. *Virchows Arch A Path Anat Histol* 373:15, 1977.

3. Schainuck LE, Striker GE, Cutler RE, et al: Structural-functional correlations in renal disease. II. The Correlations. *Human Pathol* 1:631, 1970.

4. Lehmann DH, Wilson CB, Dixon FJ: Extraglomerular immunoglobulin deposits in human nephritis. *Am J Med* 58:765, 1975.

5. Andres GA, McCluskey RT: Tubular and interstitial renal disease due to immunologic mechanisms. *Kidney Int* 7:271, 1975.

6. McCluskey RT, Colvin RB: Immunologic aspects of renal tubular and interstitial diseases. *Ann Rev Med* 29:191, 1978.

7. Andres G, Brentjens J, Kohli R, et al: Histology of human tubulo-interstitial nephritis associated with antibodies to renal basement membranes. *Kidney Int* 13:480, 1978.

7a. Mancilla-Jiminez R, Katzenstein, A-LA, Heritier F, et al: Antitubular basement membrane antibodies in renal allograft rejection. *Transplantation* 24:39, 1977.

8. Bergstein J, Litman N: Interstitial nephritis with anti-tubular-basement-membrane antibody. *N Engl J Med* 292:875, 1975.

9. Greenhill AH, Norman EM, Cornfeld J, et al: Acute renal failure secondary to acute pyelonephritis. *Clin Nephrol* 8:400, 1977.

10. Lyons H, Pinn VW, Cortell S, et al: Allergic interstitial nephritis causing reversible renal failure in four patients with idiopathic nephrotic syndrome. *N Engl J Med* 288:124, 1973.

11. Heptinstall RH: Interstitial nephritis: A brief review. *Am J Pathol* 83:214, 1976.

12. Jensen HA, Halveg AB, Saunamaki KI: Permanent impairment of renal function after methicillin nephropathy. *Br Med J* 4:406, 1971.

13. Woodroffe AJ, Thomson NM, Meadows R, et al: Nephropathy associated with methicillin administration. *Aust NZ J Med* 4:256, 1974.

14. Sheth KJ, Casper JT, Good TA: Interstitial nephritis due to phenytoin sensitivity. *J Pediat* 91:438, 1977.

15. Ooi BS, First MR, Pesce AJ, et al: IgE levels in interstitial nephritis. *Lancet* 1:1254, 1974.

16. Faarup P, Christensen E: IgE-containing plasma cells in acute tubulo-interstitial nephropathy. *Lancet* 2:718, 1974.

17. Dobrin RS, Vernier RL, Fish AJ: Acute eosinophilic interstitial nephritis and renal failure with bone marrow-lymph node granulomas and anterior uveitis: a new syndrome. *Am J Med* 59:325, 1975.

18. Baldwin DS, Levine BB, McCluskey RT, et al: Renal failure and interstitial nephritis due to penicillin and methicillin. *N Engl J Med* 279:1245, 1968.

19. Appel GB, Neu HC: The nephrotoxicity of antibiotics (first of three parts). *N Engl J Med* 296:663, 1977.

20. Medley CR, McKenzie PE, Dunn DE, et al: Cloxacillin-induced acute interstitial nephritis. *Aust NZ J Med*, in press.

21. Robson M, Levi J, Dolberg L, et al: Acute tubulointerstitial nephritis following sulfadiazine therapy. *Israel J Med Sci* 6:561, 1970.

22. Case records of the Massachusetts General Hospital. *N Engl J Med* 293:1308, 1975.

23. Ramgopal Y, Edward C, Bhathena D: Acute renal failure associated with rifampicin. *Lancet* 1:1195, 1973.

23a. Walker RG, Thomson NM, Dowling JP, et al: Minocycline-induced acute interstitial nephritis. *Br Med J* 1:524, 1979.

24. Gelbert DR, Weinstein AB, Fajardo LF: Allopurinol-induced interstitial nephritis. *Ann Int Med* 86:196, 1977.

25. Sloth K, Thomsen AC: Acute renal insufficiency during treatment with azathioprine. *Acta Med Scand* 189:145, 1971.

26. Ortino J, Botella J: Recurrent acute renal failure induced by phenazone sensitivity. *Lancet* 2:1473, 1973.

27. Smith K: Acute renal failure in phenindione sensitivity. *Br Med J* 2:24, 1965.

28. Russell GE, Bing RF, Walls J, et al: Interstitial nephritis in a case of phenylbutazone sensitivity. *Br Med J* 2:1322, 1978.

29. Schrier RW, Bulger RJ, Vanarsdel PP: Nephropathy associated with penicillin and homologues. *Ann Int Med* 64:116, 1966.

30. More RH, McMillan GL, Duff GL: The pathology of sulfonamide allergy in man. *Am J Pathol* 22:702, 1946.

31. Councilman WT: Acute interstitial nephritis. *J Exp Med* 3:393, 1898.

32. Kannerstein M: Histologic kidney changes in the common acute infectious diseases. *Am J Med Sci* 205:65, 1942.

33. Meuhrcke RC: *Acute Renal Failure: Diagnosis and Management.* St Louis, C V Mosby Co, 1969.

34. Case records of the Massachusetts General Hospital. *N Engl J Med* 298:1014, 1978.

35. Guignard JP, Torrado A: Interstitial nephritis and toxoplasmosis in a 10-year-old child. *J Pediat* 85:381, 1974.

36. Lee S, Kjellstrand CM: Renal disease in infectious mononucleosis. *Clin Nephrol* 9:236, 1978.

37. Sitprija V, Evan S: The kidney in human Leptospirosis. *Am J Med* 49:780, 1970.

38. Levinsky NG: Pathophysiology of acute renal failure. *N Engl J Med* 296:1453, 1977.

39. Oken DE: Local mechanisms in the pathogenesis of acute renal failure. *Kidney Int* 10(Suppl 6):S94, 1976.

40. Olsen S: Renal histopathology in various forms of acute anuria in man. *Kidney Int* 10(Suppl 6):S2, 1976.

41. Brentjens JR, Sepulveda M, Baliah T, et al: Interstitial immune complex nephritis in patients with systemic lupus erythematosus. *Kidney Int* 7:342, 1975.

42. Case records of the Massachusetts General Hospital. *N Engl J Med* 294:100, 1976.

43. Richmond J, Sherman RS, Diamond HD, et al: Renal lesions associated with malignant lymphomas. *Am J Med* 32:184, 1962.

44. Schwarze E-W: Pathoanatomical features of the kidney in myelomonocytic and chronic lymphocytic leukemia. *Virchows Arch A Path Anat Histol* 368:243, 1975.

45. Kanfer A, Vandewalle A, Morel-Maroger L, et al: Acute renal insufficiency due to lymphomatous infiltration of the kidneys. *Cancer* 38:2588, 1976.

46. Siegel MB, Alexander L, Weintraub L, et al: Renal failure in Burkitt's lymphoma. *Clin Nephrol* 7:279, 1977.

47. Grossman ME, Bia MJ, Goldwein MI, et al: Giant kidneys in Waldenström's macroglobulinemia. *Arch Intern Med* 137:1613, 1977.

48. Lundberg WB, Cadman ED, Finch SC, et al: Renal failure secondary to leukemic infiltration of the kidneys. *Am J Med* 62:636, 1977.

49. Talal N, Zisman E, Schnur PH: Renal tubular acidosis, glomerulonephritis and immunologic factors in Sjögren's syndrome. Arthritis Rheum 11:774, 1968.

50. Mason AMS, Golding PL: Hyperglobulinaemic renal tubular acidosis: a report of nine cases. *Br Med J* 3:143, 1970.

51. Ford PM: A naturally occurring human antibody to loops of Henle. *Clin Exp Immunol* 14:569, 1973.

52. Cochrane AMG, Tsantoulos DC, Moussouros A, et al: Lymphocyte cytotoxicity for kidney cells in renal tubular acidosis of autoimmune liver disease. *Br Med J* 2:276, 1976.

53. Bennington JL, Beckwith JB: Tumors of the kidney, renal pelvis and ureter, in *Atlas of Tumor Pathology, Armed Forces Institute of Pathology*, second series, fascicle 12, 1975, p 163.

54. Longcope WT, Frieman DG: A study of sarcoidosis: based on a combined investigation of 160 cases including 30 autopsies from the Johns Hopkins Hospital and Massachusetts General Hospital. *Medicine (Balt)* 31:1, 1952.

55. Lofgren S, Snellman B, Lindgren AGH: Renal complications in sarcoidosis: functional and biopsy studies. *Acta Med Scand* 159:295, 1957.

56. Turner MC, Shin ML, Ruley RJ: Renal failure as a presenting sign of diffuse sarcoidosis in an adolescent girl. *Am J Dis Child* 131:997, 1977.

57. King B, Esparza AR, Kahn SI, et al: Sarcoid granulomatous nephritis occurring as isolated renal failure. *Arch Intern Med* 136:241, 1976.

58. Mayaud C, Kanfer A, Kourlsky O, et al: Interstitial nephritis after methicillin. *N Engl J Med* 292:1132, 1975.

58a. Steinmuller DR, Bolton K, Stilmant MM, et al: Chronic interstitial nephritis and mixed cryoglobulinemia associated with drug abuse. *Arch Pathol Lab Med* 103:63, 1979.

59. Abdou NI, Napombejara C, Sagawa A, et al: Malakoplakia: evidence for monocyte lysosomal abnormality correctable by cholinergic agonist in vitro and in vivo. *N Engl J Med* 297:1413, 1977.

60. Bowers JH, Cathey WJ: Malakoplakia of the kidney with renal failure. *Am J Clin Pathol* 55:765, 1971.

61. Galla JH, Bhathena D: Malakoplakia of the kidney: apparent improvement following medical management. *Clin Nephrol* 9:35, 1978.

62. Hill J W, Seedat YK: The diagnosis of malakoplakia of the kidney by percutaneous renal biopsy. *S Afr Med J* 46:953, 1972.

63. Osborn DE, Castro JE, Ansell ID: Malakoplakia in a cadaver renal allograft: a case study. Human Pathol 8:341, 1977.

64. Ravel R: Magalocytic interstitial nephritis. *Am J Clin Pathol* 47:781, 1967.

65. Murray T, Goldberg M: Chronic interstitial nephritis: etiologic factors. *Ann Int Med* 82:453, 1975.

66. Hall PW III, Dammin GJ: Balkan nephropathy. *Nephron* 22:281, 1978.

67. Smith CA, Graham JB: Congenital medullary cysts of the kidney with severe refractory anemia. *Am J Dis Child* 69:369, 1945.

68. Fanconi G, Hanhart E, Von Albertini A, et al: Die familiäre junvenile nephronophthise. *Helo Paediat Acta* 6:1, 1951.

69. Mongeau JG, Worthen HG: Nephronophthisis and medullary cystic disease. *Am J Med* 43:345, 1967.

70. Gardner KD: Evolution of clinical signs in adult-onset cystic disease of the renal medulla. *Ann Intern Med* 74:47, 1971.

71. van Collenburg JJM, Thompson MW, Huber J: Clinical, pathological and genetic aspects of a form of cystic disease of the renal medulla: familial juvenile nephronophthisis (FJN). *Clin Nephrol* 9:55, 1978.

72. Coles GA, Robinson K, Branch RA: Familial interstitial nephritis. *Clin Nephrol* 6:513, 1976.

73. Spence HM, Singleton R: What is sponge kidney disease and where does it fit in the spectrum of cystic disorders? *J Urol* 63:37, 1971.

74. Sherman FE, Studnicki FM, Fetterman GH: Renal lesions of familial juvenile nephronophthisis examined by microdissection. *Am J Clin Pathol* 55:391, 1971.

75. Collan Y, Sipponen P, Haapanen E, et al: Hereditary nephronophthisis with a life span of three decades: light and electron microscopical, immunohistochemical, clinical and family studies. *Virchows Arch A Path Anat Histol* 376:195, 1977.

23
Transplantation

To the patient with chronic renal failure, a functioning transplanted kidney means freedom from the rigors of dialysis and fluid restriction. To the physician, the procedure means continued access to long-term dialysis for other patients with progressive kidney damage. Transplantation and long-term dialysis are, therefore, mutually contributory in the management of end-stage renal disease. This was not always so. The early results of transplantation were so disastrous that its routine use seemed an impossible dream (1). Yet within only 30 years, the procedure has become a standard and relatively safe component of nephrology. This remarkable change occurred less because of dramatic advances in technology than as a result of improved methods for the selection and the treatment of rejection (2). With the increasing success of transplantation, the use of the procedure has spread from highly specialized units to most large medical centers. This move has brought the general pathologist into intimate contact with the transplant team, for renal biopsy is an important tool in the diagnosis of declining graft function. This chapter provides a brief and practical approach to the interpretation of morphologic changes that occur in rejection and in other conditions that may impair graft performance (Table 23-1).

Table 23-1. Morphologic Changes in Failing Transplanted Kidneys

Rejection
  Hyperacute
  Acute:
    cellular, vascular
  Chronic:
    vascular, transplant glomerulopathy

Perfusion nephropathy

Glomerulonephritis and other disease
  Recurrent
  De novo

Acute medical and surgical complications

REJECTION

The major cause of graft failure is rejection of the foreign tissue by defense mechanisms of the host. A variety of interrelated systems are involved in rejection, and interpretation of the morphologic changes requires some knowledge of these systems (3,4).

Pathogenesis and Classification

Early experimental studies of rejection revealed progressive graft failure with massive mononuclear inflammatory cell infiltration. The rejection process was noted to be accentuated with increasing genetic differences between donor and recipient and accelerated in second grafts between the same animals or species. These studies convinced early workers that cellular mechanisms were predominant in rejection and that humoral factors played a minor role. Experience with human transplantation has modified this interpretation. There is now clear evidence of several distinct, but often coexisting, patterns of humoral and cellular patterns of rejection (Table 23-1). In either humoral or cellular rejection, two major groups of tissue antigens are the principal determinants of immune activity. The ABO and other blood group antigens, which are expressed on endothelial as well as erythrocyte membranes, are absolute barriers to engraftment. Grafts from people with different ABO characteristics from those of the recipient encounter circulating antibodies, which attach to the endothelium and cause immediate (hyperacute) rejection. The other major group of antigens is the HLA system, a series of polypeptides that are expressed on endothelial membranes and are controlled by several closely related loci on the sixth chromosome (5,6). Occasionally, presensitization of recipients to HLA antigens may evoke the formation of antibodies in sufficient concentration to cause hyperacute rejection similar to that occurring with ABO incompatibility. More commonly, a complex mixture of cellular and humoral mechanisms produces less dramatic patterns of rejection.

After anastomosis, the graft provokes an immune reaction by a series of afferent stimuli to both B and T lymphocytes. The recipient is sensitized by a variety of mechanisms, which include the passage of recipient lymphocytes through the graft and the release of donor antigens into the circulation either directly, as a result of ischemic cell damage, or via leukocytes trapped in the graft circulation during the procedure. Recognition of these antigens by macrophages in lymphoid tissue leads to the production of one or more clones of sensitized T cells. These cells are specifically localized in the graft and cause damage by an efferent series of highly complex and interrelated pathogenetic mechanisms. Briefly, different subpopulations of sensitized T cells are capable of direct cytotoxic damage to donor cells, recruitment of nonsensitized cells to cause similar damage, and the release of a variety of factors that augment the rejection reaction. These factors increase vascular permeability, attract macrophages and other inflammatory cells, stimulate lymphocyte proliferation, and activate the coagulation and complement systems. Since the sensitized lymphocytes reach the graft via the circulation, the changes of acute cellular rejection are maximal in and around the rich peritubular circulation. Simultaneously, T lymphocytes transmit antigenic information to B cells which, in turn, produce specific antibodies against the graft. Antibodies are produced in lymph nodes and by plasma cells within the graft, and, by attaching to donor antigens to form immune complexes, cause further damage by activating complement, coagulation, and other mechanisms.

The process of acute graft rejection is, therefore, extraordinarily complex. Crude subdivisions can, however, be made into predominantly cellular or vascular patterns. The cellular pattern of rejection is predominantly mediated by T lymphocytes and occurs around the peritubular capillary circulation with secondary damage to other structures. The vascular pattern may involve direct cellular damage, but is principally caused by antibody reaction with vascular endothelium. Clearly, the mechanisms of these two patterns are so interlinked that they frequently coexist in the same patient, but either may be predominant, and recognition of the major form of rejection is of considerable prognostic importance. Acute rejection is now effectively controlled in most patients by immunosuppression. This control may, however, lapse for a variety of reasons, and the morphologic features of acute rejection may suddenly appear months or even years after engraftment. Alternatively, further patterns of chronic rejection may cause destruction of the graft. Chronic rejection is characterized by prolonged and repeated endothelial damage, almost certainly by humoral mechanisms, which causes profound intimal thickening of arteries in the graft. This vascular pattern is often accompanied by striking mesangial hypertrophy, possibly caused by persistent phagocytosis of coagulation products, producing a highly characteristic pattern of chronic glomerular rejection or glomerulopathy.

The risk of rejection correlates directly with the degree of genetic dissimilarity between donor and recipient. Hence, the most favorable results can be expected from grafts between identical twins (isografts). Few patients with end-stage renal disease are fortunate enough to have an identical twin and most transplants must be between individuals showing some genetic differences (allografts). These differences can be minimized by careful matching of HLA and ABO systems, but there are probably a variety of other as yet unrecognized antigen systems, and a perfect allograft match is not possible. The chances of identity are, clearly, greater among members of a single family than between unrelated people, and the risks of rejection are, therefore, greater in unrelated and cadaver grafts than in grafts from related donors. Careful matching of HLA and ABO antigens is now routine before transplantation and is accompanied by a variety of cross-matching techniques to detect circulating antibodies in the recipient to donor antigens (5–7).

Pathologic Characteristics

Rejection affects all components of the kidney. Significant changes occur in the renal capsule, ureter, and major vessels, but this discussion includes only the lesions occurring in the cortex, since these are the major features seen in renal biopsy specimens. Recent detailed reviews of the renal and systemic effects of rejection may be consulted for further information (8–10).

HYPERACUTE REJECTION

Prompt and permanent rejection may occur within minutes or hours of revascularization. Urine flow is either never established or ceases abruptly and the diagnosis may be apparent to the surgeon by the sudden appearance of mottling, cyanosis, and diminished turgor of the graft (11). Hyperacute rejection more often affects second or subsequent rather than initial grafts in the same person, and its incidence has been reduced, but not abolished, by routine cross matching between donor and recipient. The reaction is produced by the interaction of circulating antibodies in the recipient with antigens on donor endothelial cells. The appearances, therefore, differ according to the stage at which the biopsy specimen is taken. Initially, linear immunofluorescence reactions for IgG, followed by C3, occur along glomerular and interstitial capillaries. As local immune complexes are formed, complement activation attracts polymorphs, and the combined cytotoxic effects cause endothelial swelling, vacuolation, and lysis, with exposure of underlying basement membranes. The accumulation of polymorphs in the glomerular and interstitial capillaries of biopsy specimens taken soon after revascularization has been regarded as a sign of impending vascular rejection (12), but is of little prognostic value in grafts preserved by pulsatile perfusion (see below). Endothelial changes are followed by platelet and fibrin thrombi, which are initially focal but become progressively more extensive and propagate to occlude major vessels (Figs. 23-1–23-5). The process is irregular, so that some glomerular and interstitial capillaries appear engorged while others are occluded by thrombi. Intense vasospasm is a significant component of hyperacute rejection and may secondarily cause foci of vacuolation and necrosis in muscular vessels. The changes rapidly culminate in irreversible damage with extensive hemorrhage and focal or confluent cortical necrosis, but at no stage is there a significant interstitial inflammatory infiltrate.

ACUTE REJECTION

Episodes of acute rejection usually occur within the first six weeks after transplantation but may develop at any time during the course of the graft. The episodes are characterized by the insidious or acute onset of oliguria, azotemia, fever, proteinuria, and painful swelling of the graft (13,14).

Acute Cellular Rejection

The pattern is that of a severe, acute, interstitial nephritis (Fig. 23-6). There is intense interstitial edema with congestion of peritubular capillaries and a predominantly mononuclear inflammatory infiltrate (Fig. 23-7). Inflammation is initially focal, in and around peritubular capillaries, but later becomes coalescent to form masses of cells that penetrate tubules and destroy tubular cells. The infiltrate is at first composed of immunoblasts but becomes progressively diluted as rejection proceeds by small and large lymphocytes, macrophages, and plasma cells (15). Eosinophils and polymorphs may be present in small numbers but, if conspicuous, raise the possibility of other disease. Inflammation may involve

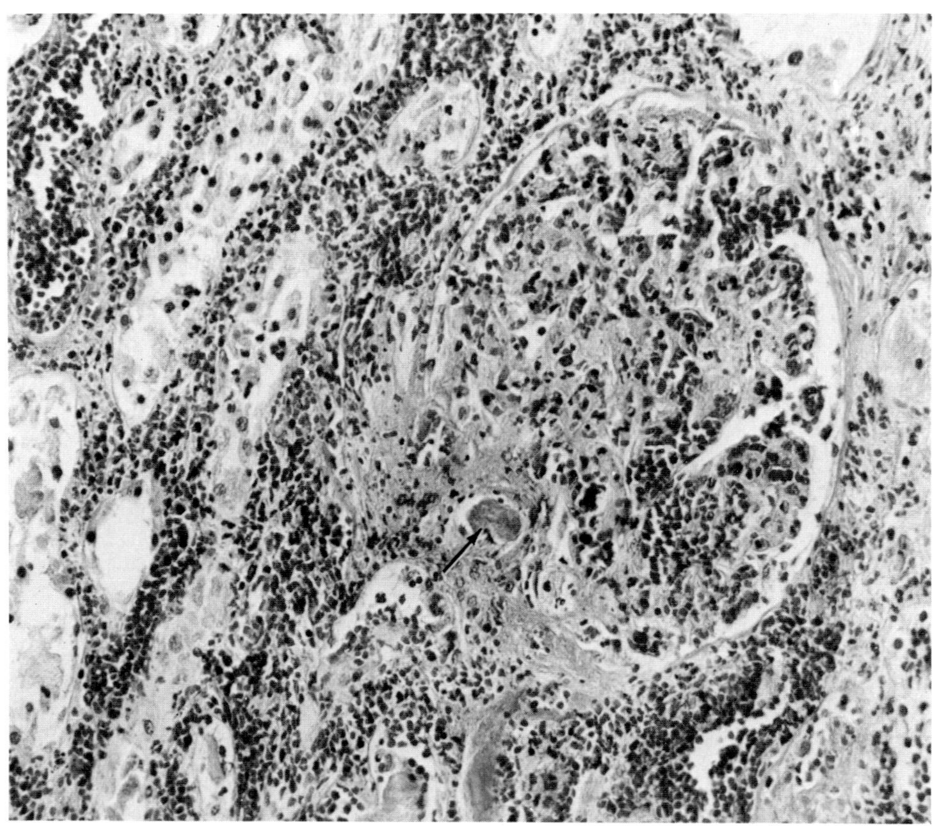

Figure 23-1. Hyperacute rejection 48 hours posttransplant. There is massive interstitial and glomerular inflammatory infiltration by polymorphonuclear leukocytes and blood stasis. The afferent arteriole is thrombosed (arrow) (H&E stain, ×240).

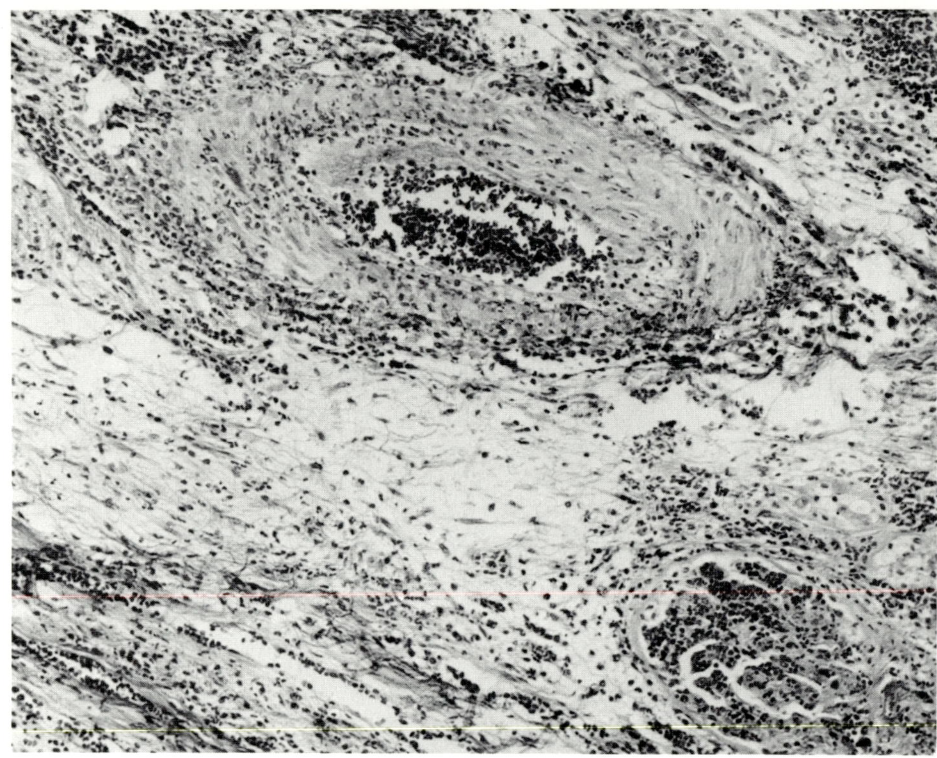

Figure 23-2. Hyperacute rejection. Same case as in Figure 23-1, showing marked interstitial edema and polymorphonuclear infiltration of the arterial wall (H&E stain, ×380).

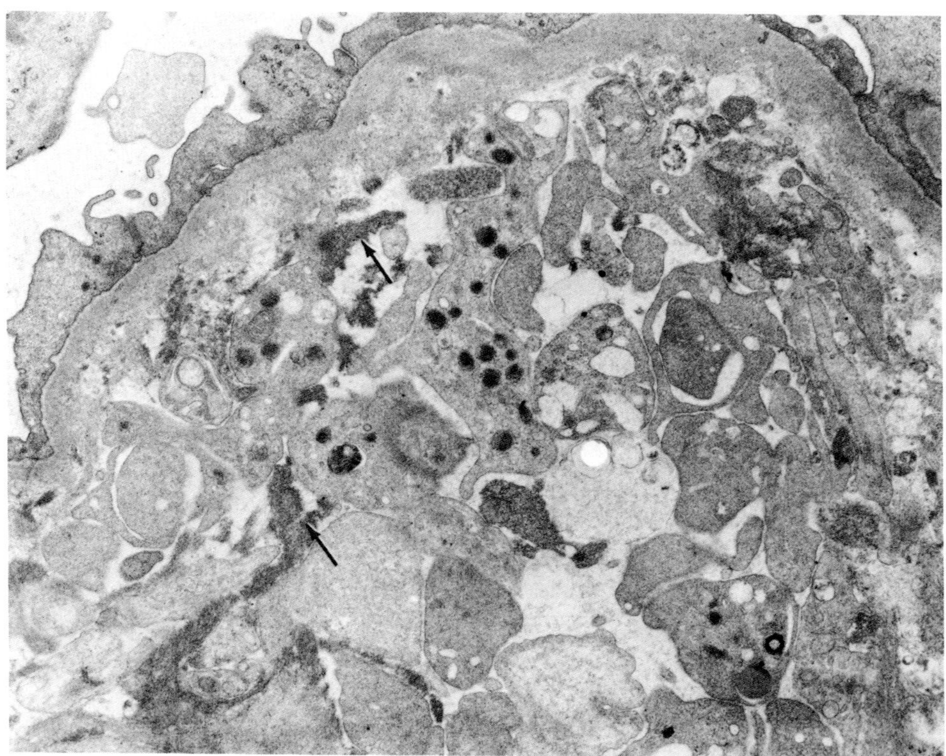

Figure 23-3. Electron micrograph in hyperacute rejection showing occlusion of the capillary loop by fibrin (arrows) and degradulated platelets. There is endothelial denudation of the basement membrane, and the foot processes are swollen and extensively obliterated, (×11,500).

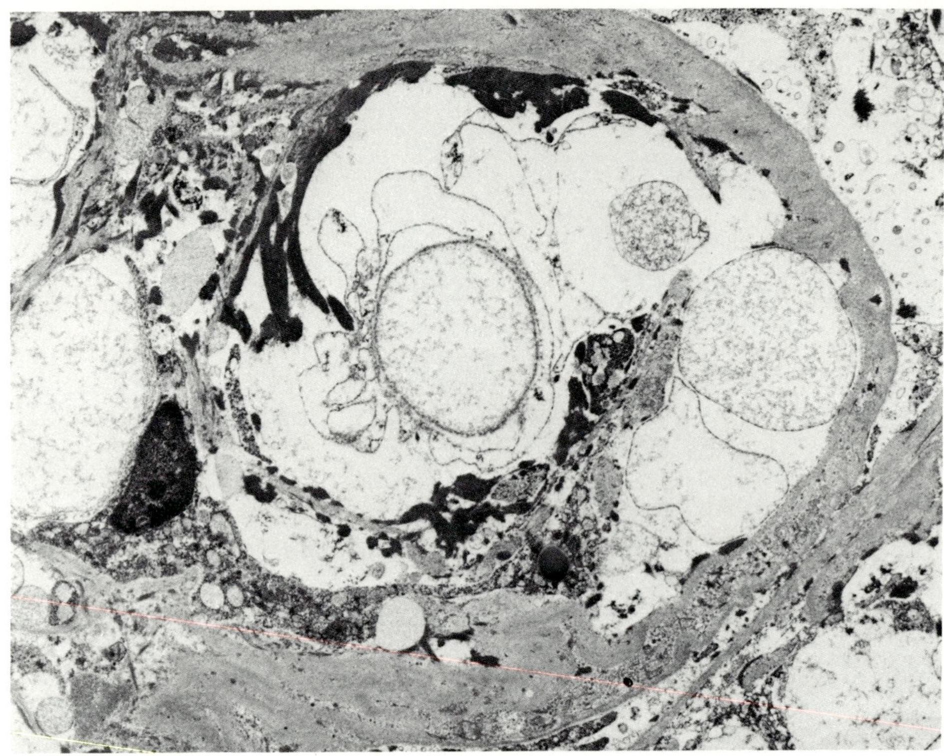

Figure 23-4. Advanced hyperacute rejection. The loop is necrotic and appears denuded of epithelial and endothelial lining. The lumen contains fibrin and cellular debris (×8,500).

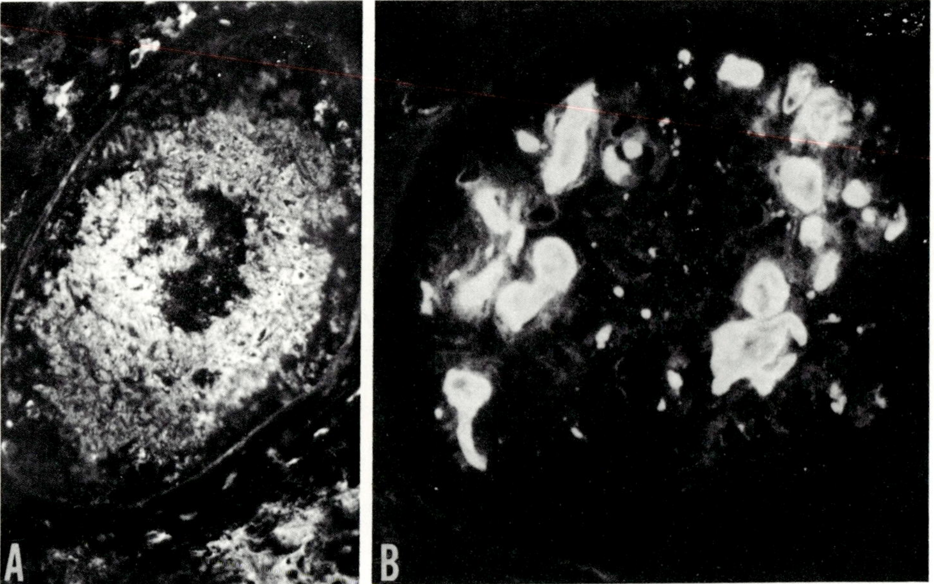

Figure 23-5. Immunofluorescent preparation demonstrating (*a*) vascular and (*b*) glomerular thrombosis in hyperacute rejection (antihuman fibrinogen, ×315).

438

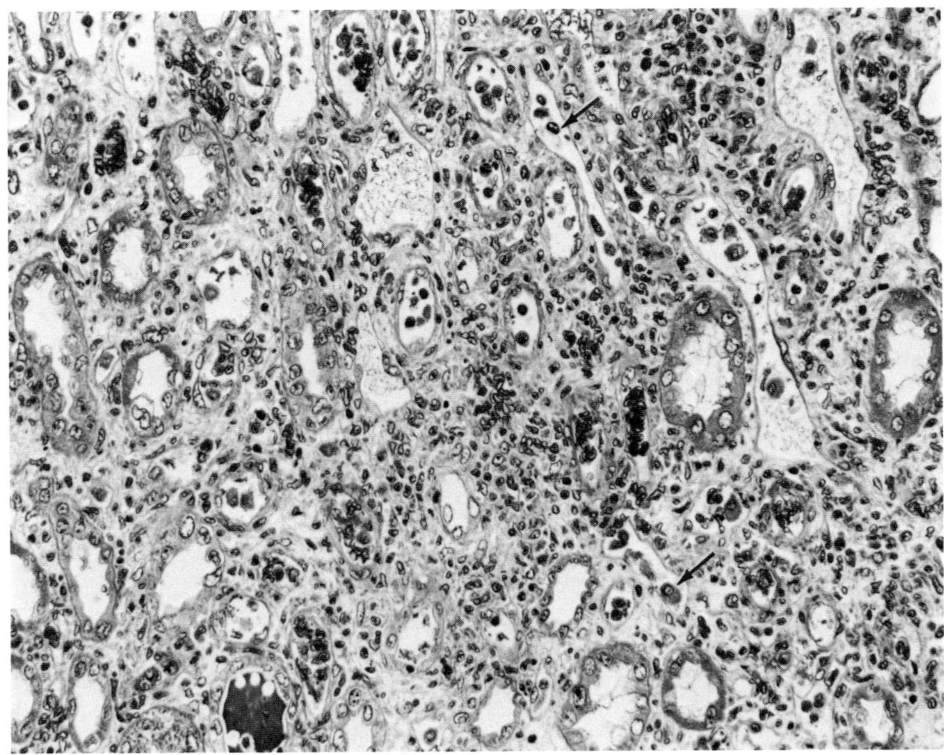

Figure 23-6. Acute interstitial rejection. Masses of predominantly immunoblasts and large lymphocytes are present in the interstitium, around the tubules and in dilated peritubular capillaries (arrows) (H&E stain, ×260).

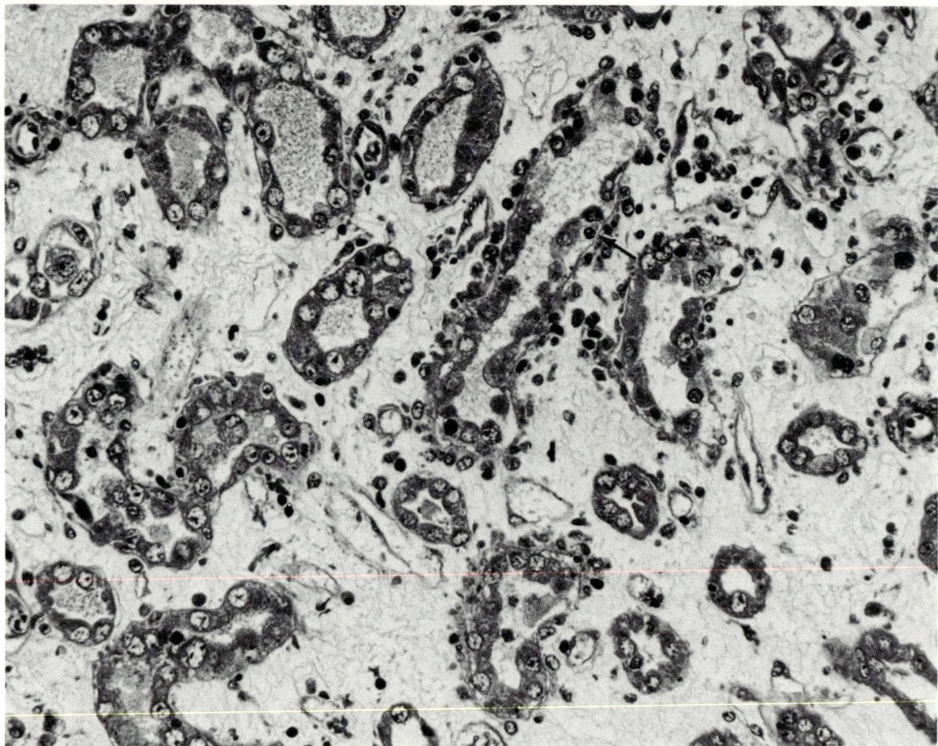

Figure 23-7. Marked interstitial edema in acute interstitial rejection. Some tubules show focal necrosis with detachment of epithelial cells (middle and right). In addition, there is peritubular mononuclear inflammatory infiltrate and dilatation of interstitial capillaries. Some inflammatory cells are located between the epithelial cells and tubular basement membrane (arrow) (H&E stain, ×300).

blood vessels other than capillaries, but significant vascular lesions are usually the result of coincident vascular rejection. Immunofluorescence studies in isolated cellular rejection are usually negative, aside from reactions for fibrin in affected vessels and for immunoglobulins in inflammatory cells.

Acute Vascular Rejection

The most severe changes occur in small arteries, veins, and arterioles, but glomerular, tubular, and interstitial damage is often prominent (16–18) (Figs. 23-8–23-12). The earliest sign of acute vascular rejection is swelling and vacuolation of endothelial cells with areas of ulceration. This is usually associated with intimal infiltration by mononuclear inflammatory cells and by changes in the media. Individual smooth muscle cells show vacuolation, caused by dilatation of smooth endoplasmic reticulum, or condensation and necrosis, producing areas of increased eosinophilia. The intimal changes can be complicated by either thrombosis or intimal proliferation. Thrombi are often small and nonocclusive but, in those cases progressing to irreversible rejection, they become obliterative and widespread with necrosis of vessel walls. Occasionally, a pattern of acute necrotiz-

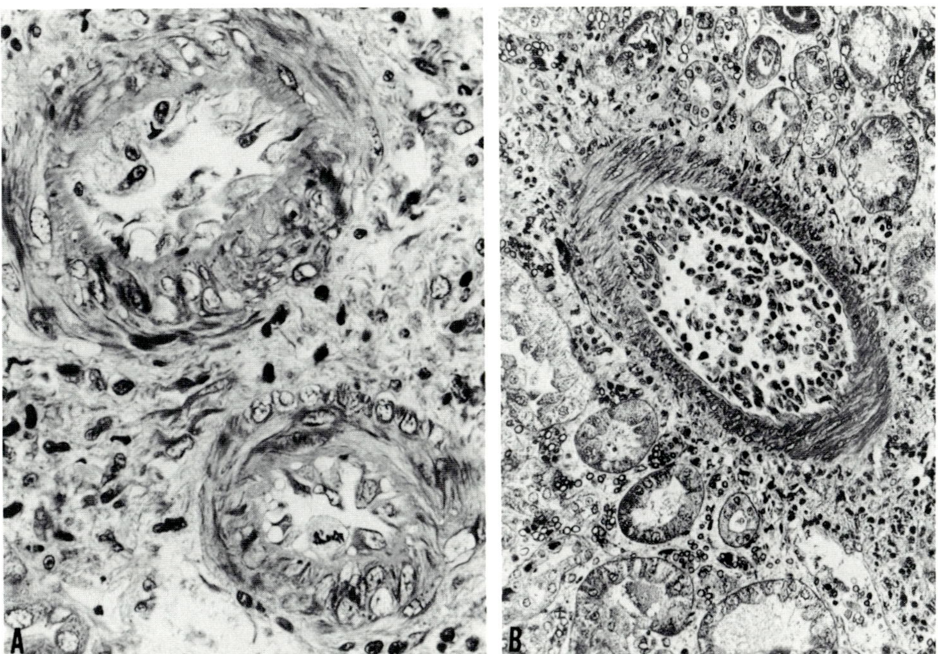

Figure 23-8. Acute vascular rejection. (*a*) The endothelial cells are swollen and vacuolated. The vascular lumina are narrowed by early intimal proliferation. Note a mitotic figure in the lower artery. (*b*) The arterial intima is detached by extensive cellular infiltrate consisting mainly of immunoblasts (H&E stain, ×260).

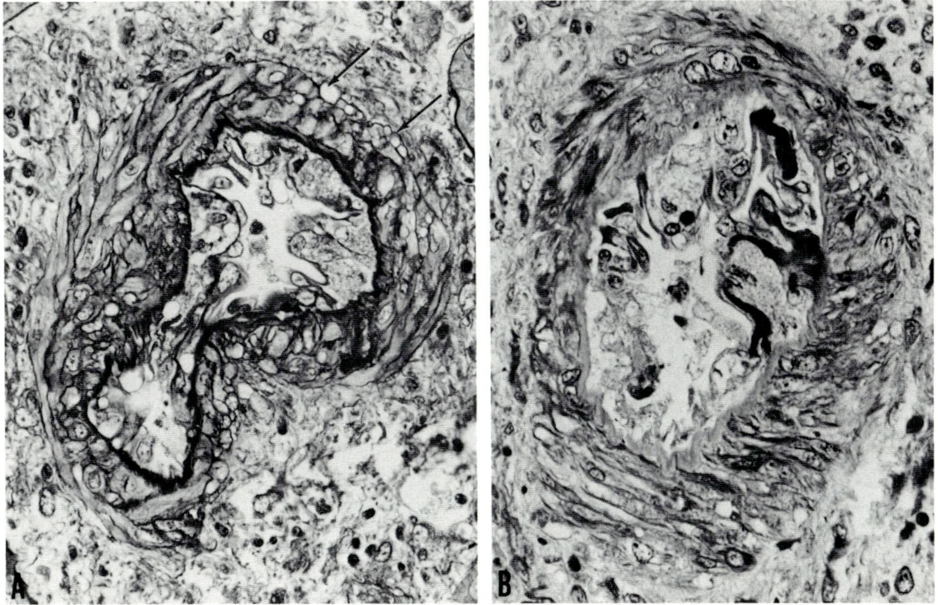

Figure 23-9. Same case as in Figure 23-8. (*a*) In addition to endothelial swelling, there is marked vacuolization of smooth muscle cells (arrows). (*b*) The intima is focally detached and degenerated (left). The darker material in contact with the endothelium represents fibrin, which appears mostly located beneath the intima (right) (H&E stain, ×465).

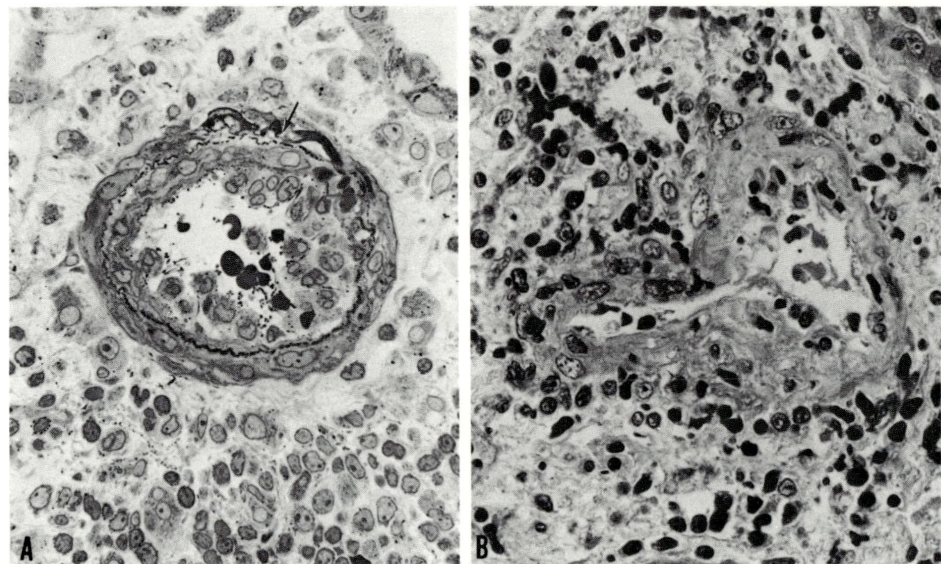

Figure 23-10. Acute vascular rejection (*a*) Small artery showing focal degeneration of the media (arrow). The intima appears infiltrated by inflammatory cells. The lumen is narrowed and contains a few strands of fibrin. The interstitium is edematous and infiltrated by mononuclear cells. (*b*) The media is focally necrotic and infiltrated by mononuclear inflammatory cells (*a*, toluidine blue stain, ×300; *b*, H&E stain, ×365).

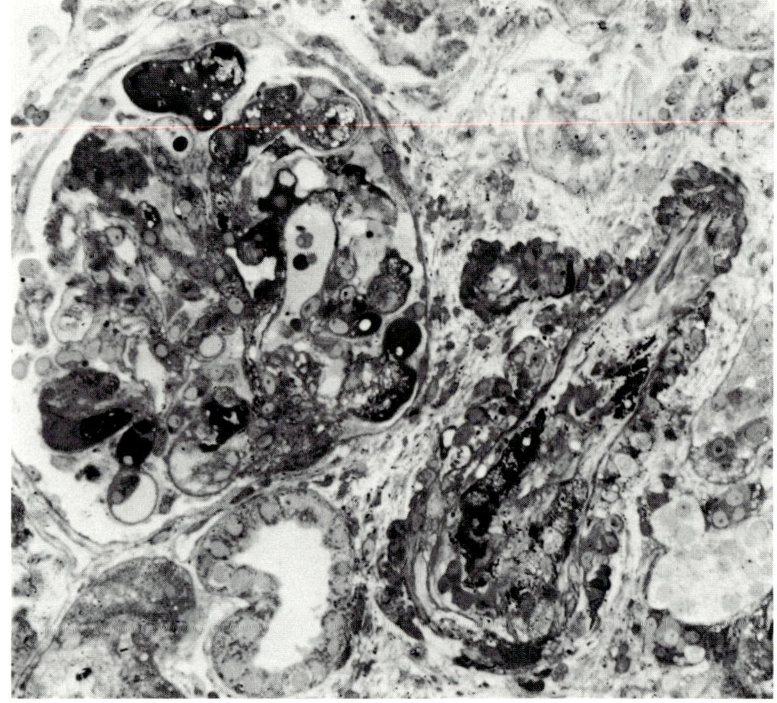

Figure 23-11. Thrombosis of the afferent arteriole and glomerular capillaries in acute vascular rejection (toluidine blue stain, ×325).

442

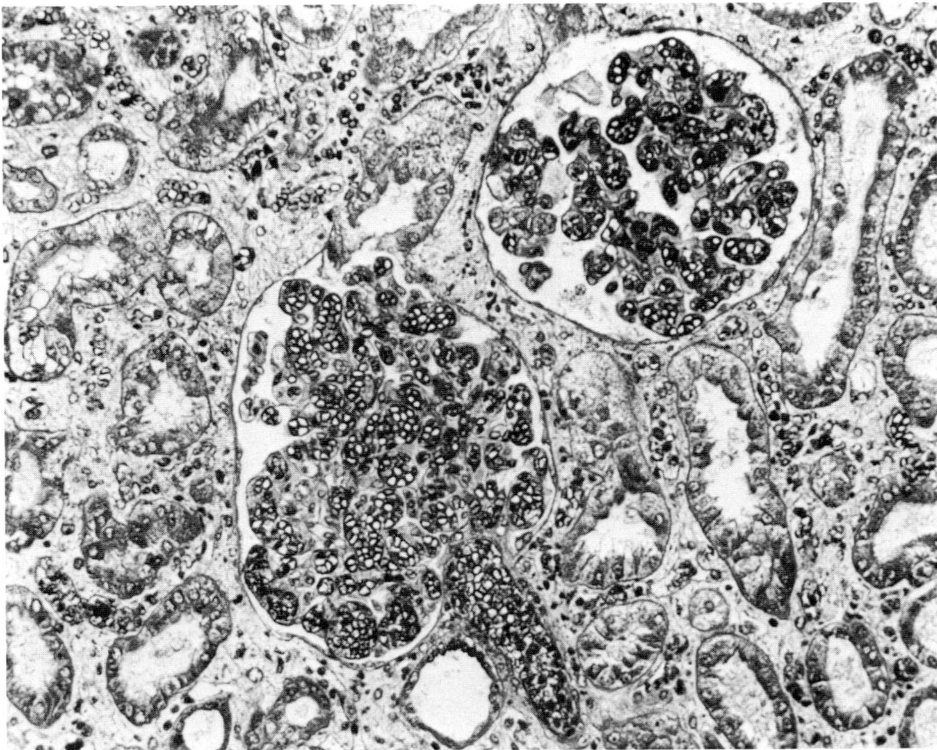

Figure 23-12. Biopsy of a case of acute vascular transplant rejection showing severe blood stasis in glomerular capillary loops and peritubular capillaries. The interstitium is edematous and the tubular epithelium shows early necrosis (H&E stain, ×300).

ing vasculitis may be seen. Probably by the incorporation of platelets and other thrombotic components, foam cells appear in the intima and are accompanied by progressive intimal fibrosis. Initially, this intimal change is mucoid and sparsely cellular, but progressive collagenization produces a fibrous collar that reduces the lumen and may obliterate the elastic lamina. Uncontrolled progression of these changes causes cortical necrosis, which may be associated with microangiopathic hemolytic anemia (19,20).

The vascular changes are associated with extensive interstitial edema, focal hemorrhage, and glomerular changes, but cellular infiltration is often inconspicuous. The glomeruli may show only ischemic collapse, but frequently are affected by endothelial and mesangial swelling, which can appear proliferative and resemble glomerulonephritis (21,22). Advancing vascular damage is associated with global or segmental occlusion by fibrin or platelet thrombi, effacement of capillary walls and, in some cases, crescents. Ultrastructurally, there is irregular vacuolation and hypertrophy of endothelial and mesangial cells with varying degrees of thrombosis and infiltration by mononuclear inflammatory cells (Fig. 23-13). The endothelium is separated from the basement membrane by patchy, lucent widening of the lamina rara interna, but no dense deposits can be seen. Immunofluorescence studies may be negative but usually show reactions

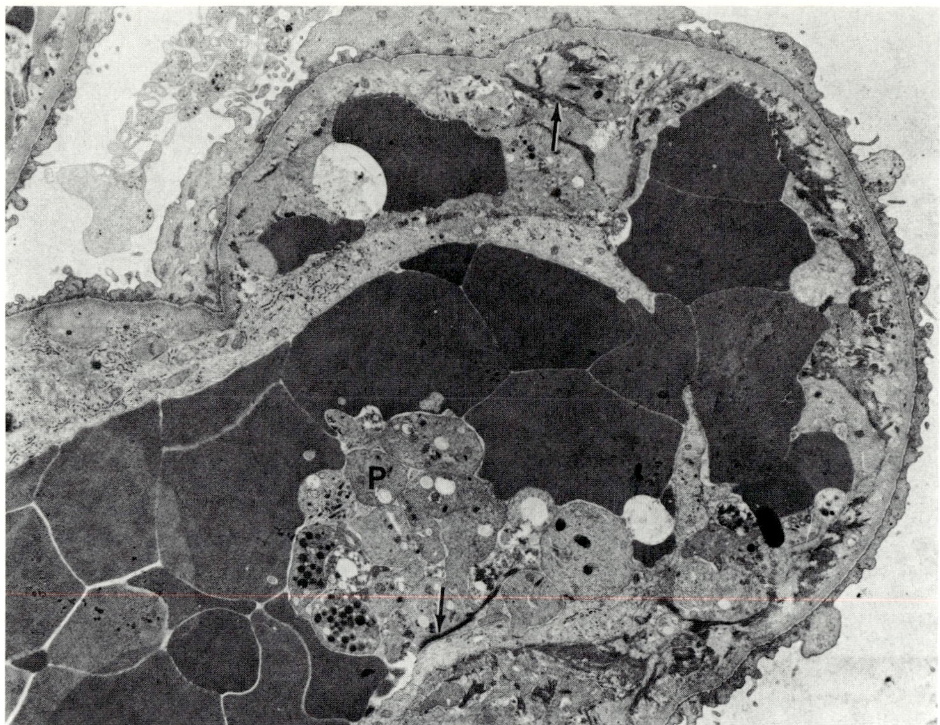

Figure 23-13. Acute vascular transplant rejection. Same case as in Figure 23-12. Severe blood stasis in glomerular capillary loop, which also contains numerous degranulated platelets (P) and fibrin (arrows). The foot processes are obliterated (×5,500).

along arterial walls, interstitial capillaries and in glomeruli for fibrin and complement, with or without IgG and IgM (Fig. 23-14). The glomerular reactions may be either granular or in an irregularly distributed linear pattern, and occur both in mesangia and along capillary walls.

CHRONIC REJECTION

Gradual deterioration in function occurs in up to a quarter of grafts surviving for more than one year (23). This deterioration may be preceded by proteinuria, sometimes with the nephrotic syndrome (24), and is usually associated with hypertension. The process may begin as early as two months after transplantation or be delayed for up to two years but, once initiated, is irreversible. Chronic rejection may take either of two morphologic patterns, although these are frequently combined. The first form resembles the late stage of acute vascular rejection, and presumably develops by similar mechanisms, while the second requires differentiation from glomerulonephritis. In both forms there is extensive tubulointerstitial scarring, but inflammatory infiltration is sparse and cellular mechanisms appear to play a minor role. The hypertension which is so common in chronic rejection has been related to increased renin production,

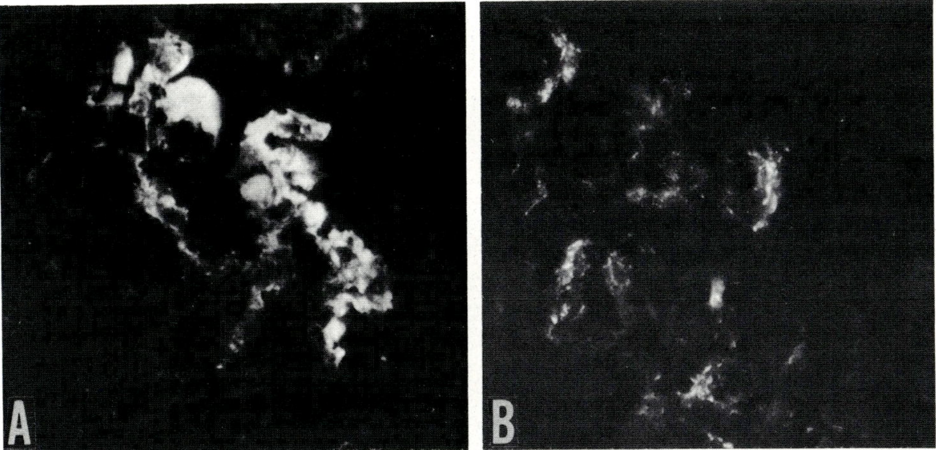

Figure 23-14. Moderate irregular granular fluorescent deposits of (*a*) IgG and (*b*) C3 in mesangium and capillary loops in acute vascular allograft rejection (×330).

and hyperplasia of the juxtaglomerular apparatus is often a prominent feature in these biopsies (25).

Chronic Vascular Rejection

The vascular changes are similar in kind to those of acute rejection but affect a wider spectrum of vessels, ranging from arterioles to the main renal artery (17,18,26). There is obliterative intimal thickening of variable type and distribution. Mucoid widening of the intima may be seen, but the usual pattern is of dense, collagenous stenosis with interruption or duplication of the elastic lamina and, often, irregular fibrosis of the media (Figs. 23-15, 23-16). Sparse mononuclear inflammatory cells are often dispersed through the intimal cushion and foam cells may be frequent. On the surface, small thrombi in various stages of organization can often be detected. Vascular involvement is irregular and almost normal vessels may coexist with others showing profound fibrous or mucoid intimal stenosis. Electron microscopy of the abnormal intima shows only abundant collagen with interspersed fibroblasts, myofibroblasts, and smooth muscle cells. Immunofluorescence microscopy usually demonstrates intimal reactions for IgM and C3, with less constant staining for fibrin and IgG (Figs. 23-17–23-19).

Transplant Glomerulopathy

Some biopsy specimens with chronic vascular rejection show only patchy ischemic glomerular collapse, whereas others demonstrate a striking glomerular lesion (Fig. 23-20). This lesion may also occur in the absence of vascular changes and typically involves glomeruli in an irregular pattern with areas of segmental scarring (15,22,26,27) (Fig. 23-21). Transplant glomerulopathy is unrelated to the original disease of the recipient, but occurs more frequently in grafts that are poorly matched or subject to vesicoureteric reflux (23,28). Affected glomeruli

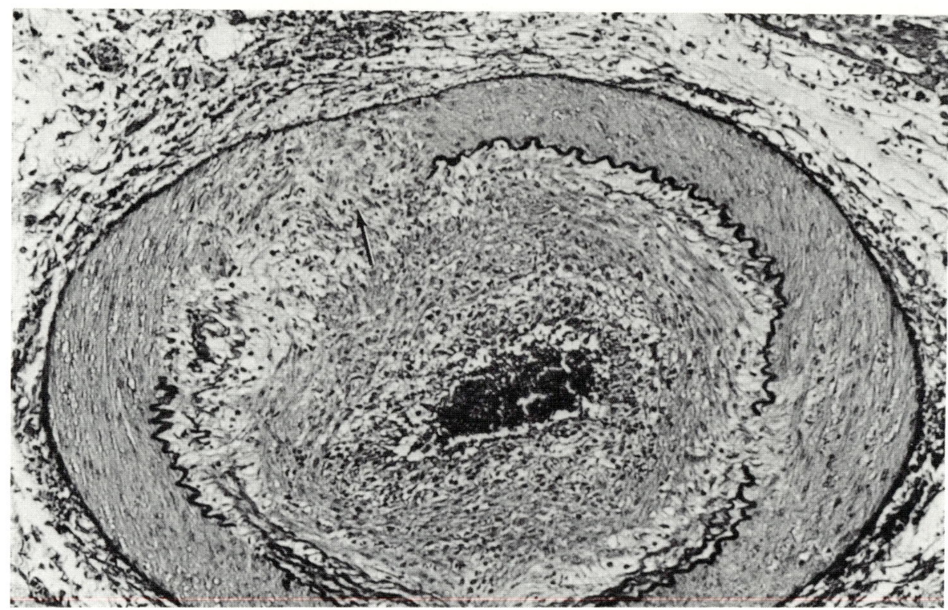

Figure 23-15. Chronic vascular rejection. The internal elastic lamina of the arcuate artery is partially split with patchy destruction (arrow). The vascular lumen is severely narrowed by fibrointimal proliferation (elastic Van Gieson stain, ×85).

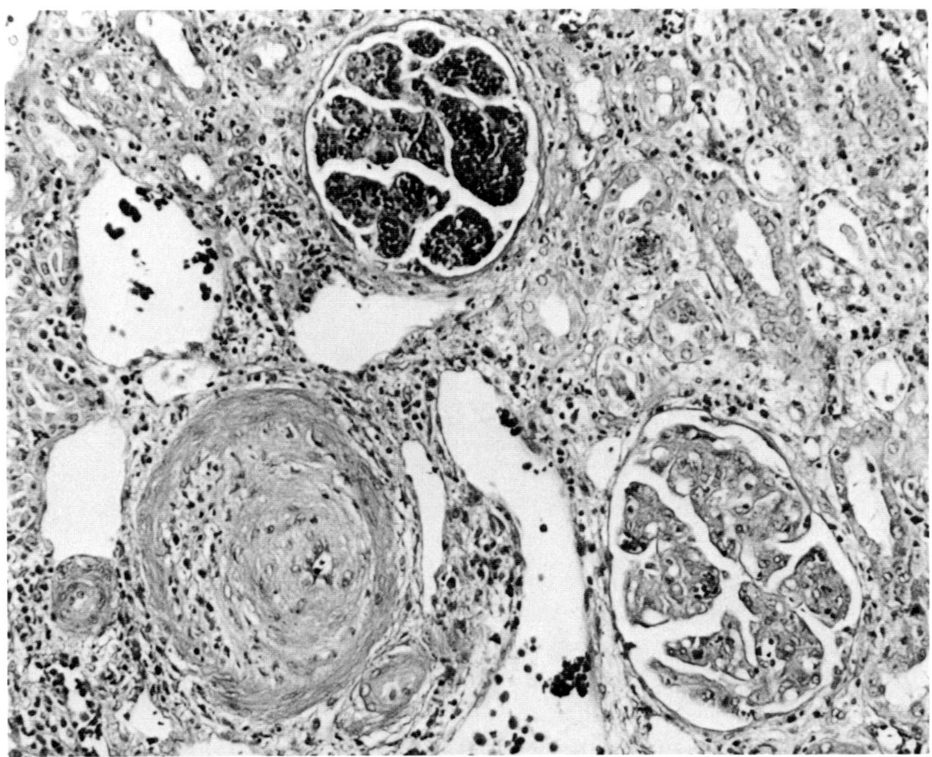

Figure 23-16. Interlobular artery showing severe fibrointimal proliferation with mononuclear inflammatory cell infiltration and narrowing of the vascular lumen. The upper glomerulus is acutely infarcted and the interstitium appears scarred and infiltrated by mononuclear cells (H&E stain, ×180).

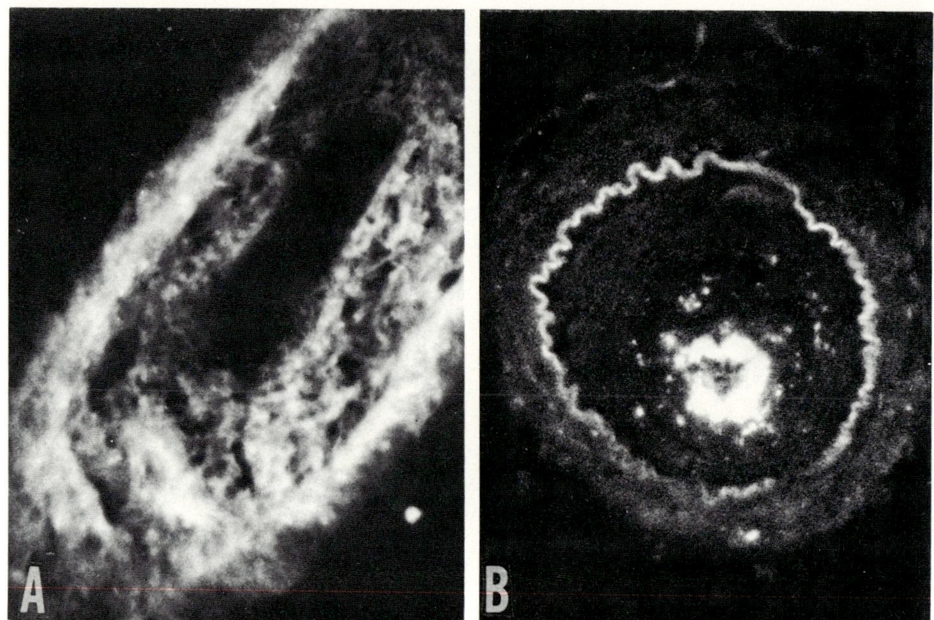

Figure 23-17. Fluorescent deposits of (*a*) fibringen and (*b*) C3 in chronic transplant vasculopathy (×400).

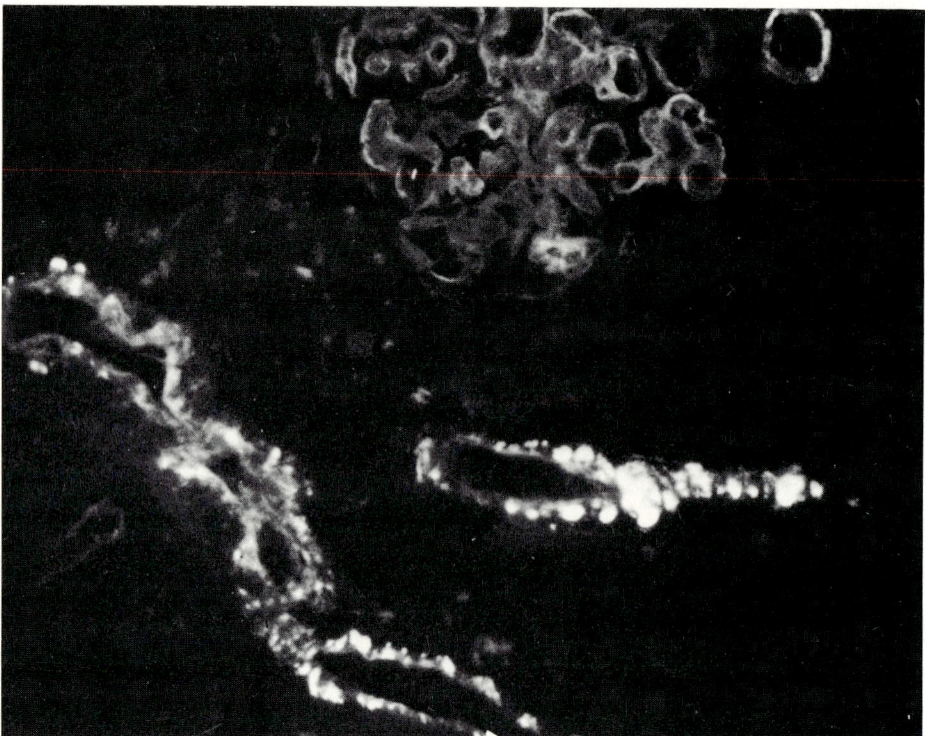

Figure 23-18. Chronic allograft rejection. The glomerular arterioles show granular deposits of C3, while linear staining is present along the glomerular capillary loops, (×225).

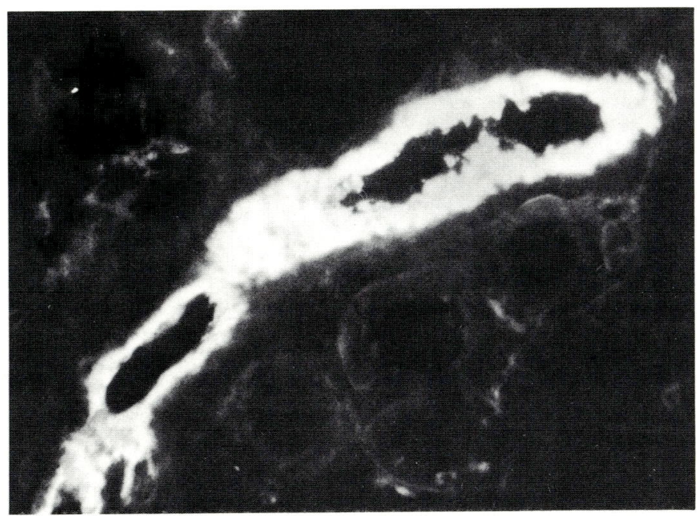

Figure 23-19. Arteriole showing homogenous staining of the entire vascular wall in a case of chronic rejection. In addition, weak focal linear staining is present along tubular basement membranes (antihuman C3, ×450).

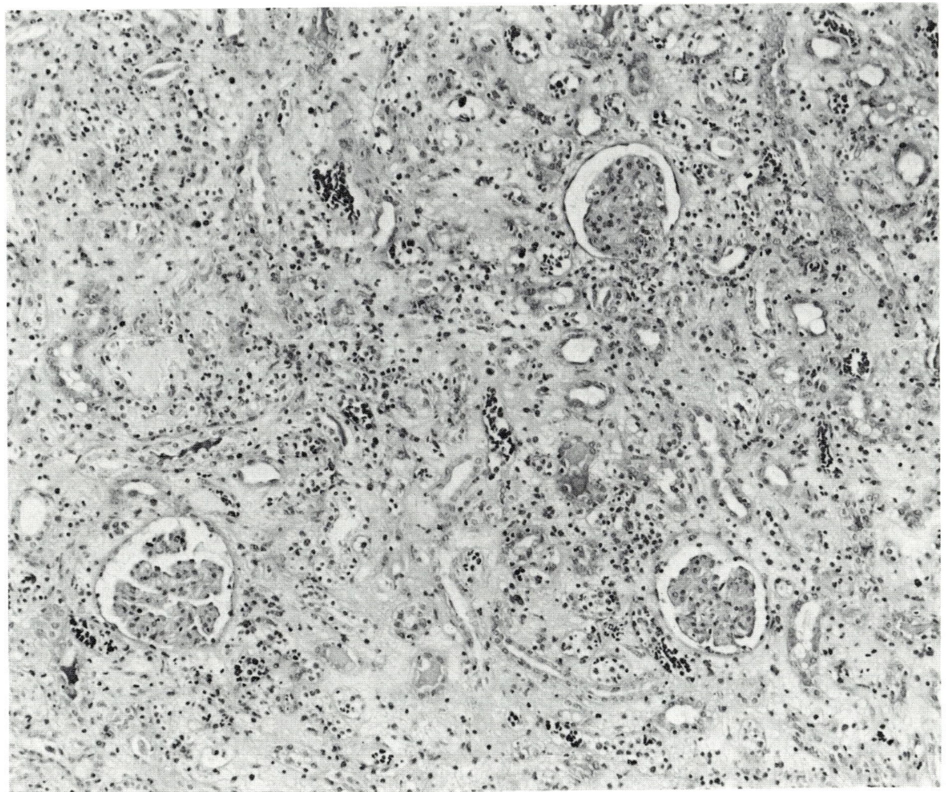

Figure 23-20. Biopsy specimen from a renal transplant patient showing changes of chronic rejection. The interstitium is scarred and contains sparse mononuclear inflammatory cells. The tubules are atrophic. The glomerular tufts are condensed, and the capillary loops show variable degree of collapse (H&E stain, ×120).

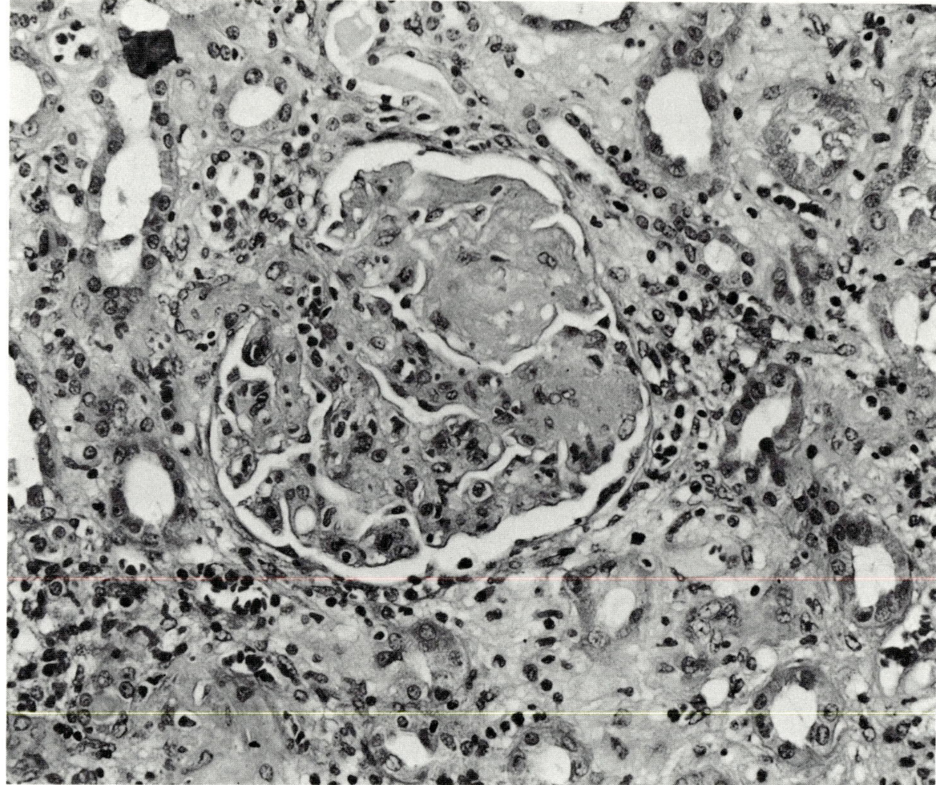

Figure 23-21. Segmental sclerosis and capillary collapse in chronic rejection glomerulopathy (H&E stain, ×480).

are enlarged with expanded, sclerotic mesangia, prominent endothelium, and thickened capillary walls. This thickening is produced by a combination of lucent subendothelial deposit, to be described below, and extensive mesangial interposition. Cellular proliferation is usually minimal, but the widespread double-contour pattern can closely resemble mesangiocapillary glomerulonephritis. There is a pronounced tendency to segmental sclerosis, with or without hyalinosis, and small crescents may be seen around sclerotic areas. The overall picture, therefore, is highly variable, with expanded glomeruli showing extensive mesangial interposition being intermixed with others exhibiting segmental sclerosis, ischemic shrinkage, or variable combinations of each pattern. Immuno-fluorescence microscopy of affected glomeruli usually demonstrates granular reactions in mesangia and along capillary walls for IgM and C3, sometimes with fibrin and IgG, but the results may be completely negative.

The ultrastructural pattern of transplant glomerulopathy is highly characteristic (22,27,29,30). There is striking widening of the lamina rara interna by electron-lucent deposit, which can considerably stenose the capillary lumen (Figs. 23-22—23-24). Strands of new basement membrane may be seen on the luminal aspect of this deposit which often contains flocculent, dense areas and dispersed fibrils. Conventional dense deposits are not common, and their pres-

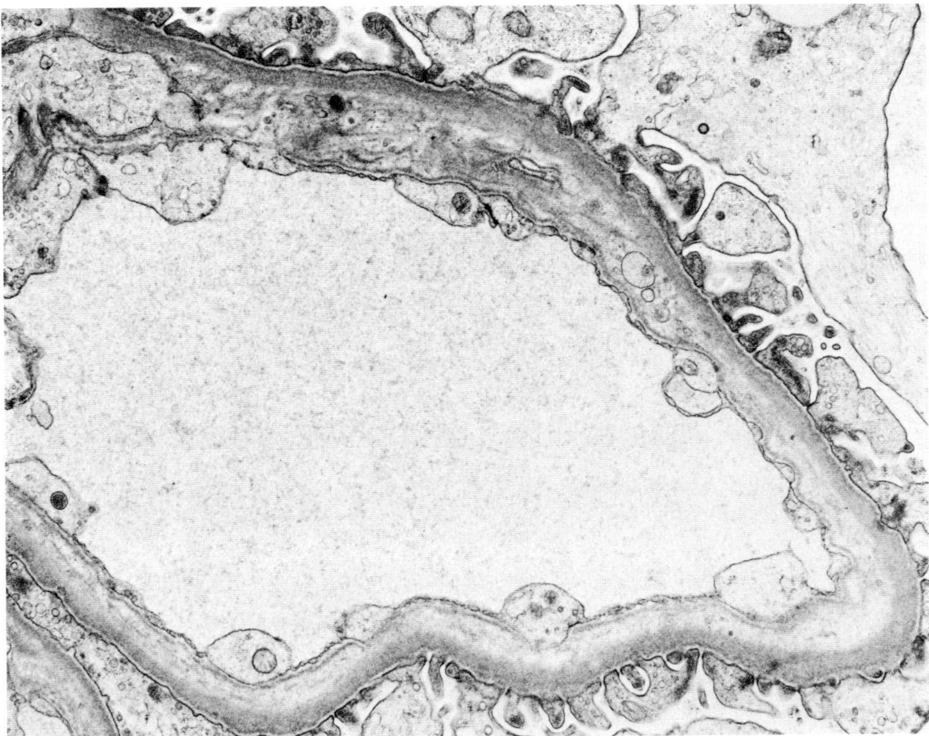

Figure 23-22. Electron micrograph of a capillary loop demonstrating widening of the lamina rara interna in chronic allograft rejection ($\times$11,000).

ence always raises the possibility of glomerulonephritis, but both subendothelial deposits and humps have been described (29,30). Mesangia are enlarged by hypertrophic cells and abundant matrix, each of these being continuous with areas of interposition between the endothelium and subendothelial deposit. There is concomitant swelling and hypertrophy of endothelial and epithelial cells. Degenerate cytoplasmic fragments occur in both subendothelial and subepithelial regions as microvesicular and striated membranous bodies, and have sometimes been confused with viral structures. These fragments are especially frequent in subepithelial areas of epithelial detachment.

PERFUSION NEPHROPATHY

A morphologic pattern similar to hyperacute rejection may occur in the absence of cytotoxic antibodies in the recipient (Figs. 23-25, 23-26). This is produced by endothelial damage during pulsatile perfusion of the graft before implantation (31,32). Endothelial injury may result from either of two postulated mechanisms, the consequences of each being intravascular coagulation and, frequently, graft failure. Focal endothelial disruption can occur from direct physical pressure

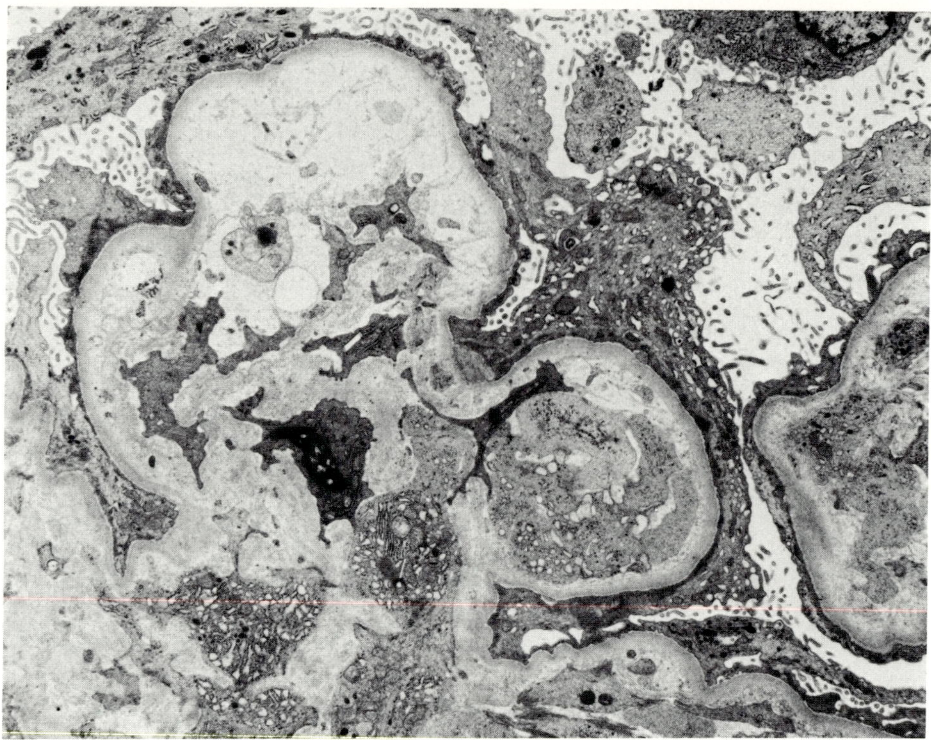

Figure 23-23. Thickening of the lamina rara interna, resultisng in almost complete vascular occlusion. The foot processes are obliterated and the epithelial cell cytoplasm appears hyperactive with prominent "villous" hyperplasia (×6,700).

during the perfusion procedure, and the denuded basement membrane could induce coagulation via the extrinsic pathway when blood flow begins (31). Alternatively, cytotoxic antibodies in the perfusate could attach to the endothelium during perfusion and induce damage by fixation of recipient complement after revascularization (33). There is, as yet, insufficient information to determine either the frequency of perfusion nephropathy or its predominant mechanism, but the survival rates of machine-perfused kidneys are significantly lower in some centers than those preserved by hypothermia alone (34). Morphologic differentiation of perfusion nephropathy from hyperacute and acute vascular rejection is impossible. Biopsy specimens taken soon after revascularization show frequent intracapillary polymorphs in each condition, and the cause of the thrombi and endothelial reaction developing later cannot be determined from morphologic examination. While the prognosis for grafts damaged by perfusion is poor, the outlook is not so uniformly disastrous as in hyperacute rejection. The possibility of perfusion nephropathy should thus be considered when acute vascular changes are demonstrated in biopsy specimens taken soon after implantation, and information about the method of preservation needs to be taken into account when the prognostic significance of these changes is assessed.

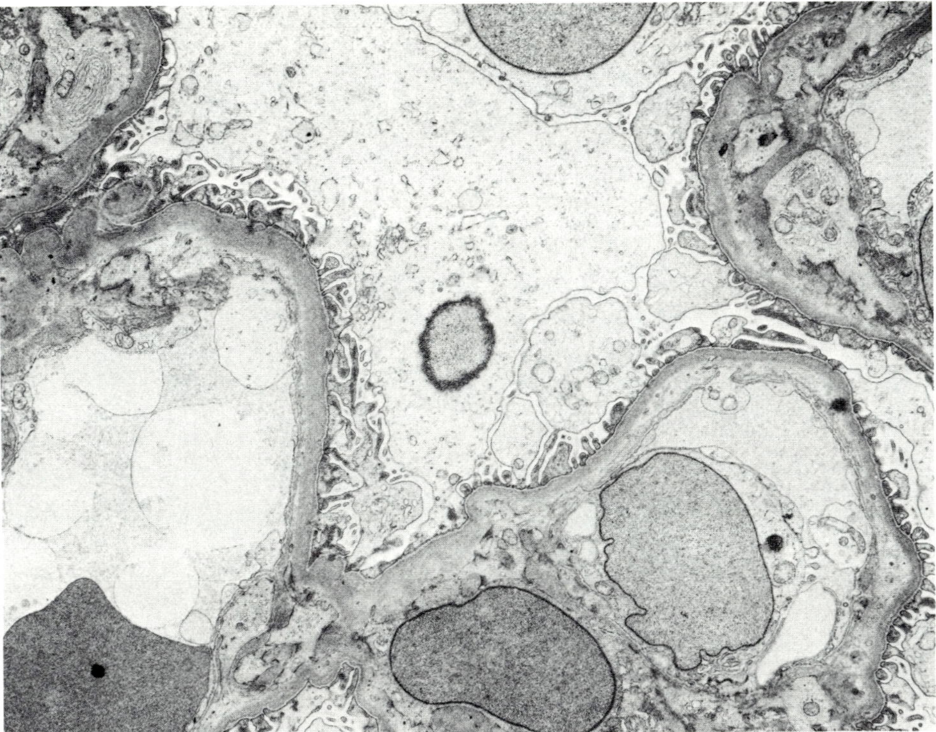

Figure 23-24. Portions of a glomerulus showing widening of the lamina rara interna and focal mesangial interposition (right upper loop). The epsithelial cell organelles are sparse, but the foot processes remain intact (×4,500).

RECURRENT OR DE NOVO DISEASE IN TRANSPLANTS

The mechanisms causing renal failure may persist to produce significant damage to the graft (see Table 23-2). Recurrent (or persistent) disease was a particular problem in isografts in the past (35), but has been reduced in frequency by conventional immunosuppression, and is common in some metabolic diseases. Crystal accumulation is, for example, inevitable in the grafts of patients with oxalosis and cystinosis, although progressive graft failure is rare in cystinosis (36,37) but usual in oxalosis (38,39). Similarly, idiopathic Fanconi syndrome has recurred in the transplanted kidney (36). The frequency of recurrent disease in diabetes mellitus and amyloidosis is, as discussed elsewhere in this book, still uncertain. The incidence of recurrent glomerulonephritis in allografts is variously quoted at 5 to 18% (40), but these figures conceal considerable variation in the behavior of individual glomerular lesions. Recurrence is almost inevitable in some conditions but rare or insignificant in others. Alternatively, the graft may be affected by mechanisms that differ from those originally causing renal failure. De novo glomerulonephritis of this type is extraordinarily rare, considering the great variety of infectious antigens and immune perturbations to which the transplant patient is subjected (40,41). Finally, unrecognized renal disease in the

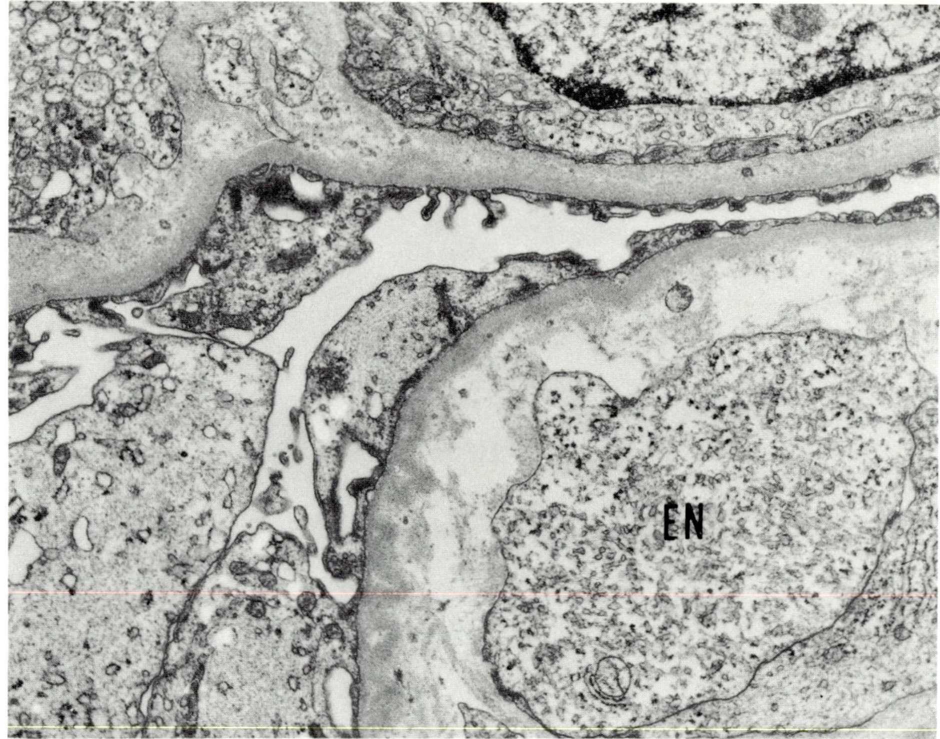

Figure 23-25. Biopsy from a perfused renal graft taken before implantation. The endothelium (EN) is focally detached from the glomerular basement membrane (×10,250).

donor might theoretically remain active in the recipient, although there is little evidence that this is a significant cause of graft failure (42).

The risks and significance of graft recurrence for most of the diseases listed in Table 23-2 are discussed elsewhere in this book and need not be repeated here. The criteria for diagnosis are the same whether the affected kidney is a transplant or native to the host, although superimposed changes of rejection may, at times, obscure the typical features. The striking similarities between the vascular lesions of rejection and those of progressive systemic sclerosis, malignant hypertension, and the hemolytic uremic syndrome are such, for example, that the diagnosis of recurrent or de novo disease must rely on a careful analysis of the clinical syndrome as well as the morphologic picture. Similarly, focal glomerulosclerosis is a relatively common and nonspecific morphologic pattern in transplant rejection (43). The most difficult diagnostic problem in the transplanted kidney is the differentiation between mesangiocapillary glomerulonephritis (type I) and transplant glomerulopathy (41,43). The extensive patterns of mesangial interposition seen in these conditions may be indistinguishable by light microscopy alone, and it is unwise to consider a diagnosis of recurrent or de novo mesangiocapillary glomerulonephritis unless the typical subendothelial deposits can be documented by electron and immunofluorescence microscopy.

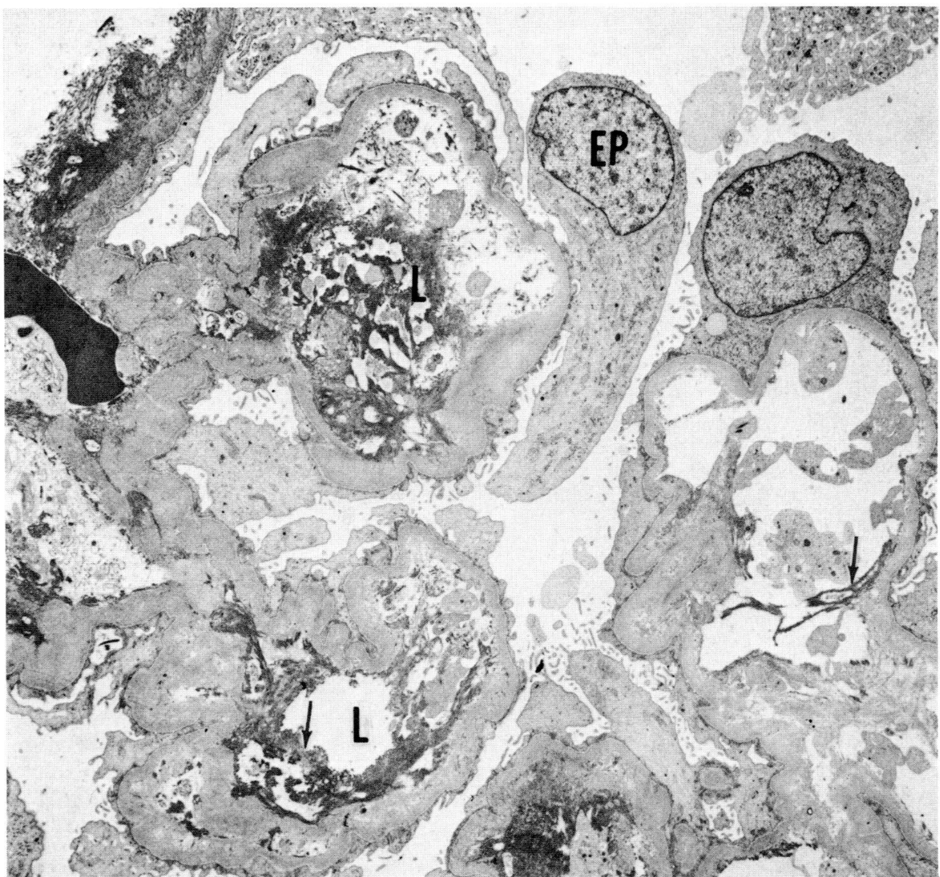

Figure 23-26. Biopsy specimen from the same kidney as in Figure 23-25, twelve hours post implantation, showing extensive endothelial denudation of glomerular capillaries. The loops contain fibrin (arrows), and cellular debris. The foot processes are focally obliterated (right loop). L, capillary lumen; EP, epithelial cell (×5,200).

DIFFERENTIAL DIAGNOSIS

Difficulty in interpretation of the morphologic changes associated with declining graft function may occur early or late in the course of the transplant. After the first few months, the major problems lie in the differentiation between chronic rejection and recurrent or de novo disease. The most perplexing decisions, and those of most prognostic significance, must be made from biopsy specimens taken to determine the cause of acute graft failure occurring soon after implantation. There are many manifestations of acute graft failure, but those most likely to lead to biopsy are recurrent glomerulonephritis, ureteric obstruction, major renal vessel occlusion, acute infection of the graft, and "prerenal" acute renal failure (13,14,44). Generally, the diagnosis of transplant rejection depends on the recognition of the features already described in this chapter, and another

Table 23-2. Glomerulonephritis and Other Diseases in Transplanted Kidneys[a]

Recurrent Disease

Diseases commonly recurring in transplants
  Focal glomerulosclerosis
  Dense deposit disease
  IgA nephropathy
  Oxalosis
  Cystinosis

Recurrent disease of uncertain frequency
  Mesangiocapillary glomerulonephritis (type I)
  Anti-basement membrane disease (glomerular and tubular)
  Amyloidosis
  Diabetic glomerulosclerosis
  Progressive systemic sclerosis

Disease rarely recurring in transplants
  Membranous nephropathy
  Henoch-Schönlein glomerulonephritis
  Hemolytic uremic syndrome
  Malignant hypertension
  Renal Fanconi syndrome
  Idiopathic crescentic glomerulonephritis
  Alport's disease (?)

De Novo Disease

  Membranous nephropathy
  Mesangiocapillary glomerulonephritis (type I)
  Acute postinfectious glomerulonephritis
  Idiopathic crescentic glomerulonephritis
  Focal glomerulosclerosis
  Epithelial cell disease
  Antibasement membrane disease (glomerular and tubular)
  Hemolytic uremic syndrome

Preexistent Disease in Donor Kidney

---

[a]See text, discussions in appropriate chapters, and refs. 40 and 41.

cause for acute renal failure is likely if these are absent (45). In assessing such biopsy specimens, it must be remembered that mild and focal edema, tubular degeneration, and mononuclear inflammatory infiltration normally occur in both autografts and isografts (10). Minor changes of this type are, therefore, of no value in differential diagnosis. The interpretation of morphologic changes in early graft biopsies is difficult, and a specific diagnosis is often impossible (46). Widespread dilatation of tubules is suggestive of obstruction or "prerenal" acute renal failure, while intense congestion may occur in either acute vascular rejection or major vessel occlusion. More constructive advice can be given to the physician when positive, rather than negative, features are recognizable. A preponderance of either polymorphs or eosinophils in an interstitial infiltrate, for example, suggests acute pyelonephritis or drug-induced interstitial nephritis. Similarly, significant glomerular proliferation suggests recurrent or de novo glomerulonephritis, although a variety of proliferative and destructive changes may occur during rejection. The diagnosis of glomerulonephritis in a transplant is, in fact, unreliable unless specific electron and immunofluorescence microscopic changes can be demonstrated. Even these studies may be confusing in some cases, since linear and granular patterns of immunofluorescence occur in rejection, and electron-dense deposits may be seen in various locations. All clinical and morphologic details must, therefore, be considered before making a specific diagnosis.

PROGNOSIS

The prognosis for the patient with a kidney transplant depends on a vast array of factors, only those directly affecting the graft having been discussed in this chapter. Systemic infection is a major hazard of the prolonged immunosuppression required for graft survival, and there is a significantly increased risk of neoplasia (47,48). The complications of immunosuppression are reduced in the fortunate but few patients receiving isografts, in whom graft survival is 90% at two years (49). The results in patients with allografts are less favorable although recent studies show a patient survival of 90% at one year for transplants from both alive, related donors and from cadavers, and a graft survival of 83% and 50%, respectively (2). The prognosis in each individual rejection episode is directly dependent on the type and severity of the morphologic changes (50). Thus, significant evidence of vascular rejection early in the course of a graft is an ominous prognostic sign, whereas cellular rejection may completely resolve, and the appearance of chronic rejection indicates inevitable graft destruction. Rejection of one graft, however, does not appear to adversely affect the outcome of further grafts, regardless of the original pattern of rejection.

SUMMARY

Progressive renal disease is no longer a sentence of death. Chronic dialysis can prolong life, and transplantation can allow a reasonably normal existence. The survival of an allograft, whether from an alive, related, or cadaver donor, depends on a balance between the graft antigens and the immunologic defense mechanisms of the recipient. This balance can be promoted by careful matching before transplantation and by therapeutic suppression of the efferent and afferent pathways of graft destruction. Any disturbance in the balance may lead to rejection, in either an abrupt and rapidly progressive or an indolent and inexorable pattern. Acute rejection is usually caused by a combination of cellular and humoral mechanisms, producing either interstitial or vascular changes, although either mechanism may predominate, while chronic rejection is principally humoral in type. The cellular and interstitial pattern of rejection is completely reversible with immunosuppressive therapy. Vascular rejection, on the other hand, is often progressive: either very rapidly with coagulation and graft necrosis (hyperacute and acute), or more slowly with irreversible stenosis and ischemic graft destruction (chronic). Each of these patterns requires differentiation from the mechanical and infective complications inherent in transplantation and from a wide variety of recurrent and de novo forms of renal disease. The pathologist is thus an important member of the transplant team, and is often called upon to provide guidance about the causes of declining graft function. This guidance can only be given by a careful analysis of the morphologic changes and a careful consideration of the clinical phenomena associated with the abnormal graft function.

REFERENCES

1. Leach G: *The Biocrats.* New York, McGraw-Hill Book Co, 1970, p 247.

2. Tilney NL, Strom TB, Vineyard GC, et al: Factors contributing to the declining mortality rate in renal transplantation. *N Engl J Med* 299:1321, 1978.

3. Najarian JS, Howard RJ, Foker JE, et al: Renal transplantation: criteria for detection and evaluation of patients and immunologic aspects of transplantation, in Brenner BM, Rector FC (eds): *The Kidney.* 1976, W B Saunders Co, Vol II, p 1745.

4. Balch CM, Diethelm AG: The pathophysiology of renal allograft rejection: a collective review. *J Surg Res* 12:350, 1972.

5. Morris PJ, Batchelor JR, Festenstein H: Matching for HLA in transplantation. *Br Med Bull* 34:259, 1978.

6. Dausset J, Rapaport FT: Immunology and genetics of transplantation, in Becker EL (ed): *Seminars in Nephrology.* New York, John Wiley and Sons, 1977, p 97.

7. Ting A, Williams KA, Morris PJ: Transplantation: Immunological monitoring. *Br Med Bull* 34:263, 1978.

8. Porter KA: Clinical renal transplantation. *Int Rev Exp Pathol* 11:73, 1972.

9. Corson JM: The pathologist and the kidney transplant. *Pathol Annu* 7:251, 1972.

10. Rowlands, DT, Hill GS, Zmijewski CM: The pathology of renal homograft rejection: a review. *Am J Pathol* 85:774, 1976.

11. Williams GM, Hume DM, Page R, et al: "Hyperacute" renal homograft rejection in man. *N Engl J Med* 279:611, 1968.

12. Kincaid-Smith P, Morris PJ, Saker BM, et al: Immediate renal-graft biopsy and subsequent rejection. *Lancet* 2:748, 1968.

13. Maher JF: A logical approach to the diagnosis of renal transplant rejection. *Am J Med* 56:275, 1974.

14. Carpenter CB: The early diagnosis of renal allograft rejection in man. *Adv Nephrol* 5:229, 1975.

15. Strom TB, Kostick R, Tilney NL, et al: A characterization of the nature and control of cellular allograft rejection. *Nephron* 22:201, 1978.

16. Busch GJ, Reynolds ES, Galvanek EG, et al: Human renal allografts: the role of vascular injury in early graft failure. *Medicine (Balt)* 50:29, 1971.

17. Mihatsch MJ, Zollinger HU, Gudat F, et al: Transplantation arteriopathy. *Pathol Microbiol* 43:219, 1975.

18. Callard P, Bedrossian J, Idatte JM, et al: The arterial lesions in the course of renal allograft rejection phenomena. *Adv Nephrol* 5:333, 1975.

19. Pillay VKG, Kurtzmann NA, Manaligod JP, et al: Selective thrombocytopenia due to localized microangiopathy of renal allografts. *Lancet* 2:988, 1973.

20. Magalhaes RL, Braun WE, Straffon RA, et al: Microangiopathic hemolytic anemia in renal transplantation: report of a successfully treated case and review of the literature. *Am J Med* 58:862, 1975.

21. Porter KA, Dossetor JB, Marchioro LT, et al: Human renal transplants. I. Glomerular changes. *Lab Invest* 16:153, 1967.

22. Rossman P, Jirka J, Malek P, et al: Glomerulopathies in human renal allografts. *Beitr Pathol Bd* 155:18, 1975.

23. Petersen VP, Olsen TS, Kissmeyer-Nielsen F, et al: Late failure of human renal transplants: an analysis of transplant disease and graft failure among 125 recipients surviving from one to eight years. *Medicine (Balt)* 54:45, 1975.

24. Cheigh J-S, Stenzel KH, Susin M, et al: Kidney transplant nephrotic syndrome. *Am J Med* 57:730, 1974.

25. Varkarakia MJ, Murphy GP: Role of juxtaglomerular apparatus in renal allograft rejection. *NY State J Med* 75:531, 1975.

26. Busch GJ, Galvanek EG, Reynolds ES: Human renal allografts: analysis of lesions in long-term survivors. *Human Pathol* 2:253, 1971.

27. Zollinger HU, Moppert J, Thiel G, et al: Morphology and pathogenesis of glomerulopathy in cadaver kidney allografts treated with antilymphocyte globulin. *Current Topics Pathol* 57:1, 1973.

28. Mathew TH, Kincaid-Smith P, Vikraman P: Risks of vesicoureteric reflux in the transplanted kidney. *N Engl J Med* 297:414, 1977.

29. Hulme B, Andres GA, Porter KA, et al: Human renal transplants. IV. Glomerular ultrastructure, macromolecular permeability and hemodynamics. *Lab Invest* 26:2, 1972.

30. Olsen S, Bohmann S-O, Petersen VP: Ultrastructure of the glomerular basement membrane in long-term renal allografts with transplant glomerular disease. *Lab Invest* 30:176, 1974.

31. Hill GS, Light GA, Perloff LJ: Perfusion-related injury in renal transplantation. *Surgery* 79:440, 1976.

32. Spector D, Limas C, Frost JL, et al: Perfusion nephropathy in human transplants. *N Engl J Med* 295:1217, 1976.

33. Filo RS, Dickson LG, Suba EA, et al: Immunological injury induced by ex vivo perfusion of canine autografts. *Surgery* 76:88, 1974.

34. Clark EA, Terasaki PI, Opelz G, et al: Cadaver-kidney transplant failures at one month. *N Engl J Med* 291:1099, 1974.

35. Glassock RJ, Feldman D, Reynolds, ES, et al: Human renal isografts: a clinical and pathological analysis. *Medicine (Balt)* 47:411, 1968.

36. Briggs WA, Kominami N, Wilson RE: Kidney transplantation in Fanconi syndrome. *N Engl J Med* 286:25, 1972.

37. Malekzadeh MH, Neustein HB, Schneider JA, et al: Cadaver renal transplantation in children with cystinosis. *Am J Med* 63:525, 1977.

38. Renal transplantation in congenital and metabolic diseases. Advisory Committee to the Renal Transplant Registry. *JAMA* 232:148, 1975.

39. Leumann EP, Wegmann W, Largiadèr F: Prolonged survival after renal transplantation in prolonged hyperoxaluria of childhood. *Clin Nephrol* 9:29, 1978.

40. McPhaul JJ Jr, Longdon RE, Thompson AL, et al: Nephritogenic immunopathologic mechanisms of human renal transplants: the problem of recurrent glomerulonephritis. *Kidney Int* 10:135, 1976.

41. Cameron JS, Turner DR: Recurrent glomerulonephritis in allografted kidneys. *Clin Nephrol* 7:47, 1977.

42. de la Rivière GB, van de Putte LBA: Preexisting glomerulonephritis in allografted kidneys: occurrence in man. *Arch Pathol Lab Med* 100:196, 1976.

43. Mathew TH, Mathews DC, Hobbs JB, et al: Glomerular lesions after transplantation. *Am J Med* 59:177, 1975.

44. Kjellstrand CM, Casali RE, Simmons RL, et al: Etiology and prognosis in acute post-transplant renal failure. *Am J Med* 61:190, 1976.

45. Finkelstein FO, Siegel NJ, Bastl C, et al: Kidney transplant biopsies in the diagnosis and management of acute rejection reactions. *Kidney Int* 10:171, 1976.

46. Zollinger HU, Mihatsch MJ, Gudat F, et al: Etiologic and prognostic significance of isolated acute renal hypoxic change (so called tubular necrosis or shock kidney) in kidney transplants. *Clin Nephrol* 6:484, 1976.

47. Lee DBN, Prompt CA, Upham AT: Medical complications of renal transplantation. I. Graft and infectious complications in recipient. *Urology* 9(suppl 4): 1977.

48. Penn I, Starzl TE: Malignant tumors arising de novo in immunosuppressed organ transplant recipients. *Transplantation* 14:407, 1972.

49. Calne RY: Renal transplantation: introduction. Urology 9(suppl 4): 1977.

50. Herbetson BM, Evans DB, Calne RY, et al: Percutaneous needle biopsies of renal allografts: the relationship between morphologic changes present in biopsies and subsequent allograft function. *Histopathol* 1:161, 1977.

Index